Orthopedic and Athletic Injury Examination Handbook

EDITION 2

Orthopedic and Athletic Injury Examination Handbook

EDITION 2

Chad Starkey, PhD, LAT
Associate Professor
Coordinator, Division of Athletic Training
College of Health and Human Services
Ohio University
Athens, OH

Sara D. Brown, MS, ATC
Clinical Associate Professor
Director, Programs in Athletic Training
College of Health and Rehabilitation
Sciences: Sargent College
Boston University
Boston, MA

Jeffrey L. Ryan, PT, MBA
Chief Clinical Operating Officer
Hahnemann Physician Practice Plan
Philadelphia, PA

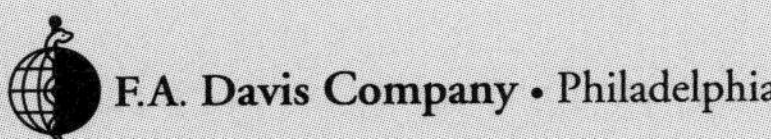
F.A. Davis Company • Philadelphia

F. A. Davis Company
1915 Arch Street
Philadelphia, PA 19103
www.fadavis.com

Printed in the United States of America

Last digit indicates print number: 10 9 8 7 6 5 4 3

Senior Acquisitions Editor: Quincy McDonald
Manager of Content Development: George W. Lang
Developmental Editor: Sarah Granlund
Art and Design Manager: Carolyn O'Brien

Library of Congress Cataloging-in-Publication Data

Starkey, Chad, 1959-
Orthopedic and athletic injury examination handbook / Chad Starkey, Sara D. Brown, Jeffrey L. Ryan. — Ed. 2.
p. ; cm.
Rev. ed. of: Orthopedic and athletic injury evaluation handbook. c2003.
Companion guide to the third edition of Evaluation of orthopedic and athletic injuries.
Includes bibliographical references and index.
ISBN-13: 978-0-8036-1722-3
ISBN-10: 0-8036-1722-4
1. Sports injuries—Handbooks, manuals, etc. 2. Orthopedics—Handbooks, manuals, etc. I. Brown, Sara D. II. Ryan, Jeffrey L., 1962- III. Starkey, Chad, 1959-. Orthopedic and athletic injury evaluation handbook. IV. Starkey, Chad, 1959-. Examination of orthopedic and athletic injuries. V. Title.
[DNLM: 1. Athletic Injuries—diagnosis—Handbooks. 2. Orthopedic Procedures—methods—Handbooks. QT 29 S795o 2010]
RD97.S833 2010
617.1'027—dc22 2009042851

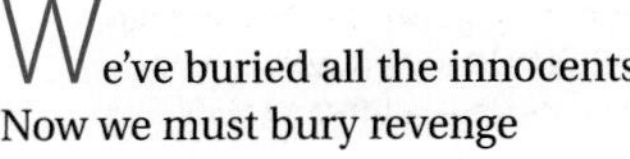

We've buried all the innocents
Now we must bury revenge

—CAS

To Tom. Lucky me.

—SDB

To Lisa and Kaley
You're smart, creative and, most of all, kind. You are an inspiration each and every day.
Thank you. I love you.

—JLR

PREFACE

Intended for use as a quick reference, the second edition of the *Orthopedic and Athletic Injury Examination Handbook* serves as a companion guide to the third edition of *Examination of Orthopedic and Athletic Injuries* (*EOAI3*). The changes in this handbook parallel those seen in *EOAI3*, with a major emphasis on instilling the need for the use of research evidence during the diagnostic process. We have made every effort to include the most up-to-date scientific evidence supporting or refuting the use of the various diagnostic procedures presented wherein.

We use the measures of interrater and intrarater reliability, positive likelihood ratios (LR+), and negative likelihood ratios (LR–) as the benchmarks for the efficacy of each procedure (Chapter 3 describes these measures and their clinical implications). Many of the common clinical procedures we describe are lacking peer-reviewed evidence. While the absence of research does not imply that the procedure is invalid, the prevalence of these missing data does demonstrate the need for research in this area. Any text that includes only information supported by research would be a very short text indeed. To aid in students understanding of manual muscle and neurological testing, we have added the muscle tables found in *EOAI3*.

As we discuss in the preface of *EOAI3*, instructors should *not* feel compelled to teach students how to perform each technique described in this handbook. Students who are finely skilled at performing fewer tests that have good reliability and diagnostic accuracy should turn out to be better clinicians than those who are able to perform a multitude of less diagnostic accuracy at a lower skill level. Moreover, an emphasis on mapping physical examination findings to identify functional limitations and the patient's description of disabilities is crucial to arrive at an effective treatment plan.

Chad Starkey
Sara D. Brown
Jeffrey L. Ryan

REVIEWERS

Paul K. Canavan, PhD, PT, ATC, CSCS
Assistant Professor
Physical Therapy and Athletic Training Education
Northeastern University
Boston, MA

Laura E. Clark, MS, ATC
Clinical Instructor and Athletic Trainer
Colorado State University – Pueblo
Pueblo, CO

Matthew J. Comeau, PhD, LAT, ATC, CSCS
Director of Graduate Athletic Training
Marshall University
School of Kinesiology
Huntington, WV

Trenton E. Gould, PhD, ATC
Assistant Professor and Director
Athletic Training Education
The University of Southern Mississippi
Hattiesburg, MS

Julie A. Rochester, MS, ATC
Associate Professor and Director
Health, Physical Education and Recreation
Northern Michigan University
Marquette, MI

CONTENTS

CHAPTER 1

The Injury Examination Process

HISTORY

Past Medical History

- **Establish general information** (age, activities, occupation, limb dominance)
- **Establish prior history of injury to area**
  - When (in years, months or days)? Number of episodes?
  - Seen by physician or other health care provider?
  - Immobilization? If so, how long?
  - Surgery? Type?
  - Limitation in activity? Duration of?
  - Residual complaints? (Full recovery?)
  - Is this a similar injury? How is it different?
- **Establish general health status** (medications, mental status, chronic or acute diseases, etc.)

History of the Present Condition

- **Establish chief complaint**
  - What is the patient's disability? What can patient not do that is impacting life?
  - What is the primary problem and the impact on ADLs and/or sport?
  - What is the duration of current problem?
  - Self-initiated treatment
  - Identify mechanism of injury
- **Establish pain information**
  - Pain location, type, and pattern. Does it change?
  - What increases and decreases pain?
  - Pattern relative to sports participation and/or occupation?
  - Pattern relative to specific sport demands
- **Establish changes in demands of activity and/or occupation**
  - Changes in activity?
  - New activity pattern?
  - New equipment?
  - Activities of daily living
- **Other relevant information**
  - Pain/other symptoms anywhere else? Altered sensations?
  - Crepitus, locking, or catching?

INSPECTION*

- **Obvious deformity**
- **Functional Assessment**
  - What functional limitations does the patient demonstrate?
  - What impairments cause the functional limitations? Which are most problematic?
- **Swelling and discoloration**
- **General posture**
- **Scars, open wounds, cuts, or abrasions**

PALPATION*

- **Areas of point tenderness**
- **Change in tissue density** (scarring, spasm, swelling, calcification)
- **Deformity**
- **Temperature change**
- **Texture**

JOINT AND MUSCLE FUNCTION ASSESSMENT

- **Active range of motion**
  - Evaluate for ease of movement, pain, available range (quantified via goniometry)
- **Manual muscle tests**
  - Evaluate for pain and weakness
- **Passive range of motion**
  - Evaluate for difference from active ROM, pain, end-feel, available range (quantified via goniometry)

JOINT STABILITY TESTS*

- **Stress Testing**
  - Evaluate for increased pain and/or increased or decreased laxity relative to opposite side
- **Joint Play**
  - Evaluate for increased pain and/or increased or decreased mobility relative to opposite side

SPECIAL TESTS*

- **Selective tissue testing**
  - Stress specific structures to identify laxity, tightness, instability, or pain.
- **Provocation/alleviation testing**
  - Identify positions or maneuvers that increase or decrease symptoms

NEUROLOGICAL ASSESSMENT*

- **Sensory**
  - Assess spinal nerve root and peripheral nerve sensory function
- **Motor**
  - Determine spinal nerve root and peripheral motor nerve function
- **Reflex**
  - Assess spinal level reflex function

VASCULAR ASSESSMENT*

- **Capillary refill**
  - Assess for adequate perfusion
- **Distal pulses**
  - Assess for adequate blood supply

CLINICAL DIAGNOSIS

- **Include all diagnoses that have not been excluded by the examination process**

DISPOSITION

- **Prognosis**
  - Predict probable short- and long-term outcome of the condition
- **Intervention**
  - Determine the patient's course of care
- **Return to activity**
  - Develop criteria for return to sport, work, and/or daily activity

* Compare bilaterally

Overview of the key elements of the examination model used throughout this text.

Box 1-1
Nagi Model of Disablement

The Nagi Model of Disablement presents a framework to identify how the patient's pathology impacts body structure, operation, and psyche (impairments); how impairments influence function (functional limitations); and how these functional limitations impact the person's life (disability). Identified functional limitations are connected to impairments. One impairment may cause other impairments that further increase functional disability.[1] Traditional evaluation models focus on the patient's pathology and tend to neglect the impact of the injury or illness on the person's ability to function on a personal and societal level.

While the examination process in this book focuses on the identification of impairments and functional limitations, doing this in the absence of understanding the resulting disability leads to ineffective treatment. Likewise, not all impairments result in functional limitations. For example, a patient may have decreased ROM in a joint without any impact on the ability to perform daily activities. In this example, a treatment approach that focuses on impairment-level treatment (increasing the ROM) will have limited impact on the patient's quality of life.

The following illustrates the primary components of the Nagi model using a sprained knee ligament as an example.

	Definition	Examples of Assessment Techniques	Measurement/Finding
Active Pathology	Interruption or interference of normal bodily processes or structure	Imaging Lab work	Ligament disruption
Impairment	Anatomical, physiological, mental or emotional abnormalities	History Pain questionnaires Instrumented testing Joint play Manual muscle tests Stress tests Special tests	Increased laxity with firm end feel Pain at rest = 3.0/10 Pain at worst = 7.5/10
Functional Limitation	Restriction of lack of ability to perform an action or activity in the manner or range considered normal (which results from impairment). How the impairment impacts the patient's ability to perform a task.	Observation during functional tasks such as walking or reaching.	Inability to walk normally
Disability	An inability or limitation in performing socially defined activities and roles expected of individuals within a social and physical environment.	Question patient regarding impact on life. What can the patient not do that he/she desires to?	Unable to participate in football practice.

Column 2 information from Nagi, SZ. Disability concepts revisited. In Pope, AM, Tarloy, AR (eds). *Prevention in Disability in America: Toward a National Agenda for Prevention.* Washington, DC: National Academy Press, 1991, p. 7.

Table 1-1 Role of the Noninjured Limb in the Examination Process

Segment	Relevance
History	**Past medical history:** Establishes preinjury health baseline and identifies conditions that can influence the current problem. **History of present condition:** Replicates the mechanism of injury, primary complaint(s), and functional limitations and disability.
Inspection	Functional assessment provides information regarding how the condition impacts the patient's ability to perform relevant tasks. Provides a reference for symmetry and color of the superficial tissues. Observation of function determines any limitation(s) between the extremities. Most meaningful when compared to baseline measures.
Palpation	Provides a reference for the comparison of bilateral symmetry of bones, alignment, tissue temperature, or other deformity as well as the presence of increased tenderness
Joint and Muscle Function Assessment	Provides a reference to identify impairments relating to available ROM, strength, and pain with movement.
Joint Stability Tests	Provides a reference for end-feel, relative laxity or hypomobility, and pain
Special Tests	Provides a reference for pathology of individual ligaments, joint capsules, and musculotendinous units, and the body's organs.
Neurologic Tests	Provides a reference for bilateral sensory, reflex, and motor function
Vascular Screening	Determines blood circulation to and from the involved extremity

History

Table 1-2 Potential Medication Effects on Musculoskeletal Healing

Medication (or medication family)	Generic Name (trade name) Example	Potential Negative Effect
Beta-blockers	Metoprolol (Lopressor) Propranolol (Inderal) Atenolol (Tenormin)	Decreased tolerance to exercise coupled with reduced perceived exertion.
Corticosteroid	Methylprednisolone (Medrol) Dexamethasone (Decadron)	Prolonged use: Muscle weakness, loss of muscle mass, tendon rupture, osteoporosis, aseptic necrosis of femoral and humeral heads, spontaneous fractures[9]
Cox-2 Inhibitors (type of NSAID)	Celecoxib (Celebrex)	Inhibit healing of soft-tissue and bone in animal models.[10]
Nonsteroidal Anti-inflammatory Drugs	Ibuprofen (Motrin) Diclofenac (Voltaren)	Delayed fracture healing or nonunion of fracture,[11] delayed soft tissue healing in animal models[10,12]
Salicylates	Aspirin	Prolonged bleeding times
Anticoagulant	Warfarin (Coumadin)	Prolonged bleeding times

Table 1-3 Referral Alerts

Finding	Possible Active Pathology or Condition
Chest pain Dizziness Shortness of breath Unexplained pain in the left arm Unexplained swelling of the ankle Unexplained weight gain	Congestive heart failure Myocardial infarction Splenic rupture
Unexplained weight loss Moles or other acute skin growths Slow to heal skin lesions Blood in the stool Unremitting night pain	Cancer
Blood in the urine Pain in the flank following the course of the ureter Low back pain associated with the above	Kidney stones Kidney/bladder infections
Loss of balance/coordination Loss of consciousness Bilateral hyperreflexia Acute hyporeflexia Inability to produce voluntary muscle contractions Unexplained general muscular weakness Bowel or bladder dysfunction	Neurologic involvement
Unexplained pain Symptoms that fail to resolve in the expected time	Unknown, warrants medical examination
Fever, chills, and/or night sweats	Systemic disease or infection
Amenorrhea Severe dysmenorrhea	Pregnancy Ectopic pregnancy

Box 1-2
Pain Rating Scales

Visual Analog Scale (VAS)

Pain as bad as it could be ——————— No pain

Using a 10-cm line, the patient is asked to mark the point that represents the current intensity of pain. The VAS value is then calculated by measuring the distance in centimeters from the right edge of the line.

Numeric Rating Scale (NRS)

No pain 0 1 2 3 4 5 6 7 8 9 10 Pain as bad as it could be

The patient is asked to circle the number from 0 (no pain) to 10 (worst pain imaginable) that best describes the current level of pain. Only whole numbers are used with this scale.

A. Where is your pain?

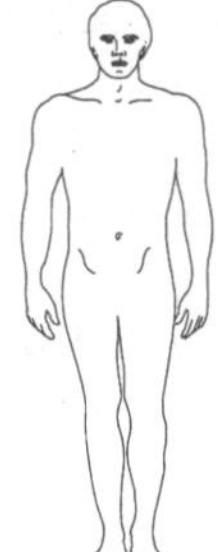

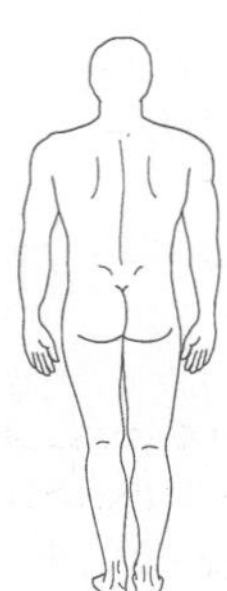

Using the above drawing, please mark the area(s) where you feel pain. Mark an "E" if the source of the pain is external or "I" if it is internal. If the source of the pain is both internal and external, please mark "B".

B. Pain rating index

Many different words can be used to describe pain. From the list below, please circle those words that best describe the pain you are currently experiencing. Use only one word from each category. You do not need to mark a word in every category -- **Only mark those words that most accurately describe your pain.**

1. Flickering, Quivering, Pulsing, Throbbing, Beating, Pounding

2. Jumping, Flashing, Shooting

3. Pricking, Boring, Drilling, Stabbing

4. Sharp, Cutting, Lacerating

5. Pinching, Pressing, Gnawing, Cramping, Crushing

6. Tugging, Pulling, Wrenching

7. Hot, Burning, Scalding, Searing

8. Tingling, Itchy, Smarting, Stinging

9. Dull, Sore, Hurting, Aching, Heavy

10. Tender, Taut, Rasping

11. Tiring, Exhausting

12. Sickening, Suffocating

13. Fearful, Frightful, Terrifying

14. Punishing, Grueling, Cruel, Vicious, Killing

15. Wretched, Blinding

16. Annoying, Troublesome, Miserable, Intense, Unbearable

17. Spreading, Radiating, Penetrating, Piercing

18. Tight, Numb, Drawing, Squeezing, Tearing

19. Cool, Cold, Freezing

20. Nagging, Nauseating, Agonizing, Dreadful, Torturing

McGill Pain Questionnaire

Pain assessment instruments such as the McGill Pain Questionnaire are often used for patients who have complex pain problems. Part A of the questionnaire identifies the area(s) of pain and if the pain is deep or superficial. Part B provides descriptors that are used to determine the intensity and nature of the patient's pain. A visual analog or numeric rating scale is often included as a part of the questionnaire.

Figures from Starkey C. *Therapeutic Modalities* (ed 3), 2004. Philadelphia: FA Davis.

Inspection

Bilateral Inspection

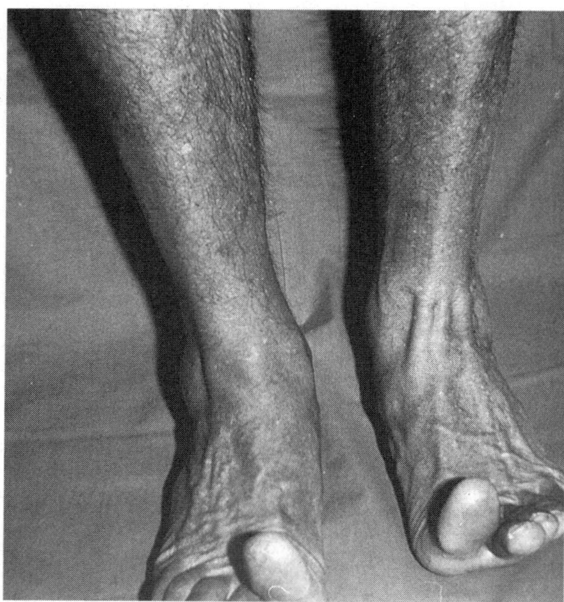

FIGURE 1-1 ■ What's wrong with this picture? (The answer is given in the legend of Figure 1-2.) The patient has few complaints other than decreased strength during dorsiflexion of the right ankle. There is no history of trauma to the body area. Carefully examine both ankles to determine the cause of these complaints.

Volumetric Measurement

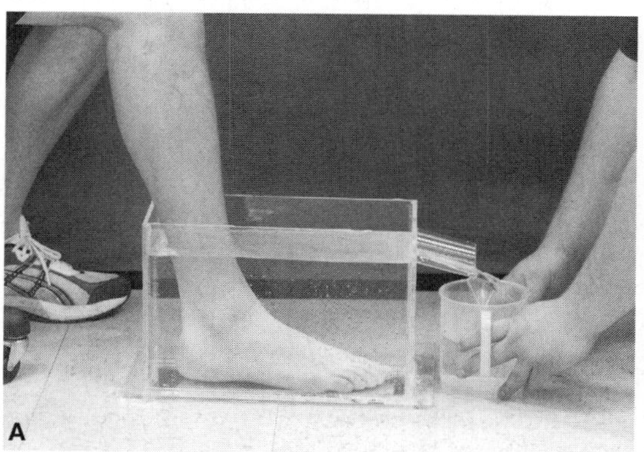

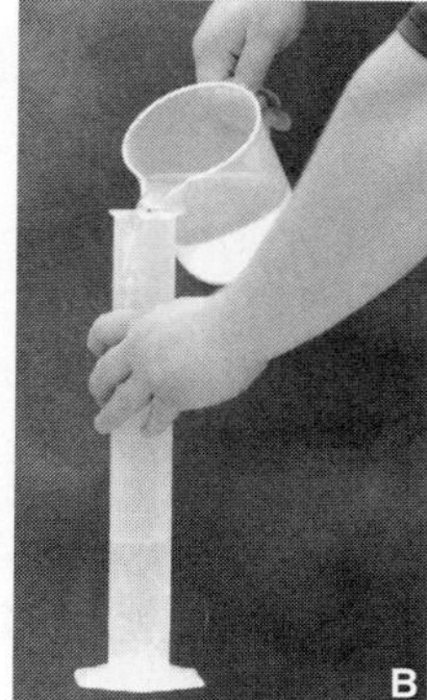

FIGURE 1-2 ■ Volumetric measurement. **(A)** The tank is filled with water up to the specified level and the limb is gently immersed. **(B)** The overflow water is collected and poured into a calibrated beaker to determine the mass (volume) of the limb. This measurement is obtained by either reading a graduate cylinder or, more accurately, by weighing the water expelled. Volumetric measurement of limb volume is most commonly used as a research tool, but can provide important clinical information. **Answer to Figure 1-1:** The right tibialis anterior tendon is ruptured. Note the absence of its tendon as it crosses the joint line.

Special Test 1-1
Girth Measurement

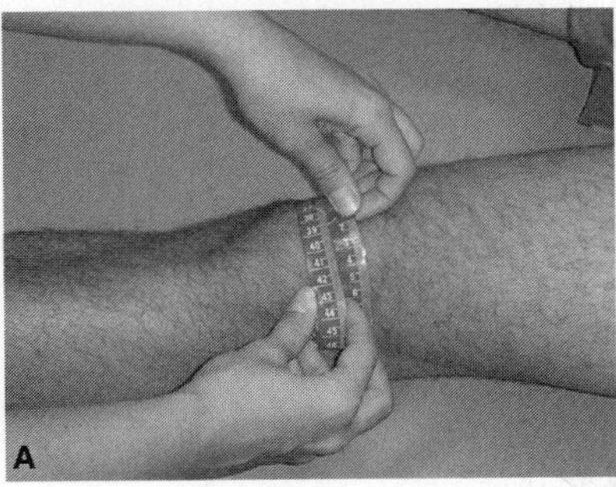

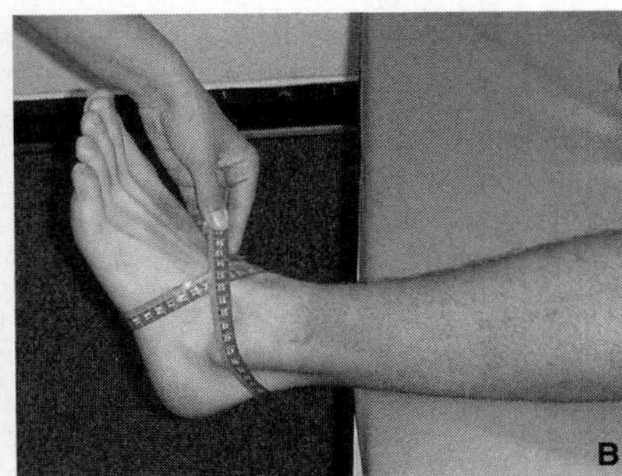

Girth measurements provide a quantifiable and reproducible measure of a limb's atrophy or hypertrophy. For a more precise measure, refer to Figure 1-2.

Patient Position	Supine
Position of Examiner	Standing to access the body part
Evaluative Procedure	**1.** To determine capsular swelling, identify the joint line using prominent bony landmarks. To determine muscular atrophy, make incremental marks (e.g., 2, 4, and 6 inches) from the joint line **(A)**. **2.** Do not use a measuring tape made of cloth (cloth tapes tend to stretch and cause the markings to fade). **3.** Lay the measuring tape symmetrically around the body part, being careful not to fold or twist the tape. **4.** To measure ankle girth use a figure-8 technique. Position the tape across the malleoli proximally and around the navicular and the base of the fifth metatarsal distally **(B)**. **5.** Pull the tape snugly and read the circumference in centimeters or inches. **6.** Take three measurements and record the average. **7.** Repeat these steps for the uninjured limb. **8.** Record the findings in the patient's medical file.
Positive Test	A significant difference in the girth between the two limbs based on factors such as lower or upper extremity, side dominance, and so on.
Implications	Increased girth across the joint line: Edema Increased girth across muscle mass: Hypertrophy or edema Decreased girth across muscle mass: Atrophy
Evidence	There is a strong positive correlation (0.90) between figure-8 and volumetric ankle measurements.

Palpation

Table 1-4 Possible Causes of Changes in Tissue Density

Tissue Feel	Possible Cause
Spongy, boggy over a joint	Synovitis
Hard, warm	Blood accumulation
Dense thickening	Scar tissue formation
Dense/viscous	Pitting edema
Increased muscle tone	Muscle spasm, muscle hypertrophy
Hard	Bone or bony outgrowth (exostosis)

Table 1-5 Joint Motion Description by Body Area

Body Area	Common Descriptors	Atypical Descriptors
Cervical Spine	Flexion Extension Rotation	Lateral or side bending (lateral flexion) Capital flexion Capital extension
Shoulder Complex	Flexion Extension Abduction Adduction Internal rotation External rotation	Horizontal abduction Horizontal adduction Elevation
Elbow/Forearm	Flexion Extension	Pronation Supination
Wrist/Hand	Flexion Extension	Radial deviation Ulnar deviation
Fingers	Flexion Extension Abduction Adduction	Opposition Apposition
Thumb (CMC joint)	Flexion Extension Abduction Adduction	Opposition Apposition
Lumbar Spine	Flexion Extension Rotation	Lateral or side bending (lateral flexion)

Table 1-5 Joint Motion Description by Body Area—cont'd

Body Area	Common Descriptors	Atypical Descriptors
Hip	Flexion Extension Abduction Adduction Internal rotation External rotation	
Knee	Flexion Extension Internal rotation External rotation	
Ankle/Foot		Plantarflexion Dorsiflexion Pronation Supination Inversion Eversion
Toes	Flexion Extension Abduction Adduction	

Abduction = Lateral movement of a body part away from the midline of the body. In the feet, the movement is in reference to the midline of the foot.

Adduction = Medial movement of a body part toward the midline of the body. In the feet, the movement is in reference to the midline of the foot.

Eversion = The movement of the plantar aspect of the calcaneus away from the midline of the body.

Extension = The act of straightening a joint and increasing its angle. Ankle extension is referred to as plantarflexion.

Flexion = Bending a joint and decreasing its angle. Ankle flexion is referred to as dorsiflexion.

Inversion = The movement of the plantar aspect of the calcaneus toward the midline of the body.

Pronation = (1) The combined motion of eversion, abduction, and dorsiflexion of the foot and ankle. (2) Movement at the radioulnar joints allowing for the palm to be turned downward.

Supination = (1) The combined motion produced by inversion, adduction, and plantarflexion of the foot and ankle. (2) Movement at the radioulnar joints allowing for the palm to turn upward, as if holding a bowl of soup.

Goniometry

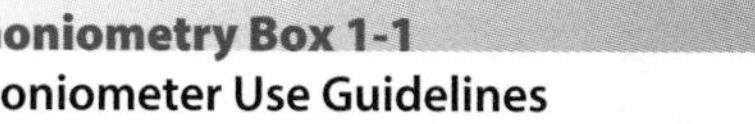

Goniometry Box 1-1
Goniometer Use Guidelines

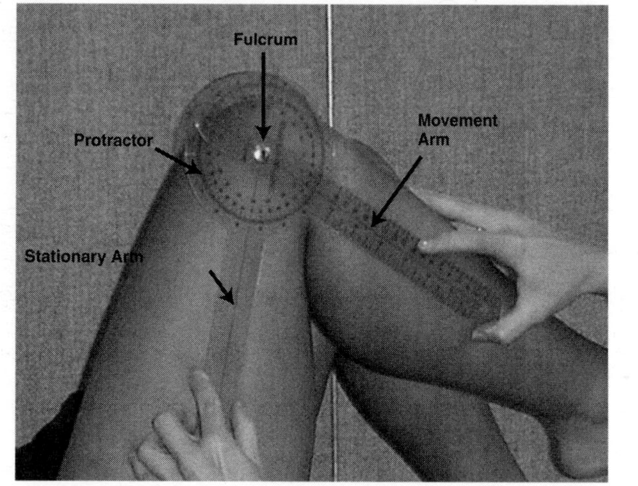

With proper training and practice, goniometers can yield accurate and quantifiable measures of a patient's active and passive ROM. Each joint has different landmarks for the fulcrum, stationary arm, and movement arm.

Goniometer Segments

Protractor: Measures the arc of motion in degrees. Full-circle goniometers have a 360° protractor; half-circle goniometers have a 180° protractor.

Fulcrum: The center of the axis of rotation of the goniometer

Stationary arm: The portion of the goniometer that extends from, and is part of, the protractor

Movement arm: The portion of the goniometer that moves independently from the protractor around an arc formed by the fulcrum

Procedure	**1.** Select a goniometer of the appropriate size and shape for the joint being tested. **2.** Position the joint in its starting position. **3.** Identify the center of the joint's axis of motion. **4.** Locate the proximal and distal landmarks running parallel to the joint's axis of motion. **5.** Align the fulcrum of the goniometer over the joint axis. **6.** Align the stationary arm along the proximal body segment and the movement arm along the distal segment. **7.** Read and record the starting values from the goniometer. **8.** Move the distal joint segment through its ROM. **9.** Reapply the goniometer as described in Steps 5 and 6. **10.** Read and record the ending values from the goniometer.
Recording Results	There are several different methods and documentation forms for recording goniometric data. Most systems use the neutral position as "0" and document the amount of motion from this point. For example, 10° of knee extension and 120° of knee flexion would be recorded as: **10°–0°–120°** In a case where the patient is unable to obtain the starting ("0") position, zero is the first number cited or is omitted. For example a limitation in the ROM, lacking 10° of knee extension would be recorded as: **0°–10°–120°** or **10°–120°** Avoid the use of negative numbers.

Manual Muscle Testing

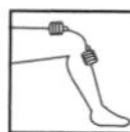

Manual Muscle Test 1-1
Muscle Testing Guidelines

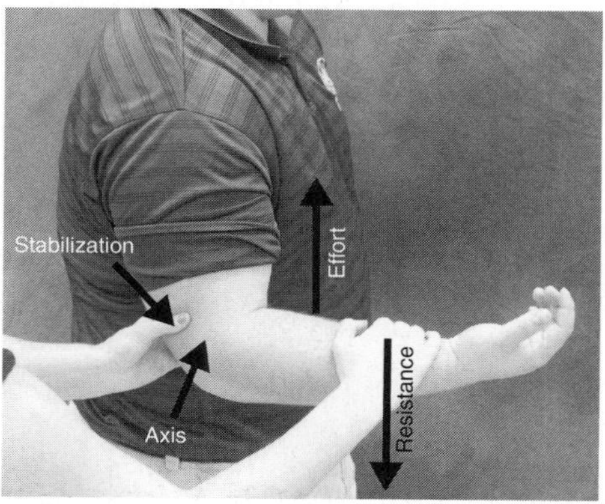

These procedures are used when attempting to isolate an individual muscle or muscle group (manual muscle test). Specific techniques are described in the appropriate chapters throughout this text.

Patient Position	Position the patient so that the muscle(s) tested must work against gravity.
Position of Examiner	As needed to stabilize proximal to the joint being tested and provide resistance distal to the joint.
Evaluative Procedure	**1.** Provide stabilization proximal to the joint to isolate the joint to the motion/muscle(s) being tested. Do not apply resistance at this point. **2.** Instruct the patient to perform the requested motion, such as elbow flexion with the forearm supinated. **3.** While the patient is attempting the motion, palpate the muscle(s) to ensure that it is contracting. **4.** If the patient is able to complete the ROM against gravity, a starting grade of "Fair" or "3" is assigned. **5.** Position the joint in the mid-ROM and apply resistance. Instruct the patient, "Don't let me move you." Gradually increase the resistance. **6.** Apply resistance as far away as possible from the target joint without crossing the distal joint. **7.** Ensure that the muscles distal to the joint being tested are relaxed. **8.** If the patient is unable to complete the ROM against gravity, reposition the body part to a gravity-eliminated position and request that the patient attempt to perform AROM again.
Positive Test	Weakness and/or pain compared to the contralateral side
Implications	See Table 1-6.

ROM = Range of motion; AROM = active range of motion.

Table 1-6 Grading Systems for Manual Muscle Tests

Verbal	Numerical	Clinical Finding
Normal	5/5	The patient can resist against maximal pressure. The examiner is unable to break the patient's resistance.
Good	4/5	The patient can resist against moderate pressure.
Fair	3/5	The patient can move the body part against gravity through the full ROM.
Poor	2/5	The patient can move the body part in a gravity-eliminated position through the full ROM.
Trace	1/5	The patient cannot produce movement, but a muscle contraction is palpable.
Zero	0/5	No contraction is felt.

Passive Range of Motion

Table 1-7 Physiological (Normal) End-Feels to PROM

End-Feel	Structure	Example
Soft	Soft tissue approximation	Knee flexion (contact between soft tissue of the posterior leg and posterior thigh)
Firm	Muscular stretch	Hip flexion with the knee extended (passive elastic tension of hamstring muscles)
	Capsular stretch	Extension of the metacarpophalangeal joints of the fingers (tension in the palmar capsule)
	Ligamentous stretch	Forearm supination (tension in the palmar radioulnar ligament of the inferior radioulnar joint, interosseous membrane, oblique cord)
Hard	Bone contacting bone	Elbow extension (contact between the olecranon process of the ulna and the olecranon fossa of the humerus)

Table 1-8 Pathological (Abnormal) End-Feels to PROM

End-Feel	Description	Example
Soft	Occurs sooner or later in the ROM than is usual or occurs in a joint that normally has a firm or hard end-feel; feels boggy	Soft tissue edema Synovitis
Firm	Occurs sooner or later in the ROM than is usual or occurs in a joint that normally has a soft or hard end-feel	Increased muscular tone. Capsular, muscular, ligamentous shortening
Hard	Occurs sooner or later in the ROM than is usual or occurs in a joint that normally has a soft or firm end-feel; feels like a bony block	Osteoarthritis Loose bodies in joint Myositis ossificans Fracture
Spasm	Joint motion is stopped by involuntary or voluntary muscle contraction.	Inflammation Strain Joint instability
Empty	Has no real end-feel because end of ROM is never reached owing to pain; no resistance felt except for patient's protective muscle splinting or muscle spasm	Acute joint inflammation Bursitis Abscess Fracture Psychogenic origin

Stress Testing

Table 1-9 Grading System for Ligamentous Laxity

Grade	Ligamentous End-Feel	Damage
I	Firm (normal)	Slight stretching of the ligament with little, if any, tearing of the fibers. Pain is present, but the degree of laxity roughly compares with that of the opposite extremity.
II	Soft	Partial tearing of the fibers. There is increased play of the joint surfaces upon one another or the joint line "opens up" significantly when compared with the opposite side.
III	Empty	Complete tearing of the ligament. The motion is excessive and becomes restricted by other joint structures, such as secondary restraints or tendons.

Joint Play

Joint Mobility Scale

0 = ankylosed
1 = considerably decreased
2 = slightly decreased
3 = normal
4 = slightly increased
5 = considerably increased
6 = dramatically increased, pathological

Neurologic Screening

The Body's Dermatomes

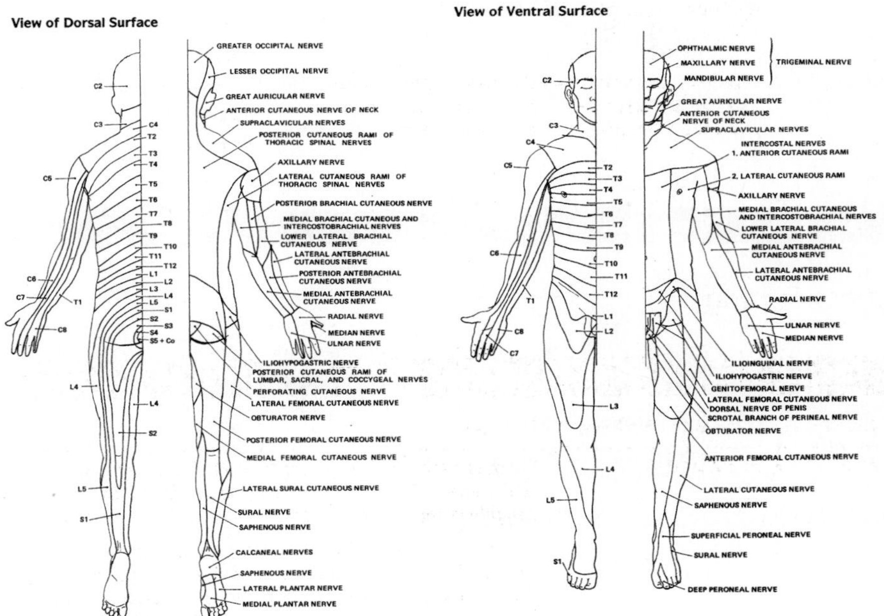

Cutaneous innervation of the back of the body. Dermatomes are on the left, and peripheral nerves are on the right.

Cutaneous innervation of the front of the body. Dermatomes are on the left, and peripheral nerves are on the right.

FIGURE 1-3 ■ These charts describe the area of skin receiving sensory input from each of the nerve roots. Note that there are many different dermatome references. (From Rothstein, JM, Roy, SH, and Wolf, SL: *The Rehabilitation Specialist's Handbook*. ed 2. Philadelphia: FA Davis, 1998.)

Two-point Discrimination Tests

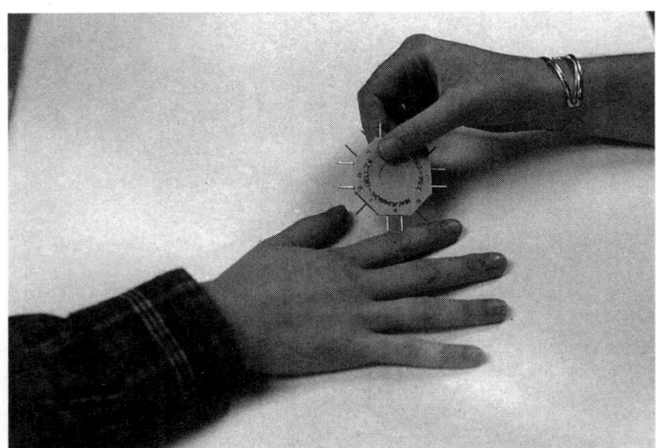

FIGURE 1-4 ■ This examination procedure is used to determine the amount of sensory loss. Normal results are that the patient can distinguish points that are at most 4 to 5 mm apart.

Table 1-10 Deep Tendon Reflex Grading

Grade	Response
0	No reflex elicited
1+	Hyporeflexia: Reflex elicited with reinforcement (precontracting the muscle)
2+	Normal response
3+	Hyperreflexia (brisk)
4+	Hyperactive with clonus

Lower Quarter Screen

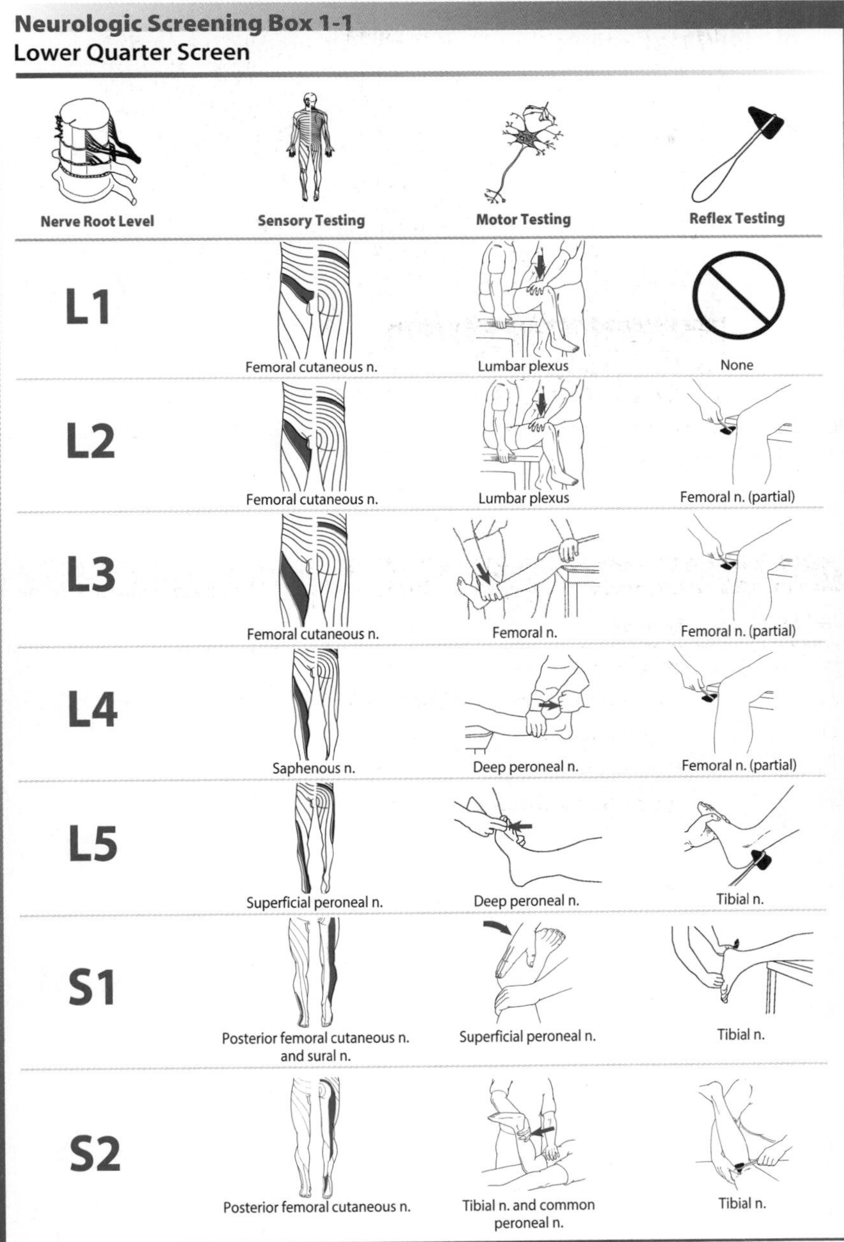

Upper Quarter Screen

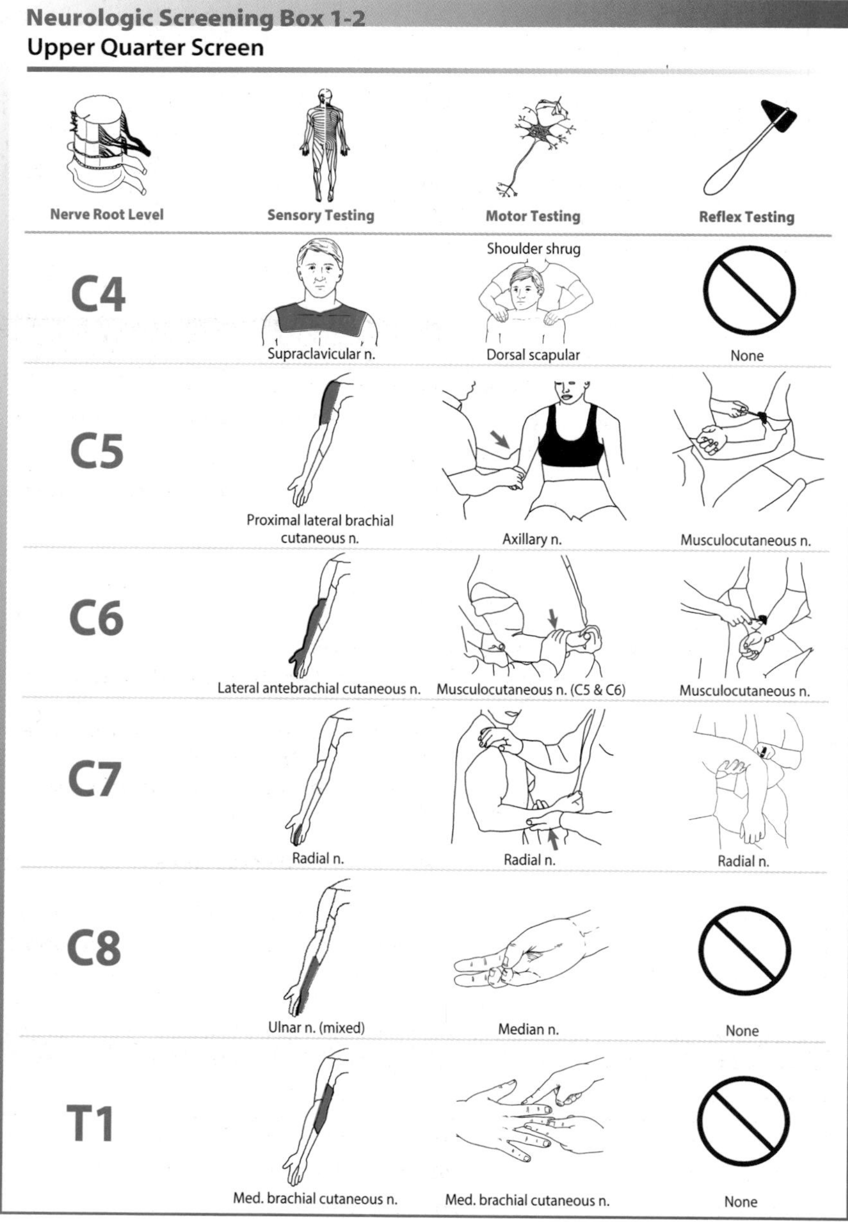

Neurologic Screening Box 1-2
Upper Quarter Screen

Nerve Root Level	Sensory Testing	Motor Testing	Reflex Testing
C4	Supraclavicular n.	Shoulder shrug Dorsal scapular	None
C5	Proximal lateral brachial cutaneous n.	Axillary n.	Musculocutaneous n.
C6	Lateral antebrachial cutaneous n.	Musculocutaneous n. (C5 & C6)	Musculocutaneous n.
C7	Radial n.	Radial n.	Radial n.
C8	Ulnar n. (mixed)	Median n.	None
T1	Med. brachial cutaneous n.	Med. brachial cutaneous n.	None

Vascular Screening

Special Test 1-2
Capillary Refill Testing

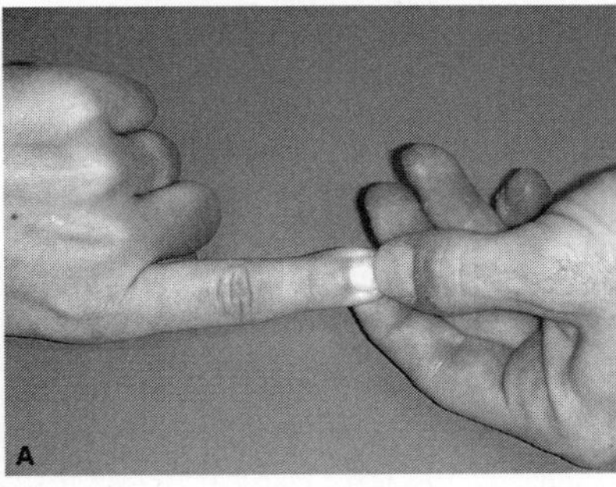

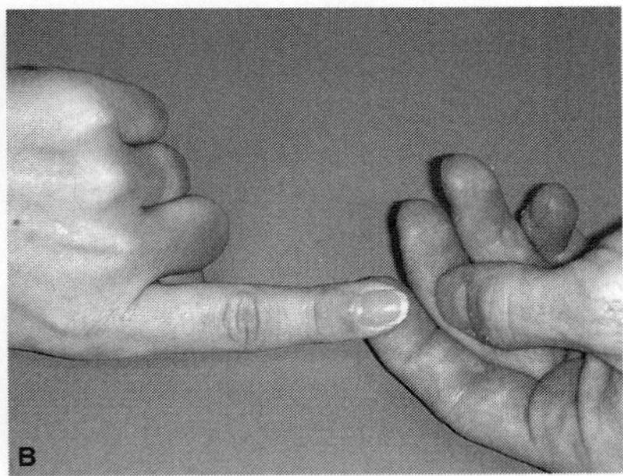

The capillary refill test provides gross information on the quality and quantity of blood flow to the extremities.

Patient Position	***Fingers:*** Sitting or lying supine. The extremity is placed in a gravity-neutral position (horizontal). ***Toes:*** Lying supine.
Position of Examiner	In front of or beside the patient.
Evaluative Procedure	Observe the color of the nail bed. Squeeze the fingernail so that the nail bed turns white or a lighter shade and hold for 5 sec. **(A)** Release the pressure and note the speed of the refill as indicated by the baseline color returning to the nail bed. **(B)** Repeat using the other fingers or toes and then perform on the opposite extremity.
Positive Test	Markedly slow or absent return of the nail's natural color.
Implications	***Unilateral:*** Occlusion of an artery or arteriole supplying the finger. ***Bilateral:*** Possible systemic cardiovascular compromise or disease.

Table 1-11 Signs of Vascular Inhibition in the Extremities

Arterial Deficiency	Venous Inhibition
Decreased pulse	Edema in the distal extremity
Decreased capillary refill	Noticeable "pitting" after removing the socks
Cyanotic color	Dark discoloration

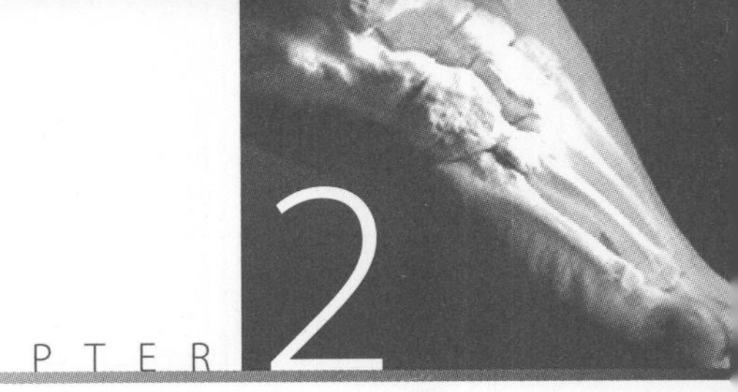

CHAPTER 2

Examination and Management of Acute Pathologies

On-Field Triage

In order of their importance, the immediate examination must rule out:

- Inhibition of the cardiovascular and respiratory systems (ABCs)
- Life-threatening trauma to the head or spinal column
- Profuse bleeding
- Fractures
- Joint dislocation
- Peripheral nerve injury
- Other soft tissue trauma

Emergency Planning

Box 2-1
Emergency Action Plan (EAP) Checklist*

Emergency Action Plan

The following elements are recommended in the development of a comprehensive EAP for sudden cardiac arrest (SCA) in athletics. Actual requirements and implementation may vary depending on the location, school, or institution.

I. **Development of an EAP**
- Establish a written EAP for each individual athletic venue.
- Coordinate the EAP with the local EMS agency, campus public safety officials, on-site first responders, administrators, athletic trainers, school nurses, and team and consulting physicians.
- Integrate the EAP into the local EMS response.
- Determine the venue-specific access to early defibrillation (less than 3 to 5 minutes from collapse to first shock recommended).

II. **Emergency Communication**
- Establish an efficient communication system to activate EMS at each athletic venue.
- Establish a communication system to alert on-site responders to the emergency and its location.
- Post the EAP at every venue and near telephones, including the role of the first responder, a listing of emergency numbers, and street address and directions to guide the EMS personnel.

III. **Emergency Personnel**
- Designate an EAP coordinator.
- Identify who will be responsible and trained to respond to a SCA (likely first responders include athletic trainers, coaches, school nurses, and team physicians).
- Train targeted responders in CPR and AED use.
- Determine who is responsible for personnel training and establish a means that training has occurred.
- Identify the medical coordinator for on-site AED programs.

IV. **Emergency Equipment**
- Use on-site or centrally located AED(s) if the collapse-to-shock time interval for conventional EMS is estimated to be more than 5 minutes.
- Notify EMS dispatch centers and agencies of the specific type of AED and the exact location of the AED on school grounds.

- Acquire pocket mask or barrier-shield device for rescue breathing.
- Acquire AED supplies (scissors, razor, towel, and consider an extra set of AED pads).
- Consider bag-valve masks, oxygen delivery systems, oral and nasopharyngeal airways, and advanced airways (e.g., endotracheal tube, Combitube, or laryngeal mask airway).
- Consult with a physician regarding emergency cardiac medications (e.g., aspirin, nitroglycerin).
- Determine who is responsible for checking equipment readiness and how often and establish a means of documentation.

V. Emergency Transportation

- Determine transportation route for ambulances to enter and exit each venue.
- Facilitate access to SCA victim for arriving EMS personnel.
- Consider on-site ambulance coverage for high-risk events.
- Identify the receiving medical facility equipped in advanced cardiac care.
- Ensure that medical coverage is still provided at the athletic event if on-site medical staff accompany the athlete to the hospital.

VI. Practice and Review of Emergency Action Plan

- Rehearse the EAP at least annually with athletic trainers, athletic training students, team and consulting physicians, school nurses, coaches, campus public safety officials, and other targeted responders.
- Rehearse mock SCA scenarios.
- Establish an evaluation system for the EAP rehearsal, and modify the EAP if needed.

VII. Postevent Catastrophic Incident Guidelines

- Establish a contact list of individuals to be notified in case of a catastrophic event.
- Determine the procedures for release of information, aftercare services, and the postevent evaluation process.
- Identify local crisis services and counselors.
- Prepare an incident report form to be completed by all responders and the method for system improvement.

*EMS indicates emergency medical services; CPR, cardiopulmonary resuscitation; and AED, automated external defibrillator.

Adapted from: Drezner, JA, et al: Inter-association task force recommendations on emergency preparedness and management of sudden cardiac arrest in high school and college athletic programs. *J Athl Train*, 42:143, 2007.

Sport-Specific Rules

Table 2-1 Rules Affecting Examination During Athletic Competition

Sport	Rule(s)
Baseball	Hard casts must be properly padded. Players are permitted to wear only one elbow pad that does not exceed 10 inches in length.[7]
Basketball	An injured player must temporarily leave the contest if the athletic trainer or other staff member comes onto the court requiring a stoppage in play.[8] Equipment deemed dangerous to others by the officiating crew is prohibited.[8] Pre-event approval of protective equipment is required.
Field Hockey	Protective equipment that increases the size of the goalkeeper is not allowed.[9]
Football	No equipment that would endanger others such as metal is allowed. Hard equipment must be covered with thick foam padding; therapeutic/preventative knee braces must be covered or worn under clothing.[10] After an injury timeout, the injured player must leave for at least one down.[10]
Ice Hockey	Use of pads or protectors made of metal or any hard substance that could cause injury is prohibited.[11]
Soccer	Athletic trainers or other staff may not enter the field unless instructed by an official. Casts, knee braces, and other hard braces must be properly padded.[12]
Softball	Casts, braces, splints, and/or prostheses may be worn provided they are well-padded and not distracting.[13]
Tennis	Time-limited medical and bleeding timeouts may be used to treat the athlete.[14]
Wrestling	Two injury timeouts may be given for a cumulative maximum of 90 seconds for the entire match. A third nonbleeding injury will end the match. Bleeding timeouts do not count as an injury timeout, but the number and length of time allowed to treat the wound are left to the official's discretion. No more than two attendants may be allowed on the mat during these timeouts.[15]
All Sports	Athletes who have an open wound must be removed from competition until the bleeding is controlled and the wound appropriately covered. Uniforms that are saturated with blood must be changed.

Refer to current national governing agencies and individual conference rules regarding competitor safety.

Critical Findings

Table 2-2 Conditions Warranting Termination of the Evaluation

Segment	Findings that Warrant Immediate Physician Referral
History	Reports of the inability to feel or move one or more limbs (confirm with neurologic screen) Reports of significant chest pain Reports of difficulty breathing (e.g., anaphylaxis, pneumothorax)
Inspection	Obvious fracture Obvious joint dislocation Prolonged loss of consciousness Cyanosis Unequal chest expansion
Palpation	Disruption in the contour of bone, indicating a fracture or joint dislocation Malalignment of joint structures
Joint and Muscle Function Assessment	Inability of the muscle to produce torque
Joint Stability Tests	Gross joint instability
Neurologic Tests	Sensory dysfunction Motor dysfunction Pathologic changes in reflex Inability to maintain balance, loss of coordination, and other signs and symptoms of brain injury
Vascular Screening	Diminished or absent pulse Pooling of venous blood, suggesting inhibition of venous return

The On-Field Examination

Primary Survey

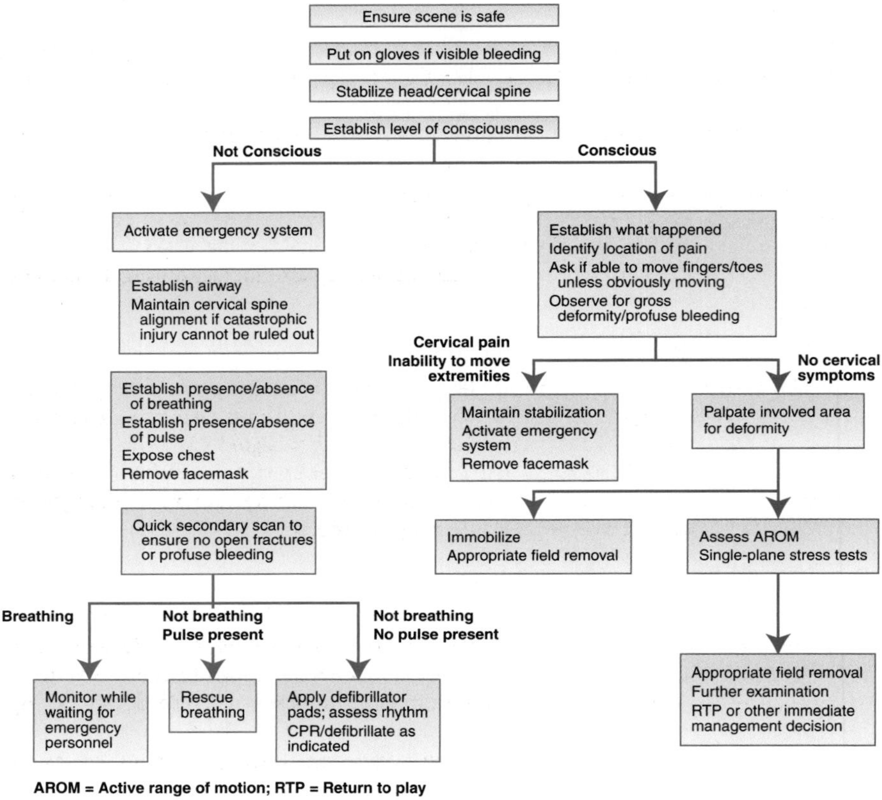

Ensure scene is safe

Put on gloves if visible bleeding

Stabilize head/cervical spine

Establish level of consciousness

Not Conscious

- Activate emergency system
- Establish airway
  Maintain cervical spine alignment if catastrophic injury cannot be ruled out
- Establish presence/absence of breathing
  Establish presence/absence of pulse
  Expose chest
  Remove facemask
- Quick secondary scan to ensure no open fractures or profuse bleeding
  - **Breathing** → Monitor while waiting for emergency personnel
  - **Not breathing, Pulse present** → Rescue breathing
  - **Not breathing, No pulse present** → Apply defibrillator pads; assess rhythm. CPR/defibrillate as indicated

Conscious

- Establish what happened
  Identify location of pain
  Ask if able to move fingers/toes unless obviously moving
  Observe for gross deformity/profuse bleeding
  - **Cervical pain, Inability to move extremities** → Maintain stabilization. Activate emergency system. Remove facemask → Immobilize. Appropriate field removal
  - **No cervical symptoms** → Palpate involved area for deformity → (Immobilize. Appropriate field removal) or (Assess AROM. Single-plane stress tests → Appropriate field removal. Further examination. RTP or other immediate management decision)

AROM = Active range of motion; RTP = Return to play

FIGURE 2-1 ■ On-field decision-making. Schematic representation of the on-field decision-making process.

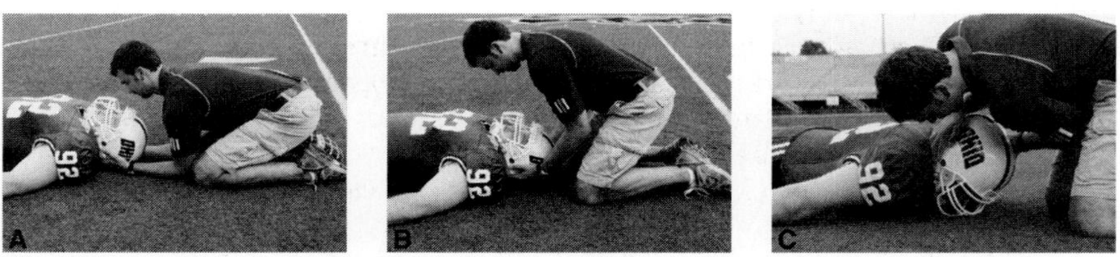

FIGURE 2-2 ■ Different c-spine stabilization techniques. **(A, B)** In-line stabilization and **(C)** prior to rolling the athlete supine.

On-Field History

- **Location of the pain:** Identify the site of pain as closely as possible. Although the athlete may be holding a particular area, do not assume that this is the only site of trauma because multiple injuries may have occurred. Ask the question, "Do you have pain anywhere else?"
- **Peripheral symptoms:** Question the athlete about the presence of pain or altered sensation that radiates into the distal extremities, suggesting spinal cord, nerve root, or peripheral nerve trauma.
- **Mechanism of the injury:** Identify the force that caused the injury (e.g., contact vs. noncontact injuries).
- **Associated sounds and symptoms:** Note any reports of a "snap" or "pop" at the time of injury that may indicate a tearing of ligaments or tendons or fracture.
- **History of injury:** Identify any relevant history of injury that may have been exacerbated by the current trauma or may influence the physical findings during the current evaluation.

On-Field Inspection

- **Position of the athlete:** Is the athlete prone, supine, or side-lying? Is a body part in an awkward position? Is any gross deformity evident? These factors take on added importance if the athlete is unconscious and must be moved to begin CPR.
- **Inspection of the injured area:** This process is an abbreviated version of the steps presented in Chapter 1, specifically observing for signs of a fracture (such as long bone angulation), joint dislocation (gross deformity), or edema.

On-Field Palpation

Palpation of the bony structures

- **Bony alignment:** Palpate the length of the injured bone to identify any discontinuity. Although fractures of long bones are often accompanied by gross deformity, those of smaller bones may present no outward signs but are exquisitely tender during palpation.
- **Crepitus:** Note any crepitus, associated with fractures, swelling, inflammation, or air entering the subcutaneous tissues.
- **Joint alignment:** If the injury involves a joint, palpate along the joint line to determine whether the joint is aligned normally.

Palpation of the soft tissues

- **Swelling:** Swelling immediately after the injury is often associated with a major disruption of the tissues. Trauma to bursae tend to swell disproportionately to the severity of the injury. Tissues that have a rich blood supply, such as the face, may present with a rapid formation of localized edema.
- **Painful areas:** Areas that are painful when palpated can indicate trauma to underlying tissue.
- **Deficit in the muscles or tendons:** Severe tearing of a muscle or tendon can result in a palpable defect. There is a "golden period" immediately after an injury that allows for defects to be palpated. After this period, edema and muscle spasm mask any underlying defect.

On-Field Joint and Muscle Function Assessment

- **Active range of motion:** The athlete is asked to move the limb through the range of motion (ROM), while the quality and quantity of movement are noted.
- **Strength assessment:** If ROM test results are normal, break pressure can be used to determine the involved muscle group's ability to sustain a forceful contraction. Similar to PROM, the more specific manual muscle tests are delayed until a more detailed examination is performed.
- **Passive range of motion:** The decision to include PROM assessment is made on a case-by-case basis and is frequently delayed until the clinical evaluation. The degree of muscular and/or ligamentous damage and capsular disruption is assessed by placing the tissues on stretch. Do not perform PROM evaluations on the field if the athlete is unable to actively move the joint.
- **Weight-bearing status (lower extremity injuries):** If the athlete is able to complete the ROM tests, the athlete can be permitted to walk off the field, with assistance if necessary. If the athlete is unable to perform these tests or signs and symptoms of a potential fracture or dislocation exist, the athlete is removed from the field in a non–weight-bearing manner.

Immediate Management

On completion of the on-field examination, a determination must be made regarding how to manage the athlete. Possible conclusions are:

- No splinting is needed: The athlete walks off under his or her own power.
- No splinting is needed: The athlete is assisted off the field.
- No splinting is needed: The athlete is transported directly to the hospital.
- Splinting is needed: The athlete walks off the field (upper extremity injury).
- Splinting is needed: The athlete is assisted off the field (lower extremity injury).
- Splinting is needed: The athlete is transported directly to the hospital.

Splinting

Box 2-2
Principles of Splinting and Immobilization

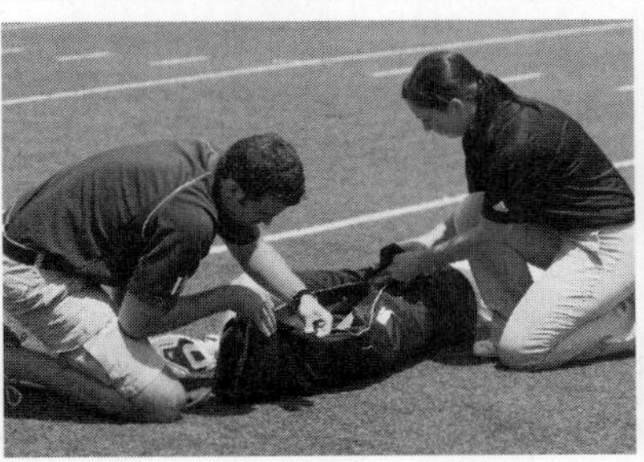

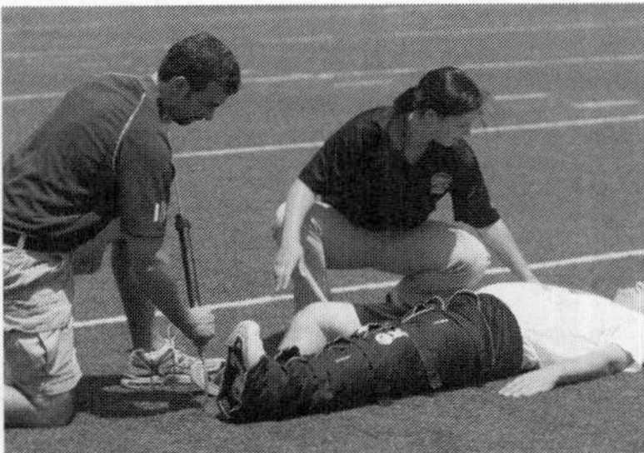

In most sports medicine settings commercial splints will be used to immobilize the body part, although upper extremity injuries can often be splinted against the torso. Regardless of the type of splint used, the splinting technique should limit motion of the involved joint and/or bone in three dimensions.

1. Unless otherwise directed by a physician, splint the extremity in the position in which it was found.
2. Establish a baseline level of sensation and skin temperature so that any changes can be noted.
3. Immobilize the joint(s) proximal and distal to the injured site.
4. Edema will most likely form soon after the injury. The splint should allow for edema and be regularly readjusted to account for swelling.[16]
5. To allow capillary refill to be checked, leave the fingers or toes uncovered when possible. Regularly assess capillary refill.
6. After immobilization, periodically question the athlete about increased pain, diminished or altered sensation, and changes in skin temperature.

Transportation

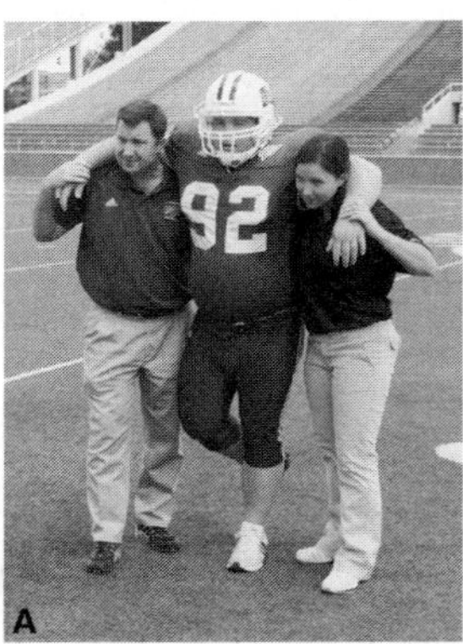
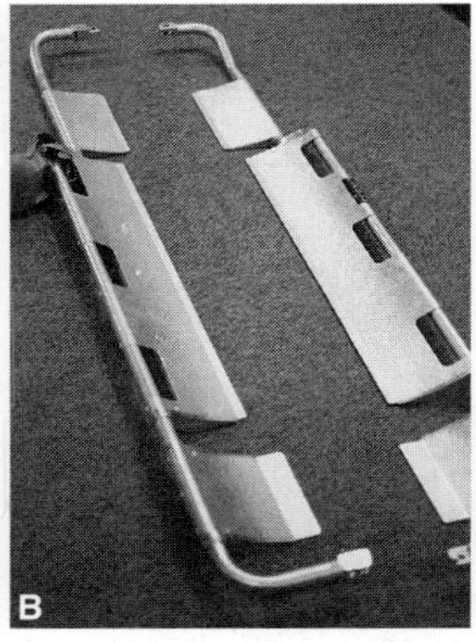
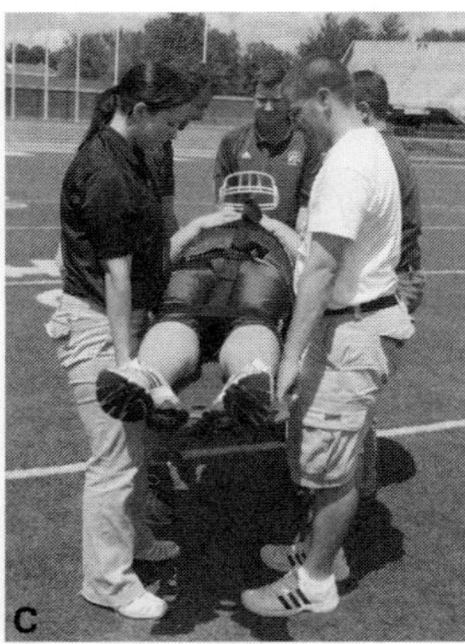

FIGURE 2-3 ■ Various athlete extraction techniques. **(A)** Assisted walking; **(B)** scoop stretcher; and **(C)** full spine board.

Return to Activity Decision Making

- **Strength and range of motion:** The athlete's strength and ROM should be approximately equal bilaterally and sufficient to protect both the injured area—and the athlete in general—from further injury.
- **Pain:** The athlete should report tolerable pain during exertional activities that does not result in noticeable change in function or worsen the condition.
- **Proprioception:** The athlete's involved extremity should demonstrate proprioceptive ability sufficient to protect the body part from further injury.
- **Functional activity progression:** Gradually increase the demands of the activity by introducing progressively more challenging tasks. For example, for a soccer player with a lower extremity injury, the functional progression would include demonstrating the ability to walk, jog, run straight ahead, change direction when jogging, and then change direction at high speed. Sport-specific skills such as dribbling are added once the athlete can complete this progression.

CHAPTER 3

Evidence-Based Practice in the Diagnostic Process

Box 3-1
Puzzlin' Evidence

Not all evidence is created equally. The data and methods used to derive conclusions are varied; some stemming from well constructed research designs to those that do not pass muster with the scientific community. The Centre of Evidence-Based Medicine has developed criteria to evaluate the quality of research. Termed "Levels of Evidence," a hierarchy of the different sources of data from which clinical decisions are made. Those at the top of the hierarchy carry more weight than the ones ranked lower:

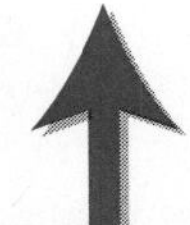

Meta-analysis: Draws a conclusion based on the statistical results of multiple studies.

Systematic review: A literature review that critiques and synthesizes high-quality research relating to a specific, focused question.

Randomized clinical trials: A research technique in which subjects are randomly assigned to an experimental or control group. The experimental group receives the treatment. The control group does not.

Cohort studies: Two groups, one that receives the treatment and one that does not, are studied forward over time to determine the impact of the treatment.

Case-control studies: Similar to a cohort study, but groups are studied from a historical perspective (backwards in time). Differences between the groups of patients are identified.

Case series: Report on a series of patients with a particular condition; no control group is used.

Case reports: A precise description and analysis of one or more clinical cases.

Expert opinion: Opinion based on general principles, animal or human-based laboratory research, physiology, and clinical experience.

Two sources may be contradictory regarding the usefulness of clinical techniques. In this case, factor in the strength of the source (based on the hierarchy above) and the weight of the recommendations. The recommendations derived from a randomized clinical trial must be given more consideration than those from a case report.

Reliability

- **Intra-rater (intra-examiner) reliability** describes the extent to which the same examiner obtains the same results on the same patient.
- **Inter-rater (inter-examiner) reliability** describes the extent to which different examiners obtain the same results for the same patient.

Table 3-1 Reliability Measures

If the reliability measure falls within this range...	...then the clinical usefulness is
Less than 0.5	Poor
0.5–0.75	Moderate
Greater than 0.75	Good

Reliability
Not Reliable — Very Reliable
Poor | Moderate | Good
0 0.1 0.2 0.3 0.4 0.5 0.6 0.7 0.8 0.9 1.0

Diagnostic Accuracy

Table 3-2 2 x 2 Contingency Table

	Gold Standard	
	Gold Standard Positive	**Gold Standard Negative**
Clinical test positive	True positive (TP)	False positive (FP)
Clinical test negative	False negative (FN)	True negative (TN)

- **True positive:** The clinical test and the gold standard are both positive.
- **False positive:** The clinical test incorrectly identifies a condition as present when, in fact, there is no pathology.
- **True negative:** The clinical test and the gold standard are both negative.
- **False negative:** The clinical procedure identifies a condition as not present when, in fact, it is present.

Diagnostic Predictive Value

- **Accuracy:** The number of correctly classified patients (True Positives + True Negatives)/ Total number of patients.
- **Positive predictive value:** How often a positive finding is correct: True Positive/True Positive + False Positive.
- **Negative predictive value:** How often a negative finding is correct: True Negative/True Negative + False Negative.

Sensitivity

- **Sensitivity:** Ability to identify the condition relative to the gold standard (true positive rate). Calculated as: True Positives/(True Positives + False Negatives).

Table 3-3 Calculating Sensitivity

	Arthroscopy	
	Arthroscopy Positive for ACL Pathology	**Arthroscopy Negative for ACL Pathology**
Clinical test positive	17 (TP)	3 (FP)
Clinical test negative	6 (FN)	14 (TN)
	Sensitivity = TP/(TP + FN) = 17/(17 + 6) = 0.74	

FN = false negative; FP = false positive; TN = true negative; TP = true positive.

- **SnNout:** In tests with a high sensitivity (Sn), a negative finding (N) effectively rules out the condition.

Specificity

- **Specificity:** Ability to identify those patients who do NOT have the disorder (true negative rate). Calculated as: True Negatives/(True Negatives + False Positives).

Table 3-4 Calculating Specificity

	Arthroscopy	
	Arthroscopy Positive for ACL Pathology	**Arthroscopy Negative for ACL Pathology**
McManus test positive	17 (TP)	3 (FP)
McManus test negative	6 (FN)	14 (TN)
	Sensitivity = TP/(TP + FN) = 17/(17 + 6) = 0.74	Specificity = TN/(TN + FP) = 14/(14 + 3) = 0.82

FN = false negative; FP = false positive; TN = true negative; TP = true positive.

- **SpPin:** In tests with a high specificity (Sp), a positive finding convincingly rules in the condition.

Likelihood Ratios

- **Positive likelihood ratio (LR+):** The change in our confidence that a condition is present when the test is positive. The higher the LR+, the more a positive test enhances the probability that the pathology is present. LR+ is calculated as: sensitivity/(1 – specificity).

Table 3-5 Interpretation of Likelihood Ratios

Positive Likelihood Ratio	Negative Likelihood Ratio	Shift in Probability Condition is Present
>10	<0.1	Large, often conclusive
5–10	0.1–0.2	Moderate but usually important
2–5	0.2–0.5	Small, sometimes important
1–2	0.5–1	Very small, usually unimportant

Table 3-6 Calculating the Positive Likelihood Ratio

	Arthroscopy	
	Arthroscopy Positive for ACL Pathology	**Arthroscopy Negative for ACL Pathology**
McManus test positive	17 (TP)	3 (FP)
McManus test negative	6 (FN)	14 (TN)
	Sensitivity = 0.74	Specificity = 0.82
	LR+ = Sensitivity/(1 – specificity) = 0.74/(1 – 0.82) ≒ 4.11	

FN = false negative; FP = false positive; TN = true negative; TP = true positive.

- **Negative likelihood ratio (LR–):** The probability that the pathology is still present even though the test was negative. The lower the LR– is, the lower is the probability that the condition exists. The LR– is calculated as: (1 – sensitivity)/specificity.

Nomogram

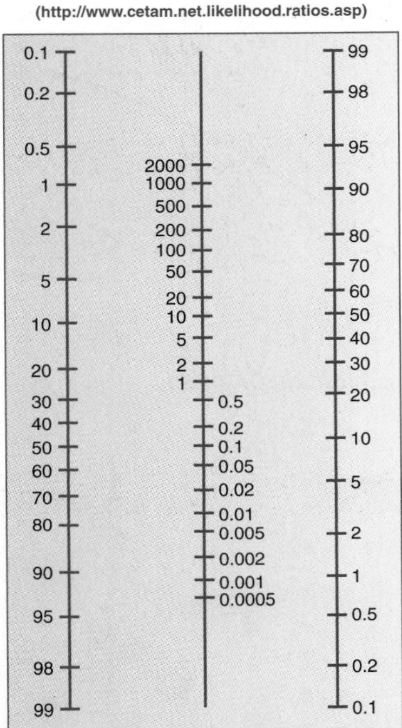

FIGURE 3-1 ■ Nomogram. The pretest probability is identified on the left side of the nomogram, the positive or negative likelihood ratio is plotted on the middle column, and a line connecting the two points is continued through the third column. The intersection in the third column indicates the change in probability that the condition exists given the results of the test.

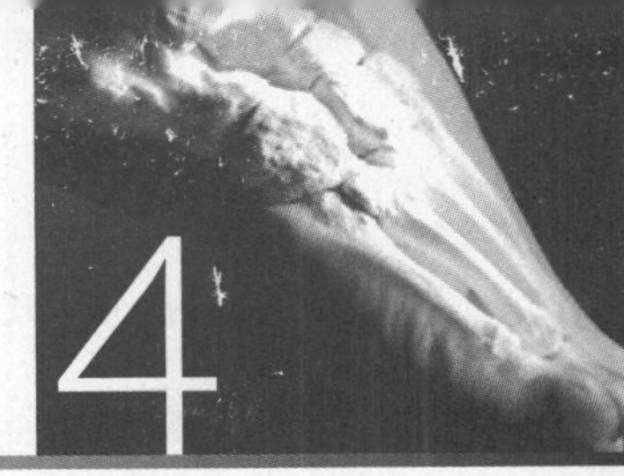

CHAPTER 4

Injury Pathology Nomenclature

Tissue Response to Stress

Physical Stress Theory

FIGURE 4-1 ■ The Physical Stress Theory. The body and specific tissues respond in a predictable manner to stresses placed upon them.

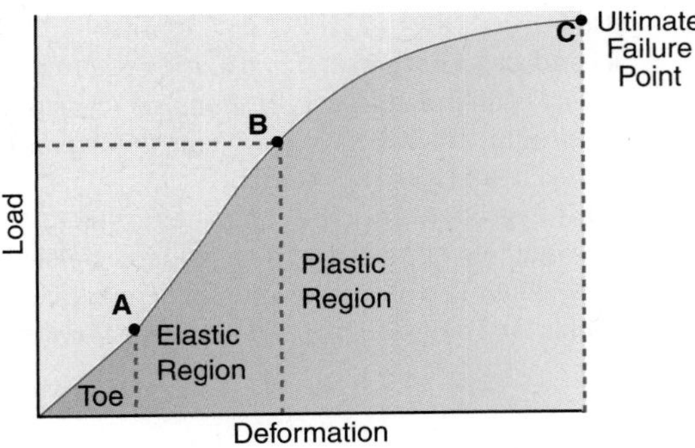

FIGURE 4-2 ■ Load-deformation curve for a connective tissue tested in tension. Initially, the crimp straightens with little force (toe region). Then, collagen fibers are stretched as the elastic region begins at **A**. After the elastic region ends **(B)**, further force application causes a residual change in tissue structure (plastic region). Continuation of load may cause the tissue to rupture at its ultimate failure point **(C)**. (From Butler, DL, et al: Biomechanics of ligaments and tendons. *Exer Sport Sci Rev* 6:144, 1978, with permission from Lippincott Williams & Wilkins.)

Forces Placed on a Joint

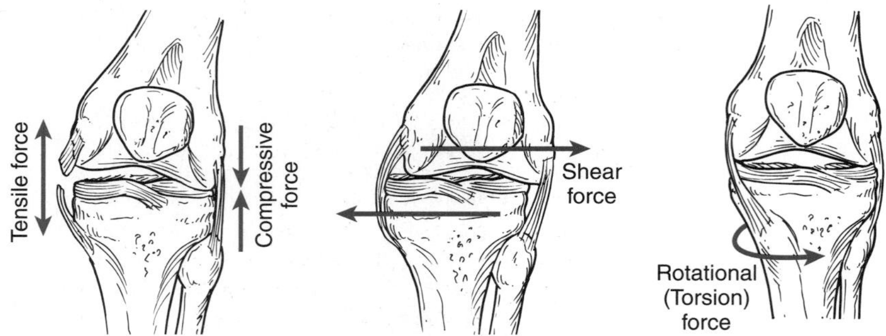

FIGURE 4-3 ■ **Tensile forces** "tear" the structure by stretching the tissue. **Compressive forces** place opposing forces on the structure. Note that tensile forces and compressive forces may occur on opposite sides of the joint. **Shear forces** place a stress perpendicular to the tissues. **Rotational forces** (torsion) place an angular stress on the tissues.

Musculotendinous Injuries

Strains

- **First-degree strains:** Stretching of the fibers and/or damage to the myofibrils, traumatizing less than 5% of the musculotendinous unit.[17] Pain increases as the muscle contracts, especially against resistance, and the site of injury is point tender. Swelling may also be present.
- **Second-degree strains:** Actual tearing of some muscle fibers, extracellular matrix, and fascia.[17] The inflammatory response is more pronounced than in first-degree strains. These injuries present with the same findings as first-degree strains but are more severe and ecchymosis may be present.
- **Third-degree strains:** The complete rupture of the muscle and blood vessels, resulting in a total loss of function and a palpable defect in the muscle that is rapidly obscured by swelling. The tissues become ischemic, causing further muscle damage and edema formation. Pain, swelling, and ecchymosis are also present.

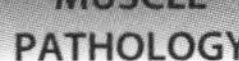

MUSCLE PATHOLOGY

Examination Findings 4-1
Muscle Strains

Examination Segment	Clinical Findings
History	***Onset:*** Acute. ***Pain characteristics:*** Pain is initially located at the site of the injury, which tends to be at or near the junction between the muscle belly and tendon. After a few days, pain becomes more diffuse and difficult to localize. The distal musculotendinous junction is most often involved. ***Mechanism:*** Strains usually result from a single episode of overstretching or overloading of the muscle but are more likely to result from eccentric loading.[17] ***Predisposing conditions:*** Imbalance in the strength of the agonist/antagonist muscle groups. History of strain to the involved muscle. Muscle tightness and improper warm-up before activity.
Inspection	Ecchymosis is evident in cases of severe muscle strains. Gravity causes the blood to pool distal to the site of trauma. Swelling may be present over or distal to the involved area. In severe acute cases or in a chronic condition a defect may be visible in the muscle or tendon. If the strain involves a muscle of the lower extremity, the patient may walk with a limp.
Palpation	Point tenderness and increased tissue density associated with spasm exists over the site of the injury, with the degree of pain increasing with the severity of the injury. A defect may be palpable at the injury site.
Joint and Muscle Function Assessment	***AROM:*** Pain is elicited at the injury site. In the case of second- or third-degree strains, the patient may be unable to complete the movement. ***MMT:*** Muscle strength is reduced. Pain increases as the amount of resistance is increased. Third-degree strains result in a total loss of function of the involved muscle. ***PROM:*** Pain is elicited at the injury site during passive motion in the direction opposite that of the muscle, placing it on stretch. Active contraction of the antagonistic muscle can also produce pain by stretching the involved muscle.
Joint Stability Tests	***Stress tests:*** Stress tests of the ligaments crossing the joint(s) serviced by the muscle should be performed. Strains may occur as the body attempts to protect against ligament injury. ***Joint play:*** Rule out hypermobility
Neurologic Screening	Use to rule out nerve entrapment that clinically appears as a strain. Tearing of muscle may also damage peripheral nerves.

Continued

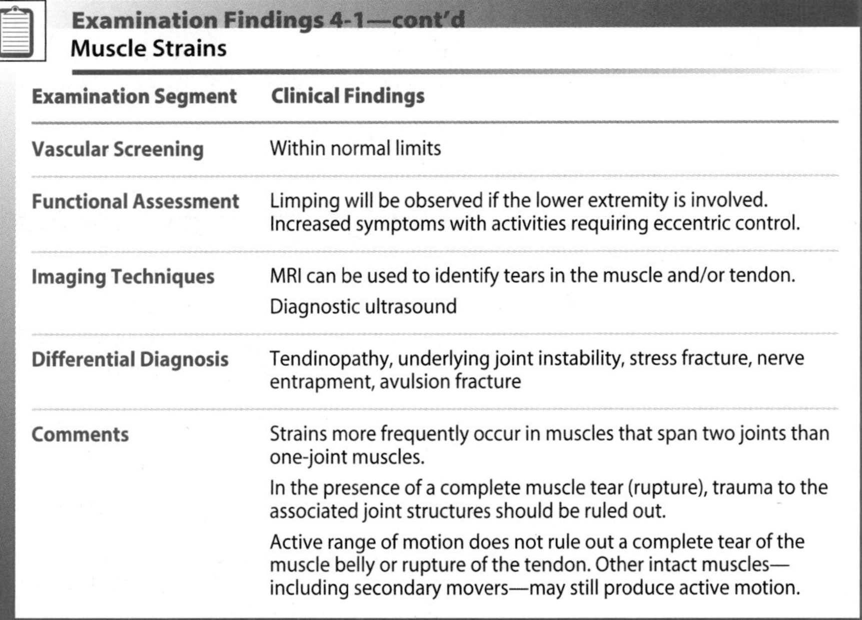

Examination Findings 4-1—cont'd
Muscle Strains

Examination Segment	Clinical Findings
Vascular Screening	Within normal limits
Functional Assessment	Limping will be observed if the lower extremity is involved. Increased symptoms with activities requiring eccentric control.
Imaging Techniques	MRI can be used to identify tears in the muscle and/or tendon. Diagnostic ultrasound
Differential Diagnosis	Tendinopathy, underlying joint instability, stress fracture, nerve entrapment, avulsion fracture
Comments	Strains more frequently occur in muscles that span two joints than one-joint muscles. In the presence of a complete muscle tear (rupture), trauma to the associated joint structures should be ruled out. Active range of motion does not rule out a complete tear of the muscle belly or rupture of the tendon. Other intact muscles—including secondary movers—may still produce active motion.

AROM = active range of motion; MMT = manual muscle test; MRI = magnetic resonance imaging; PROM = passive range of motion.

Severe Hamstring Strain

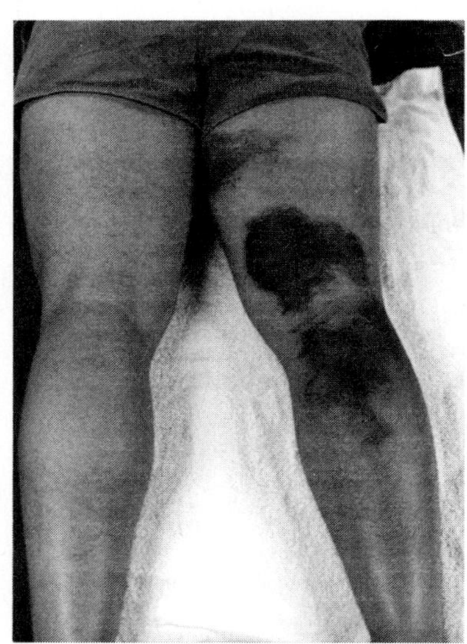

FIGURE 4-4 ■ Ecchymosis associated with a muscular strain. Gravity causes blood that has seeped into the tissues to drift inferiorly.

Tendinopathy

- **First-degree tendinopathy** is marked by pain and slight dysfunction during activity.
- **Second-degree tendinopathy** results in decreased function and pain during and after activity.
- **Third-degree tendinopathy** is characterized by constant pain that prohibits activity.

Examination Findings 4-2
Tendinopathy

Examination Segment	Clinical Findings
History	***Onset:*** Occurs gradually or is chronic. An acute inflammation may occur following a rapid increase in activity, such as running a marathon. ***Pain characteristics:*** Pain in tendon, often near the bony insertion, that increases or decreases with the level of activity. ***Other symptoms:*** Not applicable ***Mechanism:*** Results from microtraumatic forces applied to the tendon ***Predisposing conditions:*** History of muscle tightness, poor conditioning, increase in the frequency, duration, and/or intensity of activity, changes in footwear or surfaces
Inspection	Swelling may be noted, but joint effusion is rare.[18] In chronic cases, atrophy of the involved muscle may be noted. A guarding posture may be noted where the patient avoids placing stress on the tendon.
Palpation	The tendon is tender to the touch. Crepitus or thickening of the tendon may be noted.
Joint and Muscle Function Assessment	***AROM:*** Pain throughout the range of motion as force is generated within the tendon. ***MMT:*** Strength is decreased secondary to pain.[19] ***PROM:*** Pain is elicited during the extremes of the range of motion as the tendon is stretched. Pain can be elicited earlier in the ROM in more severe cases.
Joint Stability Tests	***Stress tests:*** Rule out underlying joint instability. ***Joint play:*** Rule out underlying joint hypomobility or hypermobility.
Special Tests	Specific to the involved joint
Neurologic Screening	Used to rule out neuropathy
Vascular Screening	Within normal limits

Continued

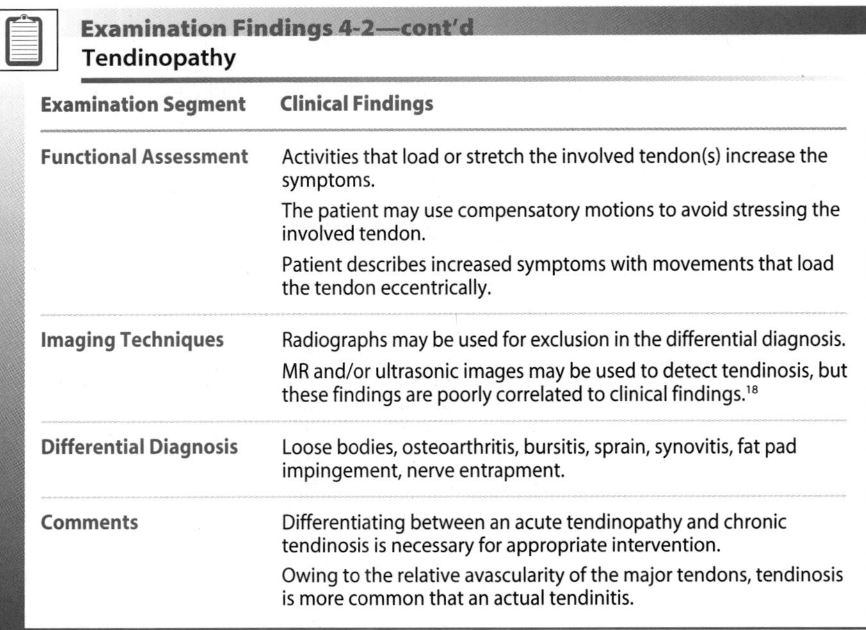

Examination Findings 4-2—cont'd
Tendinopathy

Examination Segment	Clinical Findings
Functional Assessment	Activities that load or stretch the involved tendon(s) increase the symptoms. The patient may use compensatory motions to avoid stressing the involved tendon. Patient describes increased symptoms with movements that load the tendon eccentrically.
Imaging Techniques	Radiographs may be used for exclusion in the differential diagnosis. MR and/or ultrasonic images may be used to detect tendinosis, but these findings are poorly correlated to clinical findings.[18]
Differential Diagnosis	Loose bodies, osteoarthritis, bursitis, sprain, synovitis, fat pad impingement, nerve entrapment.
Comments	Differentiating between an acute tendinopathy and chronic tendinosis is necessary for appropriate intervention. Owing to the relative avascularity of the major tendons, tendinosis is more common that an actual tendinitis.

AROM = active range of motion; MMT = manual muscle test; MR = magnetic resonance; PROM = passive range of motion.

Table 4-1 Mechanisms Leading to Tendinopathy

Mechanism	Implications
Microtrauma	Repetitive tensile loading, compression, and abrasion of the working tendons. Insufficient rest periods allow for the accumulation of the microtrauma, possibly leading to tendon failure.
Macrotrauma	A single force placed on the muscle, causing discrete tearing within the tendon or at the musculotendinous junction. This area becomes the weak link when the forces of otherwise normal activity are sufficient to cause further inflammation.
Biomechanical Alteration	The alteration of otherwise normal motion with redistribution of the forces around a joint, resulting in new tensile loads, compressive forces, or wearing of the tendons. Examples of this include running on uneven terrain or using poor technique with sporting equipment such as a tennis racquet.

Heterotopic Ossification

Examination Findings 4-3
Heterotopic Ossification

Examination Segment	Clinical Findings
History	***Onset:*** The initial trauma is a hematoma caused by a single acute or by repeated blows to the muscle. The ossification occurs gradually. ***Pain characteristics:*** Pain occurs at the site of ossification, usually the site of a large muscle mass that is exposed to blows (e.g., the quadriceps femoris or biceps brachii muscles). ***Other symptoms:*** A fever may develop. ***Mechanism:*** Calcium within the muscle fascia secondary to an abnormality in the healing process ***Predisposing conditions:*** History of heterotopic ossification
Inspection	A superficial bruise may be noted. Edema of the distal joint closest to the site injury occurs. Ecchymosis may be present.
Palpation	Acutely, the muscle is tender. As the ossification develops, it may become palpable within the muscle mass. Swelling and warmth may be felt at the site of injury.
Joint and Muscle Function Assessment	***AROM:*** As the ossification grows, the number of contractile units available to the muscle decreases. Antagonist motion is painful secondary to decreased flexibility within the affected muscle mass. ***MMT:*** Decreased secondary to pain; the ossification does not allow the muscle to contract normally ***PROM:*** Decreased secondary to pain and adhesions within the muscle
Joint Stability Tests	***Stress tests:*** Not applicable ***Joint play:*** Not applicable
Special Tests	None
Neurologic Screening	Within normal limits
Vascular Screening	Within normal limits
Functional Assessment	Compensatory motions to avoid using the muscle containing the ossification.

Continued

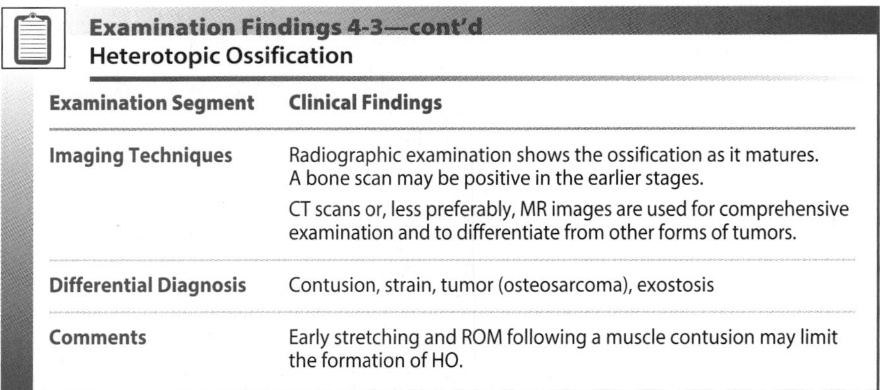

Examination Findings 4-3—cont'd
Heterotopic Ossification

Examination Segment	Clinical Findings
Imaging Techniques	Radiographic examination shows the ossification as it matures. A bone scan may be positive in the earlier stages. CT scans or, less preferably, MR images are used for comprehensive examination and to differentiate from other forms of tumors.
Differential Diagnosis	Contusion, strain, tumor (osteosarcoma), exostosis
Comments	Early stretching and ROM following a muscle contusion may limit the formation of HO.

AROM = active range of motion; CT = computed tomography; MMT = manual muscle test; MR = magnetic resonance; PROM = passive range of motion; ROM = range of motion.

Radiograph of Heterotopic Ossification

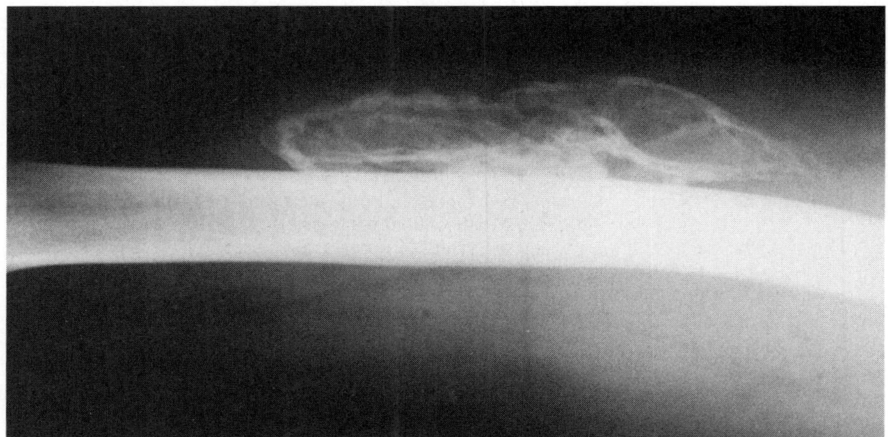

FIGURE 4-5 ■ Radiograph of heterotopic ossification. This calcification has occurred in the biceps brachii of a football lineman who sustained multiple blows to the muscle during the act of blocking.

Box 4-1
Compartment Syndromes

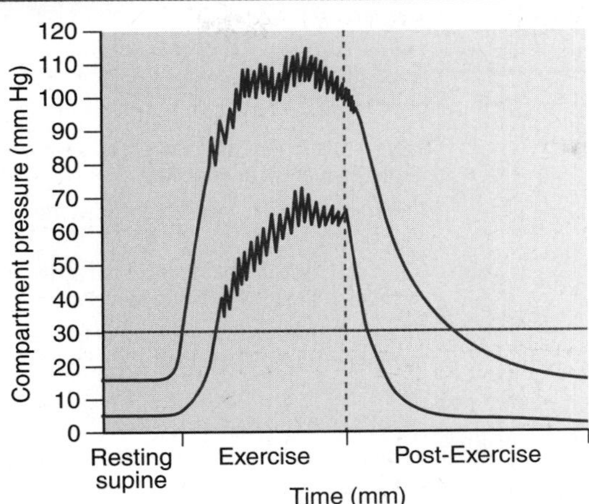

"Compartments" are areas within the extremities defined by relatively unyielding borders such as dense fascia and bone. An increase in pressure, caused by increased blood volume, excess fluid, or muscle hypertrophy can result in a disruption of distal arterial, vascular, and nerve function. Blood supply to the structures within the compartment is also compromised.

Acute compartment syndromes result from trauma such as contusions and fractures. Chronic compartment syndromes (also referred to as exertional or recurrent compartment syndromes) occur during exercise as muscles enlarge but the compartment cannot expand to accommodate the increased volume. The anatomical compartments most disposed to this condition are located in the leg and forearm.

Patients will complain of pain, numbness, and/or paresthesia in the distal extremity. The classic signs—the "five P's"—**pain, pallor** (redness), **pulselessness, paresthesia,** and **paralysis,** are indicative of late-stage compartment syndrome. Acute compartment syndromes are medical emergencies. If a pulse is absent, the extremity is in immediate danger.

Bursitis

Examination Findings 4-4
Bursitis

Examination Segment	Clinical Findings
History	***Onset:*** Acute in the case of direct trauma to the bursa; insidious in the case of overuse or infection ***Pain characteristics:*** Pain occurring at the site of the bursa ***Mechanism:*** Chemical: Calcium or other chemical deposits within the bursa activating the inflammatory response. Mechanical: Repetitive rubbing of the soft tissue over a bony prominence or a direct blow, possibly related to improper biomechanics. Septic: Viral or bacterial invasion of the bursa. ***Predisposing conditions:*** Improper biomechanics, poor padding of at-risk bursae (e.g., suprapatellar bursa, olecranon bursa).
Inspection	Local swelling of bursae can be very pronounced, especially those located over the olecranon process and patella. Chronic or septic bursitis may appear red with accompanying lymphatic streaking.
Palpation	Point tenderness is noted over the site of the bursa. Localized heat and swelling may be noted.
Joint and Muscle Function Assessment	***AROM:*** Pain may be noted. ***MMT:*** Strength limited secondary to pain. As the muscle contracts, it compresses the bursal sac. ***PROM:*** Pain is produced if the motion causes the tendon or other structure to rub across or compress the inflamed bursa.
Joint Stability Tests	***Stress tests:*** Rule out underlying instability. ***Joint play:*** Rule out underlying hypermobility.
Special Tests	None
Neurologic Screening	Within normal limits
Vascular Screening	Within normal limits
Functional Assessment	Increased pain and/or weakness with tasks that require strength of involved muscles
Imaging Techniques	T2-weighted MRI with fat suppression are used to image bursae.
Differential Diagnosis	Contusion, tendinopathy, septic joint, synovitis
Comments	Signs and symptoms of an infected bursa warrant immediate referral to a physician. Chronic bursal irritation is often associated with tendon pathology.

AROM = active range of motion; MMT = manual muscle test; MRI = magnetic resonance imaging; PROM = passive range of motion.

Joint Structure Pathology

Sprains

- **First-degree sprain:** Little or no tearing of the fibers. No abnormal motion is produced when the joint is stressed, and a normal, firm **end-point** is felt. Local pain, mild point tenderness, and slight swelling of the joint are present.
- **Second-degree sprain:** Partial tearing of the ligament's fibers has occurred, resulting in joint laxity when the ligament is stressed. A soft but definite end-point is present. Moderate pain and swelling occur and a loss of the joint's function is noted.
- **Third-degree sprain:** The ligament has been completely ruptured, causing gross joint laxity, possible instability, and an empty or absent end-point. Swelling is marked, but pain may be limited secondary to tearing of the local nerves. A complete loss of function of the joint is usually noted.

Examination Findings 4-5
Sprains

Examination Segment	Clinical Findings
History	***Onset:*** Acute ***Pain characteristics:*** Pain is localized to the site of injury with first-degree sprains. As the severity of the sprain increases, the pain radiates throughout the joint. ***Other symptoms:*** A "popping" sensation or sound may be reported by the patient. ***Mechanism:*** Sprains result from tensile forces caused by the stretching of the ligament. ***Predisposing conditions:*** A history of a sprain can predispose the ligament to further injury. Shoe wear that increases the friction between the shoe–surface interface may increase the chance of lower extremity sprains. Women have a greater risk of some knee ligament sprains, but the exact cause has not been determined.
Inspection	Acutely, localized swelling is evident with injury to superficial structures. Effusion may be visible. Ecchymosis may form at and distal to the site of injury.
Palpation	Point tenderness is noted over the ligament. The entire joint may be tender. Palpable effusion may be noted
Joint and Muscle Function Assessment	***AROM:*** Limited by pain in the direction that stresses the involved ligament (or ligaments) ***MMT:*** Isometric contractions may not produce as intense pain. Resisting ROM through the range may be painful, especially at the end. ***PROM:*** Limited by pain, especially in the direction that stresses the involved ligament (or ligaments)

Continued

Examination Findings 4-5—cont'd
Sprains

Examination Segment	Clinical Findings
Joint Stability Tests	***Stress tests:*** The ligament can be stressed by producing a force through the joint that causes the ligament to stretch. The examiner should note the amount of increased laxity compared with the opposite side, as well as the quality of the end-point. The end-point should be distinct and crisp. A soft, "mushy," or absent end-point is a sign of ligamentous damage. ***Joint play:*** Hypermobility of the involved joint
Special Tests	Based on the joint being examined
Neurologic Screening	Within normal limits
Vascular Screening	Within normal limits
Functional Assessment	Depending on severity of sprain, instability during functional movements may be present.
Imaging Techniques	Radiographs and/or CT scans to rule out fracture; stress radiographs to identify laxity. Some ligaments, such as the anterior cruciate ligament, can be visualized via MR images.
Differential Diagnosis	Strain, epiphyseal fracture, osteochondral fracture, joint subluxation/dislocation
Comments	Strains can occur simultaneously with sprains, as the muscles attempt to protect the joint.

AROM = active range of motion; CT = computed tomography; MMT = manual muscle test; MR = magnetic resonance; PROM = passive range of motion; ROM = range of motion.

Joint Dislocation

Examination Findings 4-6
Joint Dislocations

Examination Segment	Clinical Findings
History	***Onset:*** Acute ***Pain characteristics:*** At the involved joint ***Mechanism:*** Dislocation caused by a stress that forces the joint beyond its normal anatomical limits ***Predisposing conditions:*** Repeated dislocation as the joint's supportive structures are progressively stretched
Inspection	Gross joint deformity may be present and swelling is observed.
Palpation	Pain is elicited throughout the joint. Malalignment of the joint surfaces may be felt.
Joint and Muscle Function Assessment	***ROM:*** ROM is not possible because of the disruption of the joint's alignment. Other ROM tests are contraindicated in the presence of an obvious dislocation
Joint Stability Tests	Contraindicated in the presence of an obvious dislocation
Special Tests	Contraindicated in the presence of an obvious joint dislocation.
Neurologic Screening	Sensory distribution distal to the dislocated joint must be established.
Vascular Screening	The presence of the distal pulse must be established. A lack of circulation to the distal extremity threatens the viability of the body part.
Functional Assessment	Contraindicated in the presence of an obvious joint dislocation.
Imaging Techniques	Radiographs and/or MRI are obtained to confirm and quantify the magnitude of joint disruption. Imaging may be obtained post-reduction to evaluate the integrity of joint surfaces.
Differential Diagnosis	Fracture, sprain, subluxation, tendon rupture
Comments	Dislocations of the major joints represent medical emergencies.

MRI = magnetic resonance imaging; ROM = range of motion.

PIP Dislocation

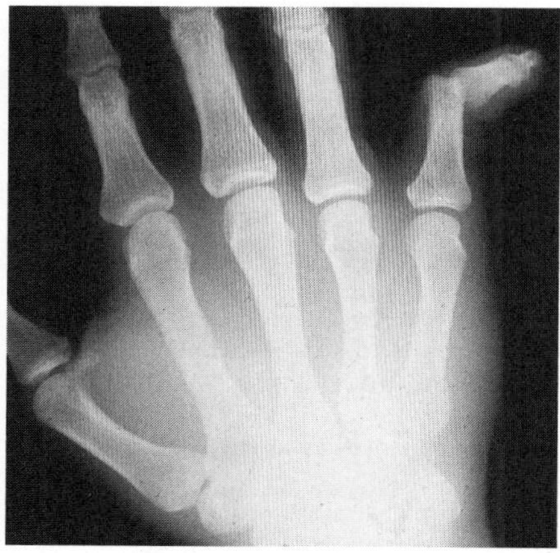

FIGURE 4-6 ■ Radiograph of a dislocation of the fifth proximal interphalangeal joint (PIP joint).

Joint Subluxation

Examination Findings 4-7
Joint Subluxations

Examination Segment	Clinical Findings
History	***Onset:*** Acute or chronic. Chronic subluxation can occur as the joint's supportive structures are progressively stretched. ***Pain characteristics:*** Pain occurs throughout the involved joint. Associated muscle spasm may involve the muscles proximal and distal to the joint. ***Other symptoms:*** Patients may not realize that their joint is actually subluxating and may report other symptoms such as pain, apprehension, or the joint "giving way." ***Mechanism:*** Joint subluxation results from a stress that takes the joint beyond its normal anatomical limits. ***Predisposing conditions:*** History of joint subluxation or dislocation; congenital hyperlaxity
Inspection	Swelling may be present. No gross bony deformity is noted because the joint relocates.
Palpation	Pain elicited along the tissues that have been stretched or compressed
Joint and Muscle Function Assessment	***AROM:*** Limited to pain possible instability The patient is unwilling or unable to move joint to the end range. ***MMT:*** Muscular strength is decreased secondary to pain and joint instability. ***PROM:*** Limited secondary to pain and instability

Examination Findings 4-7—cont'd
Joint Subluxations

Examination Segment	Clinical Findings
Joint Stability Tests	***Stress tests:*** Pain is elicited during stress testing of the involved ligament (or ligaments). Laxity of the tissues is present, particularly post-acutely. The patient may note instability and react to guard against this by contracting the surrounding musculature or pulling away, an apprehension response. ***Joint play:*** Hypermobility
Special Tests	Based on the body part being examined
Neurologic Screening	Transient paresthesia of the nerves crossing the joint may be present.
Vascular Screening	Repeated subluxations may result in occlusion of the vessels crossing the joint. Assess distal capillary refill and note for venous pooling in the distal extremity.
Functional Assessment	May describe sensation of instability with motions that stress the joint. Observation may reveal avoidance of those positions secondary to this apprehension.
Imaging Techniques	Radiographs; MRI may be used to rule out bony or soft tissue injury.
Differential Diagnosis	Sprain or damage to other supportive structures (e.g., labrum), nerve pathology

AROM = active range of motion; MMT = manual muscle test; MRI = magnetic resonance imaging; PROM = passive range of motion.

Synovitis

Examination Findings 4-8
Synovitis

Examination Segment	Clinical Findings
History	***Onset:*** Insidious; often subsequent to a previous injury to the joint ***Pain characteristics:*** Pain occurring throughout the entire joint, causing aching at rest and increased pain with activity ***Mechanism:*** Synovitis often begins after an injury to a joint. The resulting inflammatory reaction triggers inflammation within the synovium. ***Predisposing conditions:*** Underlying pathology within the joint
Inspection	The joint may appear swollen. The patient may move the joint in a guarded manner. Joints affected by synovitis do not appear red. Persistent synovitis can result in muscle atrophy secondary to pain and decreased joint ROM.
Palpation	Warmth may be felt. A "boggy" swelling is present. Diffuse soreness is usually present.
Joint and Muscle Function Assessment	***AROM:*** Limitations exist within the capsular pattern of the joint. ***MMT:*** Weakness secondary to muscle guarding ***PROM:*** Normally, this is greater than AROM but is still limited by pain.
Joint Stability Tests	***Stress tests:*** Not applicable ***Joint play:*** In the absence of underlying pathology to the capsule, joint play is normal.
Special Tests	None.
Neurologic Screening	Within normal limits
Vascular Screening	Within normal limits
Functional Assessment	Avoid maneuvers that increase stress on the joint. Antalgic gait present with lower extremity joint involvement.
Imaging Techniques	In most cases, the diagnosis of synovitis is made without the need for imaging studies.
Differential Diagnosis	Joint sepsis, sprain, osteochondral fracture
Comments	The signs and symptoms of synovitis may mimic those of an infected joint.

AROM = active range of motion; MMT = manual muscle test; PROM = passive range of motion.

Synovitis

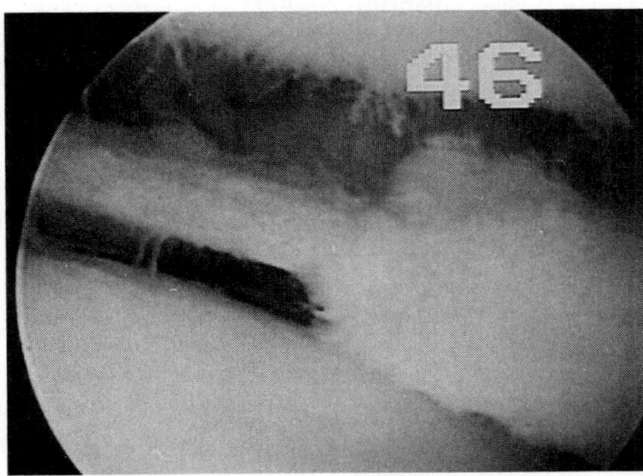

FIGURE 4-7 ■ Arthroscopic view of synovitis of the knee joint capsule. The hairlike strands emerging from the top border of the joint represent inflammation of the synovial capsule.

Articular Surface Pathology

Osteochondral Defects

Examination Findings 4-9
Osteochondral Defects

Examination Segment	Clinical Findings
History	***Onset:*** Acute or insidious ***Pain characteristics:*** Complaints of pain in the joint during weight-bearing activities. Depending on the site of the defect, the entire joint may be painful secondary to a synovial reaction (see Synovitis). Pain may be absent at rest. ***Other symptoms:*** Dislodged bony fragments may cause joint locking. ***Mechanism:*** **Acute:** A rotational or axial load placed on two opposing joint surfaces. The resulting friction results in a tearing away of the cartilage. **Chronic:** A progressive degeneration of the articular cartilage. ***Predisposing conditions:*** Joint trauma
Inspection	Effusion is present. The patient tends to hold the joint in a pain-free position.
Palpation	The joint line may be tender from the defect, but the defect itself is usually not palpable. Joint effusion Tenderness may also be caused by synovitis.

Continued

Examination Findings 4-9—cont'd
Osteochondral Defects

Examination Segment	Clinical Findings
Joint and Muscle Function Assessment	***AROM:*** Limited due to pain and swelling ***MMT:*** Strength is decreased secondary to pain if the joint is compressing the defect (position-dependent). ***PROM:*** Increased relative to the AROM but still limited by pain and swelling AROM, PROM, and MMT may be reduced secondary to a loose body lodging between the joint surfaces, creating a mechanical block against movement.
Joint Stability Tests	***Stress tests:*** Underlying instability may be a causative factor. ***Joint play:*** Hypermobility may be present.
Special Tests	Specific to the involved joint.
Neurologic Screening	Within normal limits
Vascular Screening	Within normal limits
Functional Assessment	Patient describes avoiding weight-bearing maneuvers that increase pressure on the defect. The defect may be present on standard radiographic examination. Better imaging is obtained through the use of MRI.
Imaging Techniques	The definitive diagnosis is based on MR images.
Differential Diagnosis	Sprain, synovitis
Comments	Osteochondral fractures are associated with a rapid-onset hemarthrosis.

AROM = active range of motion; MMT = manual muscle test; MRI = magnetic resonance imaging; PROM = passive range of motion.

Radiograph of an Osteochondral Defect

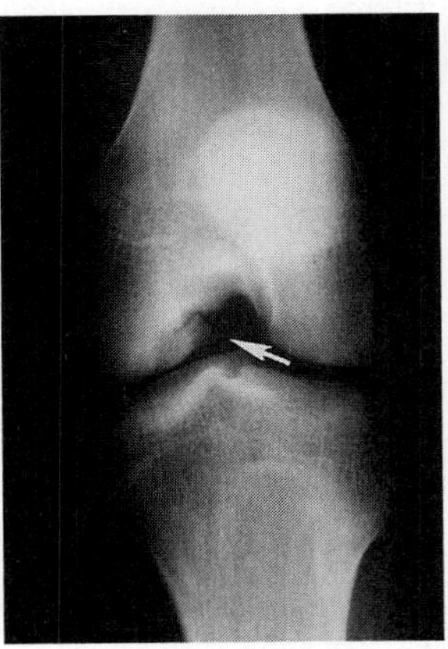

FIGURE 4-8 ■ Note the small fracture line on the medial portion of the trochanteric groove.

Table 4-2 **Progressive Stages of Osteochondral Defects**

Stage	Description
I	Soft tissue swelling Mild osteoporosis Frank fracture resulting from acute trauma
II	Microfractures begin to develop Irregular contour of the articular surface Subcortical bone begins to thin and defragment
III	Necrotic tissue is replaced by granulation tissue Structural weakness of the underlying bone alters the shape of the articular surface

Osteoarthritis

Examination Findings 4-10
Osteoarthritis

Examination Segment	Clinical Findings
History	***Onset:*** Insidious ***Pain characteristics:*** Pain occurs throughout the involved joint. ***Mechanism:*** Osteoarthritis develops secondary to trauma and irregular biomechanical stresses being placed across the joint. ***Predisposing conditions:*** For osteoarthritis, previous trauma to the joint has occurred. Certain occupations and obesity may overload the joints, causing increased forces over time.
Inspection	In chronic cases, gross deformity of the joint is noticed. Individuals with cases of shorter duration present with swelling.
Palpation	Warmth and swelling are identified in the affected joint. The articular surfaces, when and where palpable, are tender to the touch.
Joint and Muscle Function Assessment	***AROM:*** May be limited by pain, often becoming contractured as the condition progresses. ***MMT:*** Decreased secondary to pain. ***PROM:*** Pain is decreased relative to AROM.
Joint Stability Tests	***Stress tests:*** Test results may be positive if a deformity has developed, causing the stressed capsule and ligaments to elongate over time. ***Joint play:*** Distraction of the joint surfaces will reduce the pain associated with joint motion.
Special Tests	Specific to the involved joint.
Neurologic Screening	Within normal limits
Vascular Screening	Within normal limits
Functional Assessment	The patient demonstrates compensations to avoid using the involved body part. When arthritis affects the joints of the lower extremity, an antalgic gait is produced.
Imaging Techniques	AP, PA, lateral, and oblique radiographs In the lower extremity, weight-bearing views to identify decreased joint spaces will be obtained.
Differential Diagnosis	Lyme disease, juvenile rheumatoid arthritis, rheumatoid arthritis infection
Comments	The differential diagnosis of RA is made using blood markers.

AP = anteroposterior; AROM = active range of motion; MMT = manual muscle test; PA = posteroanterior; PROM = passive range of motion.

Radiograph of Osteochondritis Dissecans

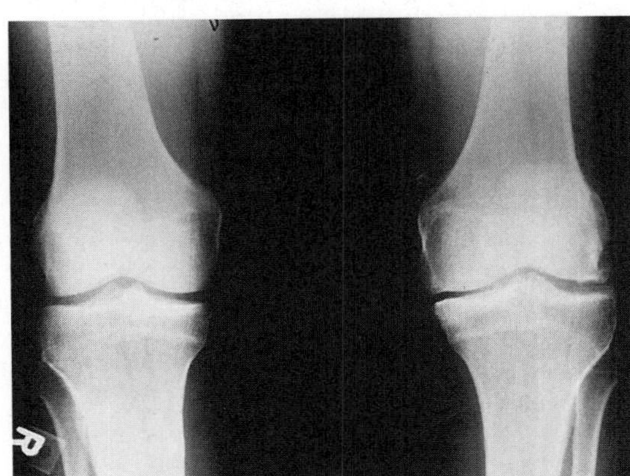

FIGURE 4-9 ■ Radiograph of a free-floating body, osteochondritis dissecans, in the joint space.

Box 4-2
Salter–Harris Classification of Epiphyseal Injuries

Fracture Configuration	Type
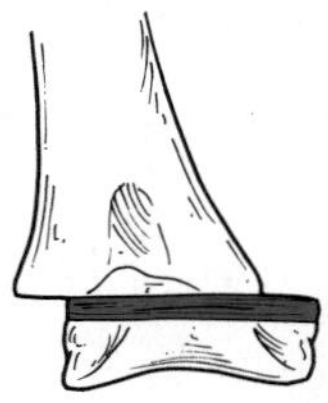	**I:** Fracture extends through the physis, separating the two segments. Common in infants.
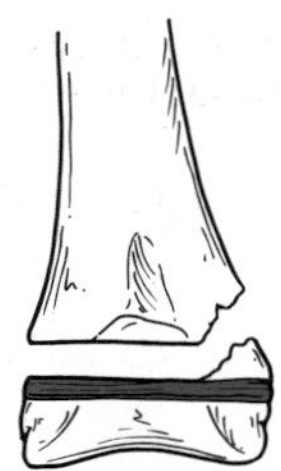	**II:** Fracture starts through the physis and ends on the shaft, creating a displaced wedge.
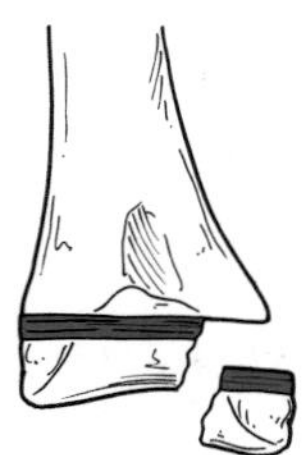	**III:** The fracture line extends perpendicularly through the joint surface and then transversely across the physis, resulting in partial displacement of the segment. Growth of the involved physis may be compromised.
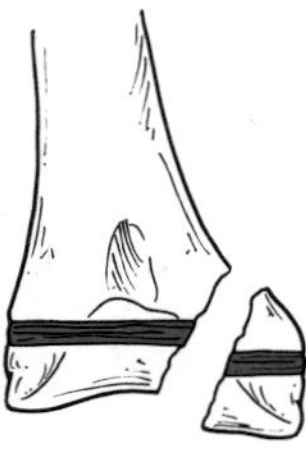	**IV:** Similar to a type III fracture, but the transverse fracture line extends across the physis into the shaft. Surgical fixation is often required and physeal growth may be affected.
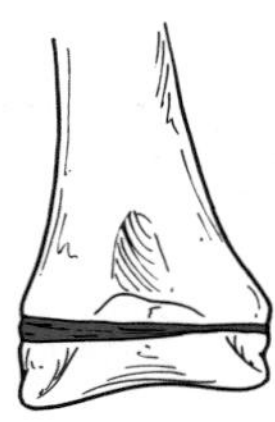	**V:** A crushing injury that compresses the physis. If undetected avascular necrosis may occur and growth may be inhibited.

Exostosis

Examination Findings 4-11
Exostosis

Examination Segment	Clinical Findings
History	***Onset:*** Insidious ***Pain characteristics:*** Exostosis involving the extremities most often results in the localization of pain and other symptoms. Spinal exostosis can result in pain being referred along the distribution of affected nerve roots. ***Mechanism:*** Exostosis is the result of repeated strain placed on a bone or the bony insertion of a tendon. May also result from repeated compressive forces. ***Predisposing conditions:*** Previous trauma to the area, osteoarthritis
Inspection	Deformity may be noted over the site of pain.
Palpation	Point tenderness is present. A large bony outgrowth may be palpable.
Joint and Muscle Function Assessment	***AROM:*** Limited secondary to pain and/or bony block ***MMT:*** Dependent on joint position ***PROM:*** Equal to AROM
Joint Stability Tests	***Stress tests:*** Within normal limits ***Joint play:*** May be restricted in direction of exostosis.
Special Tests	Not applicable
Neurologic Screening	Within normal limits
Vascular Screening	Within normal limits
Functional Assessment	Patient demonstrates avoidance of movements that add tensile stress or compress the exostosis.
Imaging Techniques	Radiograph
Differential Diagnosis	Tumor, apophysitis (e.g., Osgood Schlatter's disease)

AROM = active range of motion; MMT = manual muscle test; PROM = passive range of motion.

Radiograph of Exostosis

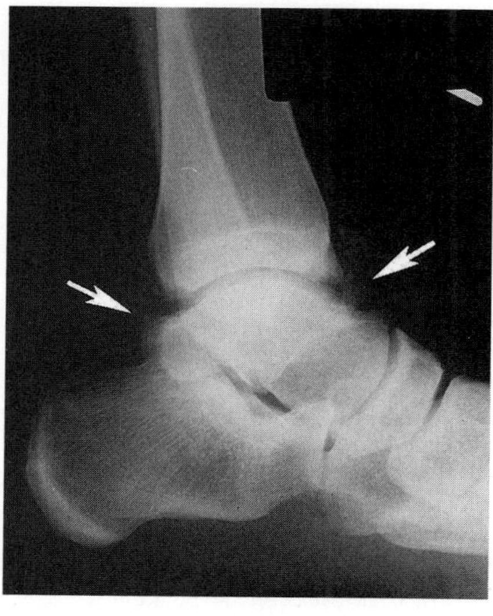

FIGURE 4-10 ■ Radiograph of exostosis of the subtalar joint. Note the bony outgrowths indicated by the arrows.

Fractures

Inspection Findings 4-1
Terminology Used to Describe the Fracture Location

Fracture	Description
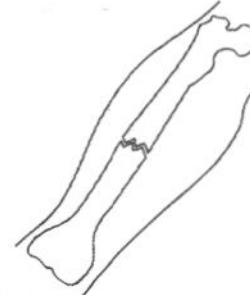	**Diaphyseal fractures** involve only the bone's diaphysis and are associated with a good prognosis for recovery.
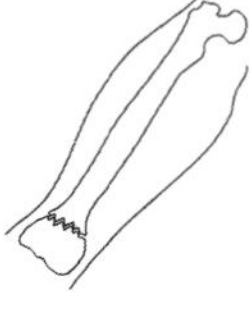	**Epiphyseal fractures** involve the fracture line crossing the bone's unsealed epiphyseal line and can have long-term consequences by disrupting the bone's normal growth. Epiphyseal fractures may mimic soft tissue injuries by resembling joint laxity during stress testing.
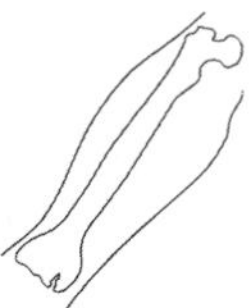	**Articular fractures** disrupt the joint's articular cartilage, which, if improperly healed, results in pain and decreased range of motion and can lead to arthritis of the joint.

Inspection Findings 4-2
Terminology Used to Describe the Relative Severity of the Fracture Line

Fracture	Description
	Incomplete fracture: Fracture line does not completely disassociate the proximal end of the bone from its distal end.
	Undisplaced fracture: Fracture line completely disassociates the two ends of the bone, but the two ends of the bone maintain their relative alignment to each other.
	Displaced fracture: Bony alignment is lost between the two segments; the surrounding tissues may be jeopardized.
	Open fracture: A bony segment of a displaced fracture protrudes the skin.

Inspection Findings 4-3
Terminology Used to Describe the Fracture Line

Fracture	Description
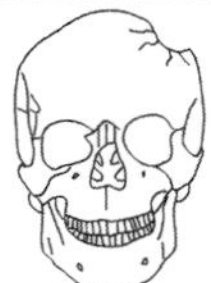	***Depressed fracture:*** Results from direct trauma to flat bones, causing the bone to fracture and depress.
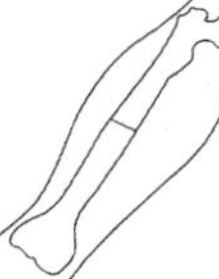	***Transverse fracture:*** Caused by a direct blow, shear force, or tensile force being applied to the shaft of a long bone and results in a fracture line that crosses the bone's long axis.
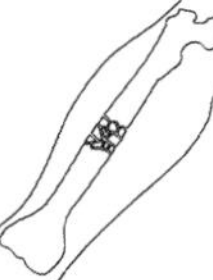	***Comminuted fracture:*** Result of extremely high-velocity impact forces that cause the bone to shatter into multiple pieces. This type of fracture often requires surgical correction.
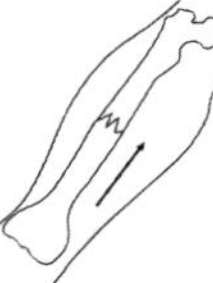	***Compacted fracture:*** Results from compressive forces applied through the long axis of the bone. One end of a fractured segment is driven into the opposite piece of the fracture, leading to a shortening of the involved bone.
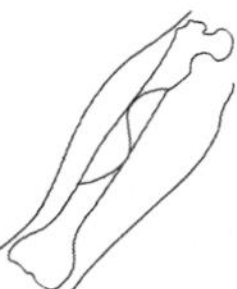	***Spiral fracture:*** The result of a rotational force placed on the shaft of a long bone, such as twisting the tibia while the foot remains fixated. The fracture line assumes three-dimensional S-shape along the length of the bone.
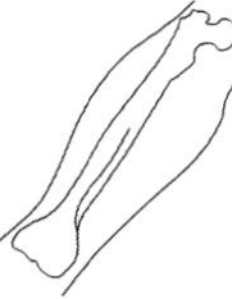	***Longitudinal fracture:*** Most commonly occur as the result of a fall and have a fracture line that runs parallel to the bone's long axis.
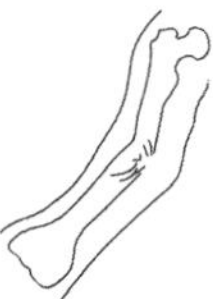	***Greenstick fracture:*** Generally specific to the pediatric and adolescent population, involve a displaced fracture on one side of the bone and a compacted fracture on the opposite side.

Stress Fractures

Examination Findings 4-12
Stress Fractures

Examination Segment	Clinical Findings
History	***Onset:*** Insidious; the patient cannot report a single traumatic event causing the pain. ***Pain characteristics:*** Pain tends to radiate from the involved bone but may become diffuse. ***Mechanism:*** Cumulative microtrauma causes stress fractures. ***Predisposing conditions:*** Overtraining, poor conditioning, amenorrhea, disordered eating, and/or improper training techniques may be noted.
Inspection	Usually no bony abnormality is noted. Soft tissue swelling and redness may be present.
Palpation	Point tenderness exists over the fracture site.
Joint and Muscle Function Assessment	All motions are generally within normal limits.
Joint Stability Tests	***Stress tests:*** Unremarkable ***Joint play:*** Unremarkable
Special Tests	Long bone compression test Percussion along the length of the bone
Neurologic Screening	Within normal limits
Vascular Screening	Within normal limits
Functional Assessment	The patient can often function normally during low-load, short-duration activity; symptoms increase as activity and duration increase, eventually leading to disability.
Imaging Techniques	Bone scans or other imaging techniques
Differential Diagnosis	Tumor, tendinopathy
Comments	Repetitive stress fractures: seek underlying cause.

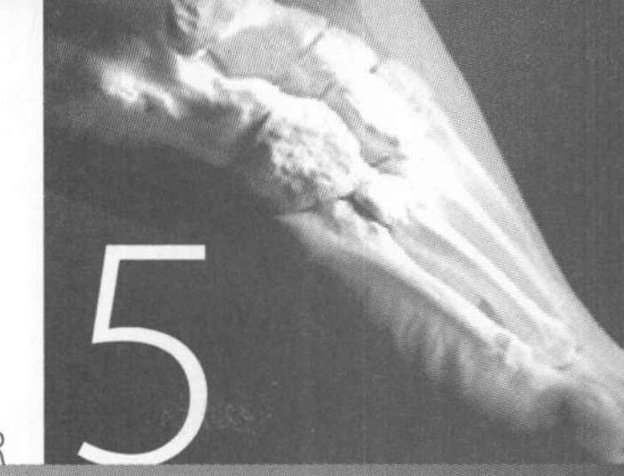

CHAPTER 5

Musculoskeletal Diagnostic Techniques

Table 5-1 Selected Diagnostic Techniques and Their Use

Technique	Best Use
Radiography	Standard: Bone lesions, joint surfaces, and joint spaces Arthrogram: Capsular tissue tears and articular cartilage lesions Angiogram: Blood vessel Myelogram: Pathologies within the spinal canal
Computed Tomography (CT)	Bony or articular cartilage lesions and some soft tissue lesions, especially when quantifying detailed lesions (e.g., size and location; useful in identifying tendinous and ligamentous injuries in varying joint positions) Angiography: Artery and/or vein pathology, including stenosis, aneurysms, and thrombi (clots)
Magnetic Resonance Imaging (MRI)	Soft tissue structures, especially ligamentous and meniscal injuries Magnetic resonance arthrography (MRA): Used to image blood vessels. Functional magnetic resonance imaging (fMRI): Assesses metabolic activity associated with brain function.
Nuclear Medicine	Bone scan: Acute bony change determination but may produce false-positive findings, especially in endurance athletes. Positron emission tomography (PET): Yields a three-dimensional image of physiological function in the body. Single photon emission computed tomography (SPECT): Produces three-dimensional images of internal structures.
Ultrasonic Imaging	Tendon and other soft tissue imaging
Electromyography	Evaluates muscle physiology at rest and with activity. Identify pathology of muscle secondary to nerve supply dysfunction or change in the muscle itself. Used in conjunction with nerve conduction study.
Nerve Conduction Study	Function of motor and sensory nerves. Nerve pathology, including axonal degeneration and neurotmesis.

Radiographs

Description: Radiographic examination uses ionizing radiation to penetrate the body. Depending on the density of the underlying tissues, the radiation is absorbed or dispersed in varying degrees. High-density tissues such as bone absorb more radiation and are therefore more difficult to penetrate than less-dense tissue. The exposure to radiation leaves an imprint on x-ray film (radiographic plate), producing the familiar radiographic image.

Patient Positioning

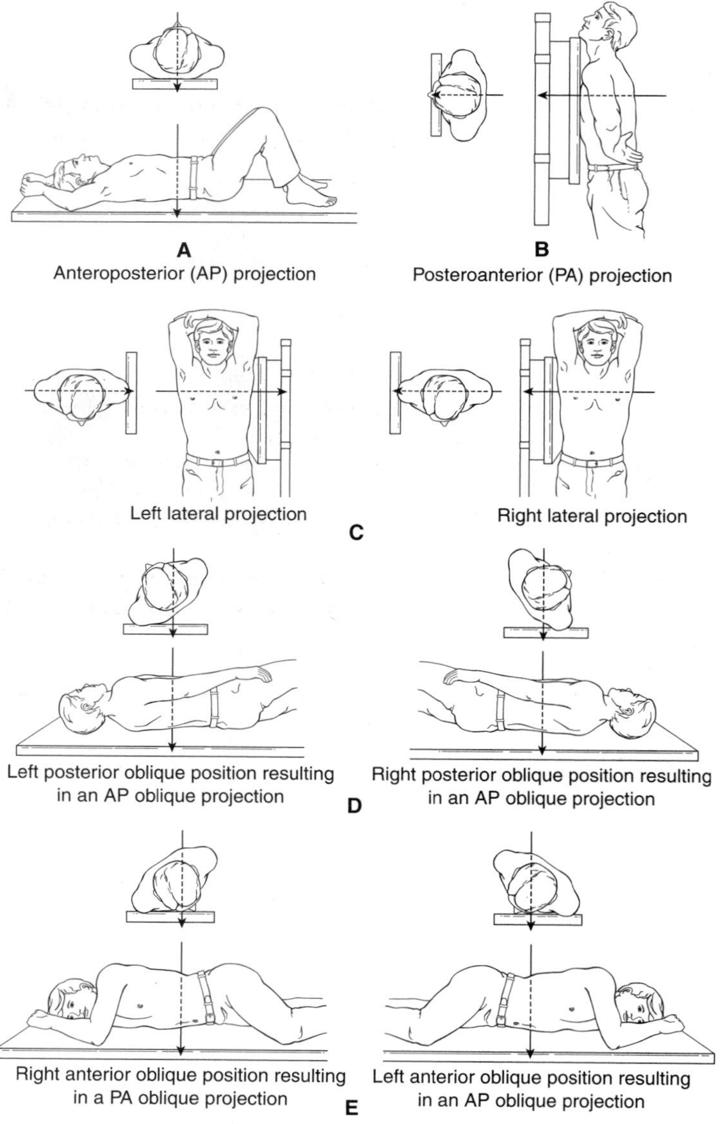

FIGURE 5-1 ■ Patient positioning for common radiographic imaging series. (Courtesy of McKinnis, L. *Fundamentals of Musculoskeletal Imaging,* 2nd ed. Philadelphia: FA Davis, 2005, p 18.)

Table 5-2 Routine Radiologic Series by Body Area

Body Area	Views
Foot	AP, lateral, oblique
Ankle	AP, AP mortise, lateral, oblique
Knee	AP, lateral, intercondylar fossa
Patellofemoral	AP, lateral, merchant
Hip	AP, lateral
Lumbar spine	AP, lateral, oblique (right and left)
Thoracic spine	AP, lateral
Cervical spine	AP, lateral, oblique (right and left), open mouth
Shoulder	AP (internally rotated), AP (externally rotated)
Elbow	AP, lateral, oblique (internal and external)
Wrist, hand, and fingers	PA, lateral, oblique

AP = anteroposterior, PA = posteroanterior.

Interpreting radiographic images using the ABCS method:

A—Alignment: The clinician observes for the normal continuity of the bones and joint surfaces and the alignment of one bone to another.

B—Bones: Bones should have normal density patterns, presenting with uniform color throughout the bone as compared bilaterally. Areas of decreased density appear as darkened areas within the bone. Fractures and abnormal bony outgrowths such as exostosis can also be visualized.

C—Cartilage: Although cartilage itself does not produce a radiographic image, the cartilage and ligamentous structures are inspected for what does not appear. The joint spaces should be smooth and uniform.

S—Soft tissue: Although soft tissue cannot be imaged, swelling within the confines of the soft tissue or between the soft tissue and the bones can be determined. In addition, the outline of soft tissues and even pockets of edema within soft tissue can be identified with adjusted exposure techniques.

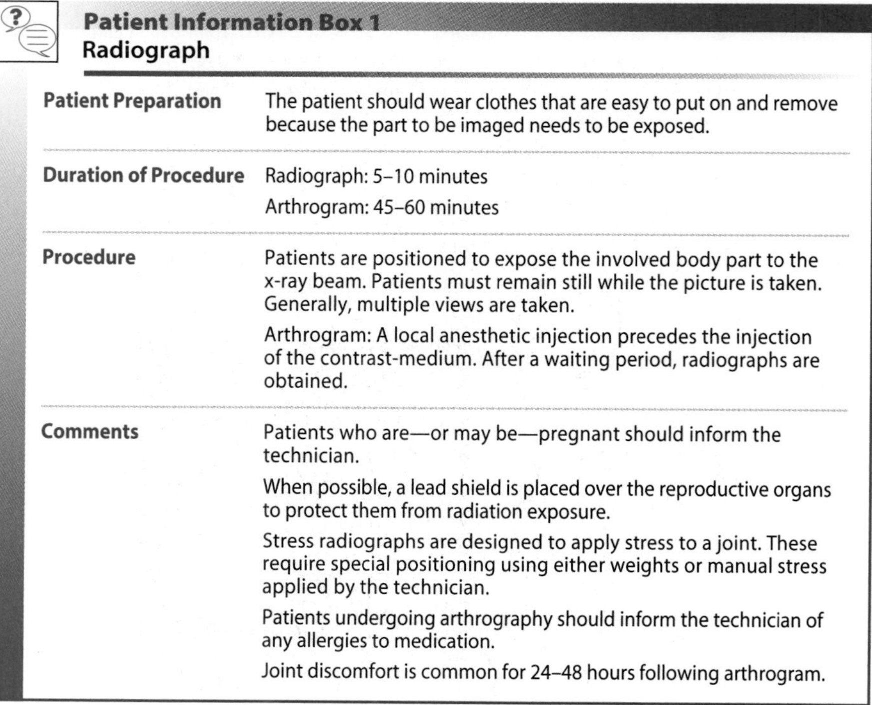

Patient Information Box 1
Radiograph

Patient Preparation	The patient should wear clothes that are easy to put on and remove because the part to be imaged needs to be exposed.
Duration of Procedure	Radiograph: 5–10 minutes Arthrogram: 45–60 minutes
Procedure	Patients are positioned to expose the involved body part to the x-ray beam. Patients must remain still while the picture is taken. Generally, multiple views are taken. Arthrogram: A local anesthetic injection precedes the injection of the contrast-medium. After a waiting period, radiographs are obtained.
Comments	Patients who are—or may be—pregnant should inform the technician. When possible, a lead shield is placed over the reproductive organs to protect them from radiation exposure. Stress radiographs are designed to apply stress to a joint. These require special positioning using either weights or manual stress applied by the technician. Patients undergoing arthrography should inform the technician of any allergies to medication. Joint discomfort is common for 24–48 hours following arthrogram.

Computed Tomography Scan

Description: CT scans are used to determine and quantify the presence of a specific pathology. The x-ray source and x-ray detectors rotate around the body and a computer determines the density of the underlying tissues based on the absorption of x-rays by the body, allowing for more precision in viewing soft tissue. This information is then used to create a two-dimensional image, or slice, of the body. These slices can be obtained at varying positions and thicknesses, allowing physicians to study the area and its surrounding anatomical relationships.

CT Scans

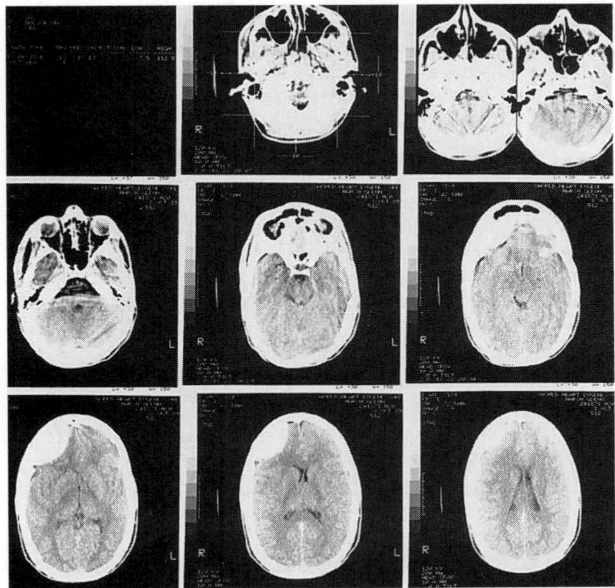

FIGURE 5-2 ■ CT scan of a cranium.

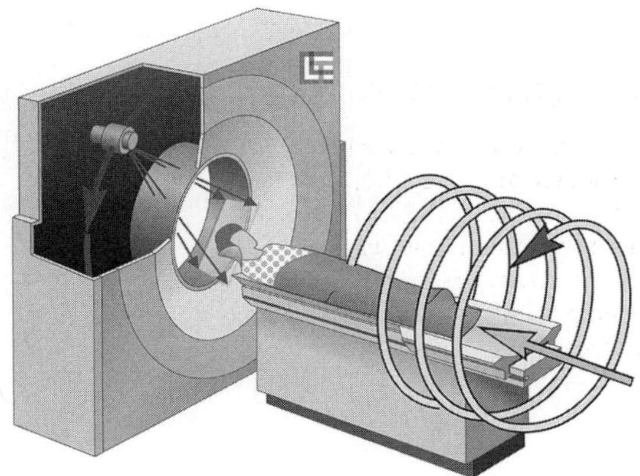

FIGURE 5-3 ■ Spiral (helical) CT scan. The patient table moves through the generator as the x-ray source rotates around the body, allowing the scan to be performed in a continuous arc. (Courtesy of McKinnis, L. *Fundamentals of Musculoskeletal Imaging*, 2nd ed. Philadelphia: FA Davis, 2005, p 119.)

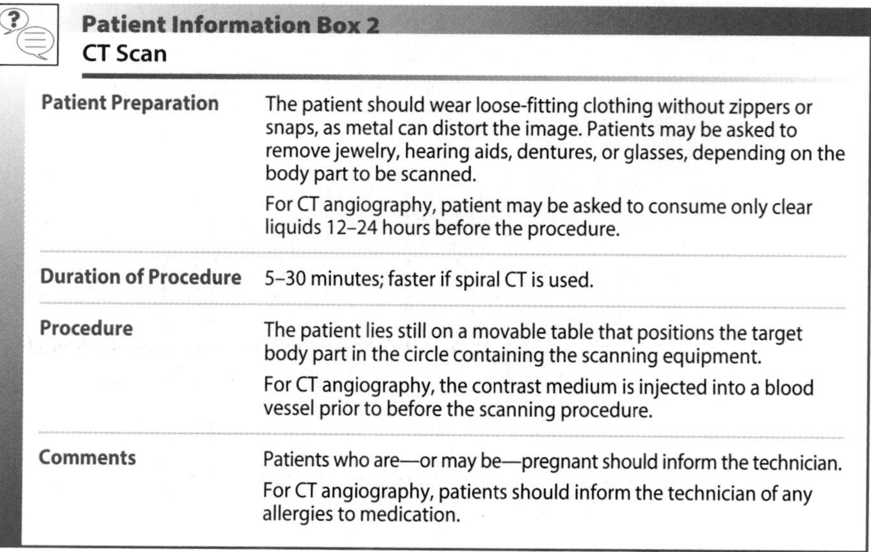

Patient Information Box 2
CT Scan

Patient Preparation	The patient should wear loose-fitting clothing without zippers or snaps, as metal can distort the image. Patients may be asked to remove jewelry, hearing aids, dentures, or glasses, depending on the body part to be scanned. For CT angiography, patient may be asked to consume only clear liquids 12–24 hours before the procedure.
Duration of Procedure	5–30 minutes; faster if spiral CT is used.
Procedure	The patient lies still on a movable table that positions the target body part in the circle containing the scanning equipment. For CT angiography, the contrast medium is injected into a blood vessel prior to before the scanning procedure.
Comments	Patients who are—or may be—pregnant should inform the technician. For CT angiography, patients should inform the technician of any allergies to medication.

Magnetic Resonance Imaging

Description: These images are obtained by placing the patient in an MRI tube that produces a magnetic field, causing the body's hydrogen nuclei to align with the magnetic axis (Fig. 5-5). The tissues are then bombarded by electromagnetic waves, causing the nuclei to resonate as they absorb the energy. When the energy to the tissues ceases, the nuclei return to their state of equilibrium by releasing energy, which is then detected by the MRI unit and transformed by a computer into images. Similar to adjusting the contrast on your television screen or computer monitor, the contrast of the MR image can be "weighted" to better identify specific types of tissues (Box 5-1). Other contrast imaging medium may be introduced into the tissues to delineate the structures further.

Box 5-1
Relative Signal Intensities of Selected Structures on Spin Echo in Musculoskeletal Magnetic Resonance Imaging

	Sequence		
	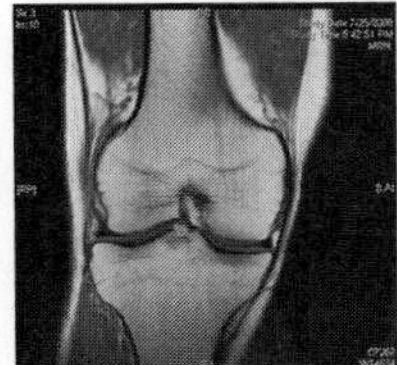	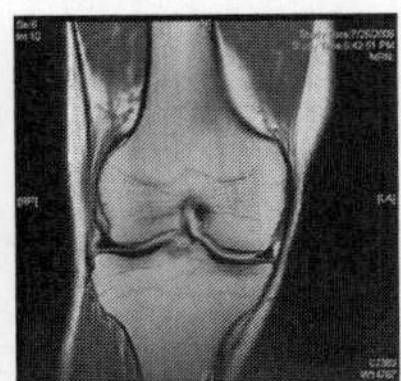	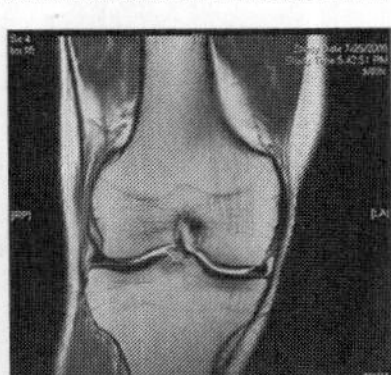
Structure	**T1-Weighted**	**Proton Density**	**T2-Weighted**
Fat*	Bright	Bright	Intermediate
Fluid**	Dark	Intermediate	Bright
Fibrocartilage***	Dark	Dark	Dark
Ligaments, Tendon****	Dark	Dark	Dark
Muscle	Intermediate	Intermediate	Dark
Bone Marrow	Bright	Intermediate	Dark
Nerve	Intermediate	Intermediate	Intermediate

*Includes bone marrow.
**Includes edema, most tears, and most cysts.
***Includes labrum, menisci, triangular fibrocartilage.
****Signal may be increased because of artifacts.

Magnetic Resonance

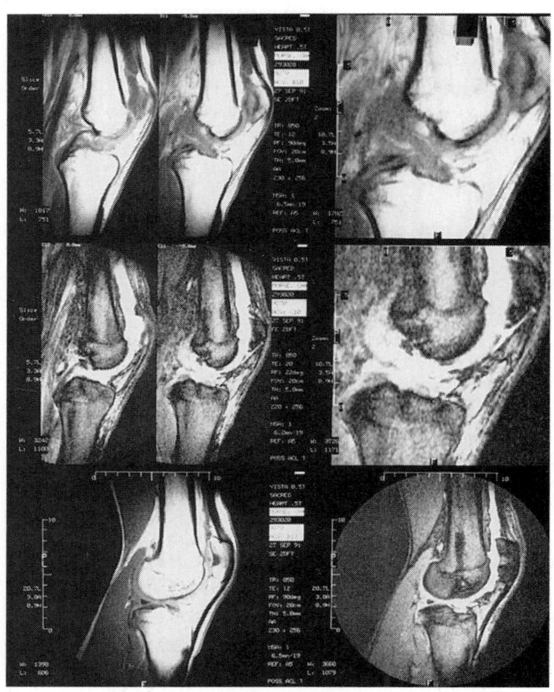

FIGURE 5-4 ■ Magnetic resonance images of the knee.

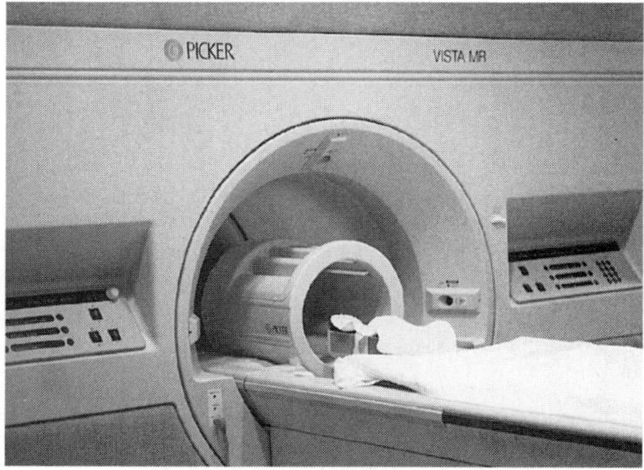

FIGURE 5-5 ■ MRI generator.

Patient Information Box 3
MRI

Patient Preparation	The patient should wear loose fitting, comfortable clothes without zippers or snaps. The facility may provide hospital scrubs or gown. Remove all jewelry and glasses, including any body piercings and jewelry before the procedure.
Duration of Procedure	15–45 minutes
Procedure	Patients are positioned on a sliding table for positioning inside the MRI tube. Patients are asked to remain still inside a tube while the images are being taken. The MR generator produces loud "clanging" noises. Many imaging centers provide ear-plugs or headphones for music during the procedure and allow the MR technologist to communicate with the patient during the procedure (and vice versa).
Comments	Patients who are claustrophobic may have increased anxiety within the enclosed tube of the MRI. A mild sedative can be administered or, if available, an open MRI can be used. Patients who have pacemakers, implanted metal (such as pins, plates, screws), or the possibility of pregnancy should inform the technician. While tooth fillings and braces are not a contraindication, their presence should be noted for accurate tuning of the MRI. Some tattoos and permanent eyeliner contain metal. If contrast medium is need, it will be administered during the procedure.

Bone Scan

Description: Bone scans are a form of nuclear medicine used to detect bony abnormalities that are not normally visible on a standard radiograph. The patient receives an injection of a radionuclide, technetium-99m (Tc-99m), a tracer element that is absorbed by areas of bone undergoing excessive remodeling, or hot spots. These areas appear as darkened spots on the image and must be correlated with clinical signs and symptoms (Fig. 5-6). Bone scans can identify common pathologies, including degenerative disease, bone tumors, and stress fractures of the long bones and the vertebrae.

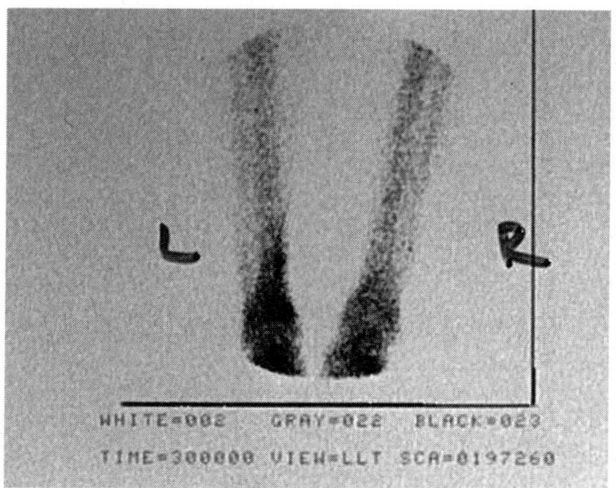

FIGURE 5-6 ■ Bone scan of the lower extremity. The darkened areas indicate "hot spots" of high uptake of the tracer element.

Patient Information Box 4
Bone Scan

Patient Preparation	The patient should wear comfortable clothing.
Duration of Procedure	Depends on type of scan and the time it takes for radioactive tracer to reach the target tissue. The imaging procedure itself takes 20–45 minutes.
Procedure	The radioactive agent is delivered into a vein. After waiting the proscribed period, the patient is asked to lie still on a table while the detector obtains and records the data.
Comments	Patients who are—or may be—pregnant should inform the technician. Patients should inform the technician of any allergies.

Diagnostic Ultrasound

Description: Diagnostic ultrasound uses sound waves having a frequency between 1 and 15 megahertz (MHz) depending on the depth and type of tissues being imaged. The frequency of the ultrasonic energy used is inversely proportional to the depth of the target tissue. A piezoelectric transducer delivers a brief pulse of ultrasonic energy into the tissues, then "listens" for a return echo. A computer interprets the strength of the returning sound wave and converts this information to display the type and depth of each structure (Fig. 5-7). The resulting image presents the tissues in cross section. Advanced units can generate color and three-dimensional images of the tissues.

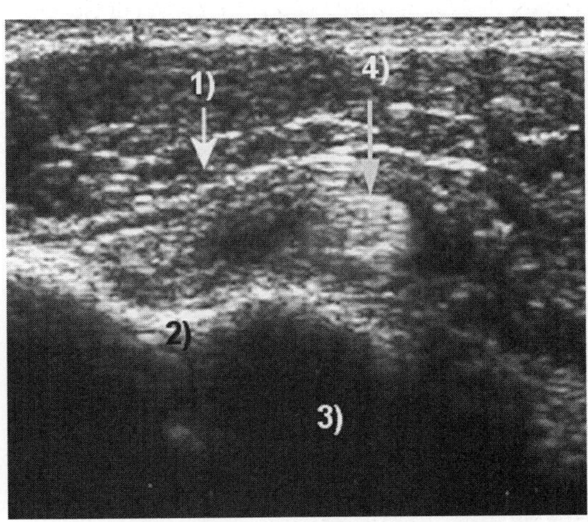

FIGURE 5-7 ■ Ultrasonic image (sonogram) showing a medial dislocation of the long head of the biceps brachii tendon. (1) pectoralis major tendon; (2) empty bicipital groove; (3) humerus; (4) displaced long head of the biceps tendon. (Courtesy of McKinnis, L. *Fundamentals of Musculoskeletal Imaging*, 2nd ed. Philadelphia: FA Davis, 2005, Figure 4-25, p 134.)

Sonogram

Patient Information Box 5
Diagnostic Ultrasound

Patient Preparation	The body part to be examined must be exposed. The patient should wear clothing that is easy to remove and put on.
Duration of Procedure	15–45 minutes
Procedure	The patient lies on a table. Gel, a coupling medium, is applied to the skin over the target and the technician runs the transducer head over the target area, capturing specific images on the computer.
Comments	Diagnostic ultrasound should not be confused with therapeutic ultrasound.

Nerve Conduction Study/Electromyography

Description: Nerve conduction studies (NCS) and electromyography (EMG) are diagnostic techniques used to detect pathology in peripheral nerves and the muscles they innervate.

Nerve conduction studies: A motor NCS is used to examine motor peripheral nerve function and detect pathology along its path. In this procedure, the peripheral nerve is stimulated with an electrical current and activity from a muscle innervated by the nerve is identified and recorded. Two primary measurements are obtained: (1) latency, the time it takes for the impulse to travel to the target muscle and (2) amplitude, the magnitude of the nerve's response (Fig. 5-8). Comparing the amplitude of the muscle's electrical activity to the initial current strength provides a measure of the nerve's health.

Electromyography: An EMG study is an invasive procedure that involves inserting a thin detecting needle electrode into the muscle. The initial electrical activity with insertion of the electrode, which follows a characteristic pattern in a healthy muscle, is noted. The electrical activity of the resting muscle is then assessed. In normal muscle, the muscle should be electrically inactive. Spontaneous activity, or depolarizations, at rest could be indicative of muscle pathology.

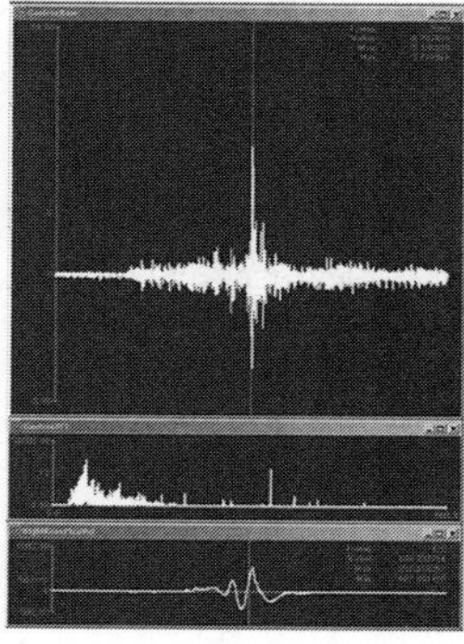

FIGURE 5-8 ■ EMG of a muscle innervated by the stimulated nerve.

Patient Information Box 6
Nerve Conduction Study/Electromyography

Patient Preparation	The body part to be examined will need to be exposed. The patient should wear clothing that is easy to remove and put on.
Duration of Procedure	30 minutes to 2 hours, depending on the extent of the examination
Procedure	NCS: The patient lies on a table. Electrodes are placed on the skin at various points along the course of the peripheral nerve. An electrical current is applied, which may be perceived as a small shock. EMG: Small, thin needle electrodes are placed in the target muscle. The patient is first asked to relax the muscle and then to contract it. The procedure is repeated in each muscle of interest.
Comments	Patients who are taking blood-thinning medications such as warfarin should inform the person conducting the test. Some patients complain of muscle soreness after the EMG procedure.

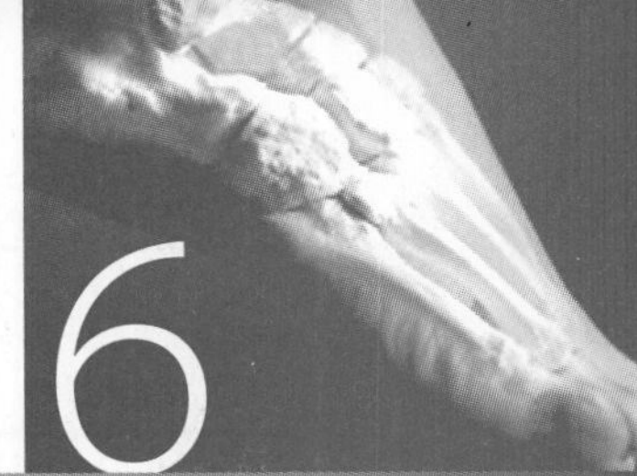

CHAPTER 6

Assessment of Posture

Box 6-1
Classifications of Body Types

	Ectomorph	Mesomorph	Endomorph
Description	Slender, thin build; relatively low body mass index	Medium, athletic build, relatively average body mass index	Stocky build; relatively high body mass index
Joint Shape	Small, flat joint surfaces	Medium joint surfaces	Large, concave-convex joint surfaces
Muscle Mass	Minimal muscle bulk, thin muscles	Medium muscle build	Thick muscle mass
Joint Mobility	Increased	Within normal limits	Decreased
Joint Stability	Decreased	Within normal limits	Increased

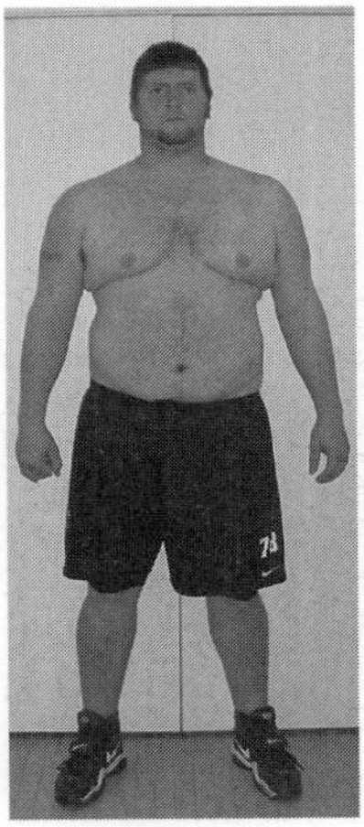

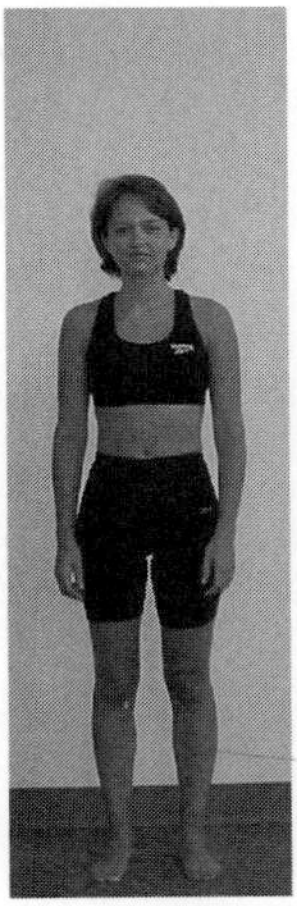

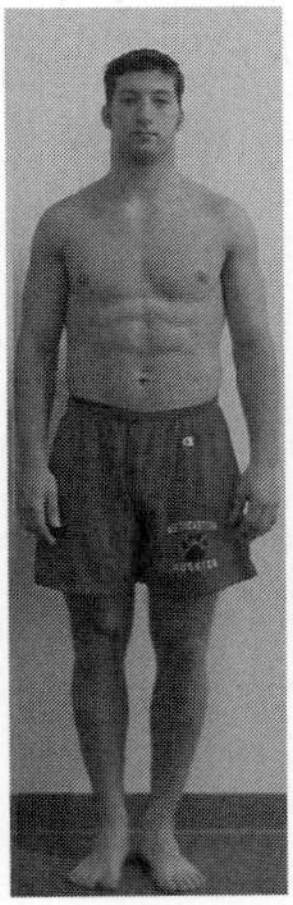

Box 6-2

Body Mass Index

Historically, the medical determination of obesity was made based on the percentage of body fat or total body weight. Depending on the measure being used, obesity is used to describe a person who is 20 to 30 percent over the average weight based on gender, age, and height. Body mass index (BMI) is an indirect estimation of the percentage of body fat.[20] The BMI, based on height and weight, is calculated by:

$$(\text{Weight [lbs.]} \times 705)/(\text{height [in.]} \times \text{height [in.]})$$

or

$$\text{Weight (kg)}/(\text{height [m]} \times \text{height [m]})$$

A BMI of 27.0 is the most commonly used threshold to define obesity. The National Center for Health Statistics proposes the following classification scheme for adult BMI. Note that there are specific formulas for children and teenagers[20]:

Underweight: <18.5

Normal: 18.5–24.9

Overweight: ≥25.0

Pre-obese: 25.0–29.9

Class I obesity: 30.0–34.9

Class II obesity: 35.0–39.9

Class III obesity: ≥40.0

BMI does not accurately describe the amount of body fat for certain groups of people, especially athletes.[21] For example, a person 6 feet tall (1.83 m) who weighs 200 lbs (90.7 kg) would have a BMI of 27.1 (90.7 kg/[1.83 m × 1.83 m]). This individual would fall into the pre-obese classification, even though he or she may have a low percentage of body fat. Therefore, obesity should be determined on a case-by-case basis taking the individual's gender, height, weight, age, BMI, percent body fat, and level of activity into consideration.

Inspection Findings 6-1
Assessment of Ideal Posture

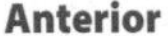

Lateral	Anterior
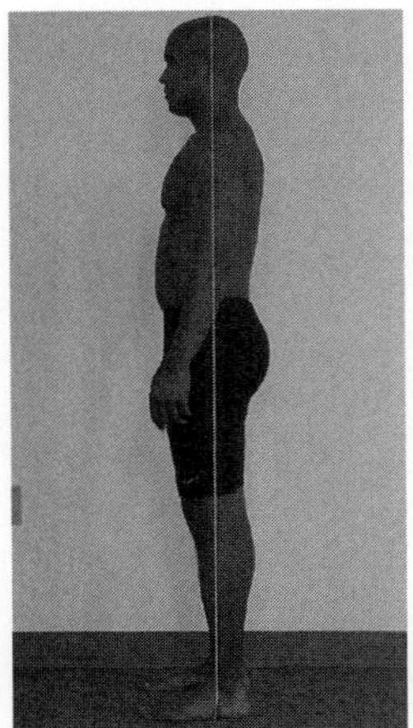	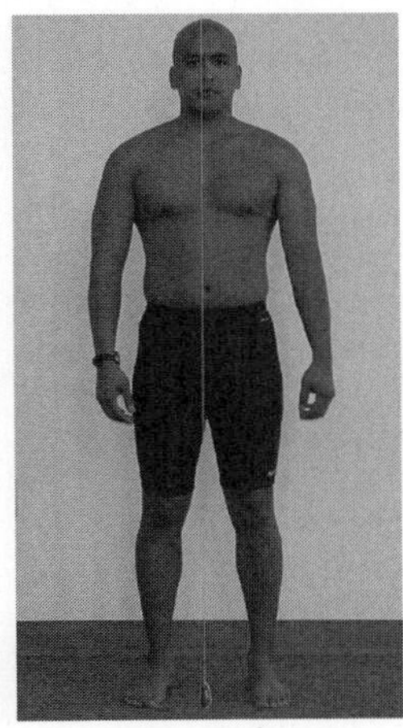
Alignment relative to plumb line: Lower extremity • Lateral malleolus: Slightly posterior • The tibia should be parallel to the plumb line and the foot should be at a 90° angle to the tibia • Lateral femoral epicondyle: Slightly anterior • Greater trochanter: Plumb line bisects	Alignment relative to plumb line: Lower extremity • Feet: Evenly spaced from plumb line • Tibial crests: Slight external rotation • Knees: Evenly spaced from plumb line • Patella: Facing anteriorly • Consistent angulation from joint-to-joint • The lateral malleoli, fibular heads, and iliac crests should be bilaterally equal
Torso	
• Midthoracic region: Plumb line bisects	• Umbilicus: Plumb line bisects, although surgical procedures may alter the alignment. • Sternum: Plumb line bisects • Jugular notch: Plumb line bisects
Shoulder	
• Acromion process: Plumb line bisects	• Acromion processes: Evenly spaced from plumb line • Shoulder heights equal or dominant side slightly lower • Deltoid, anterior chest musculature bilaterally symmetrical and defined
Head and Neck	
• Cervical bodies: Plumb line bisects • Auditory meatus: Plumb line bisects	• Head is bisected by plumb line • Nasal bridge: Plumb line bisects • Frontal bone: Plumb line bisects

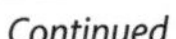

Continued

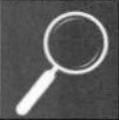

Inspection Findings 6-1—cont'd
Assessment of Ideal Posture

Posterior

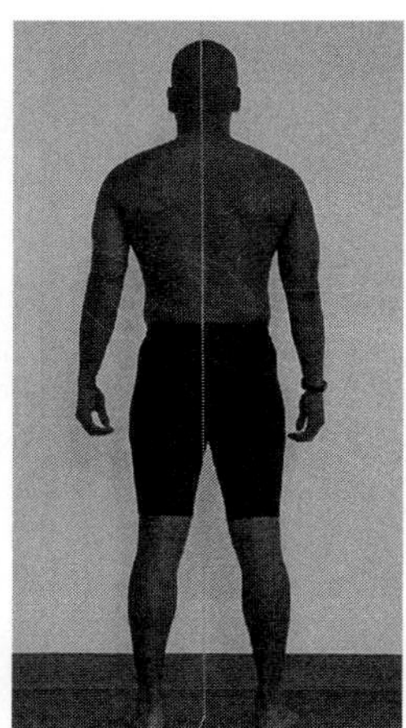

Alignment relative to plumb line:

Lower extremity

- Feet evenly spaced from plumb line
- Feet in slight lateral rotation: Lateral 2 toes are visible
- Knees evenly spaced from plumb line
- Consistent angulation from joint-to-joint

Torso

- Median sacral crests: Plumb line bisects
- Spinous processes: Plumb line bisects
- Paraspinal muscles bilaterally symmetrical

Shoulder

- Scapular borders: Evenly spaced from plumb line
- Acromion processes: Evenly spaced from plumb line
- Deltoid, posterior musculature bilaterally symmetrical
- Shoulder heights equal or dominant side slightly lower

Head and Neck

- Cervical spinous processes: Plumb line bisects
- Occipital protuberance: Plumb line bisects

Postural and Phasic Muscles

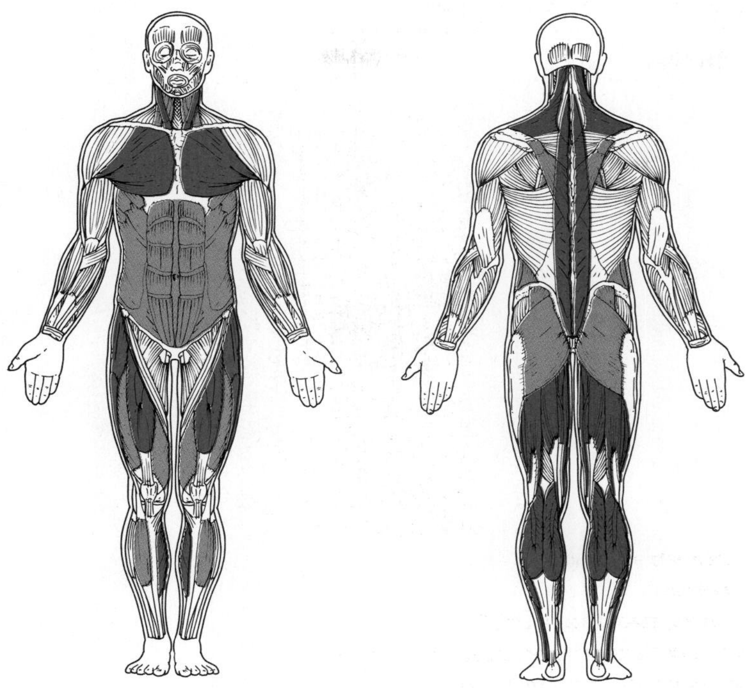

FIGURE 6-1 ■ Postural and phasic muscles.

Common Postural Muscles	Common Phasic Muscles
Sternocleidomastoid	Scalenes
Pectoralis major	Subscapularis
Upper trapezius	Lower trapezius
Levator scapula	Rhomboids
Quadratus lumborum	Serratus anterior
Iliopsoas	Rectus abdominis
Tensor fascia latae	Internal obliques
Rectus femoris	External obliques
Piriformis	Gluteus minimus
Hamstring group	Gluteus maximus
Short hip adductors	Gluteus medius
Gastrocnemius	Vastus medialis
Soleus	Vastus lateralis
Erector spinae	Tibialis anterior
Longissimus thoracic	Peroneals
Multifidus or rotatores	
Tibialis posterior	

Table 6-1 Deviations Noted from the Lateral View

Body Region	Deviation from Ideal Posture	Structural Relationships
Talocrural Joint	Dorsiflexed	Knee flexed, hip flexed
	Plantarflexed	Genu recurvatum, knee extension, hip extension
Knee Joint	Lateral epicondyle posterior to plumb line	Genu recurvatum, ankle plantarflexed, hip extended
	Lateral epicondyle anterior to plumb line	Knee flexed, hip flexed, and ankle dorsiflexed
Hip Joint	Greater trochanter posterior to plumb line	Hip flexed, anterior pelvic tilt, increased lumbar lordosis
	Greater trochanter anterior to plumb line	Hip extended, posterior pelvic tilt, decreased lumbar lordosis
Pelvic Position	Angle between ASIS, PSIS, and a horizontal line greater than 10°: Anterior pelvic tilt (see Goniometry Box 6-1)	Increased lumbar lordosis, hip flexed
	Angle between ASIS and ipsilateral PSIS less than 8°: Posterior pelvic tilt	Decreased lumbar lordosis, hip extended
Lumbar Spine	Lumbar vertebral bodies anterior to plumb line: Increased lumbar lordosis	Anterior pelvic tilt, hip flexed
	Lumbar vertebral bodies posterior to plumb line: Decreased lumbar lordosis	Posterior pelvic tilt, hip extended
Thoracic Spine	Midthorax posterior to plumb line: Increased thoracic kyphosis	Forward head posture, forward shoulder posture, shortened anterior chest musculature
	Midthorax anterior to plumb line: Decreased thoracic kyphosis	Inability to flex through thoracic spine, possible shortened thoracic paraspinal muscles
Shoulder Joint	Acromion process posterior to plumb line: Retracted shoulders or scapulae	Decreased thoracic kyphosis
	Acromion process anterior to plumb line: Rounded shoulder or protracted scapulae	Forward head posture, increased thoracic kyphosis, shortened anterior chest musculature, poor postural control of the scapula
Cervical Spine	Lower cervical vertebral bodies posterior to plumb line: Decreased cervical lordosis	Decreased lordosis
	Lower cervical vertebral bodies anterior to plumb line: Increased cervical lordosis	Forward head posture, forward shoulder posture
Head Position	External auditory meatus posterior to plumb line: Head retraction	Decreased lordosis
	External auditory meatus anterior to plumb line: Forward head posture	Forward shoulder posture, suboccipital restrictions

ASIS = anterior superior iliac spine; PSIS = posterior superior iliac spine.

Table 6-2 Postural Deviations Observed from the Anterior View

Body Region	Deviation from Ideal Posture	Structural Relationships
Feet	Internally rotated feet (pigeon toed)	Internally rotated tibia, femoral anteversion, or STJ pronation
	Externally rotated feet (duck feet)	Externally rotated tibia, femoral retroversion, or STJ supination
	Flattened medial arch	Excessive STJ and midtarsal pronation, internal tibial rotation
	High medial arch	Excessive STJ and midtarsal supination, external tibial rotation
Tibial Position	External tibial rotation: Tibial crests positioned lateral to midline	Femoral retroversion, supinated STJ, laterally positioned patella
	Internal tibial rotation: Tibial crests positioned medial to midline	Femoral anteversion, pronated STJ, laterally positioned patella
Patellar Position	Squinting patellae	Internally rotated tibia, femoral anteversion, pronated STJ
	Frog-eyed patellae	Externally rotated tibia, femoral retroversion, supinated STJ
Leg Positions	Genu varum	Increased angle of inclination of femur, femoral retroversion, supinated STJ
	Genu valgum	Decreased angle of inclination of femur, femoral anteversion, pronated STJ
	Tibial varum	Structural deformity of the tibias causing excessive STJ pronation
Pelvic Position	Asymmetrical iliac crest height	Leg length discrepancy, scoliosis
	Asymmetrical ASIS height	One ilium is rotated either anteriorly or posteriorly, leg length discrepancy, or congenital anomaly
Chest Region	Pectus carinatum: Outward protrusion of the chest and sternum	Not applicable
	Pectus excavatum: Inward position of the chest and sternum	Not applicable
Shoulder Region	Asymmetrical shoulder heights	Scoliosis
		Side dominance
Head and Cervical Spine	The head side bent or rotated; asymmetrical muscle mass of neck	Poor postural sense, overuse of one side, torticollis (congenital deformation or acute spasm of the sternocleidomastoid muscle)

ASIS = anterior superior iliac spine; STJ = subtalar joint.

Table 6-3 Postural Deviations Observed from the Posterior View

Body Region	Deviation from Ideal Posture	Structural Relationships
Calcaneal Position	Calcaneal varum	STJ and midtarsal joints in a supinated position
	Calcaneal valgum	STJ and midtarsal joints in a pronated position
Posterior Leg Musculature	Asymmetry in girth or definition of musculature	Leg side dominance
		Atrophy caused by injury or immobilization of one side
Iliac Crest Heights	Asymmetry of iliac crest heights	Possible leg length discrepancy
		Scoliosis
Back Musculature	Asymmetry between mass or definition of erector spinae musculature	Side dominance or overuse of one side of the musculature (e.g., rowing)
		Scoliosis
Spinal Alignment	The spinous processes not in vertical alignment	Structural or functional scoliosis
		Asymmetry of scapula
		Asymmetry of spinal musculature
		Asymmetry of rib cage
Scapular Position	Unequal height	Side dominance
		Scoliosis
		Muscle imbalance caused by paralysis or weakness of musculature
	Excessively protracted or asymmetrically protracted	Muscle imbalance
		Poor posture
		Scoliosis
		Forward shoulder posture
		Forward head posture

	Asymmetrically rotated	Muscle imbalance Side dominance Forward shoulder posture Forward head posture
	Winging scapula	Poor posture Muscle imbalance Muscular weakness
Shoulder Heights	Shoulder heights unequal	Scoliosis Dominant side Scapula positioning
Neck Musculature	The upper trapezius hypertrophied in relation to other periscapular muscles	Overused in normal upper extremity activities or overemphasized in weight lifting Side dominance
Head Position	The head not sitting in a vertical position in relation to the neck Side bend, rotated	Caused by muscle imbalance Poor postural, proprioceptive sense Compensation for scoliosis Torticollis (acquired or congenital)

STJ = subtalar joint.

Table 6-4 Leg Length Differences

Category Type	Description	Possible Causes
Functional or Apparent Leg Length	Leg length difference that is attributed to something other than the length of the tibia and/or femur.	Tightness of muscle or joint structures or muscular weakness in the lower extremity or spine. Examples include knee hyperextension, scoliosis, or pelvic muscle imbalances.
Structural or True Leg Length	An actual difference in the length of the femur or the tibia of one leg compared with the other	Possibly from disruption in the growth plate of one of the long bones or a congenital anomaly

Leg Length Discrepancy

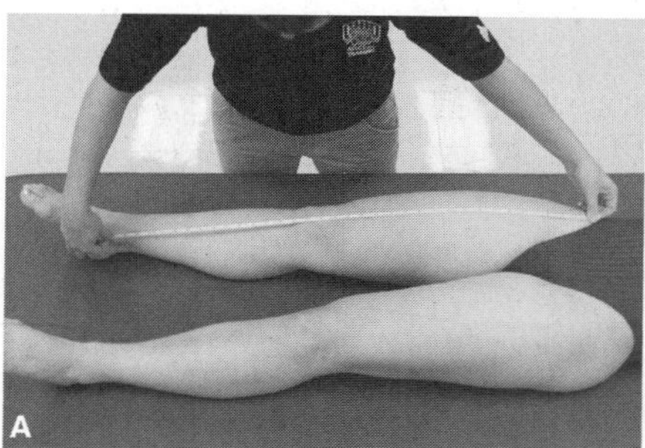

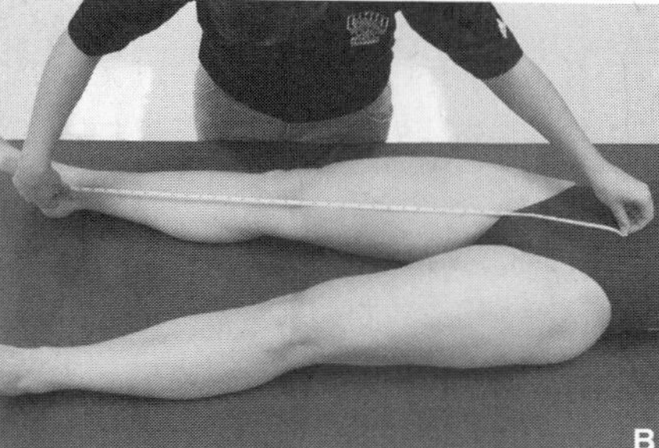

FIGURE 6-2 ■ **(A)** Test for the presence of a structural (true) leg length discrepancy. Measurements are taken from the anterior superior iliac spine to the medial malleolus. Bilateral discrepancies of greater than 10–20 mm are considered significant. **(B)** Test for the presence of a functional (apparent) leg length discrepancy. Measurements are taken from each medical malleolus to the umbilicus. This test is meaningful only if the test for a true leg length difference is unremarkable.

Special Test 6-1
Measured Block Method of Determining Leg Length Discrepancies

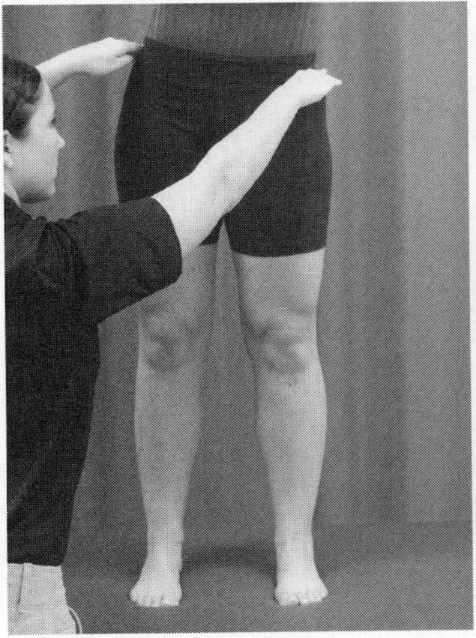
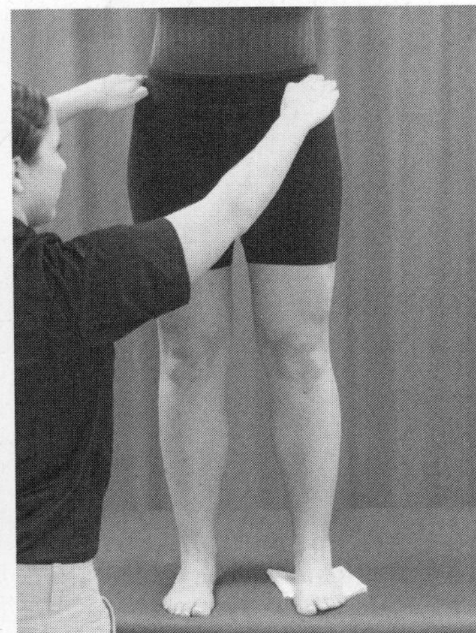

The block method of determining a leg length difference. Blocks of a known thickness are placed under the shorter extremity.

Patient Position	Standing on a firm surface with the feet shoulder-width apart and the weight evenly distributed
Position of Examiner	Standing in front of the patient
Evaluative Procedure	The starting levels of the iliac crests are noted. If heights are determined to be unequal, blocks of known thickness (measured in millimeters) are placed under the shorter leg until the iliac crests are of equal height. The leg length difference is calculated by totaling the sum of the heights of the individual blocks.
Positive Test	A leg length difference of 10–20 mm is frequently cited as the level at which treatment is considered. Patients who acquire the LLD at an early age may tolerate more difference. Patients who are athletic or must stand for much of the day may tolerate less.[22,23]
Comment	When the iliac crests are level, observe the heights of the ASIS. If the ASIS are not an equal height, then the patient has asymmetrical innominate bones.
Evidence	Intra-rater reliability Not Reliable — Very Reliable Poor / Moderate / Good 0 0.1 0.2 0.3 0.4 0.5 0.6 0.7 0.8 0.9 1.0 Inter-rater reliability Not Reliable — Very Reliable Poor / Moderate / Good 0 0.1 0.2 0.3 0.4 0.5 0.6 0.7 0.8 0.9 1.0

ASIS = anterior superior iliac spine.

The Foot Posture Index

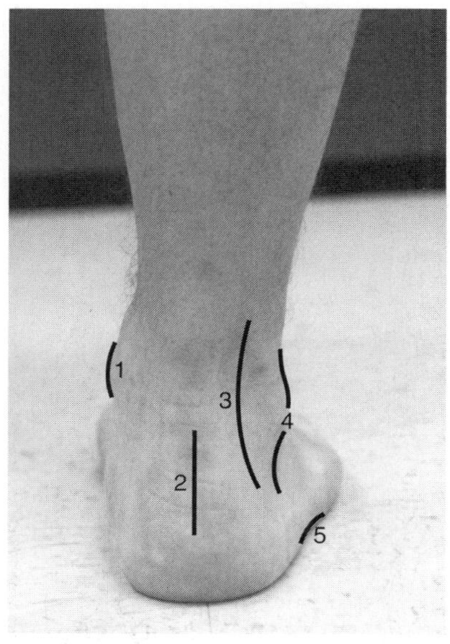

FIGURE 6-3 ■ Posterior view of a pronated foot as defined by the foot posture index. 1, talar navicular prominence; 2, calcaneal frontal plane position; 3, Helbing's sign; 4, inferior and superior lateral malleolar curves; 5, congruence of the lateral border.

The Foot Posture Index (FPI) was designed to improve the reliability and validity of classification of foot postures as supinated, neutral, or pronated and may be useful in predicting injury risk.[38,39] Using simple palpation and inspection metrics with the patient in a relaxed stance, the FPI uses a 5-point Likert scale to assess six aspects of foot position:

1. Talar head palpation
2. Curves above and below the lateral malleoli
3. Inversion or eversion of the calcaneus
4. Bulge in the region of the talonavicular joint
5. Congruence of the medial longitudinal arch
6. Abduction or adduction of the forefoot on the rearfoot

Each feature is assigned a rating from −2 to +2. Negative values reflect more supinated positioning and positive values reflect pronated positioning (Fig. 6-15). The scores are added with a composite score being used. A more pronated foot type as identified by the FPI is associated with an increased risk of medial tibial stress syndrome.[40]

Goniometry Box 6-1
Assessment of Pelvic Position

Neutral	Anterior Pelvic Tilt	Posterior Pelvic Tilt
8–10° angle between the ASIS and PSIS relative to horizontal	More than a 10° angle between the ASIS and PSIS relative to horizontal	Less than an 8° angle between the ASIS and relative to horizontal

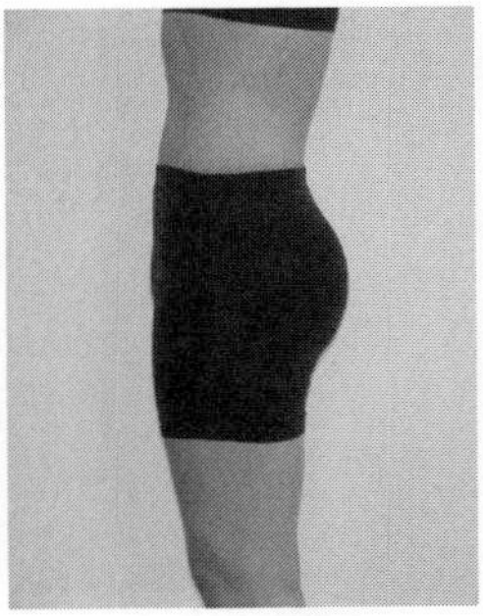

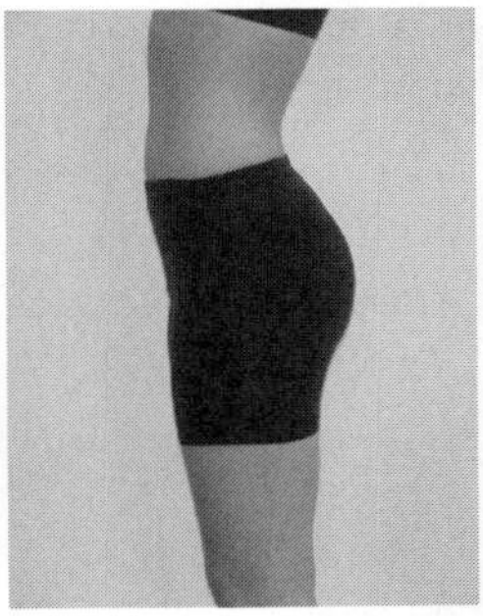

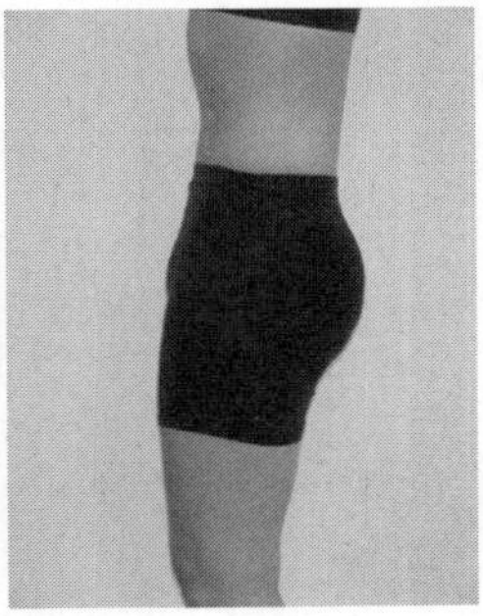

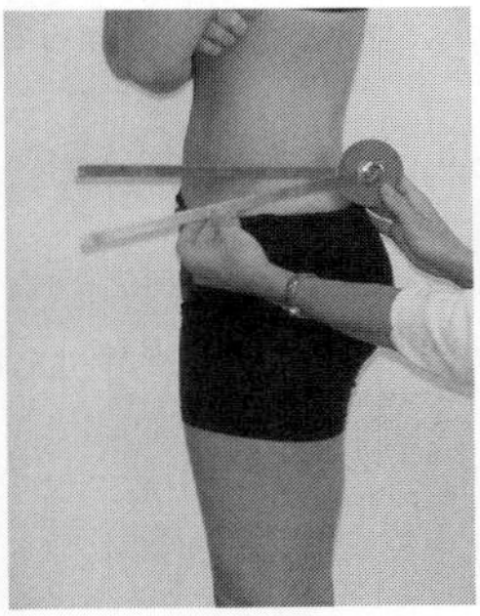

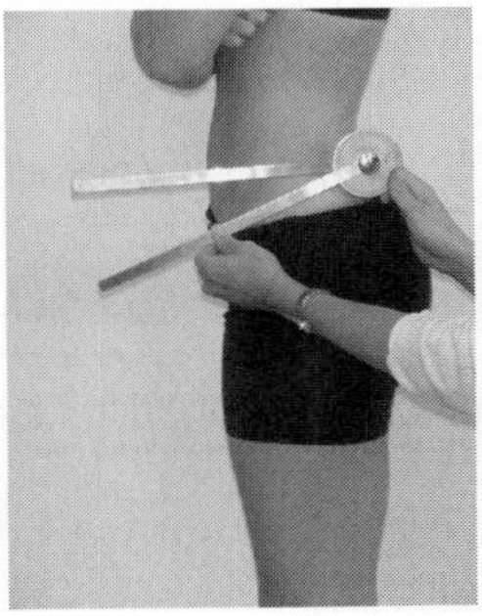

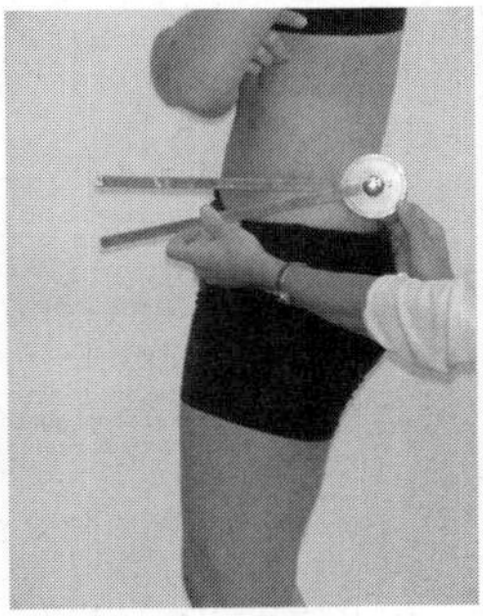

ASIS = anterior superior iliac spine; PSIS = posterior superior iliac spine.

Box 6-3
Resting Scapular Postures

Scapular Elevation/Depression

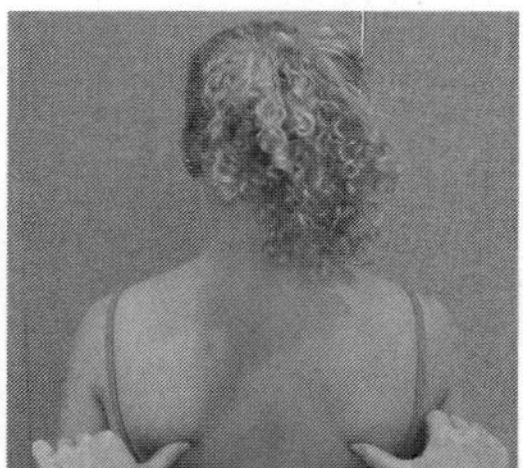

The height of the scapulae are compared using the inferior angle as a landmark. The normal height correlates to the 7–9 thoracic vertebrae.[24]

Scapular Protraction/Retraction

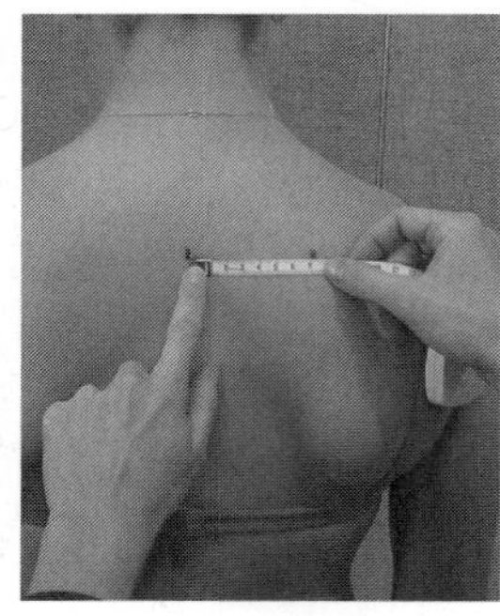

The distance from the T3 spinous process to the medial border of the scapula is measured with the patient standing. The normal value is 5–7 cm. An increased distance represents a protracted scapular position; a decreased distance, a retracted scapula.

Scapular Rotation

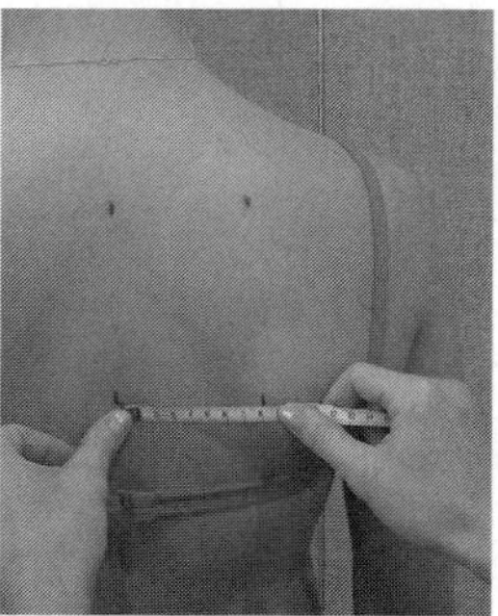

The distance from the T7 vertebrae to the inferior angle of each scapula is measured. An increased distance indicates an upwardly rotated scapula.

Scapular Winging

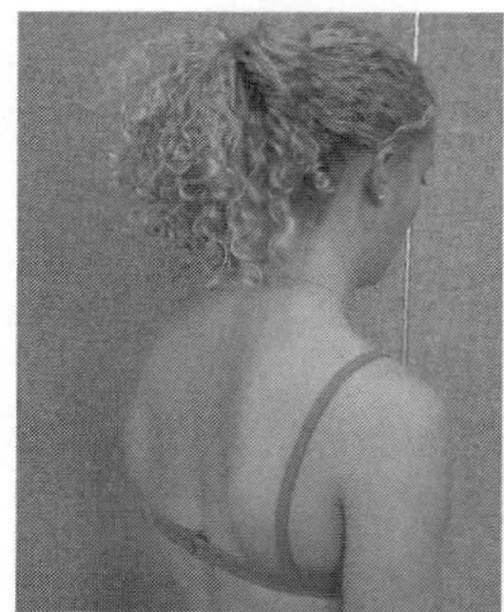

Protrusion of the medial border of scapula.

"Pseudowinging" is apparent when the inferior angle (not the entire medial border) is prominent and is associated with increased anterior tipping of the scapula.

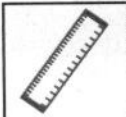

Muscle Length Box 6-1
Muscle Length Assessment for the Gastrocnemius

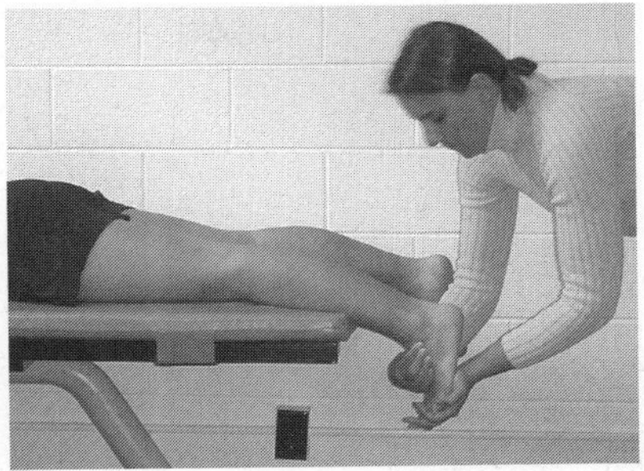

Patient Position	Prone with the foot off the edge of the table with the knee extended
Position of Examiner	One hand palpating the subtalar joint The other hand grasping the foot
Evaluative Procedure	While maintaining the subtalar joint in the neutral position, the foot is taken into dorsiflexion. ROM can be measured goniometrically by placing the axis over the lateral malleolus, the distal arm aligned parallel to the bottom of the foot, and the proximal arm aligned with the fibula.
Positive Test	Less than 10° of dorsiflexion may affect normal walking gait; less than 15° of dorsiflexion may affect normal running gait.
Implications	Tightness of the gastrocnemius can create overuse pathology at the foot, ankle, and knee.
Possible Pathologies	Plantar fasciitis, Sever's disease, Achilles tendinopathy, calcaneal bursitis, patellofemoral pathology.
Comment	The length of the soleus is assessed using dorsiflexion range of motion with the knee flexed to at least 60°.
Evidence	Inter-rater reliability Not Reliable — Very Reliable Poor / Moderate / Good 0 0.1 0.2 0.3 0.4 0.5 0.6 0.7 0.8 0.9 1.0

ROM = range of motion.

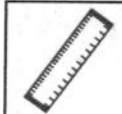

Muscle Length Box 6-2
Muscle Length Assessment for the Hamstring Group

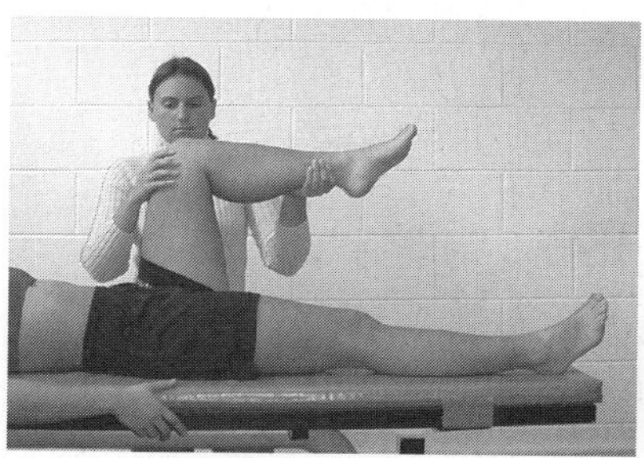

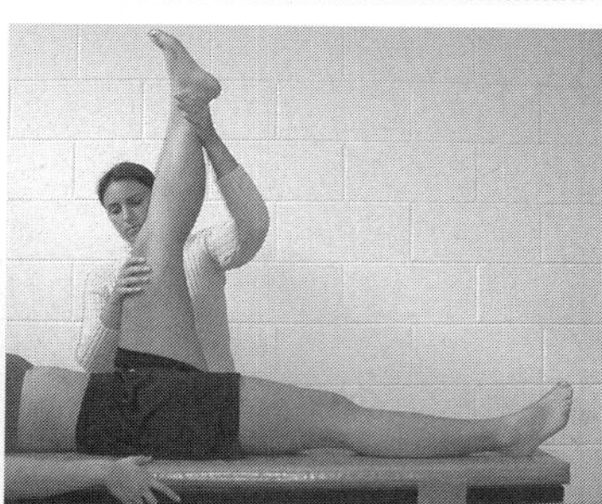

Patient Position	Supine
Position of Examiner	Standing at the side of the patient; the leg being assessed is placed in 90° of hip flexion and 90° of knee flexion (90/90 position)
Evaluative Procedure	The upper leg is stabilized in 90° of hip flexion and the lower leg is extended at the knee.
Positive Test	Lacking more than 20° of full knee extension.
Implications	Tightness of the hamstrings may affect the knee, thigh, hip, and spine.
Possible Pathologies	Muscle strains, patellofemoral dysfunction, ischial tuberosity inflammation, low back dysfunction
Evidence	Inter-rater reliability

Not Reliable — Very Reliable

Poor | Moderate | Good

0 0.1 0.2 0.3 0.4 0.5 0.6 0.7 0.8 0.9 1.0

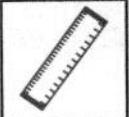

Muscle Length Box 6-3
Muscle Length Assessment of the Rectus Femoris

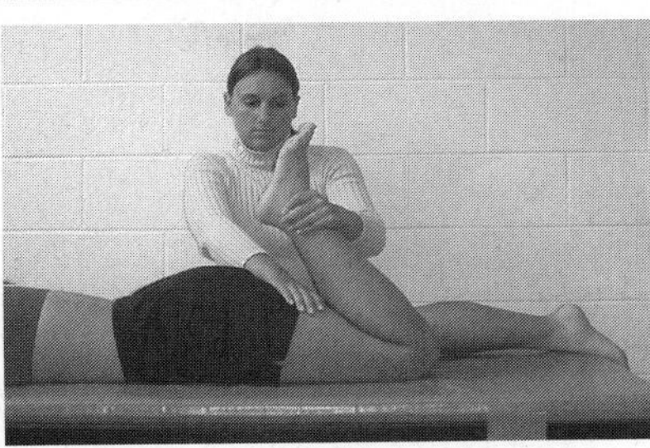

Patient Position	Prone
Position of Examiner	At the side of the patient
Evaluative Procedure	The knee is flexed. ROM can be measured using a goniometer with the axis placed over the lateral epicondyle, the distal arm aligned with the lateral malleolus, and the proximal arm aligned with the greater trochanter.
Positive Test	10° or greater difference as compared with the nonaffected side.
Implications	Tightness of the quadriceps may affect the knee, thigh, hip, and spine.
Possible Pathologies	Muscle strains, patellofemoral dysfunction, low back dysfunction
Evidence	Intra-rater reliability Not Reliable — Very Reliable Poor / Moderate / Good 0 0.1 0.2 0.3 0.4 0.5 0.6 0.7 0.8 0.9 1.0

ROM = range of motion.

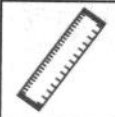

Muscle Length Box 6-4
Muscle Length Assessment of the Shoulder Adductors

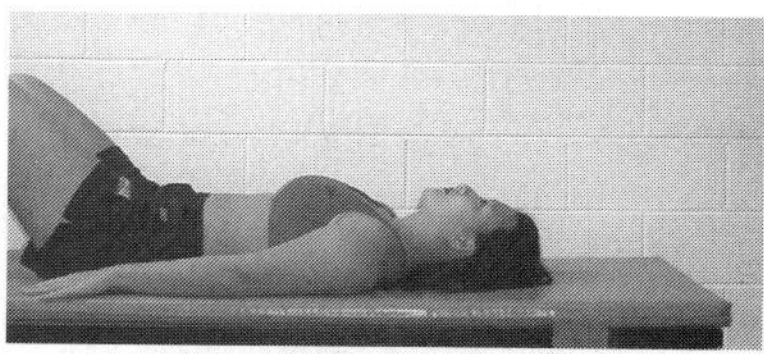

Starting Position

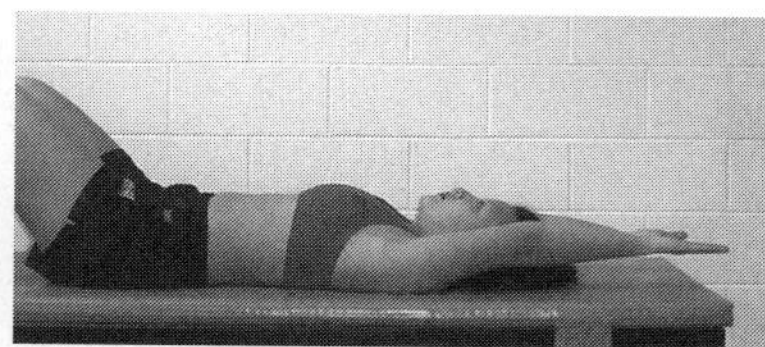

Ending Position

Patient Position	In the hook-lying position with the arms at the side
Position of Examiner	At the side of the patient
Evaluative Procedure	The patient flexes the shoulders above the head and attempts to place the arms on the table.
Positive Test	The patient cannot flex the arms above the head or the lumbar spine lifts off the table.
Implications	Shortness of the latissimus dorsi and teres major muscles

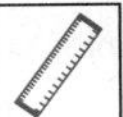

Muscle Length Box 6-5
Muscle Length Assessment of the Pectoralis Major Muscles

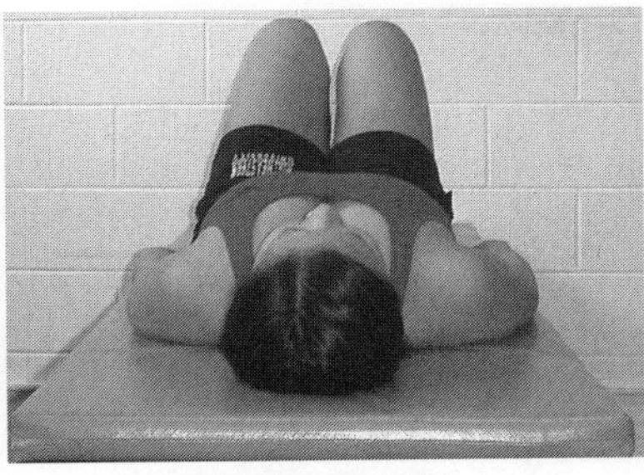

Normal Findings

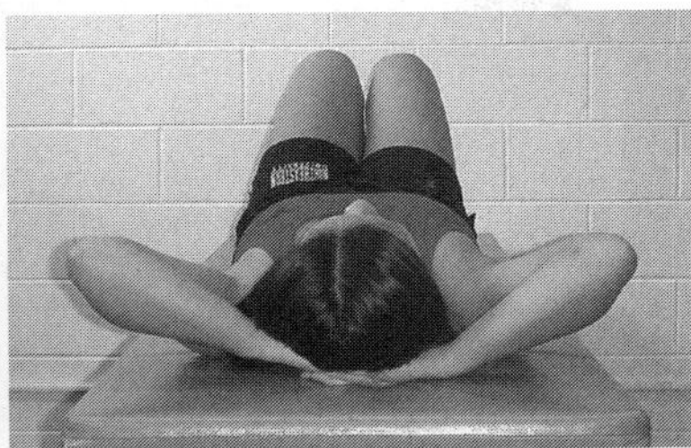

Positive Findings

Patient Position	In the hook-lying position with the arms abducted, externally rotated, with the elbows flexed and the hands locked behind the head
Position of Examiner	At the head of the patient
Evaluative Procedure	The patient attempts to position the elbows flat on the table.
Positive Test	The elbows do not rest on the table. To establish an objective baseline, measure (in centimeters) the distance from the posterior aspect of the acromion process to the tabletop.
Implications	Tight pectoralis major muscles may create rounded shoulders and subsequent forward head posture, although shortness of the pectoralis minor is most commonly implicated.

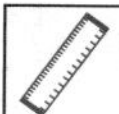

Muscle Length Box 6-6
Muscle Length Assessment of the Pectoralis Minor Muscles

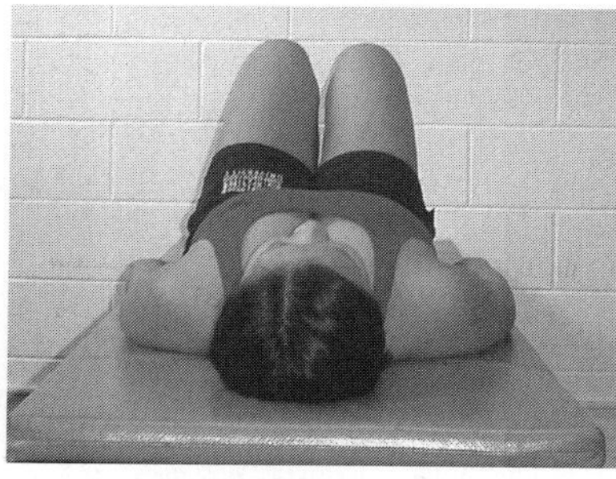

Normal Findings

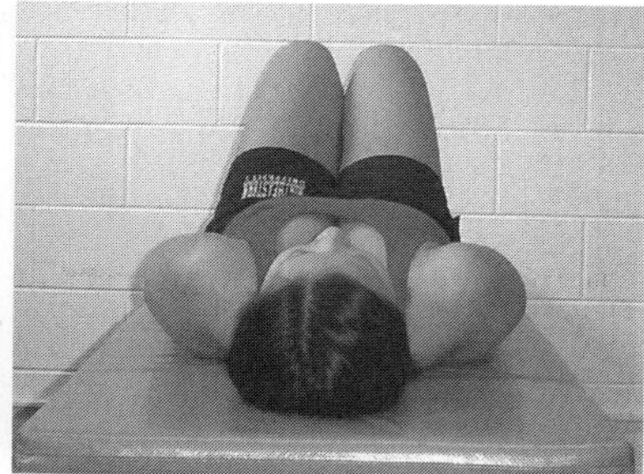

Positive Findings

Patient Position	Supine with the arms at the side
Position of Examiner	At the head of the patient
Evaluative Procedure	Observe the position of the shoulders in reference to the table.
Positive Test	The posterior shoulder does not rest on the table. To establish an objective baseline, measure (in centimeters) the distance from the posterior aspect of the acromion process to the tabletop.
Implications	Tight pectoralis minor muscles may create rounded shoulders and subsequent forward head posture.
Modifications	1. Repeat the above test, but with the patient standing to avoid falsely positioning the scapula.[24] 2. Measure from the sternoclavicular joint to the coracoid process.
Evidence	Tabletop measurement poorly correlated with more direct measurements of muscle length because of the supine positioning.[25]

Inspection Findings 6-2
Genu Recurvatum

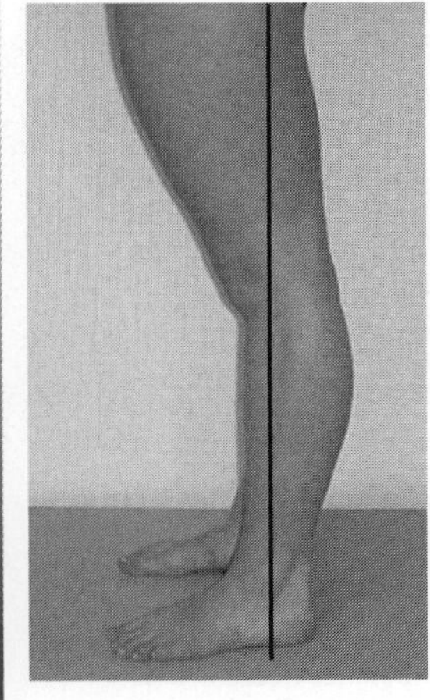

Potential Causes	Hypermobility of joints/lax ligaments (commonly seen in ectomorph body type) Combined posterior cruciate ligament and anterior cruciate ligament laxity[26] Poor postural sense
Resulting Effects	Increased stress on the ACL Increased tension on the posterior and posterolateral soft tissue structures Compressive forces on the anterior and medial compartments of the tibiofemoral joint

ACL = anterior cruciate ligament.

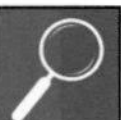

Inspection Findings 6-3
Hyperlordotic Posture

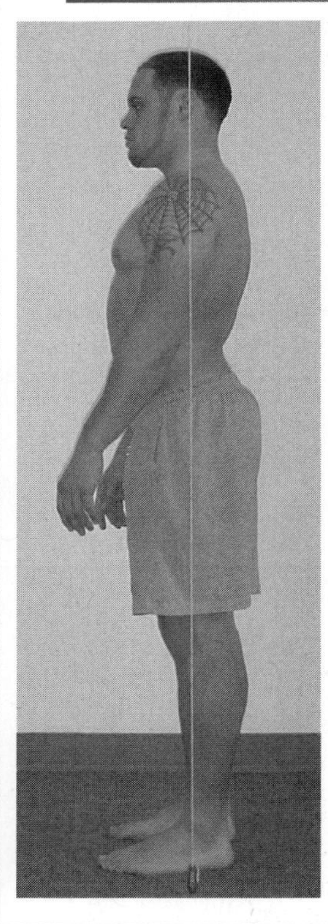

Joints Involved	Lumbar spine, pelvis, hip
Potential Cause	Tightened or shortened hip flexor muscles or back extensors Weakened or elongated hip extensors or abdominals Poor postural sense
Resulting Effects	Increased lumbar lordosis Anterior pelvic tilt Hip assuming a flexed position
Potential Associated Compressive or Distractive Forces and Pathological Conditions	Increased shear forces placed on lumbar vertebral bodies secondary to psoas tightness Increased compressive forces on lumbar facet joints Adaptive shortening of the posterior lumbar spine ligaments and the anterior hip ligaments Elongation of the anterior lumbar spine ligaments and the posterior hip ligaments Narrowing of the lumbar intervertebral foramen

Inspection Findings 6-4
Kypholordotic Posture

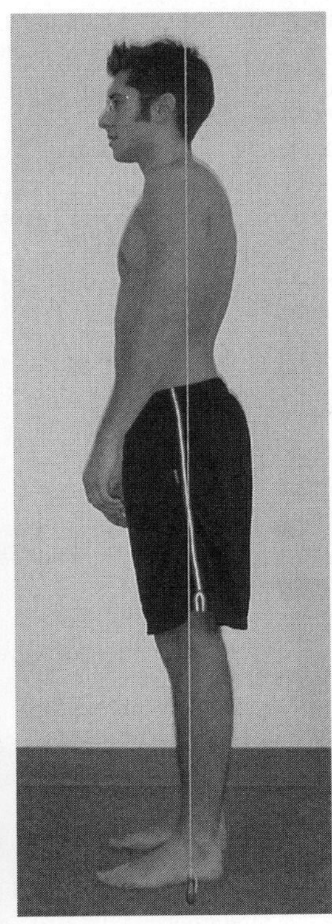

Joints Involved	Pelvis, hip joint, lumbar spine, thoracic spine, cervical spine
Potential Cause	Poor postural sense Muscle imbalance Tightened or shortened hip flexors or back extensors Weakened or elongated hip extensors or trunk flexors
Resulting Effects	Anterior pelvic tilt Flexed hip joint Increased lumbar lordosis Increased thoracic kyphosis
Potential Associated Compressive or Distractive Forces and Pathological Conditions	Adaptive shortening of anterior chest musculature Elongation of thoracic paraspinal musculature Increased compressive forces on anterior structures of thoracic vertebrae and posterior structures of lumbar vertebrae Increased tensile forces on ligamentous structures in posterior aspect of thoracic spine and anterior aspect of lumbar spine Increased compression of lumbar facet joints Increased compression of thoracic anterior vertebral bodies Forward head posture Forward shoulder posture

Inspection Findings 6-5
Swayback Posture

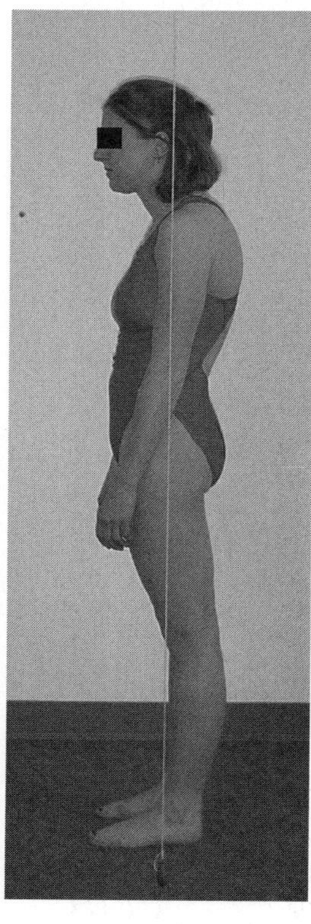

Joints Involved	Knee joint, hip joint, lumbar spine, lower thoracic spine, cervical spine
Potential Cause	Poor postural sense Tightened or shortened hip extensors Weakened or elongated hip flexors or lower abdominals Decreased general muscular strength
Resulting Effects	Genu recurvatum Extended hip joint Posterior pelvic tilt Anterior shift of the lumbosacral region Lumbar spine in neutral or minimal flexed position Increase in lower thoracic, thoracolumbar curvature (increase in lower thoracic kyphosis to cause posterior shift of trunk to compensate for anterior shift of L5/S1)
Potential Associated Compressive or Distractive Forces and Pathological Conditions	Elongation or increased tensile forces on the ligamentous structures at the anterior hip joint and posterior aspect of the lower thoracic spine Adaptively shortened or increased compressive forces on the posterior ligamentous structures at the hip joint and anterior aspect of the lower thoracic spine Increased tensile forces on the soft tissue structures of the posterior knee; compressive forces on anterior knee Increased shearing forces L5/S1 Forward head posture Forward shoulder posture

Inspection Findings 6-6
Flat Back Posture

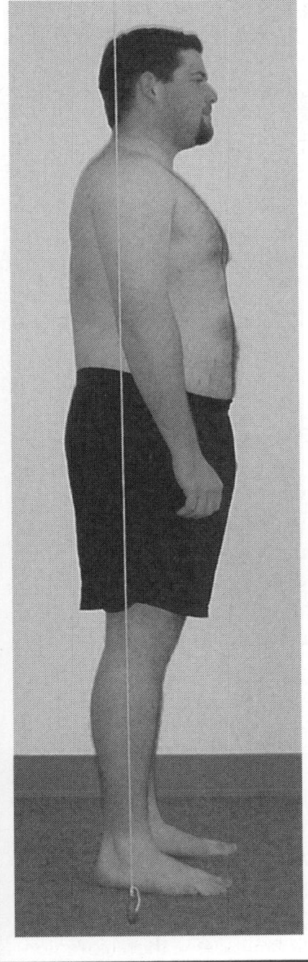

Joints Involved	Hip joint, lumbar spine, thoracic spine, cervical spine
Potential Causes	Shortened or tightened hip extensors, abdominal musculature Weakened/elongated hip flexors, back extensors Poor postural sense
Resulting Effects	Extended hip joint Posterior pelvic tilt Decreased lumbar lordosis Decreased thoracic kyphosis Flexed middle and lower cervical spine, extended upper cervical spine (FSP)
Potential Associated Compressive or Distractive Forces and Pathological Conditions	Adaptive shortening of soft tissue, compressive forces in posterior hip joint, anterior lumbar and mid-low cervical spines, posterior thoracic and upper cervical spines Elongation of soft tissue, tensile forces on the anterior hip joint, posterior lumbar and middle and lower cervical spines, anterior thoracic and upper cervical spines FHP resulting as compensation for the posterior displacement of the spine Knee flexion possibly occurring for the same reason

FHP = forward head posture; FSP = forward shoulder posture.

Inspection Findings 6-7
Scoliosis

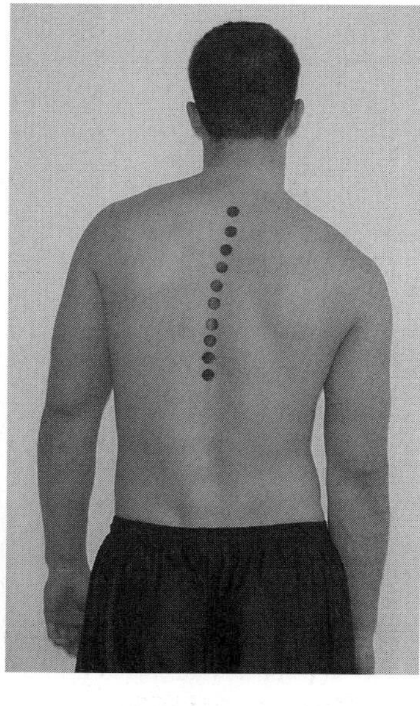

Left thoracic curve. Note the resulting asymmetrical scapular position.

Structures Involved	Thoracic and lumbar vertebrae
Potential Causes	Structural scoliosis: Anomaly of vertebrae Functional scoliosis: Muscle imbalance, leg length discrepancy
Resulting Effects	Rotation of one or more vertebrae Compression of one facet joint; distraction of the opposite facet joint Shortened or tightened trunk muscles on concave side of the curvature Weakened or elongated trunk muscles on convex side of the curvature
Potential Associated Compressive or Distractive Forces and Pathological Conditions	Disc pathology Soft tissue pathology as the body attempts to compensate and maintain head posture Sacroiliac joint dysfunction Decreased mobility of spine and chest cage Asymmetry in chest expansion with deep breathing Decreased pulmonary function (if excessive in thoracic region) If caused by limb length inequality: Degenerative changes in lumbar spine, hip, knee joints in longer limb Muscle overuse on longer limb caused by increased muscle activity SI joint dysfunction Excessive pronation of longer limb with dysfunctions associated with pronation Alteration of pattern of mechanical stresses on joint involved—structural

SI = sacroiliac.

Inspection Findings 6-8
Forward Shoulder Posture

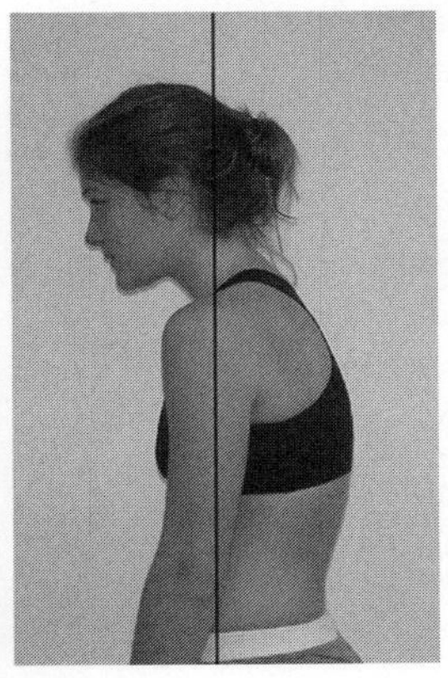

Structures Involved	Scapulothoracic articulation GH joint Thoracic spine Cervical spine
Potential Causes	Shortened or overdeveloped anterior shoulder girdle muscles (pectoralis major, pectoralis minor) Weakened or elongated interscapular muscles (mid trap, rhomboid, lower trap) Poor postural awareness Abnormal cervical and thoracic spine sagittal plane alignments[27] Postural muscle fatigue Large breast development Repetitive occupational and sporting positions
Resulting Effects	Humeral head is displaced anteriorly; decreased posterior glide Forward head posture
Potential Associated Compressive or Distractive Forces and Pathological Conditions	Thoracic outlet syndrome Abnormal scapulohumeral rhythm and scapula stability Acromioclavicular joint degeneration Bicipital tendinopathy Impingement syndrome Trigger points, myofascial pain in periscapular muscles Abnormal biomechanics of GH joint

GH = glenohumeral.

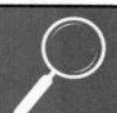

Inspection Findings 6-9
Forward Head Posture

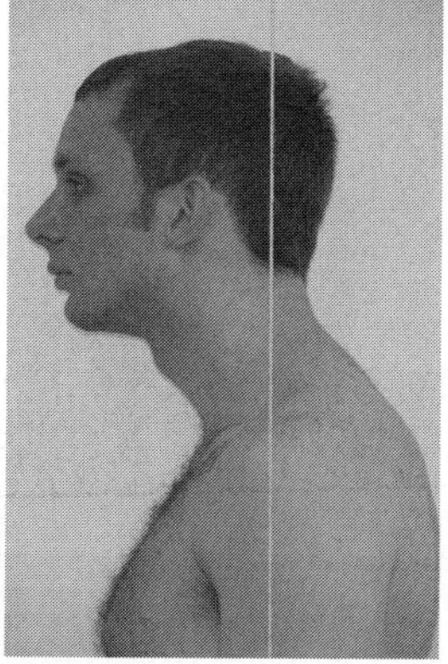

Structures Involved	Cervical spine GH joint Thoracic spine
Potential Causes	Wearing of bifocals Poor eyesight and need for glasses Muscle fatigue and weakness Poor postural sense Compensatory mechanism for other postural deviations (occupational activities and ADLs)
Resulting Effects	Flexed lower cervical spine Flattening or flexion of mid-cervical spine Extended upper cervical spine
Potential Associated Compressive or Distractive Forces and Pathological Conditions	Adaptively shortened suboccipital muscles (capital extensors), scalenes, upper trapezius, and levator scapula Elongated and weakened anterior cervical flexors and scapular depressors Hypomobile upper cervical region with compensatory hypermobility of the mid-cervical spine Abnormal shoulder (GH joint) biomechanics; decrease in shoulder elevation Temporomandibular joint dysfunction[28] Thoracic outlet syndrome involving the anterior and mid-scalene region Myofascial pain periscapular muscles and posterior cervical muscles[29] Overuse of posterior cervical and upper shoulder girdle muscles to maintain head in forward posture[29] Forward shoulder posture

ADL = activity of daily living; GH = glenohumeral.

CHAPTER 7

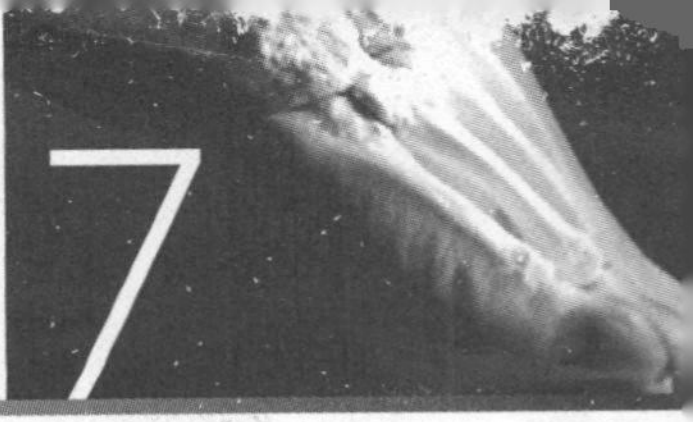

Evaluation of Gait

Phases of Gait

Phases of the Gait Cycle

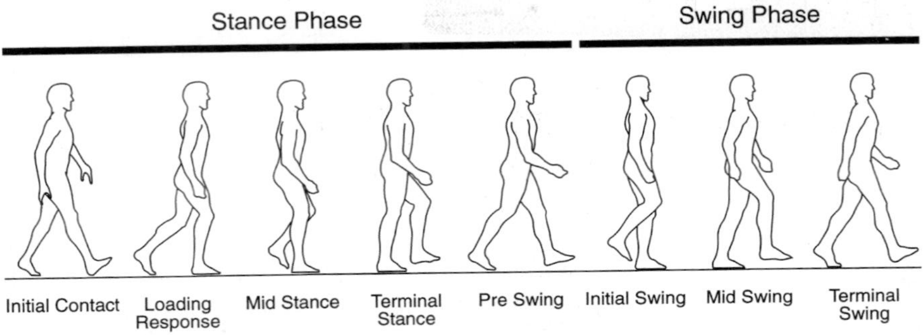

Stance Phase | Swing Phase

Initial Contact | Loading Response | Mid Stance | Terminal Stance | Pre Swing | Initial Swing | Mid Swing | Terminal Swing

FIGURE 7-1 ■ With the right (facing) limb as an example, two distinct phases occur—the weight-bearing stance phase and the non–weight-bearing swing phase. With the exception of the dual phases of double limb support, one limb is in the stance phase and the other is in the swing phase and vice versa. (Courtesy of Norkin, CC, and Levangie, PK: Joint *Structure and Function: A Comprehensive Analysis*, ed 2. Philadelphia: FA Davis, 1992.)

Box 7-1
Stance Phase of Gait

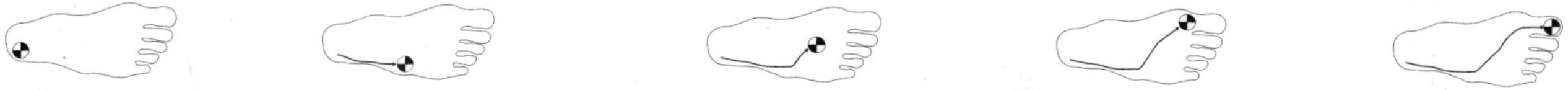

	Initial Contact	Loading Response	Midstance	Terminal Stance	Preswing
Subtalar Joint	5° Supination	10° Pronation	5° Pronation, supinating toward neutral	5° Supination	10° Supination
Talocrural Joint	Neutral or slightly plantarflexed moving in plantar flexion direction	Reaches maximum of 7° plantarflexion	Reaches maximum of 15° dorsiflexion as lower leg moves anteriorly over foot	5°–10° Dorsiflexion moving toward plantarflexion	0°–20° Plantarflexion
Knee	0° Flexion: Tibia externally rotated	20° Flexion: Tibia internally rotates, tibia begins to externally rotate as the knee extends	20° Flexion to 0°: Tibia externally rotating	5° Flexion to 0°: Tibia externally rotates	0°–40° Flexion: Tibia externally rotates
Hip	30° Flexion: Femur externally rotated	30° Flexion: Femur internally rotating to neutral	25° Flexion to 0°: Femur internally rotated, femur is abducted 5°	0°–10° Extension: Femur externally rotates and adducts	20° Extension to 0° extension: Femur externally rotates with slight abduction

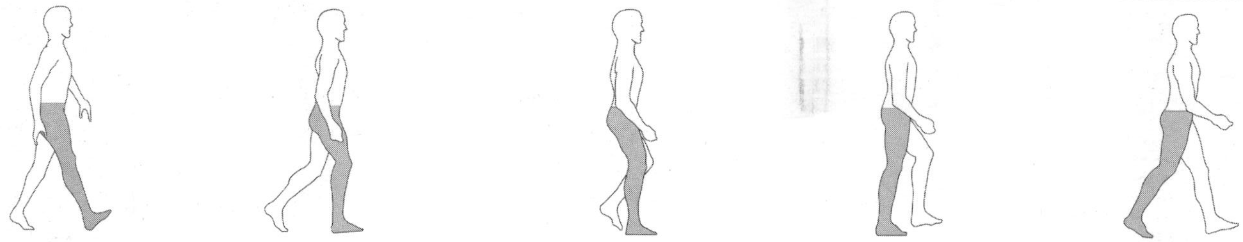

Weight-Bearing Surface

Muscle Activity				
Foot Intrinsics				
Isometric stabilization	Eccentric	Concentric	Concentric	Concentric
Plantarflexors				
Silent	Eccentric	Eccentric	Eccentric to concentric	Concentric
Dorsiflexors				
Eccentric	Eccentric	Concentric, but momentum can carry the talocrural joint through its range of motion.	Isometric	Concentric to silent
Quadriceps				
Concentric	Eccentric	Silent	Silent	Eccentric to silent
Hamstrings				
Eccentric	Isometric stabilization	Isometric	Concentric	Concentric
Hip Adductors				
Eccentric	Eccentric	Isometric	Isometric	Eccentric to control the pelvis
Gluteus Maximus				
Isometric to eccentric	Concentric	Silent	Isometric	Isometric
Gluteus Medius and Minimus				
Eccentric	Isometric or concentric	Concentric	Concentric	Isometric
Iliopsoas				
Eccentric	Isometric stabilization	Eccentric	Eccentric	Concentric

Figures modified from Levangie, PK, and Norkin, CC: *Joint Structure and Function: A Comprehensive Analysis*, ed 4. Philadelphia: FA Davis, 2005.

Table 7-1 Effects of Impairments During the Stance Phase of the Gait Cycle

	Compensation			
Impairment	**Initial Contact**	**Loading Response**	**Midstance**	**Terminal Stance**
Decreased Dorsiflexion	Increased subtalar pronation Forefoot abduction	Increased and prolonged midtarsal joint pronation		Decreased ability to toe-off Premature heel rise
Decreased First MTP Joint Motion				Decreased ability to toe-off Premature heel rise
Extrinsic Leg or Thigh Muscle Weakness	Altered position	Increased subtalar joint pronation Increased tibial rotation	Impaired supination	Impaired supination Decreased ability to toe-off
Hip	Toe-out gait			
Rotator Muscle Weakness		Increased rotation of femur and tibia		
Rearfoot Varus	Increased subtalar pronation Increased medial leg or foot stresses	Excessive pronation	Impaired supination	Incomplete resupination with decreased force at toe-off
Rearfoot Valgus	Decreased shock absorption	Decreased subtalar pronation Heel approaching the vertical position	Decreased ability to accommodate to uneven surfaces	Decreased ability to supinate
Hypomobile First Ray	Altered midfoot and forefoot position	Instability in midtarsal joints and forefoot	Altered distribution of ground reaction forces	Pain or decreased force at toe-off
Plantarflexed First Ray	First ray contacts the ground	Decreased subtalar pronation	Decreased ability to absorb shock	Increased force on first ray

Forefoot Varus	Increased pronation Toe-out gait		
Forefoot Valgus		Decreased ability to absorb shock	Decreased force at toe-off
Tarsal Coalition	Decreased or absent subtalar joint motion		
Tibial Torsion	Increased compensatory subtalar joint pronation		
Femoral Torsion	Toe-in gait Increased subtalar joint pronation secondary to internal tibial rotation		
Leg Length Discrepancy	Compensatory pronation of the longer leg with compensatory supination of the shorter leg		

MTP = metatarsophalangeal.

Box 7-2
Swing Phase of Gait

	Initial Swing	Midswing	Terminal Swing
Limb Position			
Weight-Bearing Surface	⊘	⊘	⊘
Subtalar Joint	Pronating	Neutral	5° Supination
Talocrural Joint	Reaches maximum of 20° rapid dorsiflexion for toe clearance	Neutral	Neutral
Knee	30°–70° Flexion: Tibia internally rotates	30°–0° Flexion: Tibia externally rotates	0°: Tibia externally rotates
Hip	0°–20° Flexion: Femur externally rotates to neutral	20°–30° Flexion: Femur externally rotates	30° Flexion: Femur externally rotates

Muscle Activity		
Foot Intrinsics		
Isometric stabilization	Isometric	Isometric stabilization
Plantarflexors		
Concentric, reducing muscular activity	Concentric	Isometric
Dorsiflexors		
Concentric until the foot is clear of the ground, then isometric	Isometric	Isometric
Quadriceps		
Concentric	Silent—Momentum carries the limb through the ROM	Concentric to stabilize the knee
Hamstrings		
Concentric to eccentric	Eccentric	Eccentric
Hip Adductors		
Concentric	Isometric	Eccentric
Gluteus Maximus		
Isometric	Eccentric	Eccentric
Gluteus Medius and Minimus		
Isometric	Isometric	Isometric
Iliopsoas		
Concentric	Concentric or silent	Isometric

Figures modified from Levangie, PK, and Norkin, CC: *Joint Structure and Function: A Comprehensive Analysis*, ed 4. Philadelphia: FA Davis, 2005.

Box 7-3
Quantitative Gait Analysis

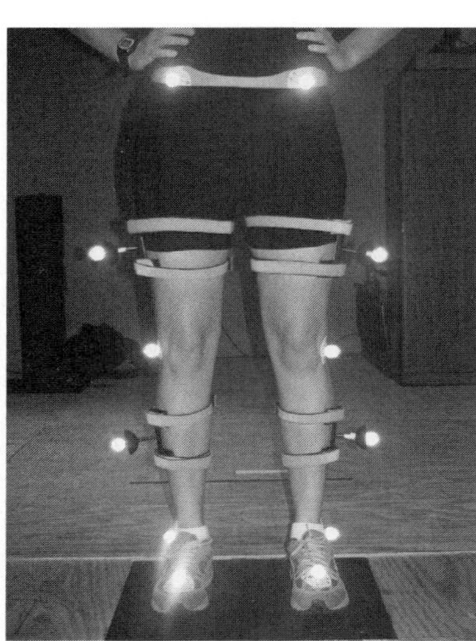

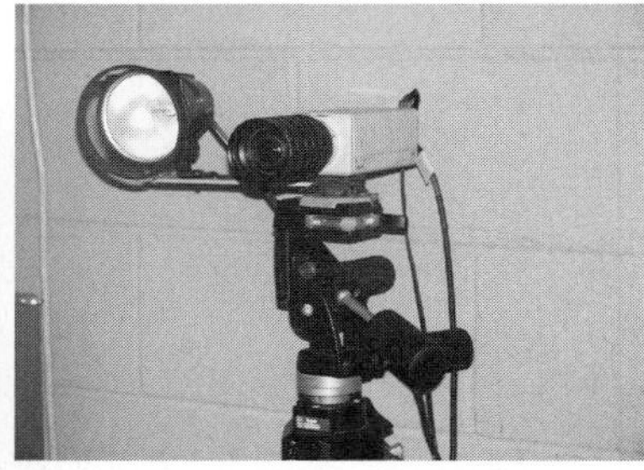

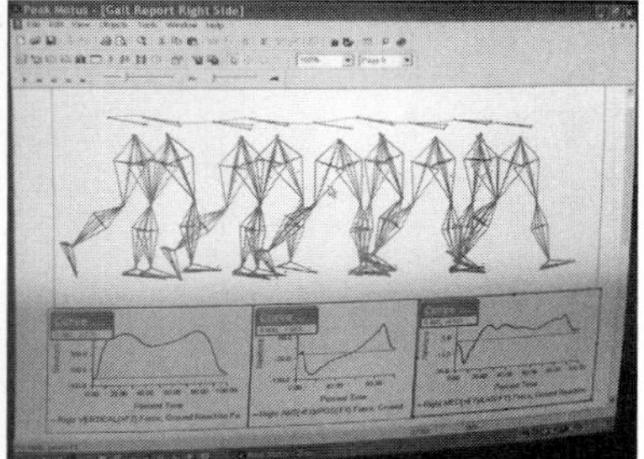

A quantitative gait analysis yields numerical results for the motion, force, and muscle activity characteristics during gait and may be conducted with simple tools such as a stopwatch and camcorder, or with a motion measurement system that may also include instrumented walkways, force plates, pressure mats, and/or electromyography (EMG) capabilities. Other more sophisticated methods include the use of (1) electromechanical instruments such as imbedding pressure-sensitive switches into the patient's shoe or inserts or applying them to the bottom of the foot and (2) optoelectronic techniques such as video capture.

Video capture requires the use of reference markers that are attached to the patient, careful calibration of the video space, a computerized digitizing process of the reference markers, and mathematical equations to yield the results. Motion measurement systems are usually housed in gait analysis laboratories. Angular kinematics, such as knee extension range of motion (ROM) or hip flexion velocity, are measured using electrogoniometry, accelerometry, or optoelectronic techniques. An electrogoniometer is a device that is attached to the body segments for a direct measure of angular displacement (ROM) of a joint. They are available in uniaxial and multiaxial designs. Accelerometers are similar. They are attached to the body segments of interest but directly measure segmental acceleration. Segmental velocities and displacements are then determined.

EMG techniques are used to measure the timing and amplitude of muscle activity, and help to describe the motor performance underlying the kinematic and kinetic characteristics of gait. Surface EMG where electrodes are attached directly to the skin over the muscles of interest is more common in clinical gait analyses. Intramuscular EMG, in which needles are inserted through the skin and into the muscles of interest, is primarily used in gait research.

EMG, force, and pressure plates are typically integrated with a motion measurement system to enable simultaneous acquisition of kinematic, kinetic, and muscle activity information. These systems are also helpful in producing gait reports.

Table 7-2 Effects of Impairments during the Swing Phase of the Gait Cycle

	Compensation		
Impairment	**Initial Swing**	**Midswing**	**Terminal Swing**
Hamstring Weakness		Decreased knee flexion leading to shortened step length	
Hip Flexor Weakness	Decreased hip flexion propulsion causing inability to achieve toe clearance; compensatory hip elevation occurs along with a shortened step length		
Hamstring Strain or Sciatic Nerve Pathology			Decreased knee extension and impaired ability to decelerate leg for contact
Leg Length Discrepancy	Hip drop when short side in swing phase		
Hip External Rotator Tightness	Toeing out		

Box 7-4
Observational Gait Analysis

Using an OGA written tool, the presence or absence of the critical events in the gait cycle can be determined. When preparing for your analysis, refer to the following OGA guidelines:

1. Prepare the area and materials ahead of time.
2. Avoid clutter in the viewing background.
3. Have the patient wear clothing that does not restrict viewing of joints.
4. Ensure that the patient is at a self-selected walking pace; otherwise, gait will be altered.
5. Position yourself in a position to view the individual segments (i.e., if you are observing for forefoot pronation and supination, then squat down so your eyes are in line with the patient's feet).
6. Observe the subject from multiple views (anterior, posterior, and both lateral views) but not from an oblique angle.
7. Look at the individual body parts first, then the whole body, then the individual parts again.
8. Conduct multiple observations or trials.
9. Conduct the analysis with the patient barefoot and wearing shoes.
10. Label all DVDs or videotapes (if used) with pertinent data.

Box 7-5

Compensatory Gait Deviations

Gluteus Maximus Gait

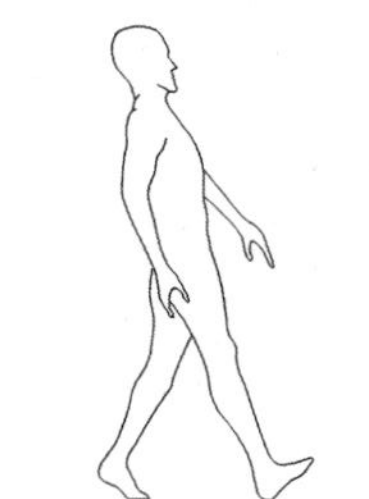

At initial contact, the thorax is thrust posteriorly to maintain hip extension during the stance phase, often causing a lurching of the trunk.

Cause: Weakness or paralysis of the gluteus maximus muscle.

Stiff Knee or Hip Gait

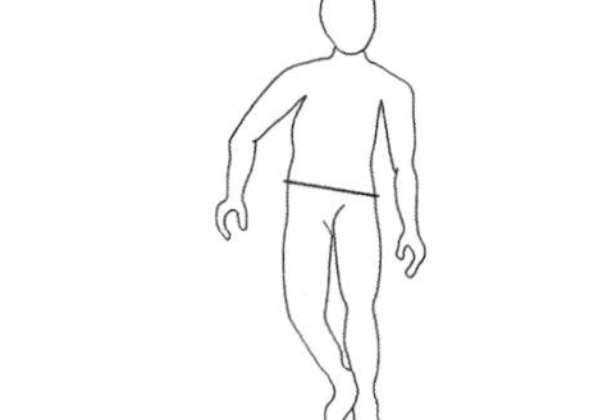

In the swing phase, the affected extremity is lifted higher than normal to compensate for knee or hip stiffness. To accomplish this, the uninvolved extremity demonstrates increased plantarflexion.

Cause: Knee pathologies such as meniscal or ligamentous tears, or hip pathologies such as bursitis or muscle strains that result in a decrease in the ROM.

Trendelenburg's Gait (gluteus medius gait)

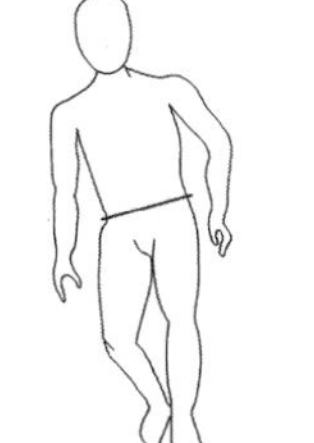

During the stance phase of the affected limb, the thorax lists toward the involved limb. This serves to maintain the center of gravity and prevent a drop in the pelvis on the affected side.

Cause: Weakness of the gluteus medius muscle.

Calcaneal Gait

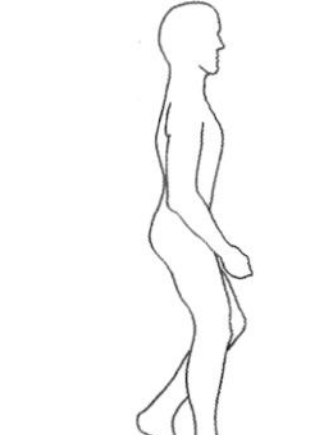

During the stance phase, increased dorsiflexion and knee flexion occur on the affected side, resulting in a decreased step length.

Cause: Paralysis or weakness of the plantarflexors or painful when weight bearing on the forefoot or toes caused by such conditions as blisters, hallux rigidus, sesamoiditis, or ankle sprains.

Psoatic Limp

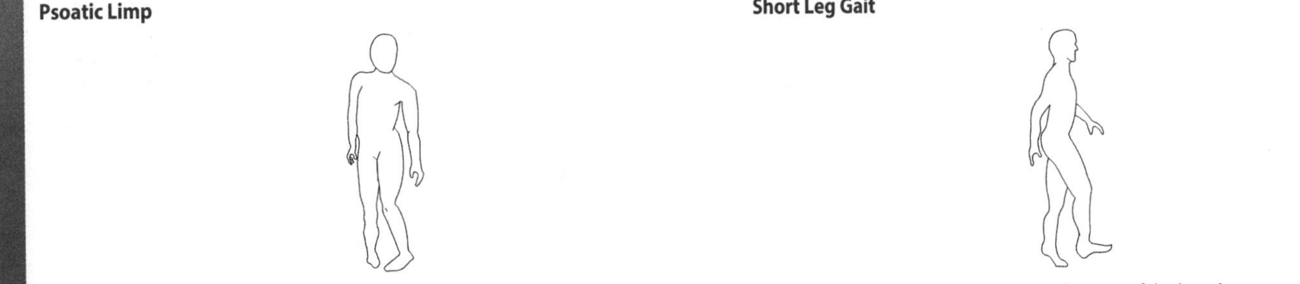

To compensate during the swing phase, lateral rotation and flexion of the trunk occurs with hip adduction. The trunk and pelvic movements are exaggerated.

Cause: Weakness or reflex inhibition of the psoas major muscle (Legg–Perthes disease).

Short Leg Gait

Increased pronation occurs in the subtalar joint of the long leg, accompanied by a shift of the trunk toward the longer extremity.

Cause: True (anatomical) leg length discrepancy; the right (facing) leg is longer.

Steppage Gait (dropfoot)

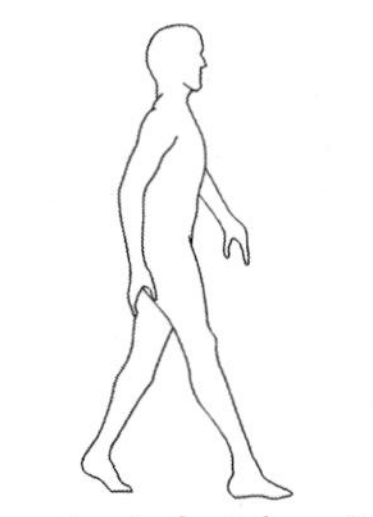

The foot slaps at initial contact, owing to foot drop. During the swing phase, the affected limb demonstrates increased hip and knee flexion to avoid toe dragging, producing a "high-step" pattern.

Cause: Weakness or paralysis of the dorsiflexors.

ROM = range of motion.
Figures modified from Levangie, PK, and Norkin, CC: *Joint Structure and Function: A Comprehensive Analysis*, ed 4. Philadelphia: FA Davis, 2005.

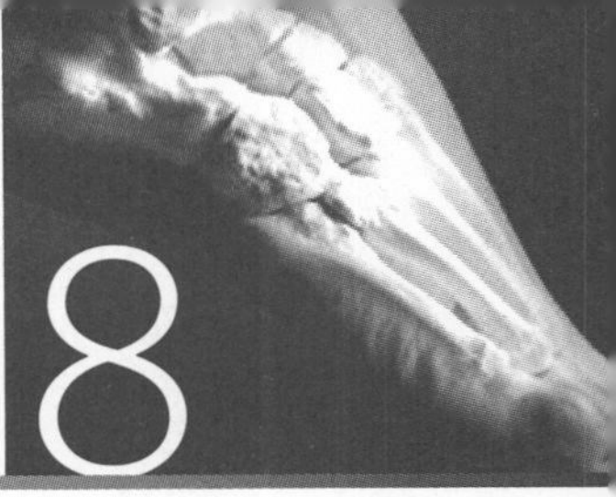

CHAPTER 8

Foot and Toe Pathologies

Examination Map

HISTORY

Past Medical History

History of the Present Condition

INSPECTION

Functional Observation

General Inspection of the Foot
General foot type classifications
Feiss line
Assessment of foot position in STNJ

Inspection of the Toes
Pathological toe postures
Posture of the first ray

Inspection of the Medial Structures
Medial longitudinal arch

Inspection of the Lateral Structures
Fifth metatarsal

Inspection of the Dorsal Structures
Long toe tendons

Inspection of the Plantar Surface
Plantar fascia
Medial calcaneal tubercle
Callus/blister formation

Inspection of the Posterior Structures
Achilles tendon
Calcaneus
Retrocalcaneal exostosis

Inspection of Foot and Calcaneal Alignment
Assessment of subtalar joint neutral
Common foot postures assessed in subtalar joint neutral
Position of first tarsometatarsal joint

PALPATION

Palpation of the Medial Structures
First MTP joint
First metatarsal
First cuneiform
Navicular
Talar head
Sustentaculum tali
Calcaneonavicular ligament
Medial talar tubercle
Calcaneus
Tibialis posterior
Flexor hallucis longus
Flexor digitorum longus
Posterior tibial pulse

Palpation of the Lateral Structures
Fifth MTP joint
Fifth metatarsal
Styloid process
Cuboid
Lateral calcaneal border
Peroneal tubercle
Peroneal tendons

Palpation of the Dorsal Structures
Rays
Cuneiforms
Navicular
Dome of the talus
Sinus tarsi
Extensor digitorum brevis
Inferior extensor retinaculum

Continued

Examination Map—cont'd

Tibialis anterior

Extensor hallucis longus

Extensor digitorum longus

Dorsalis pedis pulse

Palpation of the Plantar Structures

Medial calcaneal tubercle

Plantar fascia

Intermetatarsal neuromas

Lateral four metatarsal heads

Sesamoids

JOINT AND MUSCLE FUNCTION ASSESSMENT

Goniometry

Rearfoot inversion and eversion

First metatarsophalangeal abduction

Metatarsophalangeal flexion and extension

Active Range of Motion

Toe flexion

Toe extension

Manual Muscle Tests

Toe flexion

Toe extension

Passive Range of Motion

Toe flexion

Toe extension

Mobility of first ray

JOINT STABILITY TESTS

Stress Testing

Metatarsophalangeal and interphalangeal joints

- Valgus and varus stress testing of the MTP and IP joints

Joint Play Assessment

Intermetatarsal joints

Tarsometatarsal joints

Midtarsal joints

NEUROLOGIC EXAMINATION

L4–S2 Nerve Roots

Tarsal Tunnel Syndrome

Interdigital Neuroma

VASCULAR EXAMINATION

Dorsalis Pedis Pulse

Posterior Tibial Pulse

Capillary Refill

PATHOLOGIES AND SPECIAL TESTS

Foot Type

Navicular drop test

Pes Cavus

Plantar Fasciitis

Test for supple pes planus

Plantar Fascia Rupture

Heel Spur

Tarsal Coalition

Tarsal Tunnel Syndrome

Dorsiflexion–eversion test

Metatarsal Fractures

Acute fractures

Stress fractures

Lisfranc Injury

Phalangeal Fractures

Intermetatarsal Neuroma

Mulder sign

Hallux Rigidus

Hallux Valgus

First MTP Joint Sprains

Sesamoiditis

Table 8-1 Possible Pathology Based on the Location of Pain

	Location of Pain					
	Proximal (Calcaneus)	**Distal (Toes)**	**Plantar**	**Dorsal**	**Medial**	**Lateral**
Soft Tissue Pathology	Calcaneal bursitis	Corns	Callus	MTP sprain	Spring ligament sprain	Peroneal tendinopathy
	Retrocalcaneal bursitis	Hallux rigidus	Plantar fasciitis	Forefoot sprain	Plantar fasciitis	
					Plantar fascia rupture or sprain	
	Achilles tendinopathy	IP sprain	Plantar fascia rupture		Posterior tibial nerve entrapment (Tarsal tunnel syndrome)	
		MTP sprain	Plantar warts		Tibialis posterior tendinopathy	
		Ingrown toenail	Intermetatarsal neuroma		1st MTP sprain	
			Tarsal tunnel syndrome			
Bony Pathology	Calcaneal fracture	Phalanx fracture	Sesamoiditis	Metatarsal stress fracture	Navicular stress fracture	Cuboid fracture
	Calcaneal spur	Arthritis or inflammation	Sesamoid fracture	Lisfranc fracture/ dislocation	Bunion	Fifth metatarsal fracture (especially at the base)
	Calcaneal cyst		Heel spur	Talus fracture	Hallux rigidus	Bunionette
				Tarsal coalition	Hallux valgus	

IP = interphalangeal; MTP = metatarsophalangeal.

Inspection Findings 8-1
General Foot Type Classifications (Weight Bearing)

	Pes Planus	Neutral	Pes Cavus
		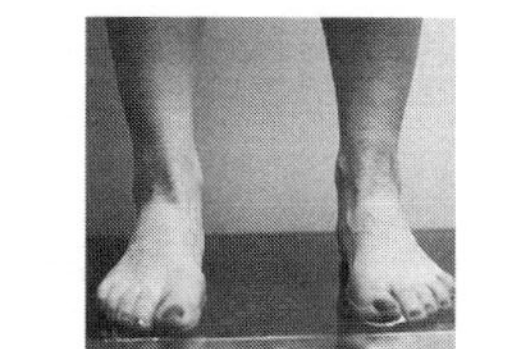	
Description	Medial bulge; abducted forefoot, everted calcaneus A medial bulge must be present at the talonavicular joint, indicating excessive talar adduction. The medial arch must be low. This is determined by the Feiss line, formed by connecting the points formed by the head of the first MT, the navicular tubercle, and the medial malleolus (see Box 4–1).	The calcaneus is slightly everted. A medial bulge is not present. Feiss line indicates that the most prominent aspect of the navicular is in line with the apex of the medial malleolus and the plantar surface of the first MTP joint.	The calcaneus must be inverted greater than 3° from perpendicular relative to the position of the ground. A medial bulge is not present. Using Feiss' line, the arch must be high.

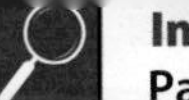

Inspection Findings 8-2
Pathological Toe Postures

	Claw Toes	Hammer Toes	Morton's Toes	Hallux Valgus
Observation				
Illustration				
Deviation	Progressive contracture of the interosseous or lumbrical muscles (or both)	Contractures of the associated toe extensors and flexors; inability of the interosseous muscles to hold the proximal phalanx in the neutral position	Although it appears that the 2nd toe is longer than the 1st, Morton's toe is formed by the 1st metatarsal being shorter than the 2nd.	Over time, there is a gradual and subluxation of the 1st MTP joint. A bunion will develop on the medial border of the 1st MTP joint. Lateral displacement of the great toe may interfere with the function of the 2nd toe[30]
Description	Hyperextension of the MTP joint and flexion of the PIP and DIP joints. Claw toes affect the lateral four toes.	Hyperextension of the MTP and DIP joints and flexion of the PIP joints of the lateral four toes	The posture of the foot is normal, but the 2nd toe extends beyond the great toe.	The 1st MTP joint exceeds an angle of 20° in the frontal plane. The 1st and 2nd toes may overlap.

DIP = distal interphalangeal; PIP = proximal interphalangeal; MTP = metatarsophalangeal.

Inspection Findings 8-3
Common Foot Postures Assessed in Subtalar Joint Neutral

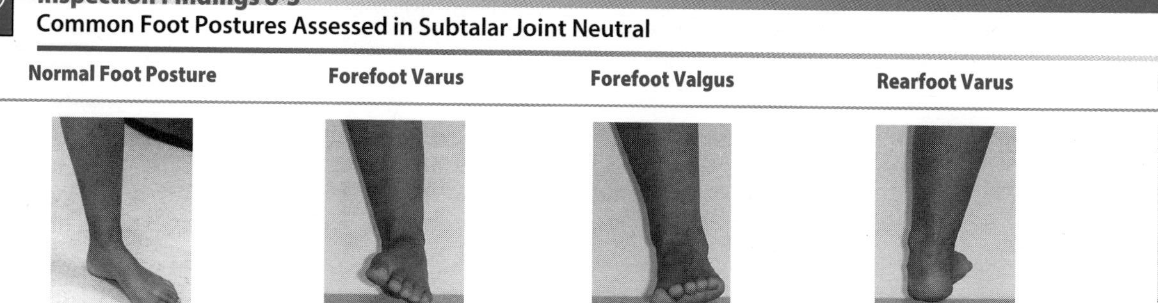

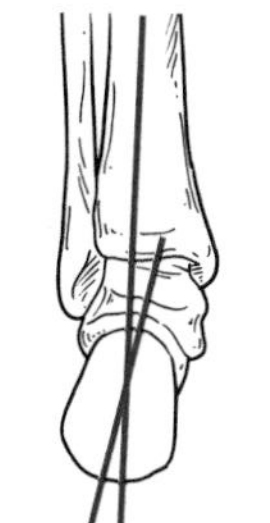

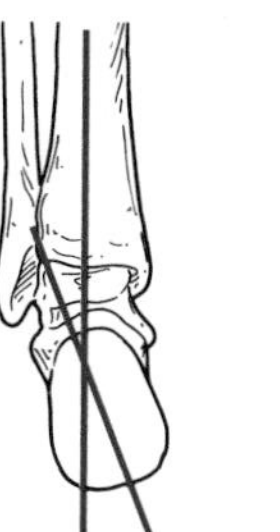

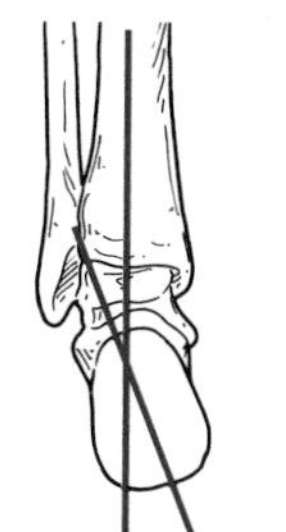

	Normal Foot Posture	Forefoot Varus	Forefoot Valgus	Rearfoot Varus	Rearfoot Valgus
Observation					
Illustration					
Posture	Calcaneus is vertical or slightly (<3º) inverted (varus) relative to the long axis of the bisected lower leg. Metatarsal heads are perpendicular to calcaneus.	Metatarsal heads are inverted relative to the rearfoot. Varus of 1–8 degrees is considered normal.[31]	Metatarsal heads are everted relative to the rearfoot. A plantarflexed first ray will also give the appearance of a forefoot valgus.	Calcaneus is inverted relative to the long axis of the bisected lower leg and may be related to a varus alignment of the tibia or a calcaneus that does not completely derotate during development.	Calcaneus is everted relative to the long axis of the tibia and can be associated with a valgus tibial alignment. Rearfoot valgus is rarely observed.

Compensation	During static weight bearing, the forefoot compensates by abducting and everting, resulting in a more planus foot. During gait, pronation is excessive and prolonged, as the 1st MT has farther to travel before contacting the ground.	During static weight bearing, the midfoot supinates as the first metatarsal contacts the ground and may give the foot a cavus appearance. During gait, the 1st MT strikes the ground prematurely, resulting in early supination, reducing the shock-absorbing capacity of the limb.	With sufficient subtalar joint mobility, the rearfoot will rapidly and excessively pronate during the early stages of gait.	The rearfoot becomes hypermobile, resulting in increased pronation.

MT = metatarsal.
Observation figures from Donatelli, RA: *Biomechanics of the Foot and Ankle*. Philadelphia: FA Davis, 1990.

PALPATION

Palpation of the Medial Structures

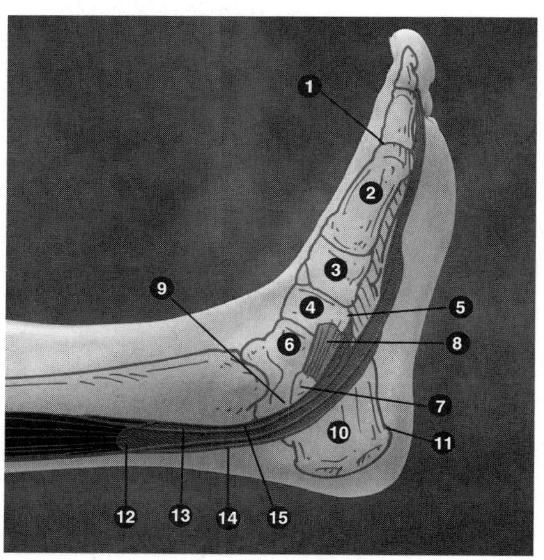

1 First MTP joint

2 First metatarsal

3 First cuneiform

4 Navicular

5 Navicular tuberosity

6 Talar head

7 Sustentaculum tali

8 Calcaneonavicular ligament

9 Medial talar tubercle

10 Calcaneus

11 Medial calcaneal tubercle

Medial tendons:

12 Flexor hallucis longus

13 Tibialis posterior

14 Flexor digitorum longus

15 Posterior tibial pulse

Palpation of the Lateral Structures

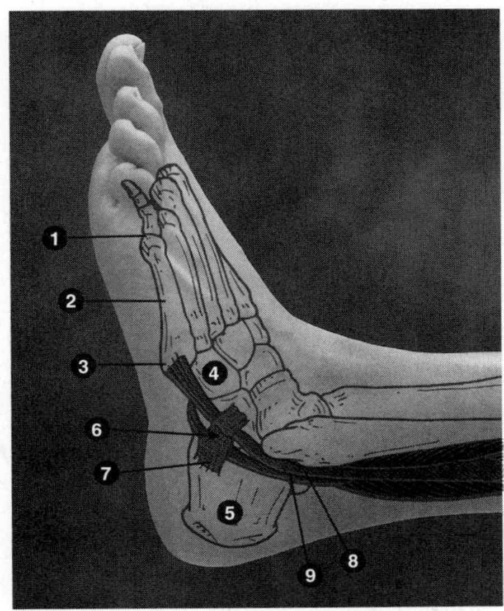

1 Fifth MTP joint

2 Fifth metatarsal

3 Styloid process

4 Cuboid

5 Lateral calcaneal border

6 Peroneal tubercle

7 Inferior peroneal retinaculum

8 Peroneus longus

9 Peroneus brevis

Palpation of the Dorsal Structures

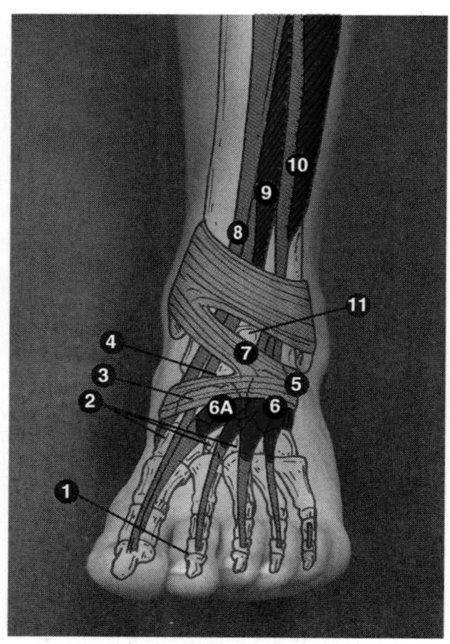

1 Rays

2 Cuneiforms

3 Navicular

4 Dome of the talus

5 Sinus tarsi

6 Extensor digitorum brevis

6A Extensor hallucis brevis

7 Inferior extensor retinaculum

8 Tibialis anterior

9 Extensor hallucis longus

10 Extensor digitorum longus

11 Dorsalis pedis pulse

Palpation of the Plantar Structures

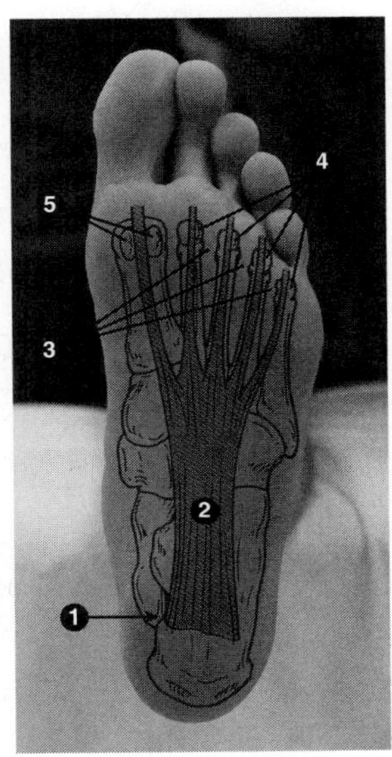

1 Medial calcaneal tubercle

2 Plantar fascia

3 Intermetatarsal neuromas

4 Lateral four metatarsal heads

5 Sesamoid bones of the great toe

Active Range of Motion

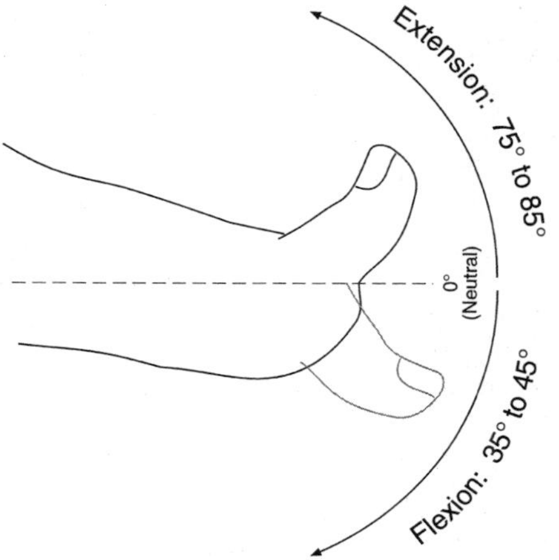

FIGURE 8-1 ■ Active range of motion for flexion and extension of the great toe's metatarsophalangeal joint. The range of motion decreases with each subsequent joint from the first MTP joint to the fifth.

Passive Range of Motion

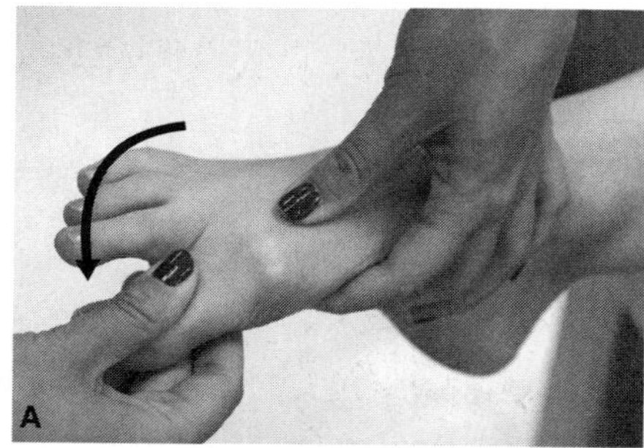

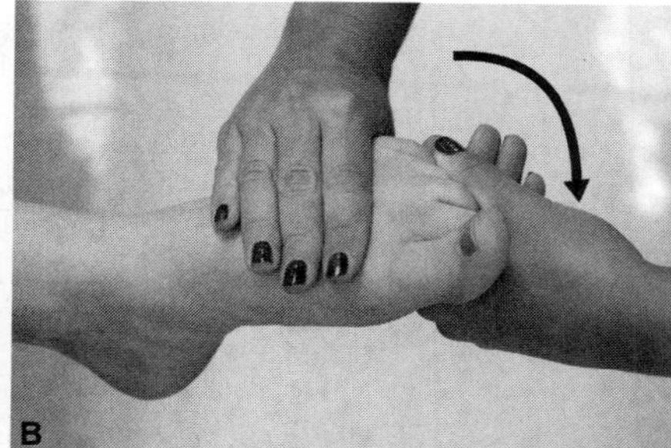

FIGURE 8-2 ■ Passive flexion of the **(A)** great toe and **(B)** lateral four toes.

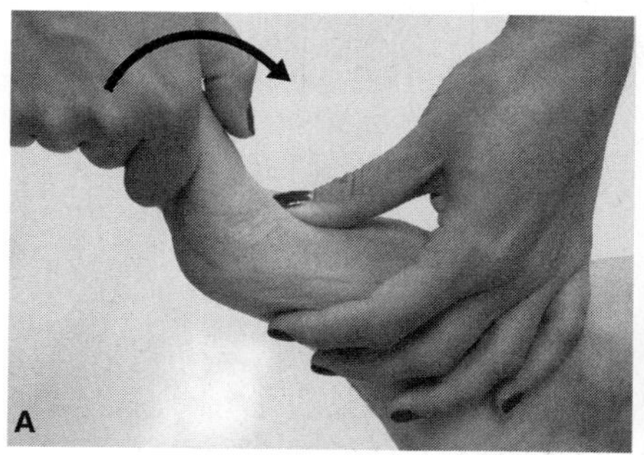

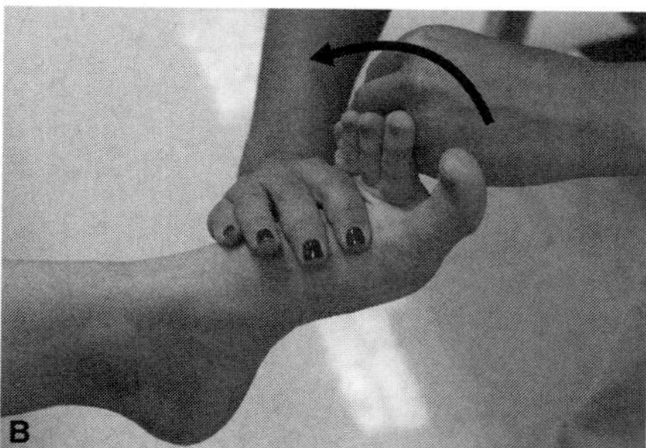

FIGURE 8-3 ■ Passive extension of the **(A)** great toe and **(B)** lateral four toes.

Table 8-2	Foot and Toe Capsular Patterns and End-Feels
Capsular Patterns	
Midtarsal joint	Dorsiflexion, plantarflexion, adduction, internal rotation
Metatarsophalangeal joint: Great toe	Extension, flexion
Metatarsophalangeal joints: 2nd–5th toes	Flexion, extension
End-feels	
Abduction at the midtarsal joints	Firm: Soft tissue stretch (intrinsic muscles, capsule, and ligaments)
Adduction at the midtarsal joints	Firm: Soft tissue stretch (intrinsic muscles, capsule, and ligaments)
Flexion of the toes	Firm: Tightness of the toe extensors
Extension of the toes	Firm: Tightness of the toe flexors
Abduction of the toes (MTP)	Firm: Soft tissue stretch (intrinsic muscles, capsule, and ligaments)
Adduction of the toes (MTP)	Firm: Soft tissue stretch (intrinsic muscles, capsule, and ligaments)

MTP = metatarsophalangeal.

Goniometry Box 8-1
Rearfoot Inversion and Eversion

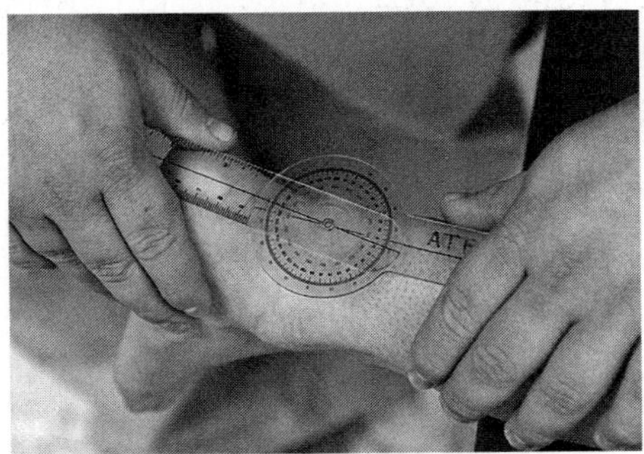

Inversion 0°–30° **Eversion 0°–5°**

Patient Position	Prone with ankle in neutral and STJ in neutral
Goniometer Alignment	
Fulcrum	The axis is centered over the Achilles tendon with the axis bisecting the malleoli.
Proximal Arm	The stationary arm is centered over the midline of the lower leg
Distal Arm	The movement arm is centered over the midline of the calcaneus.

STJ = subtalar joint.

Goniometry Box 8-2
First Metatarsophalangeal Abduction

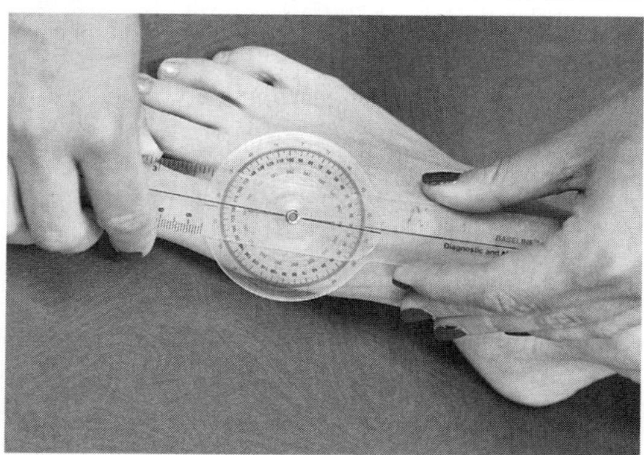

Passive Abduction

Patient Position	Supine or sitting with the STJ and ankle in neutral
Goniometer Alignment	
Fulcrum	The axis of the goniometer is placed over the dorsal aspect of the MTP joint.
Proximal Arm	The stationary arm is centered over the metatarsal being tested.
Distal Arm	The movement arm is centered over the proximal phalanx.

MTP = metatarsophalangeal; STJ = subtalar joint.

Goniometry Box 8-3
Metatarsophalangeal Flexion and Extension

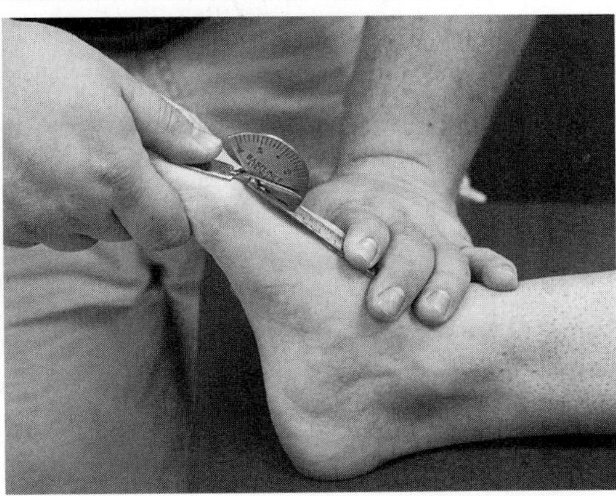

Flexion 0°–70° **Extension 0°–30°**

Patient Position	Supine with ankle in neutral
Goniometer Alignment	
Fulcrum	Position the axis of the goniometer over the dorsal aspect of the MTP joint being tested.
Proximal Arm	The stationary arm is centered on the midline of the metatarsal.
Distal Arm	The movement arm is centered on the midline of the proximal phalanx.
Comments	Place the goniometer on the plantar surface to test MTP extension.

MTP = metatarsophalangeal.

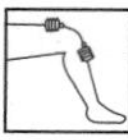

Manual Muscle Test 8-1
Toe Flexion

	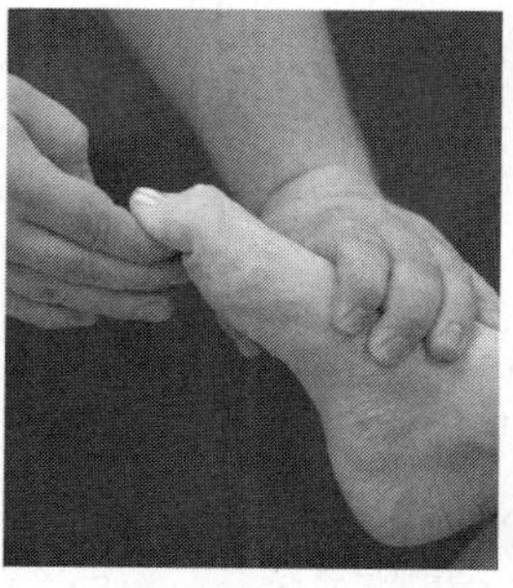 **Great Toe MTP Flexion**	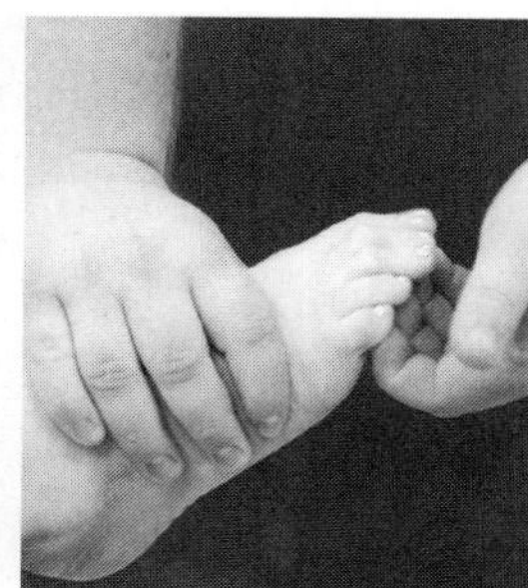 **Lateral 4 Toes Flexion**
Patient Position	Long sitting with the ankle in the neutral position	
Starting Position	The toes are in the neutral position.	
Stabilization	The forefoot is stabilized by grasping the metatarsals proximal to their heads.	
Palpation	Head of the first metatarsal, palpating the flexor hallucis longus	Not applicable (tendons are too deep to palpate).
Resistance	Along the entire length of the toe's plantar aspect	On the plantar aspect of the lateral four toes
Primary Mover(s) (Innervation)	Flexor hallucis longus: IP joint (L4, L5, S1) Flexor hallucis brevis: MTP joint (L4, L5, S1)	Flexor digitorum longus: DIP joint (L5, S1) Flexor digitorum brevis: PIP joint (L4, L5, S1) Flexor digiti minimi brevis: MTP joint of the 5th toe (S1, S2)
Secondary Mover(s) (Innervation)		Dorsal interossei: MTP joint flexion (S1, S2) Plantar interossei: MTP joint flexion (S1, S2) Lumbricals: MTP flexion (1st MTP: L4, L5, S1; 2nd to 5th: S1, S2)
Compensation/ Substitution	IP joint flexion, talocrural plantarflexion	Talocrural plantarflexion
Comments		The toe flexors collectively flex the MTP joints.

IP = interphalangeal; MTP = metatarsophalangeal.

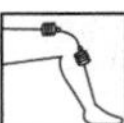

Manual Muscle Test 8-2
Toe Extension

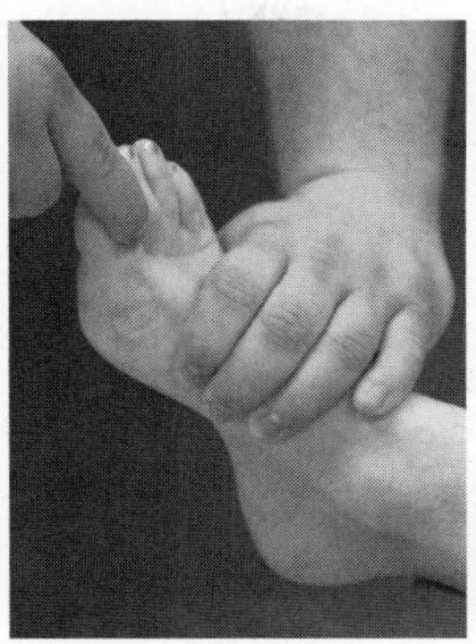

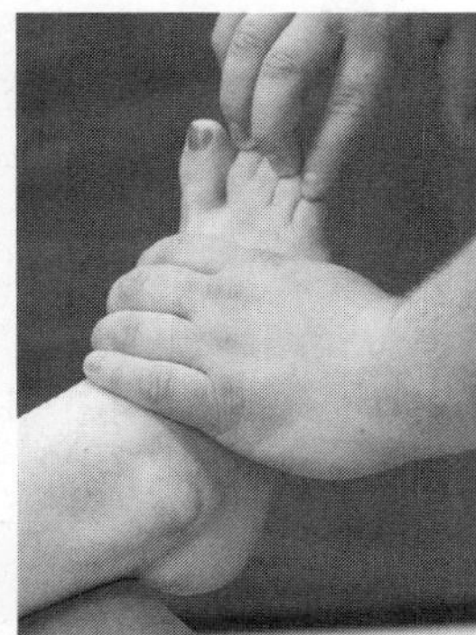

	MTP Extension	Toe Extension
Patient Position	Long sitting with the ankle in the neutral position	
Starting Position	The toes are in the neutral position.	
Stabilization	The forefoot is stabilized by grasping the metatarsals proximal to their heads.	
Palpation	Dorsal surface of the distal first metatarsal	Common extensor tendon on the proximal portion of the dorsum of the foot
Resistance	Dorsal aspect of the proximal phalanx of hallux	Dorsal aspect of the proximal phalanges of toes 2–5
Primary Mover(s) (Innervation)	Extensor hallucis longus (L4, L5, S1) Extensor hallucis brevis (L5, S1)	Extensor digitorum longus (L4, L5, S1) Extensor digitorum brevis (L5, S1) Dorsal interossei: IP joint extension (S1, S2) Plantar interossei: IP joint extension (S1, S2) Lumbricals (IP joint extension)
Compensation/ Substitution	Tibialis anterior	Tibialis anterior

Table 8-3 Intrinsic Foot and Toe Muscles

Muscle	Action	Origin	Insertion	Innervation	Root
Abductor Digiti Minimi	Flexion of the 5th MTP joint Abduction of the 5th MTP joint	Lateral portion of the calcaneal tuberosity Proximal lateral portion of calcaneus	Lateral portion of the 5th proximal phalanx	Lateral plantar	S1, S2
Abductor Hallucis	Abduction of the 1st MTP joint Assists in flexion of the 1st MTP joint Assists in forefoot adduction	Medial calcaneal tuberosity Flexor retinaculum Plantar aponeurosis	Plantar surface of the medial base of the 1st toe's proximal phalanx	Medial plantar	L4, L5, S1
Adductor Hallucis	Adduction of the 1st MTP joint Assists in flexion of the 1st MTP joint	Oblique head • Bases of 2nd through 4th metatarsals • Tendon sheath of peroneus longus Transverse head • Plantar surface of 3rd, 4th, and 5th metatarsal heads	Lateral surface of the base of the 1st toe's proximal phalanx	Lateral plantar	S1, S2
Flexor Digiti Minimi Brevis	Flexion of the 5th MTP joint	Plantar surface of the cuboid Base of the 5th metatarsal	Plantar aspect of the base of the 5th proximal phalanx	Lateral plantar	S1, S2
Flexor Digitorum Brevis	Flexion of the 2nd through 5th PIP joints Assists in flexion of the 2nd through 5th MTP joints	Medial calcaneal tuberosity Plantar fascia	Via four tendons, each having two slips, into the medial and lateral sides of the proximal 2nd through 5th phalanges	Medial plantar	L4, L5, S1

Flexor Hallucis Brevis	Flexion of 1st MTP joint	Medial side of the cuboid's plantar surface Slip from the tibialis posterior tendon	Via two tendons into the medial and lateral sides of the proximal phalanx of the first toe	Medial plantar	L4, L5, S1
Interossei, Dorsal	Abduction of the 3rd and 4th digits Assists in flexion of the MTP joints Assists in extension of the 3rd, 4th, and 5th IP joints	Via two heads to the contiguous sides of the metatarsals	Bases of proximal phalanges and associated dorsal extensor mechanism of medial second toe and the lateral 2nd, 3rd, and 4th toes.	Lateral plantar	S1, S2
Interossei, Plantar	Adduction of the 3rd, 4th, and 5th digits Assists in MTP joint flexion Assists in extension of the 3rd, 4th, and 5th IP joints	Base and medial aspect of the 3rd, 4th, and 5th metatarsals	Medial portion of the bases of the 3rd, 4th, and 5th proximal phalanges	Lateral plantar	S1, S2
Lumbricals	Flexion of the 2nd through 5th MTP joints Assists in extension of the 2nd through 5th IP joints	Tendons of flexor digitorum longus	Posterior surfaces of the 2nd through 5th toes via the flexor digitorum longus tendons	1st: Medial plantar 2nd to 5th: Lateral plantar	1st: L4, L5, S1 2nd to 5th: S1, S2
Quadratus Plantae	Modifies the flexor digitorum longus' angle of pull Assists in flexion of the 2nd through 5th MTP joints	Medial head Medial calcaneus Lateral head Lateral calcaneus	Dorsal and plantar surfaces of the flexor digitorum longus	Lateral plantar	S1, S2

IP = interphalangeal; MTP = metatarsophalangeal; PIP = proximal interphalangeal.

Table 8-4 Posterior Leg Muscles Acting on the Ankle, Foot, and Toes

Muscle	Action	Origin	Insertion	Innervation	Root
Flexor Digitorum Longus	Flexion of 2nd through 5th PIP and DIP joints Flexion of 2nd through 5th MTP joints Assists in ankle plantarflexion Assists in foot supination	Posterior medial portion of the distal two thirds of the tibia From fascia arising from the tibialis posterior	Plantar base of distal phalanges of the 2nd through 5th toes	Tibial	L5, S1
Flexor Hallucis Longus	Flexion of 1st IP joint Assists in flexion of 1st MTP joint Assists in foot supination Assists in ankle plantarflexion	Posterior distal two thirds of the fibula Associated interosseous membrane and muscle fascia	Plantar surface of the proximal phalanx of the 1st toe	Tibial	L4, L5, S1
Gastrocnemius	Ankle plantarflexion Assists in knee flexion	Medial head • Posterior surface of the medial femoral condyle • Adjacent portion of the femur and knee capsule Lateral head • Posterior surface of the lateral femoral condyle • Adjacent portion of the femur and knee capsule	To the calcaneus via the Achilles tendon	Tibial	S1, S2

Peroneus Brevis	Pronation of foot Assists in ankle plantarflexion	Distal two thirds of the lateral fibula	Styloid process at the base of the 5th metatarsal	Superficial peroneal	L4, L5, S1
Peroneus Longus	Pronation of foot Assists in ankle plantarflexion	Lateral tibial condyle Fibular head Upper two thirds of the lateral fibula	Lateral aspect of the base of the 1st metatarsal Lateral and dorsal aspect of the 1st cuneiform	Superficial peroneal	L4, L5, S1
Plantaris	Ankle plantarflexion Assists in knee flexion	Distal portion of the supracondylar line of the lateral femoral condyle Adjacent portion of the femoral popliteal surface Oblique popliteal ligament	To the calcaneus via the Achilles tendon	Tibial	L4, L5, S1
Soleus	Ankle plantarflexion	Posterior fibular head Upper one third of the fibula's posterior surface Soleal line located on the posterior tibial shaft Middle one third of the medial tibial border	To the calcaneus via the Achilles tendon	Tibial	S1, S2
Tibialis Posterior	Supination of the foot Assists in ankle plantarflexion	Length of the interosseous membrane Posterior, lateral tibia Upper two thirds of the medial fibula	Navicular tuberosity Via fibrous slips to the sustentaculum tali; cuneiforms; cuboid; and bases of the 2nd, 3rd, and 4th metatarsals	Tibial	L4, S1

DIP = distal interphalangeal; IP = interphalangeal; MTP = metatarsophalangeal; PIP = proximal interphalangeal.

Table 8-5 Anterior Leg Muscles Acting on the Ankle, Foot, Toes

Muscle	Action	Origin	Insertion	Innervation	Root
Extensor Digitorum Brevis	Extension of the 1st though 4th MTP joints Assists in extension of the 2nd, 3rd, and 4th PIP and DIP joints	Distal portion of the superior and lateral portion of the calcaneus Lateral talocalcaneal ligament Lateral portion of the inferior extensor retinaculum	To the dorsal surface of the base of the first phalanx (extensor hallucis brevis) Proximal phalanges of the 2nd, 3rd, and 4th toes and to the distal phalanges via an attachment to the extensor digitorum longus tendon	Deep peroneal	L5, S1
Extensor Digitorum Longus	Extension of the 2nd through 5th MTP joints Assists in extending 2nd through 5th PIP and DIP joints Assists in foot pronation Assists in ankle dorsiflexion	Lateral tibial condyle Proximal three fourths of anterior fibula Proximal portion of the interosseous membrane	Via four tendons to the distal phalanges of the 2nd through 5th toes	Deep peroneal	L4, L5, S1
Extensor Hallucis Longus	Extension of the 1st MTP joint Extension of the 1st IP joint Assists in ankle dorsiflexion	Middle two thirds of the anterior surface of the fibula Adjacent portion of the interosseous membrane	Base of the distal phalanx of the 1st toe	Deep peroneal	L4, L5, S1
Peroneus Tertius	Pronation of the foot Dorsiflexion of the ankle	Distal one third of the anterior surface of the fibula • Adjacent portion of the interosseous membrane	• Dorsal surface of the base of the 5th metatarsal	Deep peroneal	L4, L5, S1
Tibialis Anterior	Dorsiflexion of the ankle Supination of the foot	Lateral tibial condyle Upper one half of the tibia's lateral surface Adjacent portion of the interosseous membrane	Medial and plantar surface of the 1st cuneiform • Medial and plantar surfaces of the 1st metatarsal	Deep peroneal	L4, L5, S1

DIP = distal interphalangeal; IP = interphalangeal; MTP = metatarsophalangeal; PIP = proximal interphalangeal.

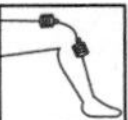

Stress Test 8-1
Valgus and Varus Stress Testing of the MTP and IP Joints

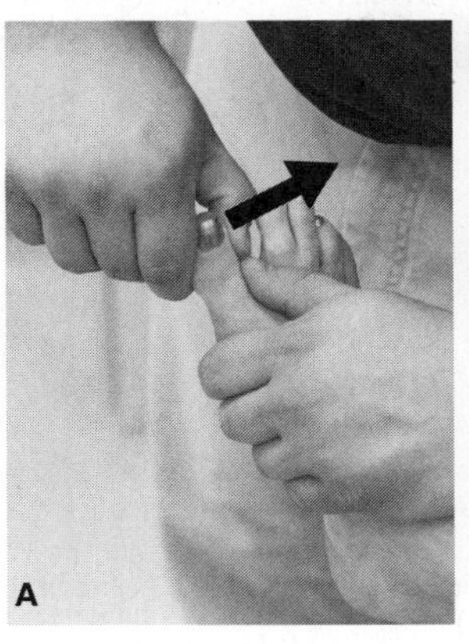

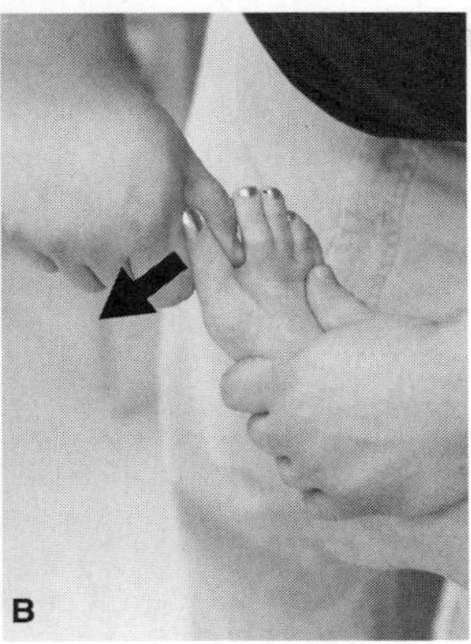

Stress testing of the toe's capsular ligaments: **(A)** Valgus stress applied to the interphalangeal joint; **(B)** varus stress applied to the metatarsophalangeal joint.

Patient Position	Supine or sitting
Position of Examiner	Standing The proximal bone stabilized close to the joint to be tested The bone distal to the joint being tested grasped near the middle of its shaft Care is necessary to isolate the joint being tested while not overlapping the test ligament.
Evaluative Procedure	***Valgus testing (A):*** The distal bone is moved laterally, attempting to open up the joint on the medial side. ***Varus testing (B):*** The distal bone is moved medially, attempting to open up the joint on the lateral side.
Positive Test	Pain or increased laxity or decreased laxity when compared with the same joint on the opposite extremity
Implications	***Valgus test (A):*** MCL sprain, avulsion fracture, or adhesions of the involved joint ***Varus test (B):*** LCL sprain, avulsion fracture, or adhesions of the involved joint
Comments	Increased joint laxity, especially with an empty end-feel, may reflect an associated fracture.
Evidence	Absent or inconclusive in the literature

IP = interphalangeal; LCL = lateral collateral ligament; MCL = medial collateral ligament; MTP = metatarsophalangeal.

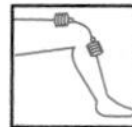

Joint Play 8-1
Intermetatarsal Glide Assessment

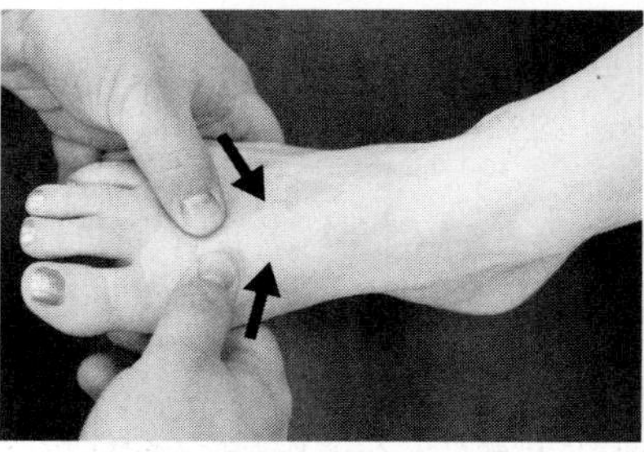

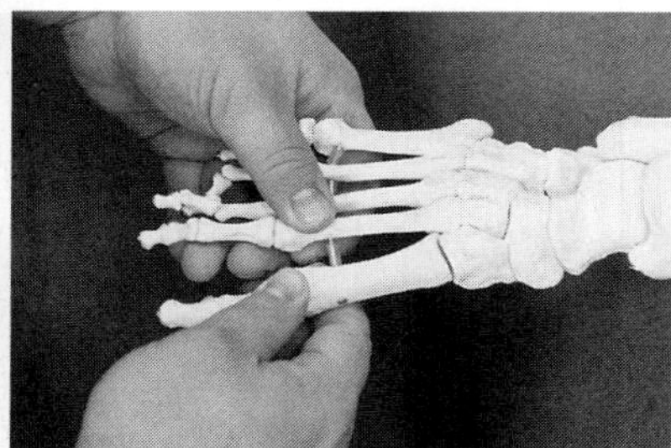

Assessment of the amount of intermetatarsal glide between the 1st and 2nd metatarsal heads. Perform this test for each of the four articulations formed between the five metatarsals.

Patient Position	Supine or sitting on the table with the knees extended
Position of Examiner	Standing in front of the patient's feet One hand grasping the first MT head; the other grasping the second MT head
Evaluative Procedure	Stabilize one of the MT heads while moving the other in a plantar and dorsal direction. This procedure is repeated by moving to the lateral MT heads until all four intermetarsal joints have been evaluated.
Positive Test	Pain or increased glide or decreased glide compared with the opposite extremity
Implications	Trauma to the deep transverse metatarsal ligament, interosseous ligament, or both Pain without the presence of laxity may indicate the presence of a neuroma
Evidence	Absent or inconclusive in the literature

MT = metatarsal.

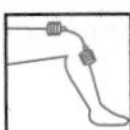

Joint Play 8-2
Tarsometatarsal Joint Play

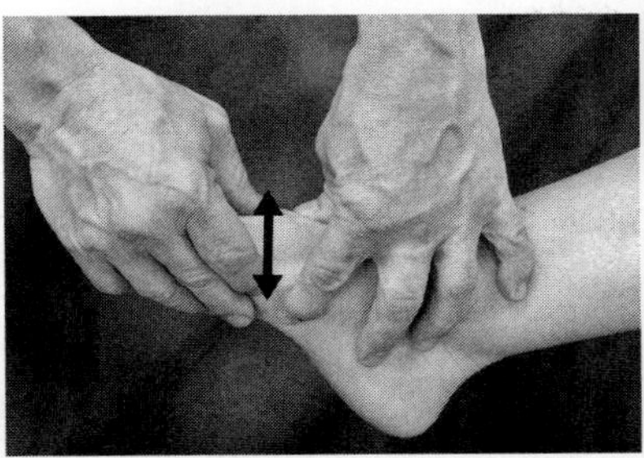

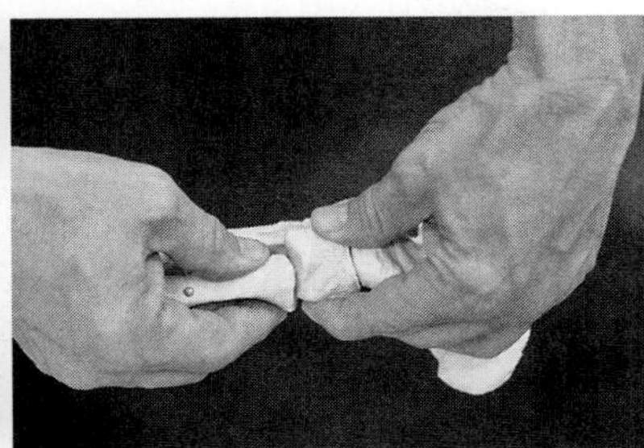

Assessment of the amount of glide between the tarsals and the base of the metatarsals. Perform this test on each of the five tarsometatarsal joints.

Patient Position	Supine or seated The foot is pronated. Knee flexed and the heel stabilized by the edge of the table
Position of Examiner	Standing or sitting in front of the patient's foot One hand grasping the proximal tarsal (e.g., cuneiform, cuboid) The opposite hand grasping the metatarsal being glided
Evaluative Procedure	The metatarsal is glided dorsally on the tarsal and then glided plantarly on the tarsal. Repeat for each joint.
Positive Test	Pain associated with movement Increased or decreased glide relative to the opposite foot
Implications	***Increased glide:*** Ligamentous laxity ***Decreased glide:*** Joint adhesions, articular change causing coalition of the joint
Modification	Wedges or balls may be needed to achieve sufficient proximal stabilization.
Evidence	Intra-rater reliability[32] Not Reliable — Very Reliable Poor / Moderate / Good 0 0.1 0.2 0.3 0.4 0.5 0.6 0.7 0.8 0.9 1.0

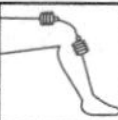

Joint Play 8-3
Midtarsal Joint Play

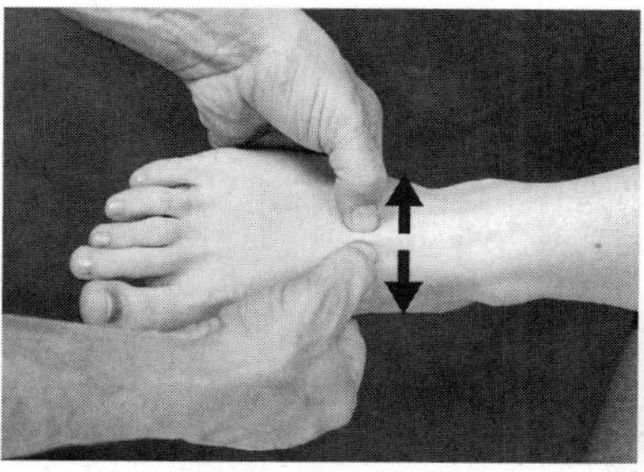

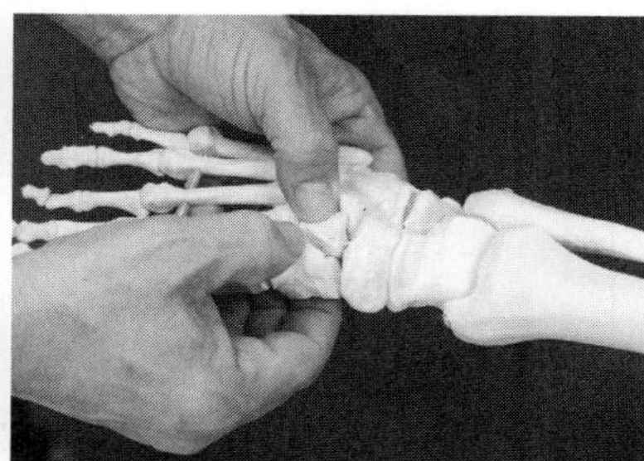

Assessment of the amount of joint glide between the tarsals

Patient Position	Supine or seated Knee flexed and the heel stabilized by the edge of the table
Position of Examiner	Standing or sitting in front of the patient's foot Grasp the plantar and dorsal aspect of one tarsal with the stabilizing hand. The opposite hand grasps the adjacent tarsal in a similar manner.
Evaluative Procedure	One tarsal is glided dorsally and then plantarly on the stabilized adjacent tarsal. Repeat for each tarsal joint.
Positive Test	Pain associated with movement Increased or decreased glide relative to the opposite foot
Implications	***Increased glide:*** Ligamentous laxity ***Decreased glide:*** Joint adhesions, articular changes causing coalition of the joint
Modification	Wedges or balls may be needed to achieve sufficient proximal stabilization.
Evidence	Absent or inconclusive in the literature

Special Test 8-1
Feiss Line

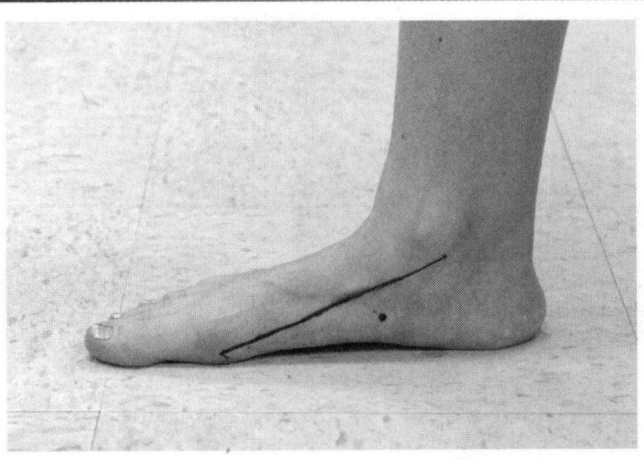

The Feiss line is used to assess static foot structure and provides a general assessment of foot type. With the patient in a weight-bearing position, a line is drawn from the plantar surface of the 1st MT head to the apex of the medial malleolus and the relative position of the navicular tubercle is noted.

Patient Position	Relaxed stance with the weight evenly distributed
Position of Examiner	Positioned at the patient's feet
Evaluative Procedure	Instruct the patient to stand with the feet shoulder-width apart and the weight evenly distributed. With the patient weight bearing, identify and mark the apex of the medial malleolus and the plantar aspect of the head of the 1st MT. Mark the position of the navicular tubercle and note its position relative to the line.
Positive Test	Tubercle above the line: Pes cavus Tubercle intersects the line: Normal Tubercle below the line: Pes planus
Implications	Cavus foot type has reduced shock-absorbing capacity. Planus foot type is often hypermobile.
Comments	The Feiss line can be assessed with the foot non–weight bearing.
Evidence	Absent or inconclusive in the literature.

MT = metatarsal.

Special Test 8-2
Assessment of Subtalar Joint Neutral

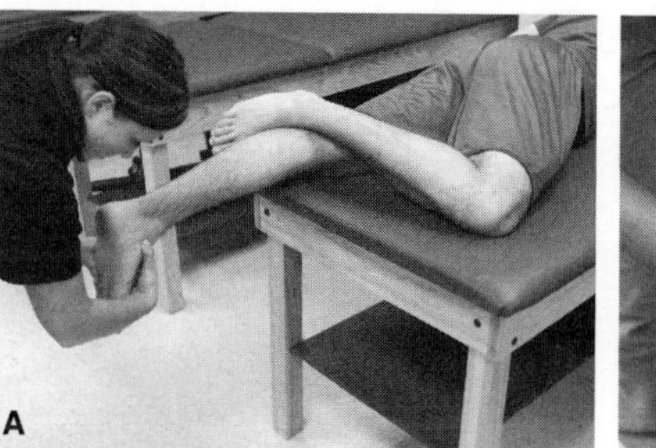

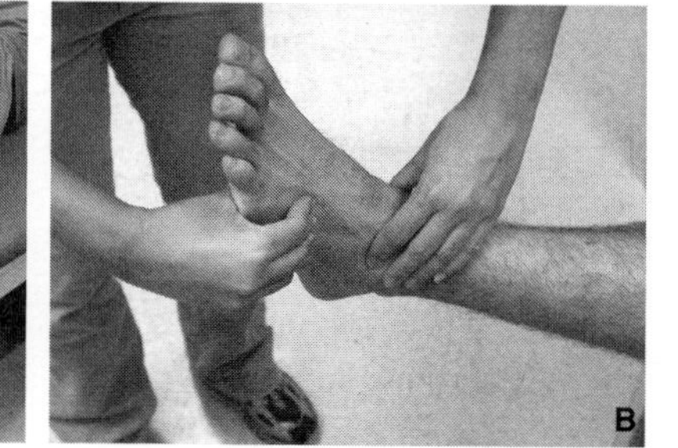

This technique positions the subtalar joint in neutral to allow standardized assessment of rearfoot and forefoot position. **(A)** Patient in the testing position. **(B)** Hand position for palpating the talus and manipulating the forefoot (patient shown supine for clarity).

Patient Position	Prone with foot off the end of the table. The nontest leg is positioned with the hip flexed, abducted, externally rotated, and the knee flexed (figure 4 position).
Position of Examiner	At the patient's feet The thumb and index finger at the anterior talocrural joint, palpating the medial and lateral aspects of talar head. The thumb and index finger of the distal hand grasp the heads of the 4th and 5th metatarsals, gently applying a dorsiflexion pressure until soft-tissue resistance is noted.[33]
Evaluative Procedure	The examiner passively supinates and pronates the foot using the distal hand while palpating talar position with the proximal hand. Neutral position is found when the talus is symmetrically aligned between the proximal thumb and forefinger. From this position, the postures of the forefoot and rearfoot are noted (see Inspection Findings 8-3). A goniometric measurement provides an objective assessment of calcaneal position with the STJ in neutral: • Align the fulcrum over the proximal calcaneus. • Position the proximal stationary arm bisecting the lower leg. • Position the distal movement arm bisecting the calcaneus.

Modification STJN can be assessed with the patient standing or sitting and the examiner kneeling in front of the patient. The assessment can also be performed with the patient in the supine position.

Comments Findings from a static foot posture assessment must be interpreted in conjunction with functional assessment.

Evidence

Non–weight bearing

Inter-rater reliability

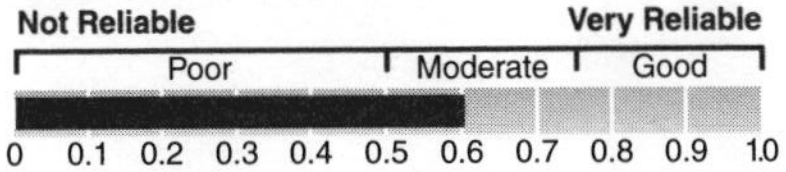

Not Reliable — Very Reliable
Poor | Moderate | Good
0 0.1 0.2 0.3 0.4 0.5 0.6 0.7 0.8 0.9 1.0

Intra-rater reliability

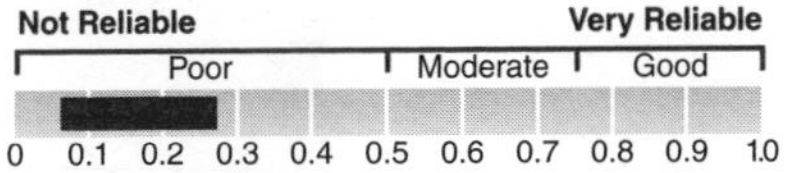

Not Reliable — Very Reliable
Poor | Moderate | Good
0 0.1 0.2 0.3 0.4 0.5 0.6 0.7 0.8 0.9 1.0

Weight bearing

Inter-rater reliability

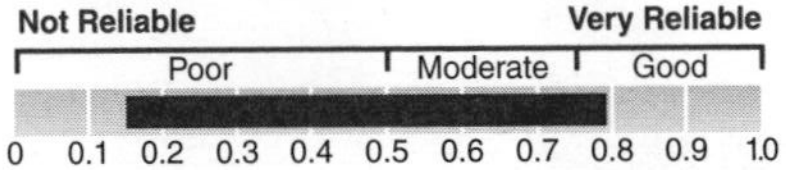

Not Reliable — Very Reliable
Poor | Moderate | Good
0 0.1 0.2 0.3 0.4 0.5 0.6 0.7 0.8 0.9 1.0

Intra-rater reliability

Not Reliable — Very Reliable
Poor | Moderate | Good
0 0.1 0.2 0.3 0.4 0.5 0.6 0.7 0.8 0.9 1.0

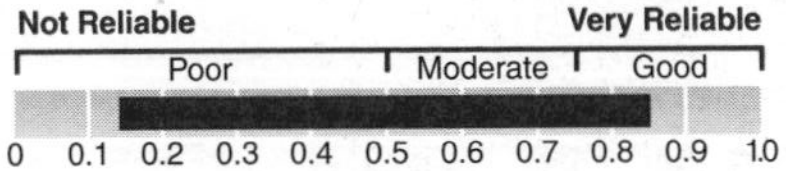

Special Test 8-3
Position and Mobility of First Tarsometatarsal Joint

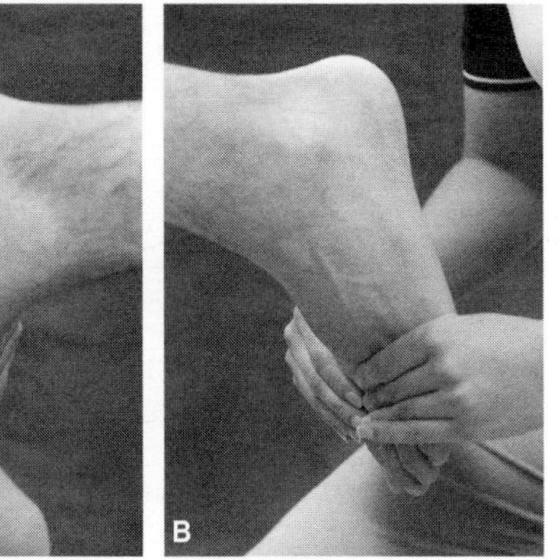

The static position and mobility of the first metatarsal can influence foot mechanics and should be assessed from a non–weight-bearing position with the subtalar joint in neutral. **(A)** Medial view. **(B)** Lateral view.

Patient Position	Prone with foot off the end of the table in subtalar joint neutral (see Special Test 8-2). The non-test leg is positioned with the hip flexed, abducted, and externally rotated and the knee flexed (figure 4 position).
Position of Examiner	Using a lumbrical grip on the lateral 4 metatarsal heads while grasping the first metatarsal head allows examination of the metatarsal position.

Evaluative Procedure	Note the resting position of the first metatarsal. Plantarflex and dorsiflex the first ray, noting the amount of mobility in each direction.
Positive Test	A rigid or stiff plantarflexed first ray cannot be brought into a neutral alignment, while a supple plantarflexed first ray has sufficient mobility to realign. A plantarflexed first ray is inferior as compared to the lateral four metatarsal heads.
Implications	A rigid plantarflexed first ray creates early supination, resulting in less shock absorption during gait. Stress fractures or sesamoid pathology may result. A hypermobile first ray may contribute to general metatarsal pain (metatarsalgia) and hallux valgus deformity.[34]
Modification	Use of a ruler for a quantitative assessment is also associated with poor inter-rater reliability (ICC = 0.05; SEM = 1.2 mm).[32]
Comments	A forefoot valgus alignment is easily confused with a plantarflexed first ray.
Evidence	Assessment of first ray mobility has poor inter-rater reliability ((κ)$\leq$ .16). The low relationship between results of the manual technique and a more reliable mechanical device indicates that the technique's validity is also suspect.[34] Mechanical measurement of dorsal first ray mobility has poor reliability (ICC = 0.05).[32]

Special Test 8-4
Navicular Drop Test

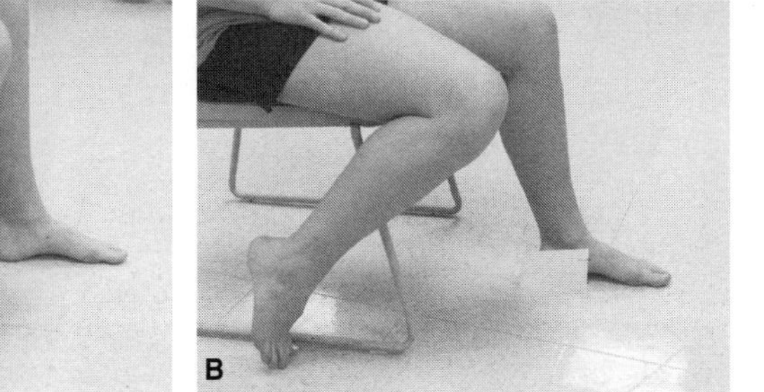

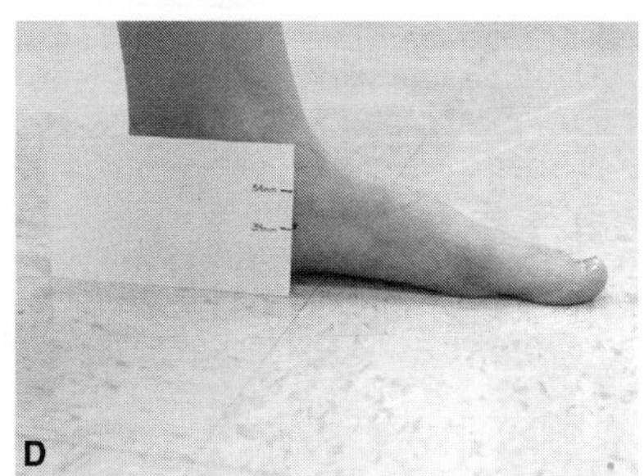

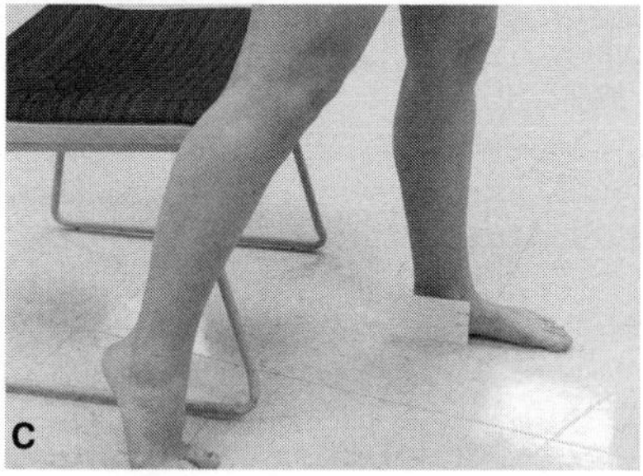

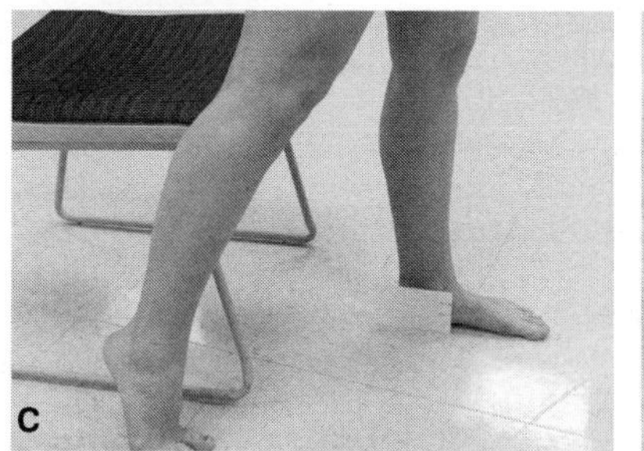

The navicular drop test is used to assess amount of pronation of the foot by measuring the height of the navicular tuberosity while the foot is non–weight bearing to weight bearing and measuring the distance of the inferior displacement. Note that the body weight should be evenly distributed between the two feet (non test leg above was moved for clarity).

Patient Position	Sitting with both feet on a noncarpeted floor
Position of Examiner	Kneeling in front of the patient

Evaluative Procedure	The subtalar joint is placed in the neutral position with the patient's foot flat against the ground, but non–weight bearing. With the patient non–weight bearing, a dot is placed over the navicular tuberosity **(A)**. While the foot is still in contact with the ground, but non–weight bearing, an index card is positioned next to the medial longitudinal arch. A mark is made on the card corresponding to the level of the navicular tuberosity **(B)**. The patient stands with the body weight evenly distributed between the two feet, and the foot is allowed to relax into pronation. The new level of the navicular tuberosity is identified and marked on the index card **(C)**. The relative displacement (drop) of the navicular is determined by measuring the distance between the two marks in millimeters **(D)**.
Positive Test	The navicular drops greater than 10 mm.[35] Normal values for restricted navicular drop have not been established.
Implications	Limited or excessive pronation
Comments	The relatively static measurement of navicular drop is associated with amount of pronation during gait.
Evidence	Highly variable intra-rater reliabilities (ICC = 0.61–0.96) have been reported and vary with the experience of the clinician.[31,36,37] Reported intra-rater reliabilities range from an ICC of 0.61[36] to 0.96.[31] The inter-rater reliability is poor (ICC = 0.57–0.73).[36,37] A strong relationship exists between excessive forefoot varus (>8°) and an increased navicular drop.[31] The low inter-rater reliability associated with the navicular drop test is related to the low reliability of assessing subtalar joint neutral. The height of the navicular in weight bearing (the second measurement of the navicular drop test) is highly correlated with radiographic measurements of navicular height in weight bearing.[38]

Special Test 8-5
Test for Supple Pes Planus Windlass Test

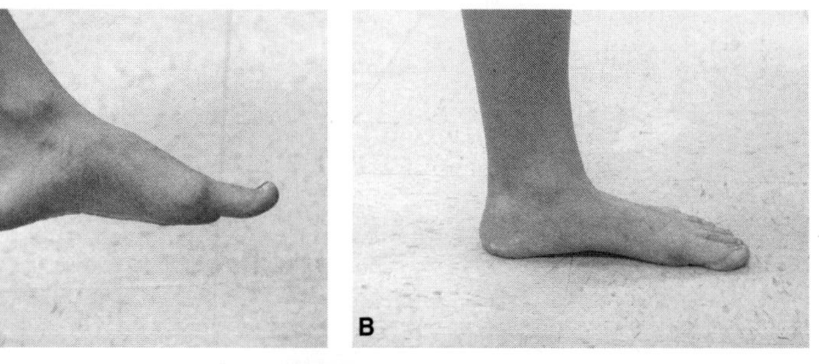

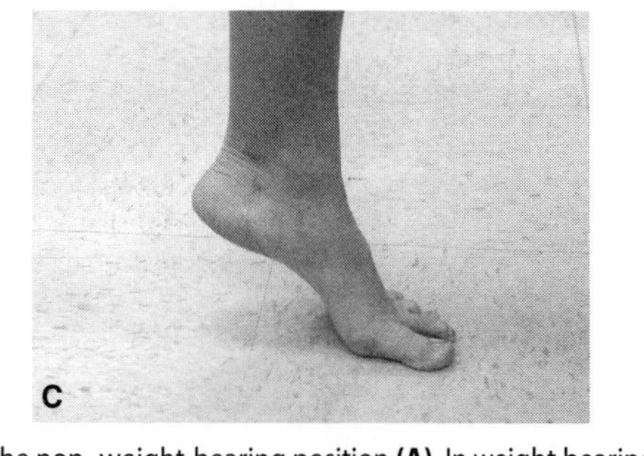

Supple pes planus. The patient displays a normal arch in the non–weight-bearing position **(A)**. In weight bearing, the arch disappears **(B)**. When the patient performs a toe raise, the arch returns by means of the windlass effect **(C)**. In the presence of plantar fasciitis **(C),** the **Windlass test** will produce pain.

Patient Position	Sitting on the edge of the examination table
Position of Examiner	Positioned at the patient's foot

Evaluative Procedure	With the patient in a non–weight-bearing position the examiner notes the presence of a medial longitudinal arch **(A)**. The examiner instructs the patient to stand so that the body weight is evenly distributed **(B)**. The patient is then asked to perform a single-leg heel raise on the limb being tested **(C)**. In the presence of supple pes planus note if the arch reappears as the patient performs a toe raise. For the **Windlass test** (used to identify plantar fasciitis), pain may be produced.
Positive Test	The presence of a medial longitudinal arch when non–weight bearing disappears when weight bearing The Windlass test is positive if pain is reproduced during part C.
Implications	If the medial longitudinal arch disappears when weight bearing, a supple pes planus is present. If no arch is present while in a non–weight-bearing position, a rigid pes planus is present. **Windlass test:** Pain during the single-leg heel raise
Comments	This test for supple pes planus is meaningful only when the medial longitudinal arch is present with the patient in a non–weight-bearing position.
Evidence	Negative likelihood ratio Not Useful — Useful Very Small · Small · Moderate · Large 1.0 0.9 0.8 0.7 0.6 0.5 0.4 0.3 0.2 0.1 0 The **windlass test** has a high specificity (1.00) but low sensitivity (0.24) indicate that a positive finding is highly related to presence of plantar fasciitis, yet a negative finding is less helpful in ruling out the condition.[39]

Special Test 8-6
Dorsiflexion–Eversion Test for Tarsal Tunnel Syndrome

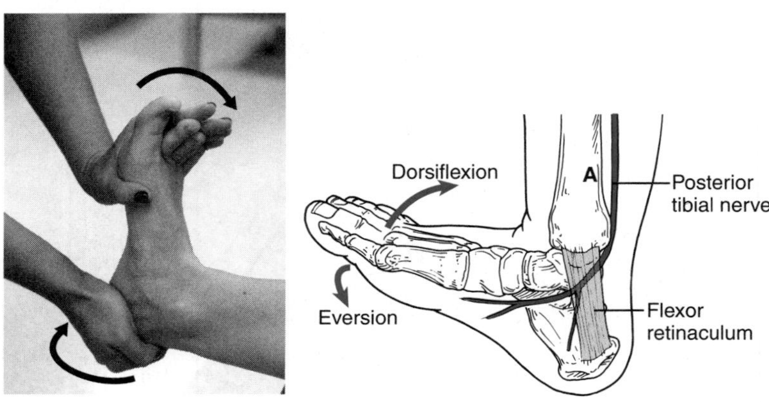

This test places tension on the posterior tibial nerve by replicating the mechanics of pes planus during gait.[40]

Patient Position	Sitting with the legs off the table
Position of Examiner	At the patient's feet
Evaluative Procedure	The examiner passively everts the heel (calcaneus and talus) while passively dorsiflexing the foot and toes. This position is held for 5 to 10 sec.
Positive Test	Provocation of pain and/or paresthesia radiating into the foot
Implications	Posterior tibial nerve dysfunction
Modification	The Tinel sign can be performed over the course of the nerve during this procedure.
Evidence	LR+ = unable to calculate; there is a high probability that the condition is present with a positive test result. LR–[40] Not Useful / Useful Very Small / Small / Moderate / Large 1.0 0.9 0.8 0.7 0.6 0.5 0.4 0.3 0.2 0.1 0

Special Test 8-7
Mulder Sign for Intermetatarsal Neuroma

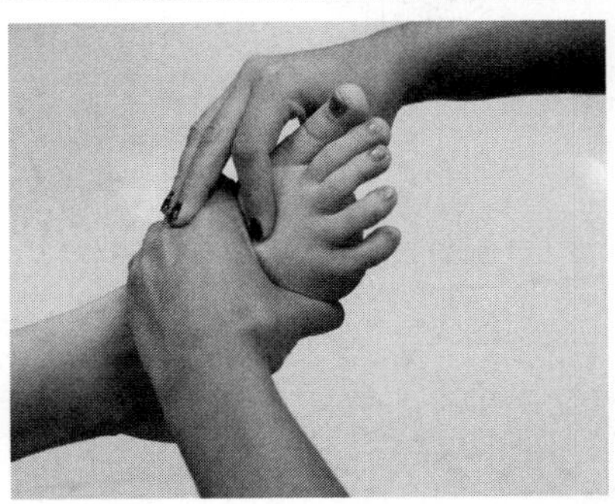

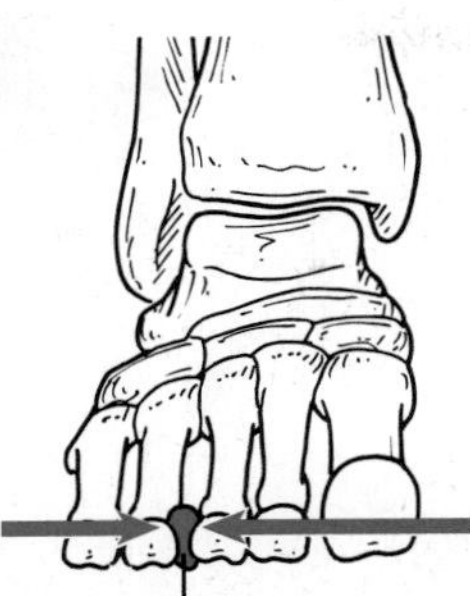

The Mulder sign involves manual compression of the transverse metatarsal arch with pressure applied over the interdigital nerve to reproduce the symptoms associated with an intermetatarsal neuroma.

Patient Position	Long or short sitting
Position of Examiner	Standing at the patient's feet
Evaluative Procedure	Position one hand along the distal fifth metatarsal and the opposite hand along the distal first metatarsal. Apply pressure to compress the transverse arch. Using the thumb and forefinger to apply pressure over the symptomatic interspace between the metatarsals.
Positive Test	A click, pain, and/or reproduction of symptoms
Implications	Intermetatarsal neuroma
Evidence	Absent or inconclusive in the literature

Intermetatarsal Neuroma

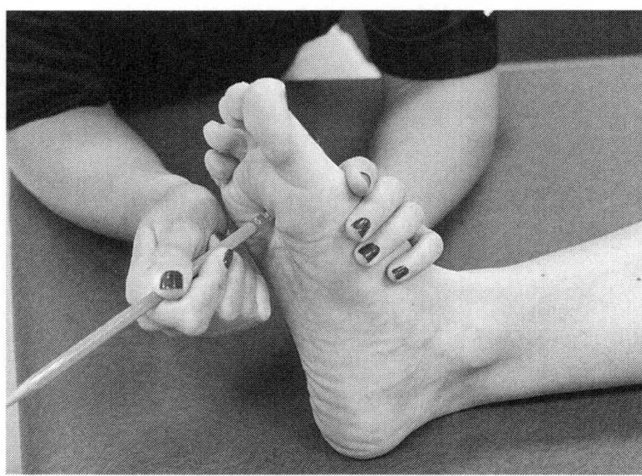

FIGURE 8-4 ■ Determining the presence of an intermetatarsal neuroma. A pencil eraser is used to apply pressure to the intermetatarsal space, compressing the nerve ending.

Long Bone Compression Test

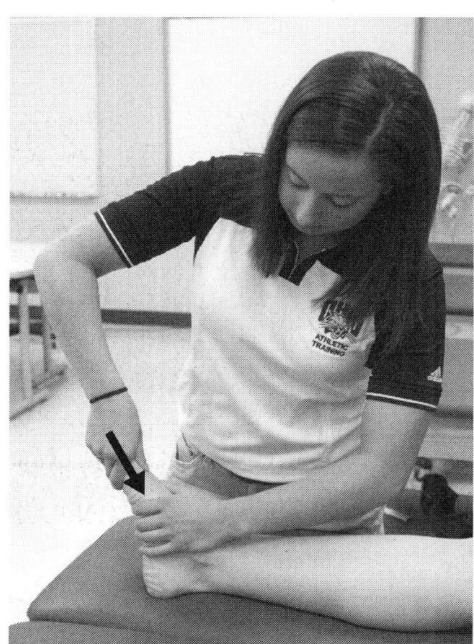

FIGURE 8-5 ■ Long bone compression test for suspected fractures of the metatarsals. A longitudinal force is placed along the shaft of the bone. In the presence of a fracture, compression of the two fragments results in pain and possibly the presence of a "false joint."

Neurologic Examination

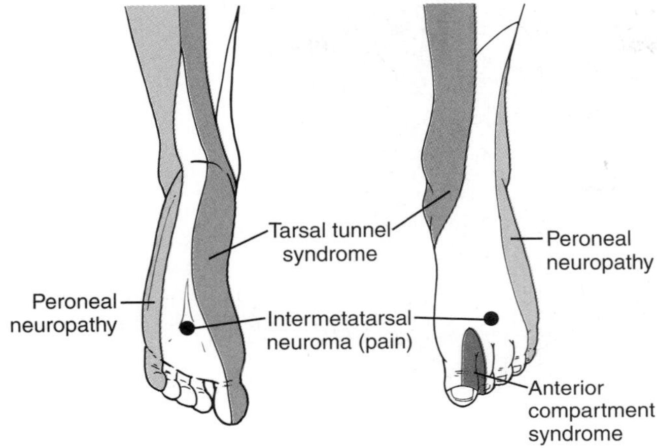

FIGURE 8-6 ■ Peripheral neurologic symptoms in the foot.

Tinel's Sign for Tarsal Tunnel Syndrome

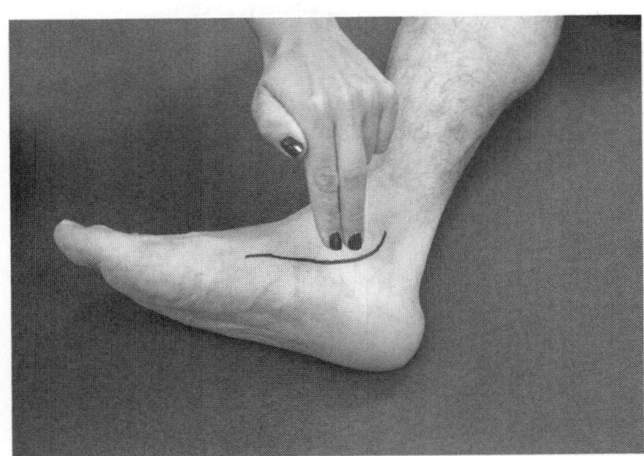

FIGURE 8-7 ■ Location of Tinel's sign for tarsal tunnel syndrome. Tapping over the path of the posterior tibial nerve causes radiating symptoms into the foot and toes.

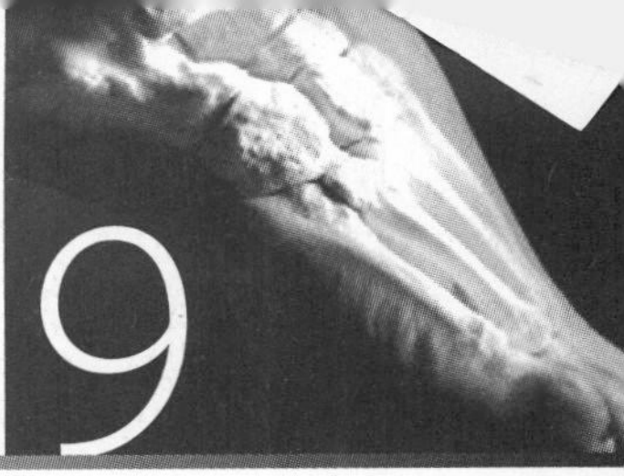

CHAPTER 9

Ankle and Leg Pathologies

Examination Map

HISTORY

Past Medical History

History of the Present Condition
Mechanism of injury

INSPECTION

Functional Observation

Inspection of the Lateral Structures
Peroneal muscle group
Distal one-third of fibula
Lateral malleolus

Inspection of the Anterior Structures
Sinus tarsi
Malleoli
Talus

Inspection of the Medial Structures
Medial malleolus
Medial longitudinal arch

Inspection of the Posterior Structures
Gastrocnemius/soleus
Achilles tendon
Bursae
Calcaneus

PALPATION

Palpation of the Fibular Structures
Common peroneal nerve
Peroneal muscle group
Fibular shaft
Anterior tibiofibular ligament
Posterior tibiofibular ligament
Interosseous membrane
Superior peroneal retinaculum

Palpation of the Lateral Ankle
Lateral malleolus
Calcaneofibular ligament
Anterior talofibular ligament
Posterior talofibular ligament
Inferior peroneal retinaculum
Peroneal tubercle
Cuboid
Base of fifth metatarsal
Peroneus tertius

Palpation of the Anterior Structures
Anterior tibial shaft
Tibialis anterior
Extensor hallucis longus
Dome of the talus
Extensor retinacula
Sinus tarsi

Palpation of the Medial Structures
Medial malleolus
Deltoid ligament
Sustentaculum tali
Spring ligament
Navicular
Navicular tuberosity
Tibialis anterior
Tibialis posterior
Flexor hallucis longus
Flexor digitorum longus

Palpation of the Posterior Structures
Gastrocnemius and soleus
Achilles tendon
Subcutaneous calcaneal bursa
Calcaneus
Subtendinous calcaneal bursa

Continued

Examination Map—cont'd

JOINT AND MUSCLE FUNCTION ASSESSMENT

Goniometry

Plantarflexion/dorsiflexion

Rearfoot inversion/eversion

Active Range of Motion

Plantarflexion

Dorsiflexion

Inversion

Eversion

Manual Muscle Tests

Dorsiflexion and supination

Eversion and pronation

Plantarflexion

Rearfoot inversion

Passive Range of Motion

Plantarflexion

Dorsiflexion

Inversion

Eversion

JOINT STABILITY TESTS

Stress Testing

Inversion stress test

Eversion stress test

Joint Play Assessment

Medial talar glide

Lateral talar glide (Cotton test)

Distal tibiofibular glide

NEUROLOGIC EXAMINATION

Lower Quarter Screen

Common peroneal nerve

Tibial nerve

VASCULAR EXAMINATION

Dorsalis pedis pulse

Posterior tibial pulse

Capillary refill

PATHOLOGIES AND SPECIAL TESTS

Ankle Sprains

Lateral ankle sprain

Distal tibiofibular syndesmosis

- Squeeze test

Medial ankle sprains

Ankle and Leg Fractures

Os trigonum injury

Achilles Tendon Pathology

Achilles tendon tendinopathy

Achilles tendon rupture

- Thompson test

Peroneal Tendon Pathology

Medial Tibial Stress Syndrome

Stress Fractures

- Bump test

Compartment Syndromes

Deep Vein Thrombosis

Table 9-1 **Possible Trauma Based on the Location of Pain**

	Location of Pain			
	Lateral	**Anterior**	**Medial**	**Posterior**
Soft Tissue	Lateral ankle ligament sprain	Extensor retinaculum sprain	Deltoid ligament	Triceps surae strain
	Syndesmosis sprain	Syndesmosis sprain	Capsular impingement	Achilles tendinopathy
	Capsular impingement	Tibialis anterior or long toe extensor strain	Tibialis posterior strain	Achilles tendon rupture
	Subluxating peroneal tendons	Tibialis anterior or long toe extensor tendinopathy	Tibialis posterior tendinopathy	Subtendinous calcaneal bursitis
	Peroneal muscle strain	Anterior compartment syndrome	Posterior tibial nerve compression (tarsal tunnel syndrome)	Subcutaneous calcaneal bursitis
	Peroneal tendinopathy	Interosseous membrane trauma		Deep vein thrombophlebitis
	Interosseous membrane trauma	Anterior tibiofibular ligament sprain		Posterior tibiofibular ligament sprain
	Peroneal nerve trauma			
Bony	Lateral ligament avulsion from malleolus, talus, and/or calcaneus	Tibial stress fracture	Medial ligament avulsion	Calcaneal fracture
		Frank tibial fracture		
	Lateral malleolus fracture	Talar fracture	Medial malleolus avulsion	Arthritis
	Fibular stress fracture	Talar osteochondritis	Medial malleolus fracture	Os trigonum trauma
	Frank fibular fracture			
	Fifth MT fracture	Arthritis	Arthritis	
	Peroneal tendon avulsion	Periostitis		
	Arthritis			

MT = metatarsal.

Table 9-2 Mechanism of Ankle Injury and the Resulting Tissue Damage

Uniplanar Motion	Tensile Forces	Compressive Forces
Inversion	Lateral structures: Anterior talofibular ligament, calcaneofibular ligament, posterior talofibular ligament, lateral capsule, and peroneal tendons; lateral malleolus fracture	Medial structures: Medial malleolus, deltoid ligament, and posterior tibial nerve, tibial artery, tibial vein.
Eversion	Medial structures: Deltoid ligament, tibialis posterior, and long toe flexors, posterior tibial nerve, tibial artery	Lateral structures: Lateral malleolus and lateral capsule
Plantarflexion	Anterior structures: Anterior capsule, long toe extensors, tibialis anterior, and extensor retinaculum Lateral structures: Anterior talofibular ligament	Posterior structures: Posterior capsule, subtendinous calcaneal bursa, subcutaneous calcaneal bursa, os trigonum, and talus fracture
Dorsiflexion	Posterior structures: Triceps surae, Achilles tendon, tibialis posterior, flexor hallucis longus, flexor digitorum longus Lateral structures: Posterior talofibular ligament, peroneal tendons	Anterior structures: Anterior capsule, syndesmosis, and extensor retinaculum, anterior talus

Pain Zones

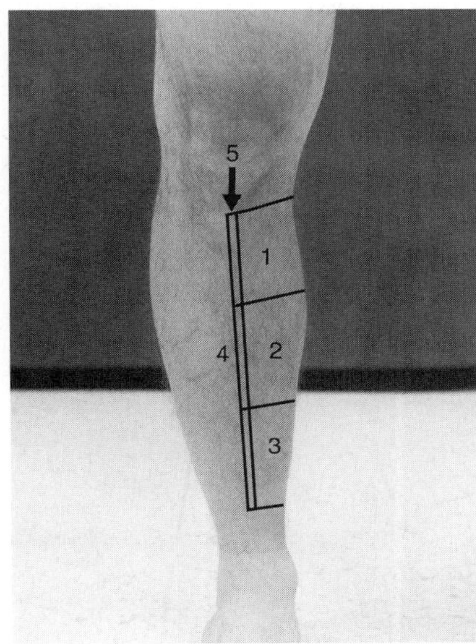

FIGURE 9-1 ■ Pain zones and anatomic correlations. *1,* Flexor digitorum longus; *2,* flexor hallucis longus; *3,* tibialis posterior; *4,* tibial crest; *5,* tibial tuberosity.

Achilles Tendon Rupture

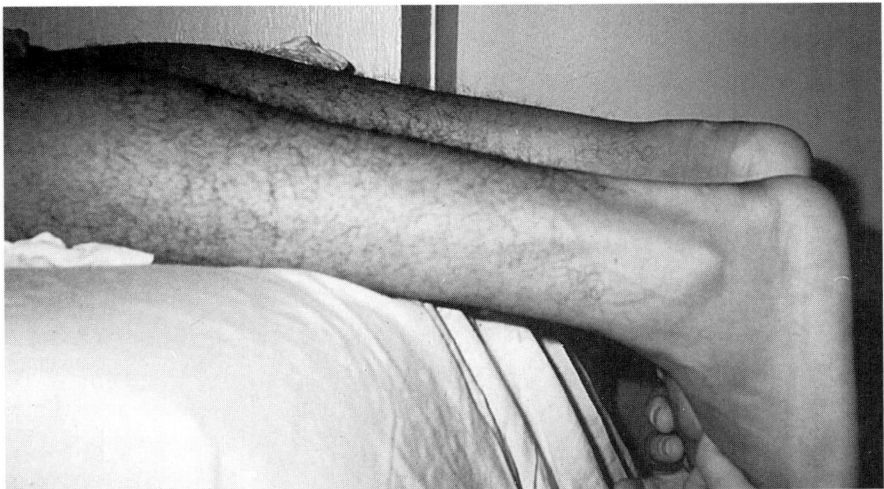

FIGURE 9-2 ■ Ruptured Achilles tendon. The patient's right (far) Achilles tendon has been ruptured. Note the depression proximal to the calcaneus and the involved swelling.

Subluxating/Dislocating Peroneal Tendons

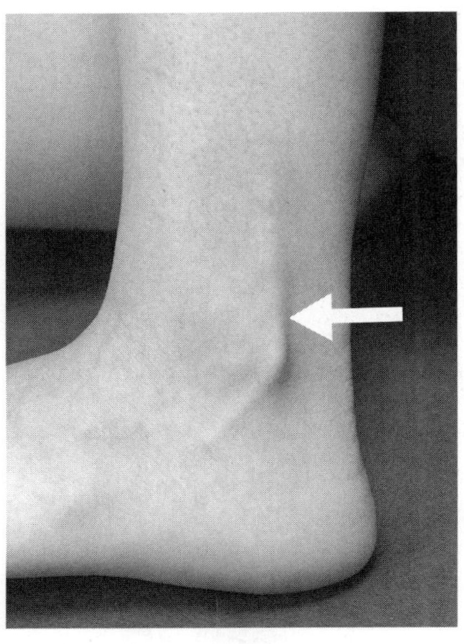

FIGURE 9-3 ■ Observable peroneal dislocation. In some instances the peroneal tendon can be observed as it subluxates from the fibular groove.

Ankle Dislocation

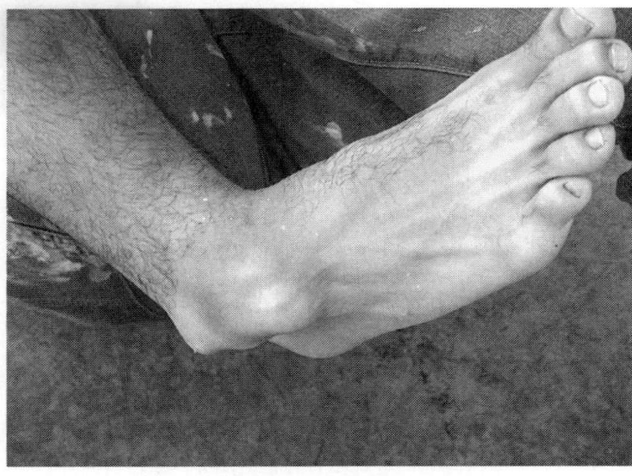

FIGURE 9-4 ■ Ankle fracture–dislocation. Note the irregular contour beneath the lateral malleolus.

PALPATION

Palpation of the Fibular Structures

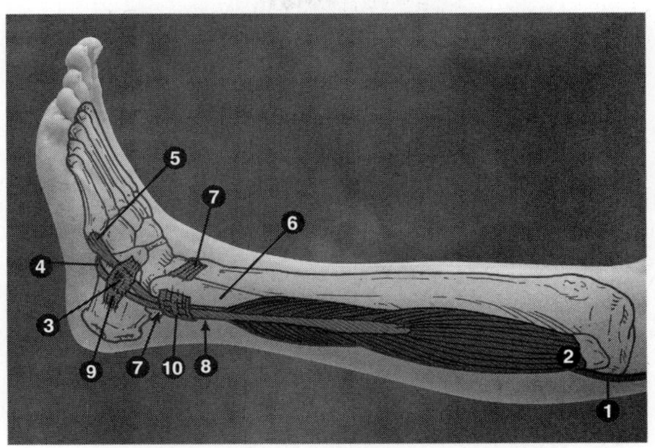

1 Common peroneal nerve

2 Peroneal muscle group

3 Peroneal tubercle

4 Peroneus longus tendon

5 Peroneus brevis tendon

6 Fibular shaft

7 Anterior and posterior tibiofibular ligaments

8 Interosseous membrane

9 Inferior peroneal retinaculum

10 Superior peroneal retinaculum

Palpation of the Lateral Ankle

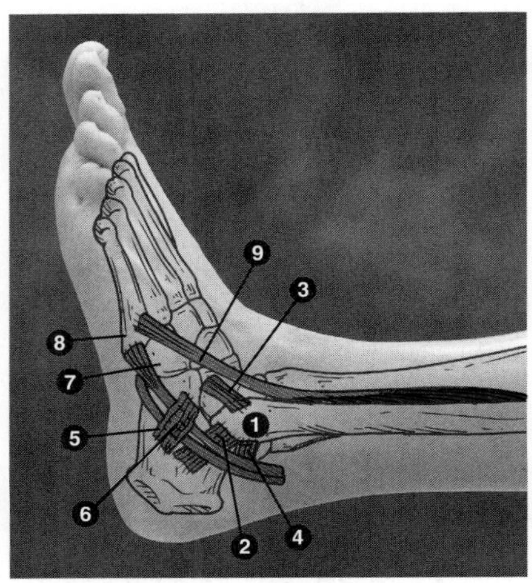

1 Lateral malleolus

2 Calcaneofibular ligament

3 Anterior talofibular ligament

4 Posterior talofibular ligament

5 Inferior peroneal retinaculum

6 Peroneal tubercle

7 Cuboid

8 Base of the fifth metatarsal

9 Peroneus tertius

Palpation of the Anterior Structures

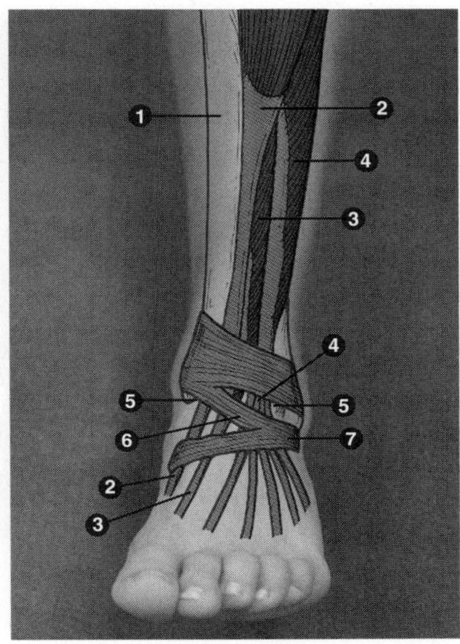

1 Anterior tibial shaft

2 Tibialis anterior

3 Extensor hallucis longus

4 Extensor digitorum longus

5 Dome of the talus

6 Inferior extensor retinaculum

7 Sinus tarsi

Palpation of the Medial Structures

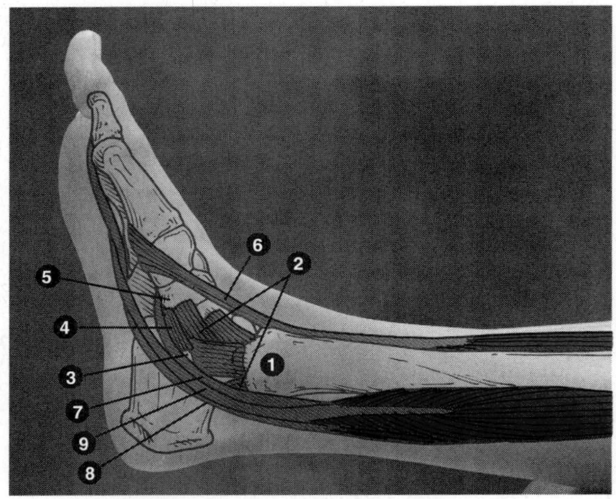

1 Medial malleolus

2 Deltoid ligament

3 Sustentaculum tali

4 Spring ligament

5 Navicular and navicular tuberosity

6 Tibialis anterior

7 Tibialis posterior

8 Flexor hallucis longus

9 Flexor digitorum longus

Palpation of the Posterior Structures

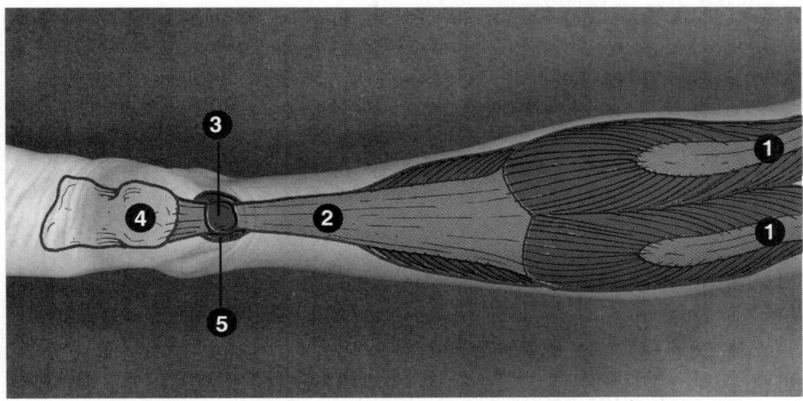

1. Gastrocnemius–soleus complex
2. Achilles tendon
3. Subcutaneous calcaneal bursa
4. Calcaneus
5. Subtendinous calcaneal bursa

Box 9-1
Modified Ottawa Ankle Rules

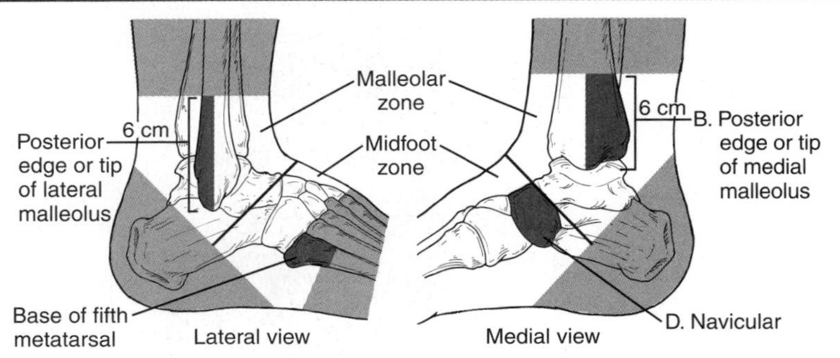

Description

The Ottawa Ankle Rules provide evaluative criteria to identify when the patient should be referred for radiographs.

Criteria for Radiographic Referral

The patient's inability to walk four steps both immediately following the injury and at the time of examination.

Ankle radiographs should be ordered if pain is elicited during palpation of Zone A or B.

Foot radiographs should be ordered if pain is elicited during palpation of Zone C or D.

Modification

Zones A and B are changed to include pain over the midline of the medial and lateral malleoli.[41,42]

Evidence

Designed to have a high sensitivity so that fractures are not missed, the Ottawa Ankle Rules have a high negative predictive value when applied to a skeletally mature population. If the rules are followed, it is highly likely that a fracture will not be missed.[43,44] The conservative nature of the rules results in a relatively low specificity (0.26–0.48), indicating that many patients are still referred for radiographs who do not have a fracture. With the modification relating to the location of the malleolar pain, the specificity is improved to 0.42–0.59.[41,42]

Table 9-3 Talocrural Joint Capsular Patterns and End-Feels

Capsular Pattern **Talocrural Joint: plantarflexion, dorsiflexion**	
Plantarflexion of the talocrural joint	Firm – soft tissue stretch
Dorsiflexion of the talocrural joint	Firm – soft tissue stretch
Capsular Pattern **Subtalar Joint: supination, pronation**	
Inversion of the subtalar joint	Firm – soft tissue stretch
Eversion of the subtalar joint	Firm – soft tissue stretch

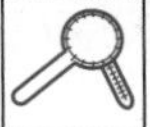

Goniometry Box 9-1
Ankle Plantarflexion/Dorsiflexion

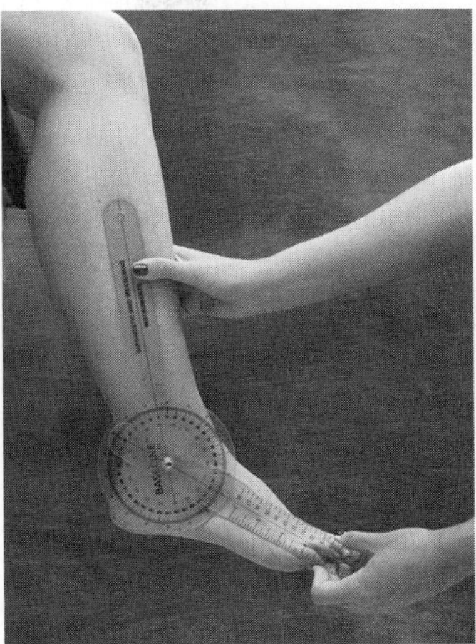

Dorsiflexion 0°–20° Plantarflexion 0°–50°

Patient Position	Sitting with the knee flexed to 90°, the ankle in anatomical position, and the foot in 0° of inversion and eversion
Goniometer Alignment	
Fulcrum	The axis is centered over the lateral malleolus.
Proximal Arm	The stationary arm is aligned with the long axis of the fibula.
Distal Arm	The movement arm is aligned parallel with the bottom of the foot.
Modification	Dorsiflexion may be measured with the patient prone and the knee flexed to 90°.
Comment	Avoid extending the toes or twisting the foot. Measuring dorsiflexion with the knee extended assesses for limitation in dorsiflexion secondary to gastrocnemius tightness, which may be clinically useful. Measurements are relative to the ankle at 90° (anatomical position).

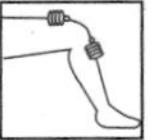

Manual Muscle Test 9-1
Dorsiflexion and Supination

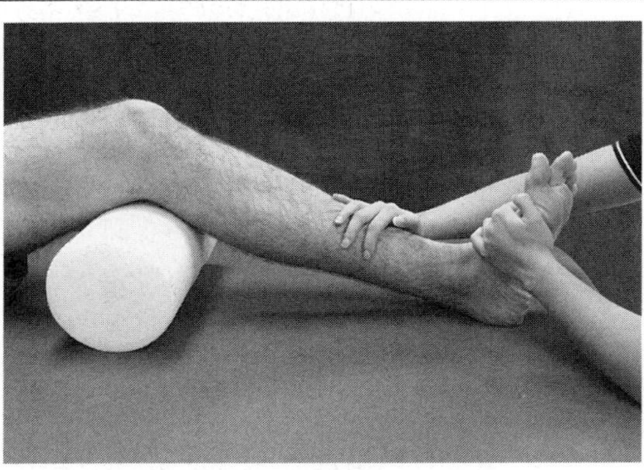

Patient Position	Seated
Starting Position	The knee is flexed. The foot is positioned in plantarflexion and eversion.
Stabilization	Distal tibia, preventing knee extension and femoral external rotation
Palpation	Muscle belly of anterior tibialis or its tendon (the most medial tendon on the anterior aspect of the talocrural joint)
Resistance	Medial aspect of the dorsum of the foot
Primary Mover(s) (Innervation)	Tibialis anterior (L4, L5, S1)
Secondary Mover(s) (Innervation)	Extensor hallucis longus (L4, L5, S1) Extensor digitorum longus (L4, L5, S1) Peroneus tertius (negligible contribution) (L4, L5, S1)
Substitution	Knee extension Toe extension
Comment	Ensure that the toes are relaxed to reduce the contribution of extensor hallucis longus and extensor digitorum longus.

Isolating the Soleus

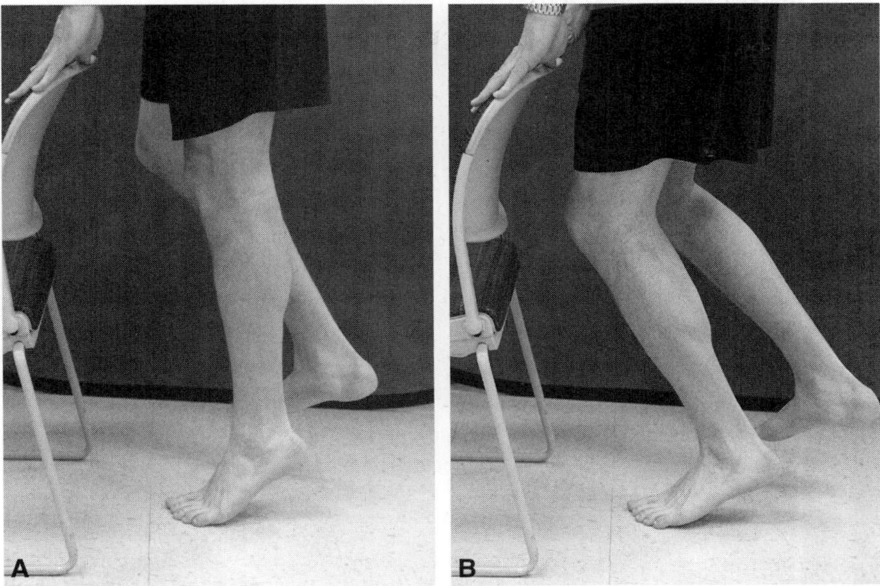

FIGURE 9-5 ■ Heel-raise test for plantarflexion. **(A)** With the knee extended to include the gastrocnemius. **(B)** With the knee flexed to isolate the soleus muscle.

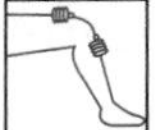

Manual Muscle Test 9-2
Eversion and Pronation

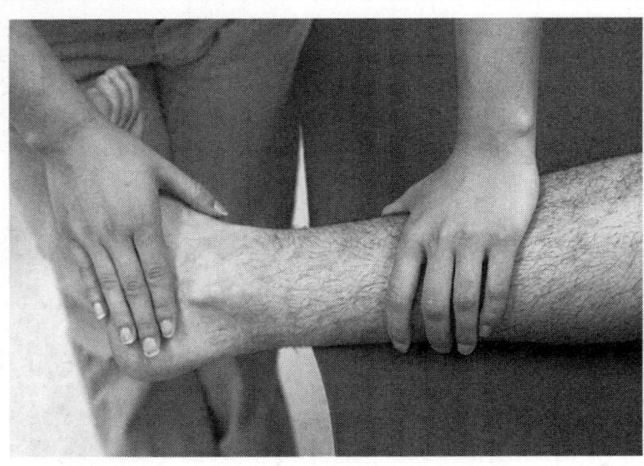

Patient Position	Side-lying on the side opposite the limb being tested The opposite hip is flexed
Starting Position	The test foot is off the end of the table in slight plantarflexion.
Stabilization	Lower leg
Palpation	Posterior aspect of the lateral malleolus; proximal portion of the fibula
Resistance	Lateral border of the foot
Primary Mover(s) (Innervation)	Peroneus longus (L4, L5, S1) Peroneus brevis (L4, L5, S1)
Secondary Mover(s) (Innervation)	Extensor digitorum longus (L4, L5, S1)
Substitution	Plantarflexors Toe extension
Comment	Avoid toe extension to decrease the contribution of the extensor digitorum longus.

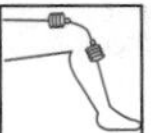

Manual Muscle Test 9-3
Plantarflexors

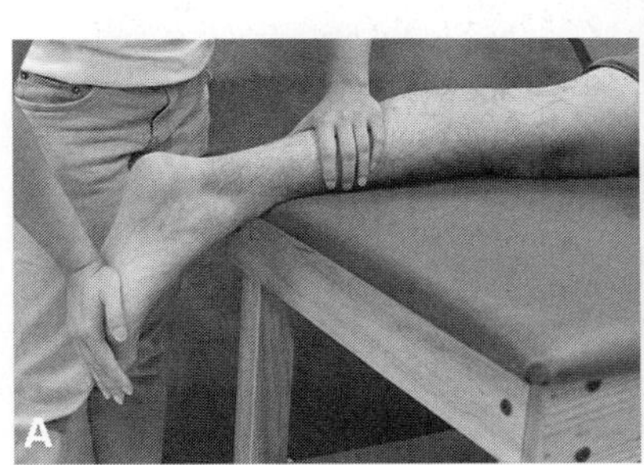

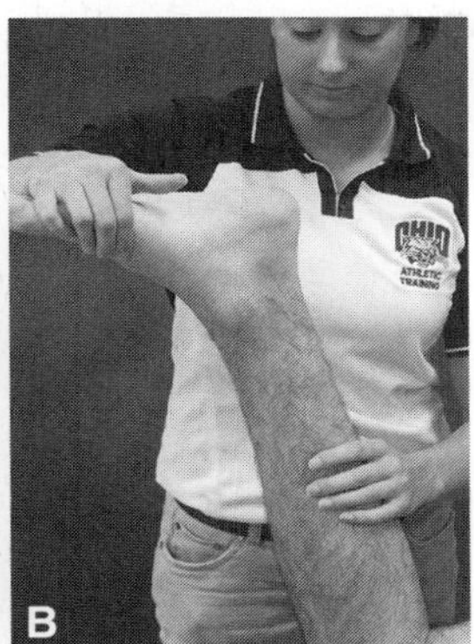

Patient Position	Prone
Starting Position	*Gastrocnemius:* **(A)** The knee is extended with the foot off the table *Soleus*: **(B)** The knee is flexed past 30°
Stabilization	Proximal to the ankle
Palpation	*Gastrocnemius:* Posterior leg just distal to the knee joint line. *Soleus*: Midleg anterior to the gastrocnemius
Resistance	Plantar aspect of the rear- and midfoot
Primary Mover(s) (Innervation)	Gastrocnemius (S1, S2) Soleus (S1, S2)
Secondary Mover(s) (Innervation)	Flexor digitorum longus (L5, S1) Flexor hallucis longus (L4, L5, S1) Tibialis posterior (L4, L5, S1)
Substitution	Hamstrings: Avoid knee flexion
Comment	Avoid toe flexion to reduce the contribution of flexor hallucis longus and flexor digitorum longus. Avoid inversion to reduce the contribution of tibialis posterior. Because the plantarflexors are a strong muscle group, single-leg heel raises may provide a better indicator of strength.

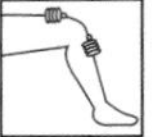

Manual Muscle Test 9-4
Rearfoot Inversion

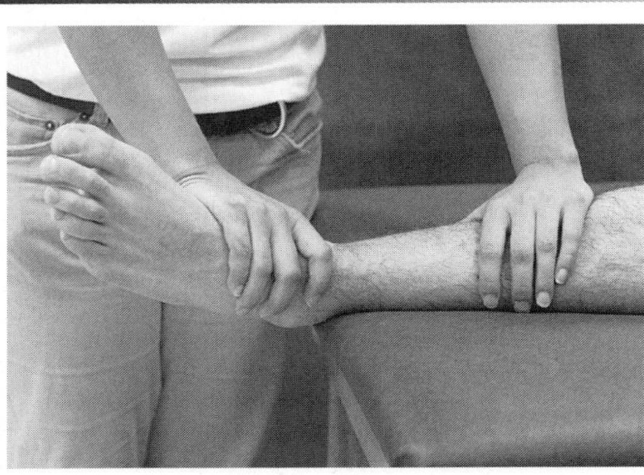

Patient Position	Side-lying on the side opposite being tested The opposite hip is flexed.
Starting Position	The test foot is off the end of the table with the ankle in the resting position.
Stabilization	Medial aspect of the distal leg
Palpation	Posterior margin of the medial malleolus
Resistance	Medial border of the foot (navicular, medial cuneiform)
Primary Mover(s) (Innervation)	Tibialis posterior (L4, L5, S1)
Secondary Mover(s) (Innervation)	Flexor digitorum longus (L5, S1) Flexor hallucis longus (L4, L5, S1)
Substitution	Plantarflexors Toe flexors
Comment	Avoid toe flexion to reduce the contribution of flexor hallucis longus and flexor digitorum longus.

Table 9-4 Muscles Acting on the Foot and Ankle

Muscle	Action	Origin	Insertion	Nerve	Root
Extensor Digitorum Longus	Extension of the 2nd through 5th MTP joints Assists in extending the 2nd through 5th PIP and DIP joints Assists in STJ and midtarsal pronation* Assists in ankle dorsiflexion	Lateral tibial condyle Proximal three-fourths of anterior fibula Proximal portion of the interosseous membrane	Via four tendons to the distal phalanges of the 2nd through 5th toes	Deep peroneal	L4, L5, S1
Extensor Hallucis Longus	Extension of the 1st MTP joint Extension of the 1st IP joint Assists with dorsiflexion Assists with supination**	Middle two-thirds of the anterior surface of the fibula Adjacent portion of the interosseous membrane	Base of the distal phalanx of the 1st toe	Deep peroneal	L4, L5, S1
Flexor Digitorum Longus	Flexion of the 2nd through 5th PIP and DIP joints Flexion of the 2nd through 5th MTP joints Assists in ankle plantarflexion Assists in STJ and midtarsal supination**	Posterior medial portion of the distal two-thirds of the tibia From fascia arising from the tibialis posterior	Plantar base of distal phalanges of the 2nd through 5th toes	Tibial	L5, S1
Flexor Hallucis Longus	Flexion of the 1st IP joint Assists in 1st MTP joint flexion Assists in STJ and midtarsal supination** Assists in ankle plantarflexion	Posterior distal two thirds of the fibula Associated interosseous membrane and muscular fascia	Plantar surface of the proximal phalanx of the 1st toe	Tibial	L4, L5, S1

Continued

Table 9-4 Muscles Acting on the Foot and Ankle—cont'd

Muscle	Action	Origin	Insertion	Nerve	Root
Gastrocnemius	Ankle plantarflexion Assists in knee flexion	Medial head • Posterior surface of the medial femoral condyle • Adjacent portion of the femur and knee capsule Lateral head • Posterior surface of the lateral femoral condyle • Adjacent portion of the femur and knee capsule	To the calcaneus via the Achilles tendon	Tibial	S1, S2
Peroneus Brevis	STJ and midtarsal pronation* Assists in ankle plantarflexion	Distal two-thirds of the lateral fibula	Styloid process at the base of the 5th metatarsal	Superficial peroneal	L4, L5, S1
Peroneus Longus	STJ and midtarsal pronation* Assists in ankle plantarflexion	Lateral tibial condyle Fibular head Upper two thirds of the lateral fibula	Lateral aspect of the head of the 1st metatarsal Lateral and dorsal aspect of the 1st cuneiform	Superficial peroneal	L4, L5, S1
Peroneus Tertius	STJ and midtarsal pronation* Assists in ankle dorsiflexion	Distal one third of the anterior surface of the fibula Adjacent portion of the interosseous membrane	Dorsal surface of the base of the 5th metatarsal	Deep peroneal	L4, L5, S1
Plantaris	Ankle plantarflexion Assists in knee flexion	Distal portion of the supracondylar line of the lateral femoral condyle Adjacent portion of the femoral popliteal surface Oblique popliteal ligament	To the calcaneus via the Achilles tendon	Tibial	L4, L5, S1

Soleus	Ankle plantarflexion	Posterior fibular head Upper one-third of the fibula's posterior surface Soleal line located on the posterior tibial shaft Middle one-third of the medial tibial border	To the calcaneus via the Achilles tendon	Tibial	S1, S2
Tibialis Anterior	Ankle dorsiflexion STJ and midtarsal supination**	Lateral tibial condyle Upper one-half of the tibia's lateral surface Adjacent portion of the interosseous membrane	Medial and plantar surfaces of the 1st cuneiform Medial and plantar surfaces of the 1st metatarsal	Deep peroneal	L4, L5, S1
Tibialis Posterior	Assists in ankle plantarflexion STJ and midtarsal supination**	Length of the interosseous membrane Posterior, lateral tibia Upper two-thirds of the medial fibula	Navicular tuberosity Via fibrous slips to the sustentaculum tali, cuneiforms, cuboid, and bases of the 2nd, 3rd, and 4th metatarsals	Tibial	L4, L5, S1

DIP = distal interphalangeal; IP = interphalangeal; MTP = metatarsophalangeal; PIP = proximal interphalangeal; STJ = subtalar joint.

*Calcaneal eversion.
**Calcaneal inversion.

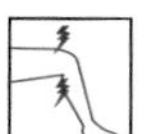

Stress Test 9-1
Anterior Drawer Test

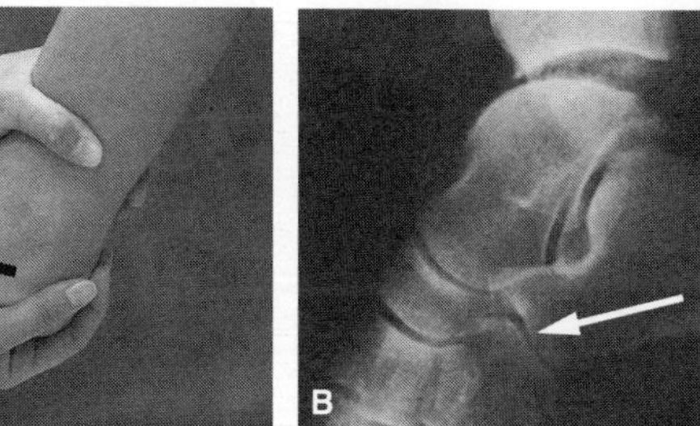

(A) Anterior drawer test to assess the integrity of the anterior talofibular ligament. **(B)** Radiographic view of a positive anterior drawer test. Note the anterior displacement of the talus relative to the tibia. (**B** Courtesy of Donatelli, RA: *Biomechanics of the Foot and Ankle*. Philadelphia: FA Davis, 1990.)

Patient Position	Sitting over the edge of the table with the knee flexed to prevent gastrocnemius tightness from influencing the outcome of the test
Position of Examiner	Sitting in front of the patient One hand stabilizes the leg, taking care not to occlude the mortise. The other hand cups the calcaneus while the forearm supports the foot in a position of slight plantarflexion (10°–20° from the anatomical position).[45,46]
Evaluative Procedure	The calcaneus and talus are drawn forward while providing a stabilizing force to the tibia.
Positive Test	The talus slides anteriorly from under the ankle mortise compared with the opposite side (assuming it is normal). There may be an appreciable "clunk" as the talus subluxates and relocates, or the patient may describe pain.
Implications	Sprain of the anterior talofibular ligament and the associated capsule

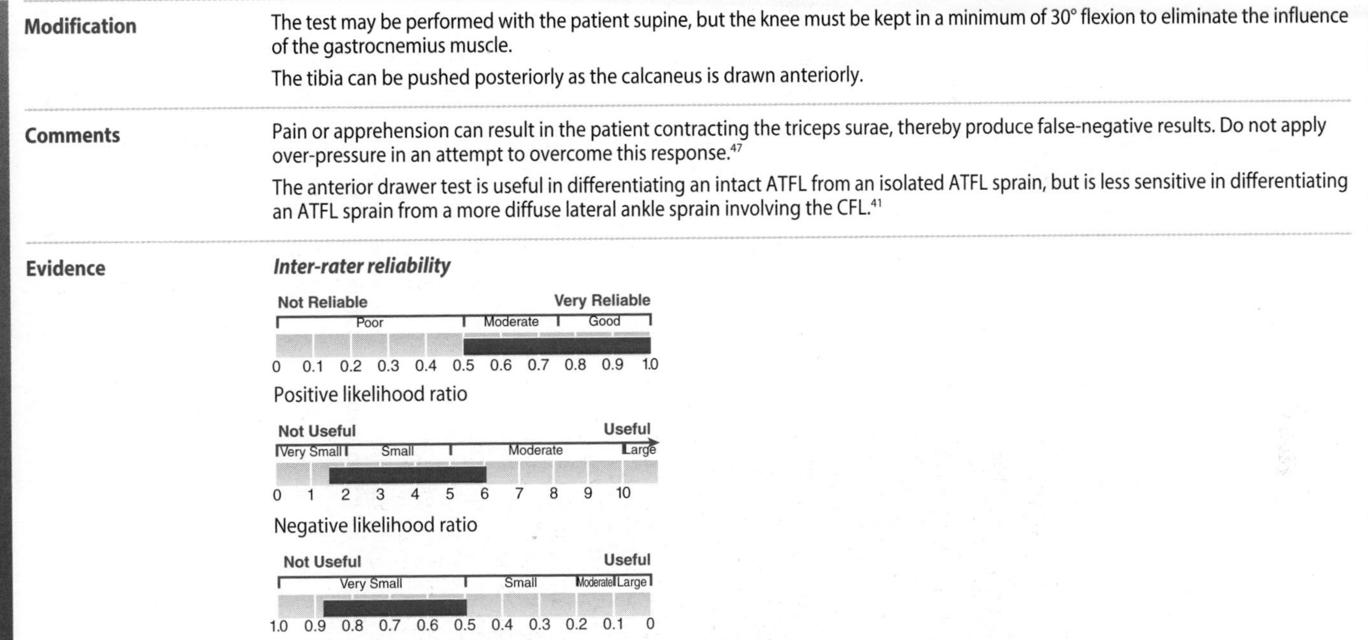

Modification	The test may be performed with the patient supine, but the knee must be kept in a minimum of 30° flexion to eliminate the influence of the gastrocnemius muscle. The tibia can be pushed posteriorly as the calcaneus is drawn anteriorly.
Comments	Pain or apprehension can result in the patient contracting the triceps surae, thereby produce false-negative results. Do not apply over-pressure in an attempt to overcome this response.[47] The anterior drawer test is useful in differentiating an intact ATFL from an isolated ATFL sprain, but is less sensitive in differentiating an ATFL sprain from a more diffuse lateral ankle sprain involving the CFL.[41]
Evidence	***Inter-rater reliability*** Not Reliable / Very Reliable Poor / Moderate / Good 0 0.1 0.2 0.3 0.4 0.5 0.6 0.7 0.8 0.9 1.0 Positive likelihood ratio Not Useful / Useful Very Small / Small / Moderate / Large 0 1 2 3 4 5 6 7 8 9 10 Negative likelihood ratio Not Useful / Useful Very Small / Small / Moderate / Large 1.0 0.9 0.8 0.7 0.6 0.5 0.4 0.3 0.2 0.1 0

ATFL = anterior talofibular ligament; CFL = calcaneofibular ligament.

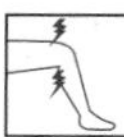

Stress Test 9-2
Inversion (Talar Tilt) Stress Test

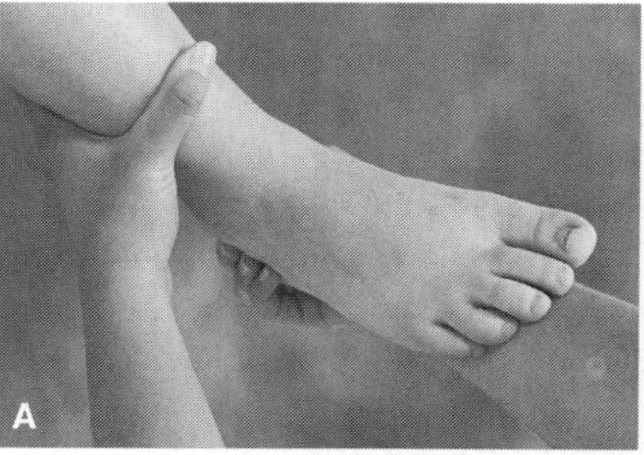

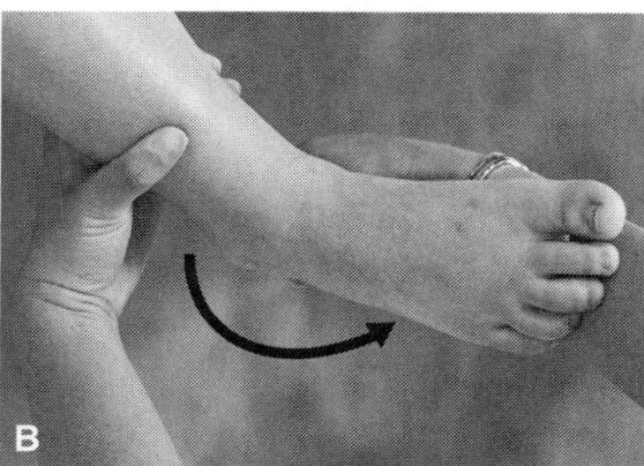

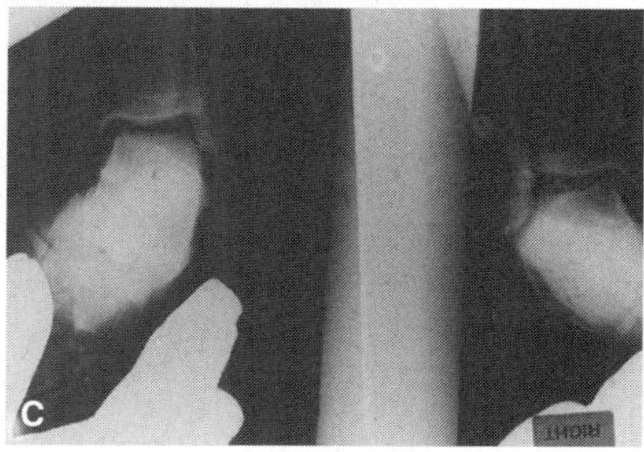

(A, B) Inversion stress test (talar tilt test) to check the integrity of the calcaneofibular ligament. **(C)** Radiograph of an inversion stress.

Patient Position	Supine or sitting with legs over the edge of a table
Position of Examiner	In front of the patient One hand grasps the calcaneus and talus as a single unit and maintains the foot and ankle in 10° of dorsiflexion to isolate the calcaneofibular ligament.[41] The opposite hand stabilizes the leg; the thumb or forefinger is placed along the calcaneofibular ligament so that any gapping of the talus away from the mortise can be felt.
Evaluative Procedure	The hand holding the calcaneus provides an inversion stress by rolling the calcaneus medially, causing the talus to tilt.
Positive Test	The talus tilts or gaps excessively (i.e., greater than 10°) compared with the uninjured side; or pain is produced.
Implications	Involvement of the calcaneofibular ligament, possibly along with the anterior talofibular and posterior talofibular ligaments
Modification	Inversion can be assessed with the ankle in different positions in the ROM to stress specific ligaments.
Comments	When the severity of injury is being based on the relative laxity, a history of injury and residual laxity to the uninvolved ankle mask the magnitude of the current trauma.[41,45]
Evidence	Specificity of 0.68 for combined ATFL and CFL sprains.[41]

ATFL = anterior talofibular ligament; CFL = calcaneofibular ligament; ROM = range of motion.

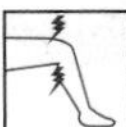

Stress Test 9-3
Eversion (Talar Tilt) Stress Test

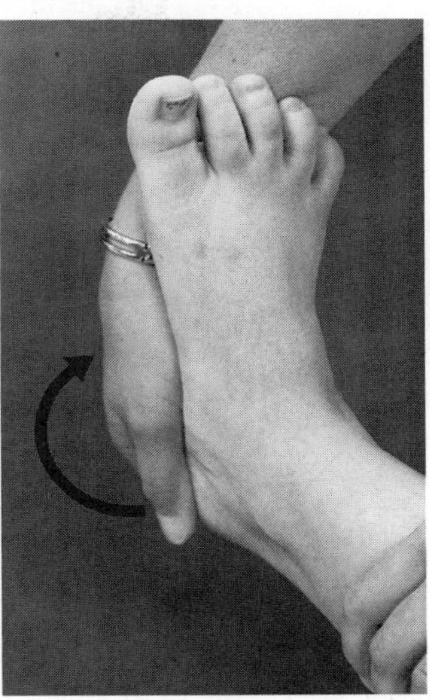

Eversion stress test to determine the integrity of the deltoid ligament, especially the tibiocalcaneal ligament.

Patient Position	Supine or sitting with legs over the edge of a table
Position of Examiner	In front of the patient One hand grasps the calcaneus and talus as a single unit and maintains the ankle in a neutral position.
Evaluative Procedure	The opposite hand stabilizes the leg. The thumb or forefinger may be placed along the deltoid ligament so that any gapping of the talus away from the mortise can be felt. The hand holding the calcaneus rolls it laterally, tilting the talus and causing a gap on the medial side of the ankle mortise.
Positive Test	The talus tilts or gaps excessively as compared with the uninjured side, or pain is described during this motion.
Implications	Deltoid ligament sprain
Comments	Pain at the distal syndesmosis may indicate a distal tibiofibular sprain.
Evidence	Absent or inconclusive in the literature

Joint Play 9-1
Subtalar Joint Play

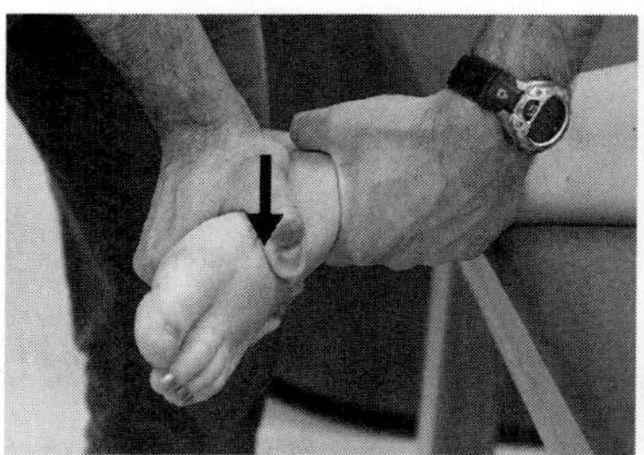

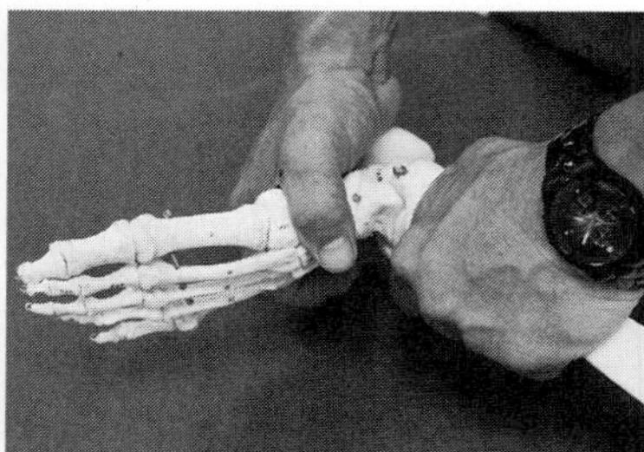

After stabilizing the talus in the mortise, the amount of medial and lateral movement at the subtalar joint is assessed (lateral glide shown).

Patient Position	***Medial glide:*** Side-lying on test limb. STJ in neutral. ***Lateral glide:*** Side-lying on non-test limb. STJ in neutral. A towel may be placed under the distal tibia.
Position of Examiner	Stabilizing talus in the mortise The opposite hand cups the calcaneus.
Evaluative Procedure	Force is applied to move the talus medially and laterally.
Positive Test	Increased or decreased medial or lateral translation of the talus relative to the opposite side.
Implications	Results are compared relative to the opposite (uninjured) ankle: Hypomobile medial glide is associated with decreased pronation/calcaneal eversion. Hypomobile lateral glide is associated with decreased supination/calcaneal inversion.
Comments	Hypermobile medial glide is commonly associated with lateral ankle sprains.[48]
Evidence	Absent or inconclusive in the literature

STJ = subtalar joint.

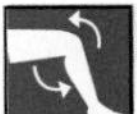

Joint Play 9-2
Cotton Test (Lateral Talar Glide)

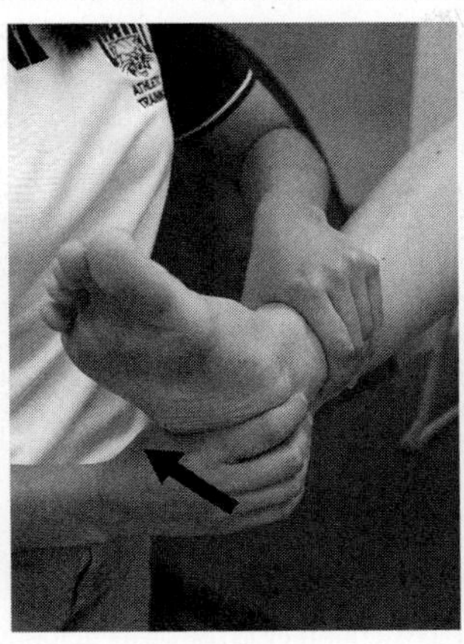

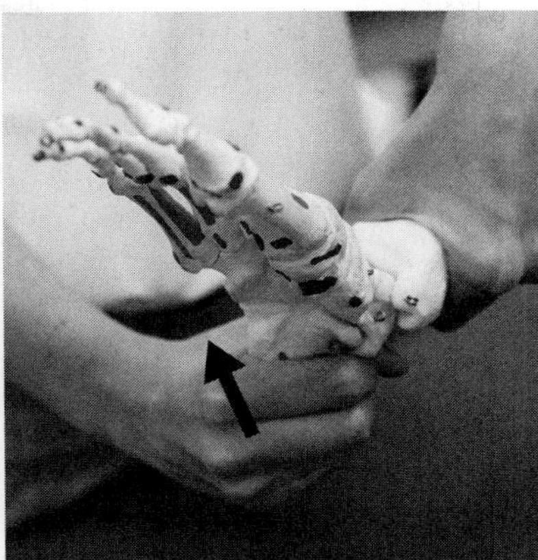

The Cotton test assesses the amount of lateral translation of the talus within the ankle mortise.

Patient Position	Supine or short sitting with the ankle in the neutral position
Position of Examiner	One hand grasps the ankle mortise just proximal to the tibiotalar joint line, stabilizing the distal leg, but do not compress the distal tibiofibular syndesmosis. The opposite hand cups the calcaneus and talus.
Evaluative Procedure	Force is applied to move the talus laterally.
Positive Test	Increased lateral translation of the talus relative to the opposite side Pain[49]
Implications	Distal tibiofibular syndesmosis sprain
Comments	There is a relationship between an arthroscopically confirmed diagnosis tibiofibular syndesmosis sprain and a positive Cotton test.[49]
Evidence	Absent or inconclusive in the literature

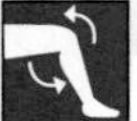

Joint Play 9-3
Distal Tibiofibular Joint Play

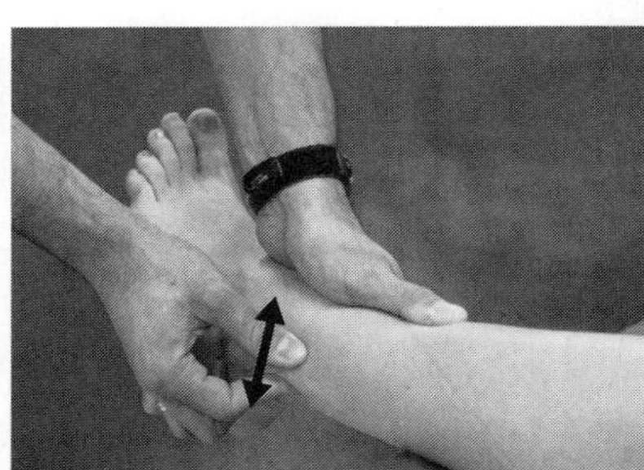

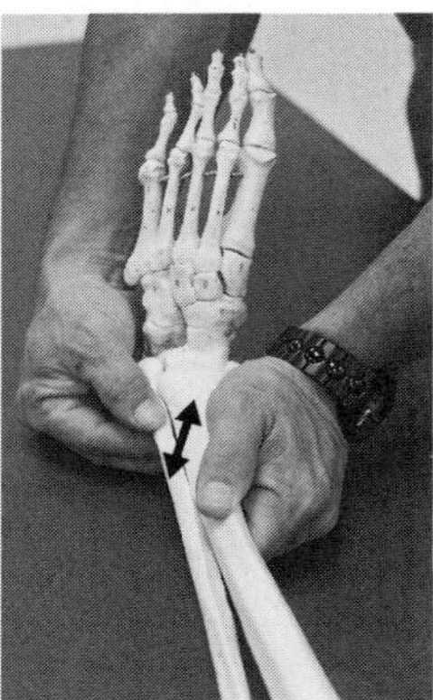

This joint play test identifies the amount of anterior–posterior play in the distal tibiofibular syndesmosis.

Patient Position	Supine or short sitting with the ankle relaxed into plantar flexion
Position of Examiner	Grasping the fibula at the lateral malleolus and stabilizing the tibia
Evaluative Procedure	Pressure is applied obliquely to move the fibula anteriorly and then posteriorly relative to the tibia.
Positive Test	Pain arising from the syndesmosis or increased motion relative to the uninvolved side[50]
Implications	Sprain of the distal tibiofibular syndesmosis
Modification	The distal fibula can be compressed ("squeezed") to identify lateral play based on the amount of movement.
Comments	Pain is a more reliable indicator of syndesmotic trauma than increased motion.[50]
Evidence	Absent or inconclusive in the literature

Special Test 9-1
External Rotation Test (Kleiger's Test)

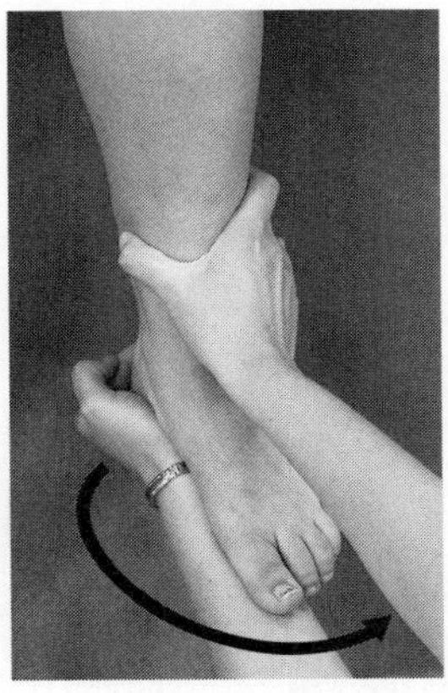

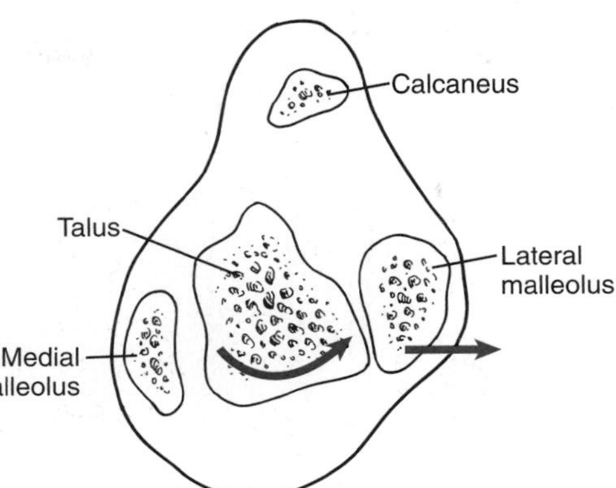

External rotation (Kleiger's) test for determination of rotatory damage to the deltoid ligament or the distal tibiofibular syndesmosis. The implication is based on the area of pain that is elicited. Externally rotating the talus (1) places a lateral force on the fibula (2), spreading the syndesmosis and stretching the deltoid ligament (3).

Patient Position	Sitting with legs over the edge of the table
Position of Examiner	In front of the patient One hand stabilizes the leg in a manner that does not compress the distal tibiofibular syndesmosis. The other hand grasps the medial aspect of the foot while supporting the ankle in a neutral position.
Evaluative Procedure	The foot and talus are externally rotated, while maintaining a stable leg. To stress the syndesmosis, place the ankle in dorsiflexion. To stress the deltoid ligament, place the ankle in neutral position or slightly plantarflexed.
Positive Test	***Deltoid ligament involvement:*** Medial joint pain. The examiner may feel displacement of the talus away from the medial malleolus. ***Syndesmosis involvement:*** Pain is described in the anterolateral ankle at the site of the distal tibiofibular syndesmosis.
Implications	Medial pain is indicative of trauma to the deltoid ligament. Pain in the area of the anterior or posterior tibiofibular ligament should be considered syndesmosis pathology unless determined otherwise (e.g., malleolar fracture). Fracture of the distal fibula
Comments	Pain arising from the distal tibiofibular syndesmosis during this test is associated with a prolonged recovery time.[48]
Evidence	***Inter-rater reliability*** Not Reliable — Very Reliable Poor — Moderate — Good 0 0.1 0.2 0.3 0.4 0.5 0.6 0.7 0.8 0.9 1.0

Special Test 9-2
Squeeze Test

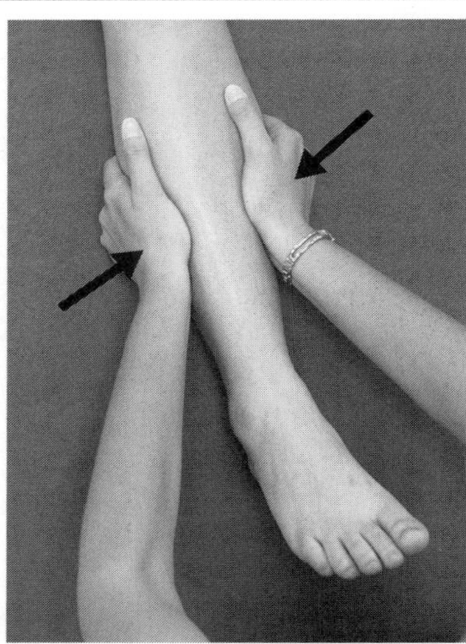

Squeeze test to identify fibular fractures or syndesmosis sprains. Pressure is applied transversely through the leg away from the site of pain.

Patient Position	Lying with the knee extended
Position of Examiner	Standing next to, or in front of, the injured leg; the evaluator's hands cupped behind the tibia and fibula away from the site of pain
Evaluative Procedure	Gently squeeze (compress) the fibula and tibia, gradually adding more pressure if no pain or other symptoms are elicited. Progress toward the injured site until pain is elicited.
Positive Test	Pain is elicited, especially when it is away from the compressed area.
Implications	**(A)** Gross fracture or stress fracture of the fibula when pain is described along the fibular shaft **(B)** Syndesmosis sprain when pain is described at the distal tibiofibular joint
Comments	Avoid applying too much pressure too soon into the test. Pressure should be applied gradually and progressively. The test is infrequently positive, even in the presence of other clinical findings indicative of a syndesmosis sprain. Its usefulness is limited.[49]
Evidence	***Inter-rater reliability*** Not Reliable — Very Reliable Poor — Moderate — Good 0 0.1 0.2 0.3 0.4 0.5 0.6 0.7 0.8 0.9 1.0

Special Test 9-3
Thompson Test for Achilles Tendon Rupture

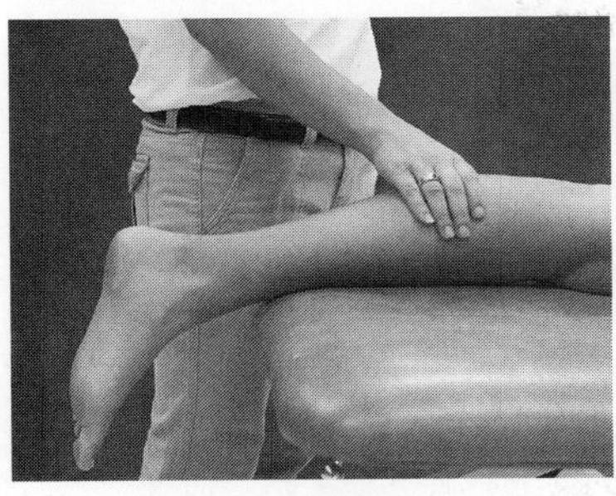

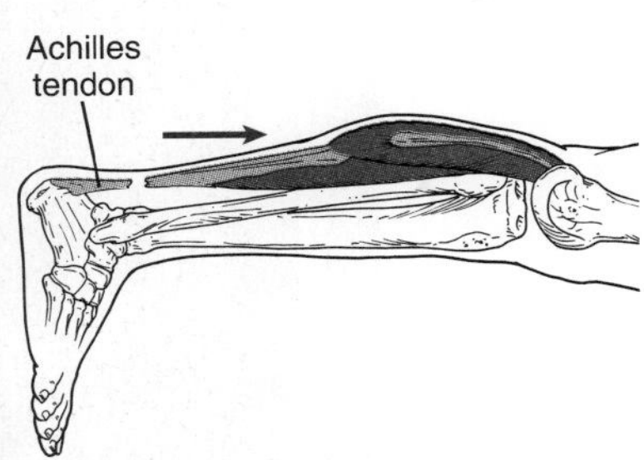

Thompson test for an Achilles tendon rupture. When the Achilles tendon is intact, squeezing the calf muscle results in slight plantarflexion. A positive Thompson test occurs when the calf is squeezed but no motion is produced in the foot, indicating a tear of the Achilles tendon.

Patient Position	Prone, with the foot off the edge of the table
Position of Examiner	At the side of the patient with one hand over the muscle belly of the calf musculature
Evaluative Procedure	The examiner squeezes the calf musculature while observing for plantarflexion of the foot.
Positive Test	When the calf is squeezed, the foot does not plantarflex.
Implications	The Achilles tendon has been ruptured.
Modification	None
Evidence	Positive likelihood ratio[51]

Not Useful — Useful
Very Small | Small | Moderate | Large
13.7
0 1 2 3 4 5 6 7 8 9 10

Negative likelihood ratio

Not Useful — Useful
Very Small | Small | Moderate | Large
1.0 0.9 0.8 0.7 0.6 0.5 0.4 0.3 0.2 0.1 0

Special Test 9-4
Bump Test for Leg Stress Fractures

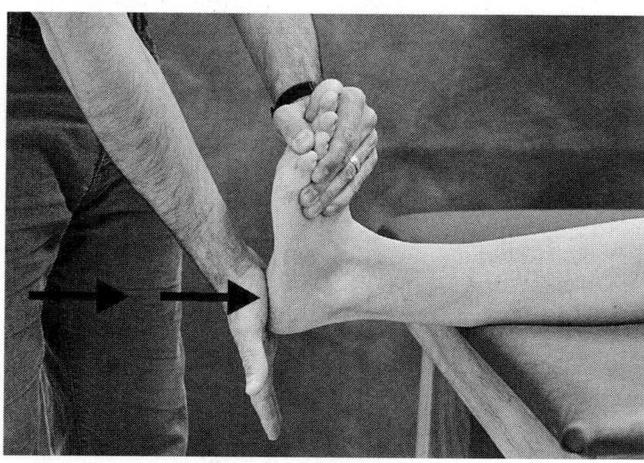

Bump test to identify stress fractures of the leg or talus. The examiner's hand is bumped against the patient's foot. The subsequent shock elicits pain in areas of stress fractures. Note that this test is not definitive and should not be used in the presence of an obvious fracture.

Patient Position	Sitting with the involved leg off the end of the table and the knee straight, or lying supine The ankle in its neutral position
Position of Examiner	Standing in front of the heel of the involved leg The posterior portion of the leg is stabilized with the nondominant hand.
Evaluative Procedure	Bumps the calcaneus using the palm of the dominant hand
Positive Test	Pain emanating from fracture of the calcaneus, talus, fibula, or tibia
Implications	Possible advanced stress fracture
Evidence	Inconclusive or absent in the literature

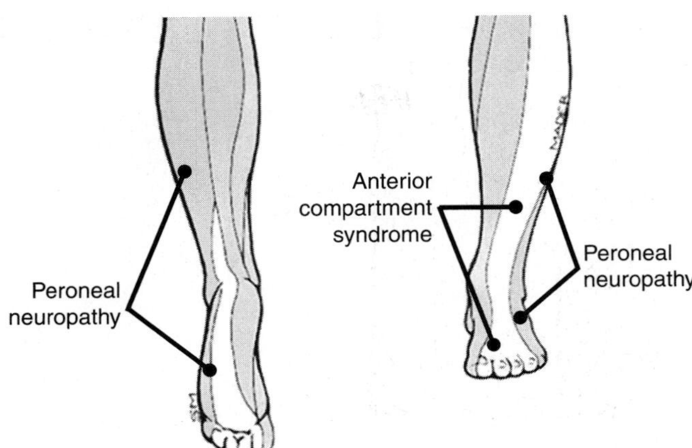

FIGURE 9-6 ■ Local neuropathies of the ankle and leg. These findings should also be matched with those of a lower quarter neurologic screen.

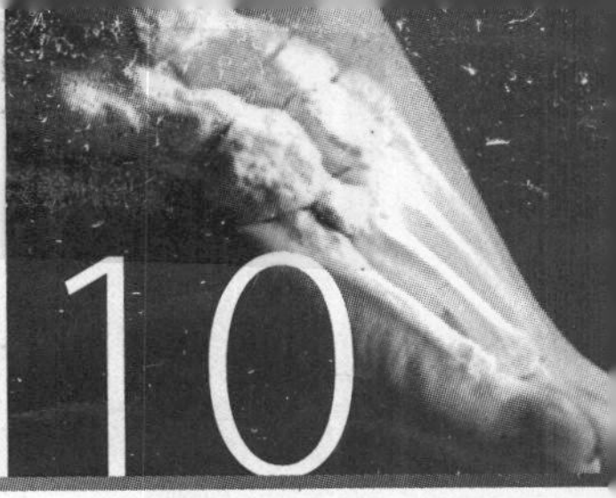

CHAPTER 10

Knee Pathologies

Examination Map

HISTORY

Past Medical History

History of the Present Condition

Mechanism of Injury

INSPECTION

Functional Assessment

Girth Measurements

Inspection of the Anterior Structures

Patella

Patellar tendon

Quadriceps muscle group

Tibiofemoral alignment

Tibial tuberosity

Inspection of the Medial Structures

General medial aspect

Vastus medialis

Inspection of the Lateral Structures

General lateral structure

Fibular head

Posterior sag of tibia

Hyperextension

Inspection of the Posterior Structures

Hamstring muscle group

Popliteal fossa
- Baker's cyst

PALPATION

Palpation of the Anterior Structures

Patella

Patellar tendon

Tibial tuberosity

Quadriceps tendon

Quadriceps muscle group
- Vastus medialis
- Rectus femoris
- Vastus lateralis

Sartorius

Palpation of the Medial Structures

Medial meniscus and joint line

Medial collateral ligament

Medial femoral condyle and epicondyle

Medial tibial plateau

Pes anserine tendon and bursa

Semitendinosus

Gracilis

Palpation of the Lateral Structures

Joint line

Fibular head

Lateral collateral ligament

Popliteus

Biceps femoris

Iliotibial band

Palpation of the Posterior Structures

Popliteal fossa

Hamstring muscle group
- Biceps femoris
- Semimembranosus
- Semitendinosus

Determination of Intracapsular versus Extracapsular Swelling

JOINT AND MUSCLE FUNCTION ASSESSMENT

Goniometry

Flexion

Extension

Continued

Examination Map—cont'd

Active Range of Motion

Flexion

Extension

Manual Muscle Tests

Knee extension

Knee flexion

Isolating the sartorius

Passive Range of Motion

Flexion

Extension

JOINT STABILITY TESTS

Stress Testing

Anterior instability

- Anterior drawer test
- Lachman's test
- Prone Lachman's test

Posterior instability

- Posterior drawer test
- Godfrey's test

Medial instability

- Valgus stress test: 0° flexion
- Valgus stress test: 25° flexion

Lateral instability

- Varus stress test: 0° flexion
- Varus stress test: 25° flexion

Joint Play Assessment

Proximal tibiofibular syndesmosis

NEUROLOGIC EXAMINATION

Lower Quarter Screen

Common Peroneal Nerve

VASCULAR EXAMINATION

Distal Capillary Refill

Distal Pulse

Posterior tibial artery

Dorsal pedal artery

PATHOLOGIES AND SPECIAL TESTS

Uniplanar Knee Sprains

Medial collateral ligament

- Valgus stress test

Lateral collateral ligament

- Varus stress test

Anterior cruciate ligament

- Anterior drawer test
- Lachman's test
- Prone Lachman's test
- Quadriceps active test

Rotational Knee Instabilities

Anterolateral rotatory instability

- Pivot shift test
- Jerk test
- Slocum drawer test
- Crossover test
- Slocum ALRI test
- Flexion–rotation drawer test

Anteromedial rotatory instability

- Slocum drawer test
- Crossover test
- Lachman's test
- Valgus stress test

Posterolateral rotatory instability

- External rotation (dial) test
- External rotation recurvatum test
- Posterolateral drawer test
- Reverse-pivot shift
- Dynamic posterior shift test

Meniscal tears

- McMurray's test
- Apley's compression/distraction test
- Thessaly test

Osteochondral lesions

- Wilson's test

Iliotibial band friction syndrome

- Noble's compression test
- Ober's test

Popliteus Tendinopathy

Tibiofemoral Joint Dislocations

Table 10-1 Possible Pathology Based on the Location of Pain

	Location of Pain			
	Lateral	**Anterior**	**Medial**	**Posterior**
Soft Tissue	LCL sprain	ACL sprain (emanating from "inside" the knee)	MCL sprain	PCL sprain
	Lateral joint capsule sprain	Patellar tendinopathy*	Medial joint capsule sprain	Posterior capsule sprain
	Superior tibiofibular syndesmosis sprain	Patellar tendon rupture (partial or complete)*	Medial patellar retinaculum irritation*	Gastrocnemius strain
	Lateral patellar retinaculum irritation*	Patellar bursitis*	Pes anserine bursitis or tendinopathy	Hamstring strain
	Biceps femoris strain	Patellofemoral joint dysfunction*	Semitendinosus strain	Popliteus tendinopathy
	Biceps femoris tendinopathy	Quadriceps contusion	Semitendinosus tendinopathy	Popliteal cyst
	Popliteal tendinopathy	Fat pad irritation*	Semimembranosus strain	Medial/lateral meniscal tear (posterior horn)
	IT band friction syndrome	Quadriceps tendon rupture*	Semimembranosus tendinopathy	
	Lateral meniscus tear		Medial meniscus tear	
Bony	Fibular head fracture	Patellar fracture	Osteochondral fracture	
	Osteochondral fracture	Tibial plateau fracture	Osteochondritis dissecans	
	Osteochondritis dissecans	Sinding–Johansson–Larsen disease*	Medial femoral condyle contusion	
	Lateral femoral condyle contusion	Osgood-Schlatter disease (in adolescents)*	Medial tibial plateau	
	Lateral tibial plateau	Patellar dislocation or subluxation*	Contusion	
	Contusion	Chondromalacia	Epiphyseal fracture in pediatric patients	
	Epiphyseal fracture in pediatric patients			

ACL = anterior cruciate ligament; IT = iliotibial; LCL = lateral collateral ligament; MCL = medial collateral ligament; PCL = posterior cruciate ligament.

*Patellofemoral disorders.

Table 10-2 Mechanism of Knee Injuries and the Resultant Soft Tissue Damage

Force Placed on the Knee	Tensile Forces	Compressive Forces
Valgus	Medial structures: MCL, medial joint capsule, pes anserine muscle group, medial meniscus	Lateral meniscus
Varus	Lateral structures: LCL, lateral joint capsule, IT band, biceps femoris	Medial meniscus
Anterior Tibial Displacement	ACL, IT band, LCL, MCL, medial and lateral joint capsules	Posterior portion of the medial and lateral meniscus
Posterior Tibial Displacement	PCL, meniscofemoral ligament(s), popliteus, medial and lateral joint capsules	Anterior portion of the medial and lateral meniscus
Internal Tibial Rotation	ACL, anterolateral joint capsule, posteromedial joint capsule, posterolateral joint capsule, LCL	Anterior horn of the medial meniscus Posterior horn of the lateral meniscus
External Tibial Rotation	Posterolateral joint capsule, anteromedial joint capsule, MCL, PCL, LCL, ACL	Anterior horn of the lateral meniscus Posterior horn of the lateral meniscus
Hyperextension	ACL, posterior joint capsule, PCL	Anterior portion of the medial and lateral meniscus
Hyperflexion	ACL, PCL	Posterior portion of the medial and lateral meniscus

ACL = anterior cruciate ligament; IT = iliotibial; LCL = lateral collateral ligament; MCL = medial collateral ligament; PCL = posterior cruciate ligament.

Box 10-1
Classification of Rotational Knee Instabilities

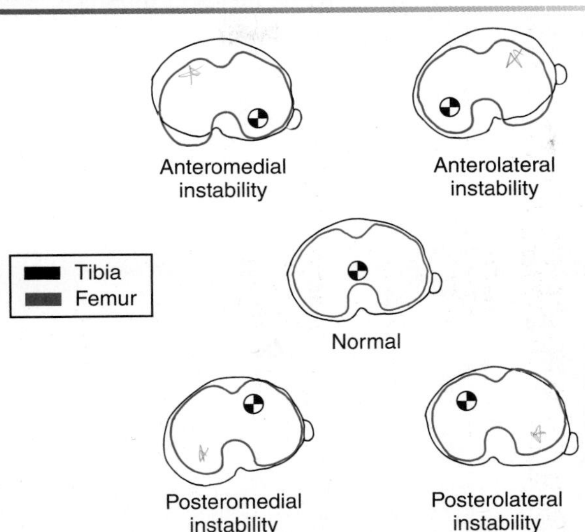

The tibial articulating surface is shown in black lines, and the femoral articular surfaces in pink lines. The type of instability is described based on the displacement of the tibia relative to the femur. Note that the axes of rotation are approximated.

Instability	Tibial Displacement	Pathologic Axis	Structural Instability
Anteromedial	Medial tibial plateau subluxates anteriorly.	Posterolateral, resulting in abnormal external tibial rotation	ACL, anteromedial capsule, MCL, pes anserine, medial meniscus, posteromedial capsule
Anterolateral	Lateral tibial plateau subluxates anteriorly.	Posteromedial, resulting in abnormal internal tibial rotation	ACL, anterolateral capsule, LCL, IT band, biceps femoris, lateral meniscus, popliteus, posterolateral capsule
Posteromedial	Medial tibial plateau subluxates posteriorly.	Anterolateral, resulting in abnormal internal tibial rotation	Posterior oblique ligament, MCL, semimembranosus, anteromedial capsule
Posterolateral	Lateral tibial plateau subluxates posteriorly.	Anteromedial, resulting in abnormal external tibial rotation	Posterolateral complex, LCL, biceps femoris

ACL = anterior cruciate ligament; IT = iliotibial; LCL = lateral collateral ligament; MCL = medial collateral ligament.

Special Test 10-1
Girth Measurements

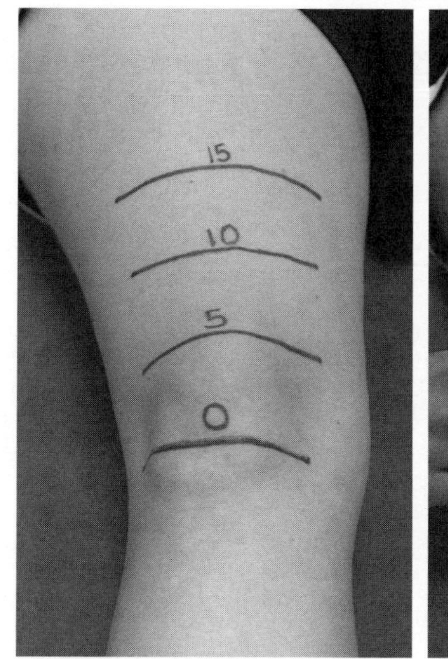

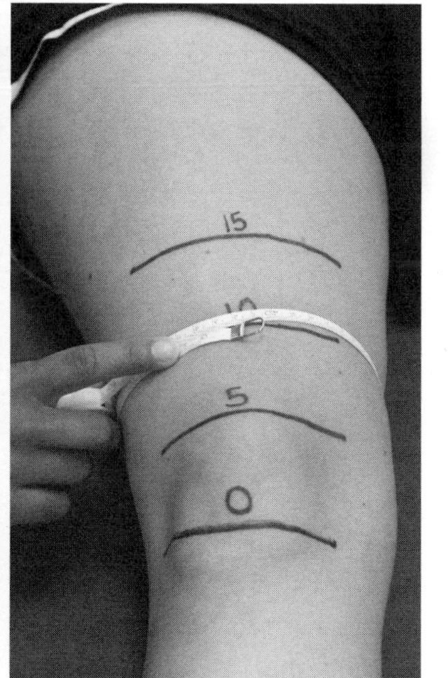

The girth about the knee is determined by identifying the joint line (0 mark) and measuring above and below the joint line. Measurements are made around the joint line and then at consistent intervals up the quadriceps group.

Patient Position	Supine or standing (the patient should be in the same position each time a measurement is taken)
Position of Examiner	Standing next to the patient

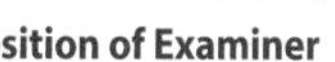

Evaluative Procedure	The joint line is identified and measured at the 0-inch mark. Measurements are taken at 5-, 10-, and 15-cm intervals above the joint line. Measurements are taken at 15 cm below the joint line.
Positive Test	A difference of ±1 cm compared bilaterally
Implications	Increased girth on the injured side across the joint line: Edema Decreased muscular girth on the injured side: Atrophy
Modification	The measurement increments can be increased for taller individuals and decreased for shorter people.
Comments	Standardization of the measurements is required for accurate results (e.g., the patient in the same position, same landmarks). The muscular girth of the dominant leg may be naturally hypertrophied relative to the nondominant leg. In the case of migrating edema, ankle and calf girth measurements should also be taken. There is only a slight to moderate relationship between strength and girth in the overall population.
Evidence	Intra-rater reliability: **Not Reliable** **Very Reliable** Poor Moderate Good 0 0.1 0.2 0.3 0.4 0.5 0.6 0.7 0.8 0.9 1.0 Inter-rater reliability: **Not Reliable** **Very Reliable** Poor Moderate Good 0 0.1 0.2 0.3 0.4 0.5 0.6 0.7 0.8 0.9 1.0

Osgood-Schlatter Disease

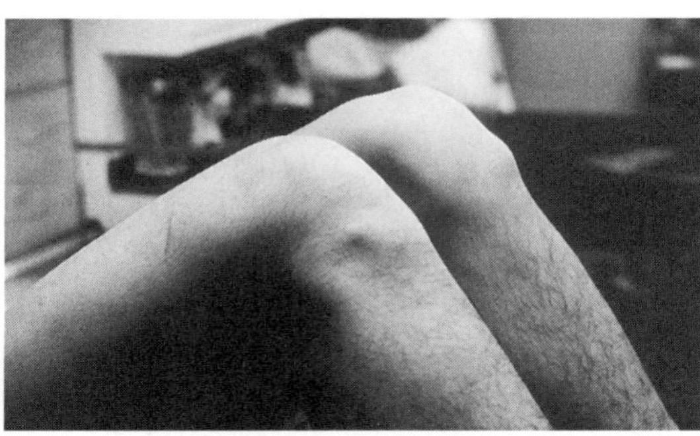

FIGURE 10-1 ■ Residual enlargement of the tibial tuberosity caused by Osgood–Schlatter disease in youth.

Posterior Tibial Sag

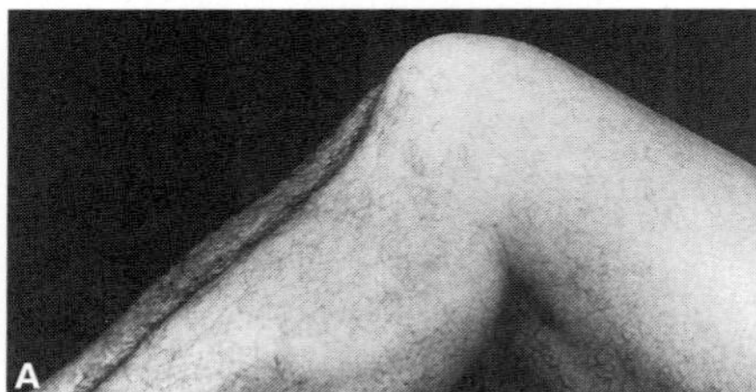

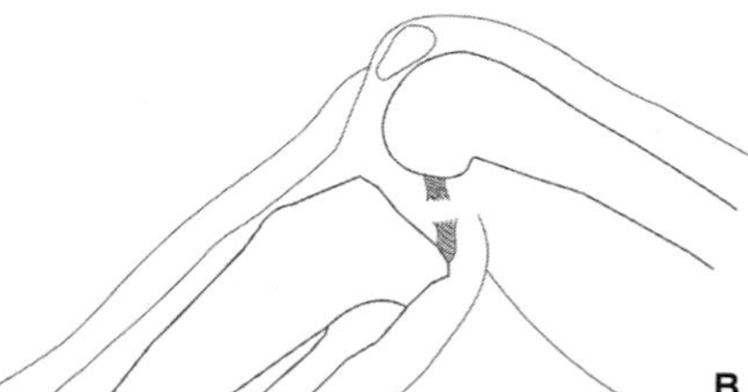

FIGURE 10-2 ■ **(A)** Posterior tibial sag indicating posterior cruciate ligament deficiency. Note the downward displacement of the tibia. **(B)** Illustration showing the posterior displacement of the tibia that is caused by tearing of the posterior cruciate ligament (the anterior cruciate ligament has been removed for clarity).

Inspection Findings 10-1
Tibiofemoral Alignment

Normal	Genu Valgum	Genu Varum	Genu Recurvatum
Description	Tibiofemoral angle of greater than 185°	Tibiofemoral angle of less than 175°	Tibiofemoral extension greater than 0°
Potential Causes	Degeneration of the medial meniscus Structural or acquired hip abnormalities Excessive foot pronation	Degeneration of the lateral meniscus Structural or acquired hip abnormalities Excessive foot supination	Rupture of the ACL or PCL
Consequences	Increased compressive forces on the medial joint structures Increased tensile forces on the lateral joint structures Increased foot pronation Internal tibial rotation Medial patellar position Internal femoral rotation	Increased tensile forces on the medial joint structures Increased compressive forces on the lateral joint structures Increased foot supination External tibial rotation Lateral patellar position External femoral rotation	Increased strain on the ACL and/or PCL Increased contact pressure between the patella and femur

ACL = anterior cruciate ligament; PCL = posterior cruciate ligament.

PALPATION

Palpation of the Anterior Structures

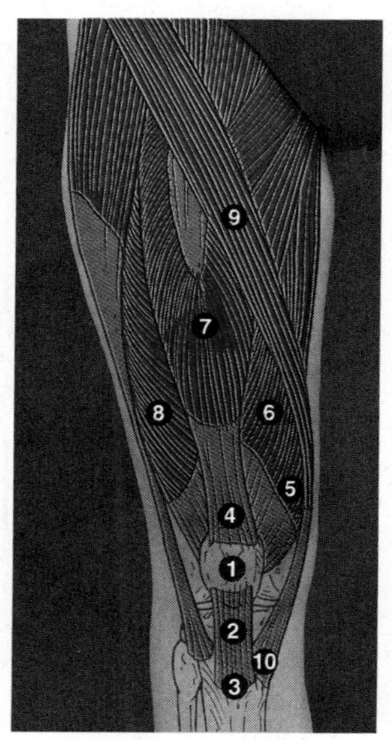

1 Patella

2 Patellar tendon

3 Tibial tuberosity

4 Quadriceps tendon

Quadriceps muscle group

5 Vastus medialis oblique

6 Vastus medialis

7 Rectus femoris

8 Vastus lateralis (the vastus intermedius is not directly palpable)

9 Sartorius

10 Pes anserine tendon

Palpation of the Medial Structures

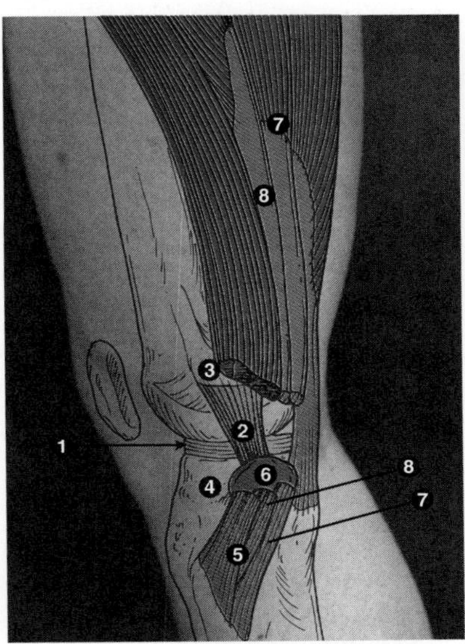

1 Medial meniscus and joint line

2 Medial collateral ligament

3 Medial femoral condyle and epicondyle

4 Medial tibial plateau

5 Pes anserine tendon bursa

6 Pes anserine bursa

7 Semitendinous tendon

8 Gracilis

Palpation of the Lateral Structures

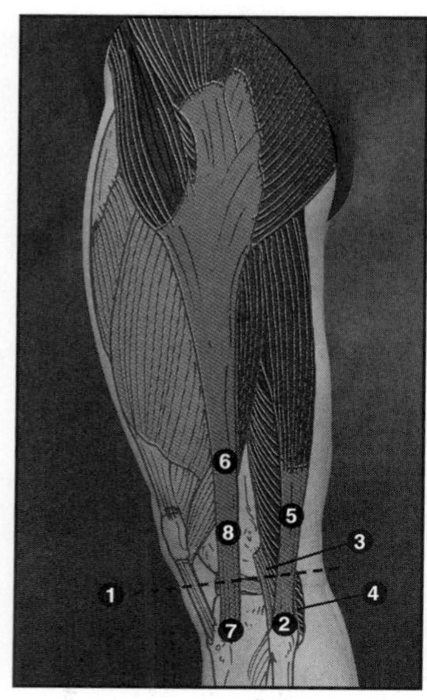

1 Joint line

2 Fibular head

3 Lateral collateral ligament

4 Popliteus

5 Biceps femoris

6 Iliotibial band

7 Gerdy's tubercle

8 Lateral femoral condyle

Palpation of the Posterior Structures

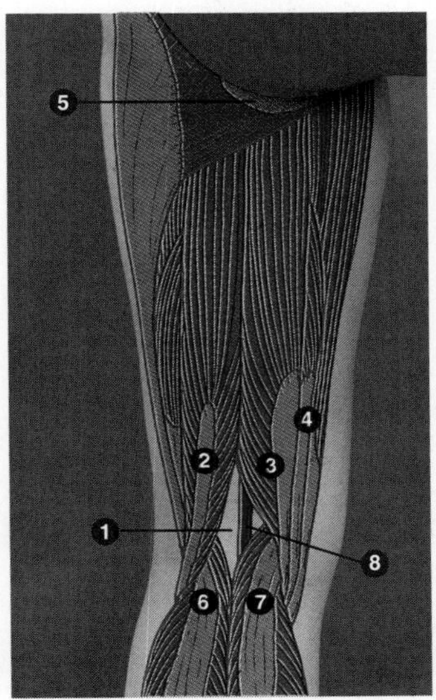

1 Popliteal fossa

Hamstring muscle group

2 Biceps femoris

3 Semimembranosus

4 Semitendinosus

5 Ischial tuberosity

6 Lateral head of the gastrocnemius

7 Medial head of the gastrocnemius

8 Popliteal artery

Table 10-3 Knee Capsular Pattern and End-Feels

Capsular Pattern: Flexion, Extension

End-Feels:	
Extension	Firm: Stretch of the posterior capsule; ACL; PCL
Flexion	Soft: Soft tissue approximation between the triceps surae and the hamstrings. Firm: Stretch of the rectus femoris.
Internal tibial rotation	Firm: Capsular stretch; LCL; IT band
External tibial rotation	Firm: Capsular stretch; MCL; LCL; Pes anserine

ACL = anterior cruciate ligament; IT = iliotibial; LCL = lateral collateral ligament; MCL = medial collateral ligament; PCL = posterior cruciate ligament.

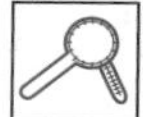

Goniometry Box 10-1
Knee Flexion/Extension

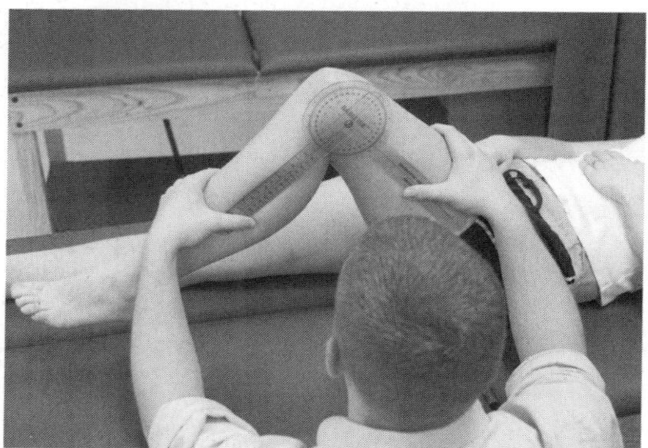

Flexion (0° to 135°–145°)/Extension (0°–10°)

Patient Position	Lying supine. Knee flexion and extension may also be measured with the patient supine and a bolster placed under the distal femur.
Goniometer Alignment	
Fulcrum	Centered over the lateral femoral epicondyle
Proximal Arm	The stationary arm is centered over the midline of the femur, aligned with the greater trochanter.
Distal Arm	The movement arm is centered over the midline of the fibula, aligned with the lateral malleolus.
Comments	Knee flexion can be assessed with the patient prone and using the same landmarks to assess the length of the two-joint rectus femoris muscle.

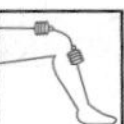

Manual Muscle Test 10-1
Knee Extension

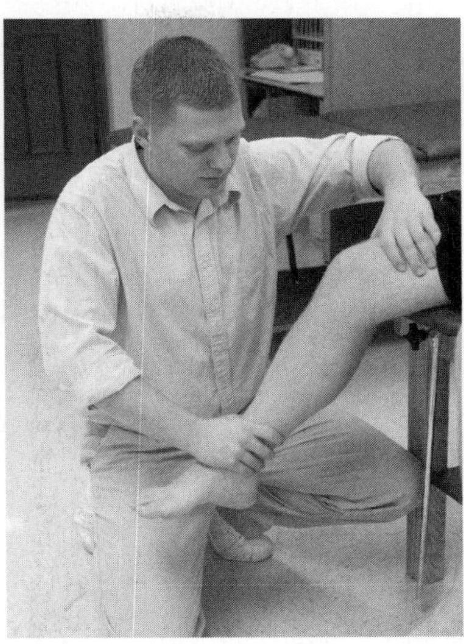

Patient Position	Seated
Starting Position	Knee flexed
Stabilization	Distal femur
Palpation	Proximal to the patella
Resistance	Distal tibia, proximal to the ankle
Primary Mover(s) (Innervation)	Vastus lateralis (L2, L3, L4) Vastus medialis (L2, L3, L4) Vastus intermedius (L2, L3, L4) Rectus femoris (L2, L3, L4)
Secondary Mover(s) (Innervation)	Not applicable
Substitution	Ankle dorsiflexion Hip extension

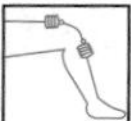

Manual Muscle Test 10-2
Knee Flexion

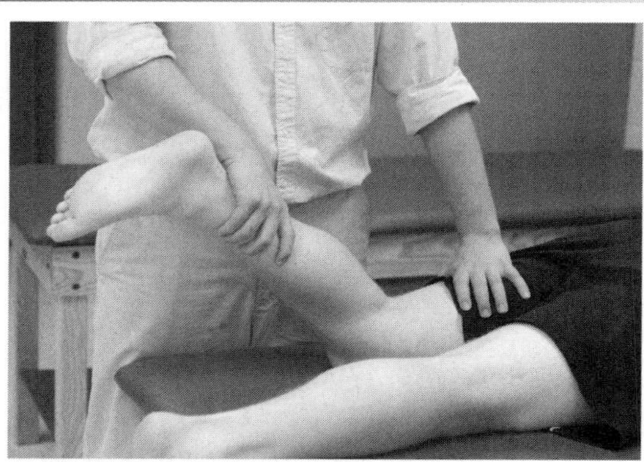

Patient Position	Prone
Starting Position	Knee extended
Stabilization	Femur
Palpation	Mid-belly of medial and lateral hamstrings
Resistance	Distal tibia
Primary Mover(s) (Innervation)	**Biceps femoris:** Long head—tibial (S1, S2, S3); short head—common peroneal (L5, S1, S2) **Semimembranosus:** Tibial (L5, S1) **Semitendinosus:** Tibial (L5, S1, S2)
Secondary Mover(s) (Innervation)	Gastrocnemius
Substitution	Hip flexion Ankle plantarflexion
Comments	Internally rotating the leg will emphasize contributions from the semimembranosus and semitendinosus. Externally rotating the leg will emphasize contribution from the biceps femoris.

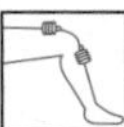

Manual Muscle Test 10-3
Isolating the Sartorius

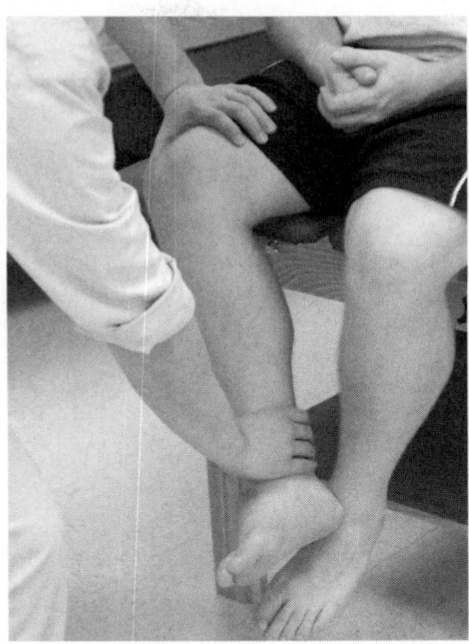

Patient Position	Seated
Starting Position	The heel of the leg being tested is positioned over the anterior talocrural joint with the patient sitting over the edge of the table.
Stabilization	Distal femur
Palpation	Just inferior to the anterior superior iliac spine
Resistance	Medial aspect of the distal tibia and medial ankle The patient attempts to slide the heel up the opposite tibia while the clinician resists hip flexion, hip abduction, hip external rotation, and knee flexion.
Primary Mover(s) (Innervation)	Sartorius (L2, L3)
Secondary Mover(s)	Secondary movers include the hamstring muscle group, hip external rotators, gracilis, and hip flexors.
Substitution	Hip flexion without external rotation or abduction indicates substitution by the rectus femoris and/or iliopsoas.[51]

Table 10-4 Muscles Acting on the Knee

Muscle	Action	Origin	Insertion	Innervation	Root
Biceps Femoris	Knee flexion External tibial rotation Long head • Hip extension • Hip external rotation	Long head • Ischial tuberosity • Sacrotuberous ligament Short head • Lateral lip of the linea aspera • Upper two-thirds of the supracondylar line	Lateral fibular head Lateral tibial condyle	Long head • Tibial Short head • Common peroneal	Long head S1, S2, S3 Short head L5, S1, S2
Gastrocnemius	Assists knee flexion Ankle plantarflexion	Medial head • Posterior surface of the medial femoral condyle • Adjacent portion of the femur and knee capsule Lateral head • Posterior surface of the lateral femoral condyle • Adjacent portion of the femur and knee capsule	To the calcaneus via the Achilles tendon	Tibial	S1, S2
Gracilis	Knee flexion Internal tibial rotation Hip adduction	Symphysis pubis Inferior ramus of the pubic bone	Proximal portion of the antero-medial tibial flare	Obturator (posterior)	L3, L4
Popliteus	Open chain • Internal tibial rotation • Knee flexion Closed chain External femoral rotation Knee flexion	Lateral femoral condyle Oblique popliteal ligament	Posterior tibia superior to the soleal line Fascia covering the soleus	Tibial	L4, L5, S1

Muscle	Action	Origin	Insertion	Nerve	Root
Rectus Femoris	Knee extension Hip flexion	Anterior inferior iliac spine Groove located superior to the acetabulum	To the tibial tubercle via the patella and patellar ligament	Femoral	L2, L3, L4
Sartorius	Knee flexion Internal tibial rotation Hip flexion Hip abduction Hip external rotation	Anterior superior iliac spine	Proximal portion of the antero-medial tibial flare	Femoral	L2, L3
Semimembranosus	Knee flexion Internal tibial rotation Hip extension Hip internal rotation	Ischial tuberosity	Posteromedial portion of the tibia's medial condyle	Tibial	L5, S1
Semitendinosus	Knee flexion Internal tibial rotation Hip extension Hip internal rotation	Ischial tuberosity	Medial portion of the tibial flare	Tibial	L5, S1, S2
Vastus Intermedius	Knee extension	Anterolateral portion of the upper two-thirds of the femur Lower one-half of the linea aspera	To the tibial tubercle via the patella and patellar ligament	Femoral	L2, L3, L4
Vastus Lateralis	Knee extension	Proximal intertrochanteric line Greater trochanter Gluteal tuberosity Upper one-half of the linea aspera	To the tibial tubercle via the patella and patellar ligament	Femoral	L2, L3, L4
Vastus Medialis	Knee extension Oblique portion • Patellar stabilization	Longus portion • Distal one-half of the intertrochanteric line • Medial portion of the linea aspera Oblique portion • Tendons from adductor longus and adductor magnus	To the tibial tubercle via the patella and patellar ligament	Femoral	L2, L3, L4

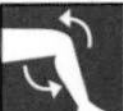

Joint Play 10-1
Proximal Tibiofibular Syndesmosis

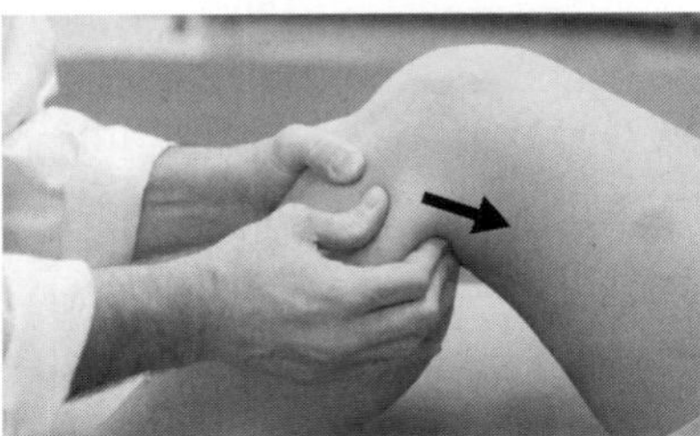

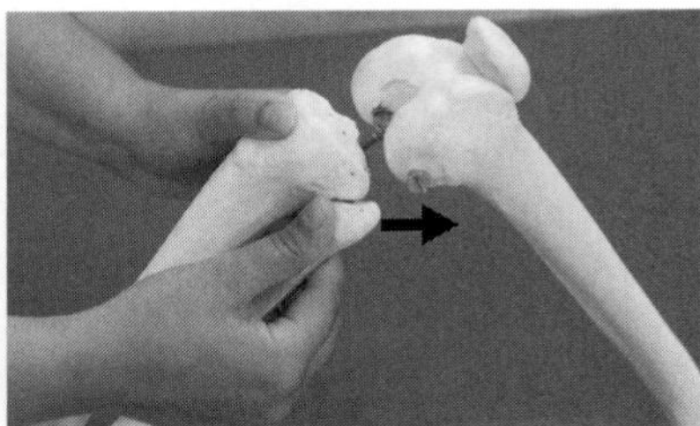

The fibular head is manually manipulated to determine its anterior/posterior stability.

Patient Position	Lying supine with the knee passively flexed to approximately 90°
Position of Examiner	Standing lateral to the involved side
Evaluative Procedure	One hand stabilizes the tibia while the other hand grasps the fibular head. While stabilizing the tibia, the examiner attempts to displace the fibular head anteriorly and then posteriorly.
Positive Test	Any perceived movement of the fibula on the tibia compared with the uninvolved side and/or pain elicited during the test
Implications	An anterior fibular shift indicates damage to the proximal posterior tibiofibular ligament; posterior displacement reflects instability of the anterior tibiofibular ligament of the proximal tibiofibular syndesmosis.
Comments	Damage to the common peroneal nerve is frequently associated with a proximal tibiofibular syndesmosis sprain.
Evidence	Inconclusive or absent in the literature

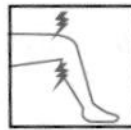

Stress Test 10-1
Anterior Drawer Test for Anterior Cruciate Ligament Instability

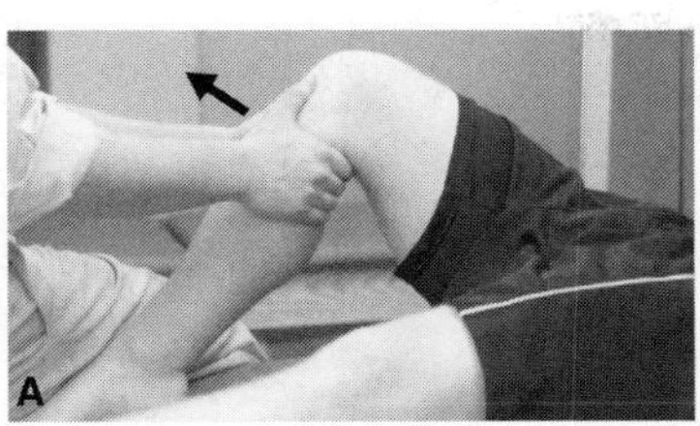

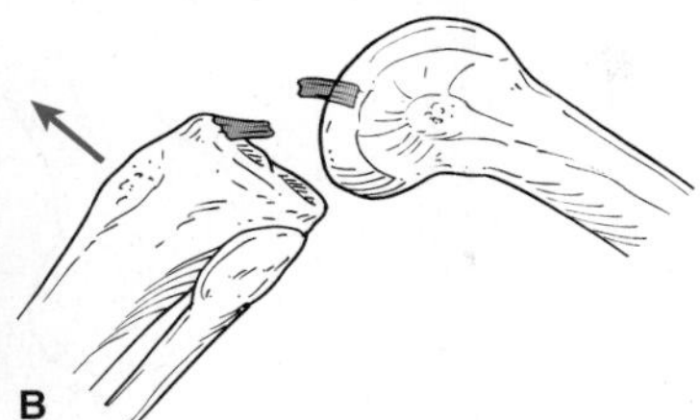

The anterior drawer test for anterior cruciate laxity **(A)**. Schematic representation of tibial displacement in a positive test **(B)**. The anterior drawer test is also used to identify interior joint play.

Patient Position	Lying supine Hip flexed to 45° and the knee to 90°
Position of Examiner	Sitting on the examination table in front of the involved knee, grasping the tibia just below the joint line of the knee. Thumbs are placed along the joint line on either side of the patellar tendon. The index fingers are used to palpate the hamstring tendons to ensure that they are relaxed.
Evaluative Procedure	The tibia is drawn anteriorly.
Positive Test	An increased amount of anterior tibial translation compared with the opposite (uninvolved) limb or the lack of a firm end-point
Implications	A sprain of the anteromedial bundle of the ACL or a complete tear of the ACL
Modification	The patient is seated to remove the posterior sag of the tibia that would be caused by PCL injury. The examiner is kneeling with the patient's lower leg stabilized between the examiner's knees. The tibia is translated anteriorly.
Comments	The hamstring muscle group must be relaxed to ensure proper test results. Too much flexion can result in false-negative result due to tibial plateau and the posterior horns of the menisci contacting the femoral condyle.
Evidence	Positive likelihood ratio Not Useful — Useful Very Small — Small — Moderate — Large 87.9 0 1 2 3 4 5 6 7 8 9 10 Negative likelihood ratio Not Useful — Useful Very Small — Small — Moderate — Large 1.0 0.9 0.8 0.7 0.6 0.5 0.4 0.3 0.2 0.1 0

ACL = anterior cruciate ligament; PCL = posterior cruciate ligament.

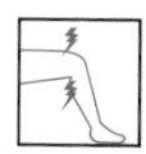

Stress Test 10-2
Lachman's Test for Anterior Cruciate Ligament Laxity

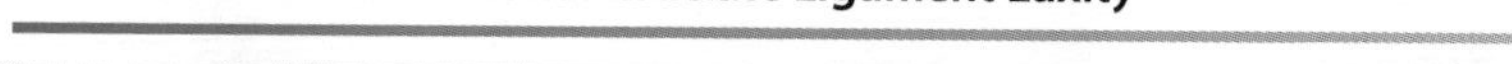

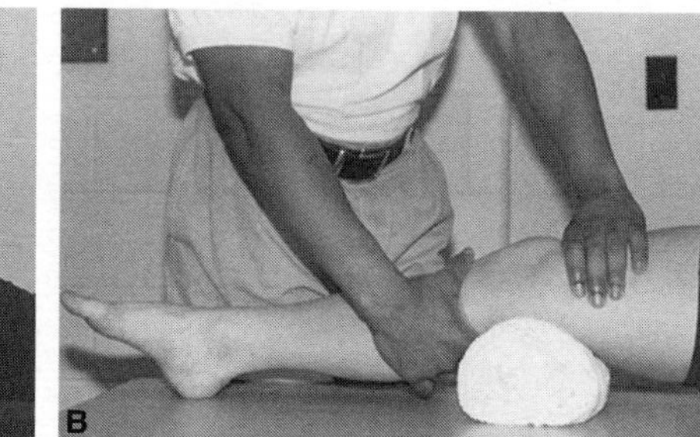

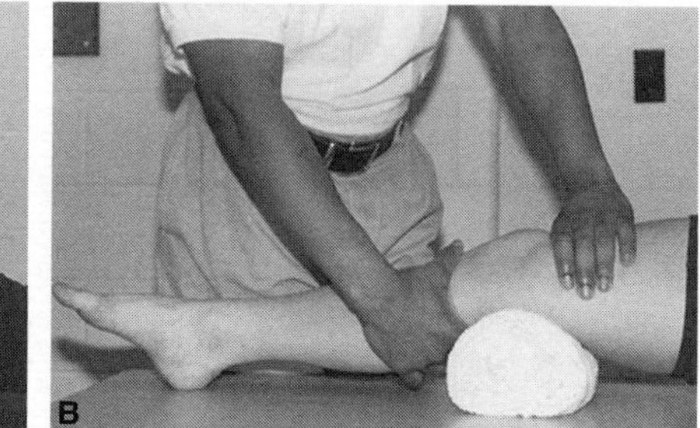

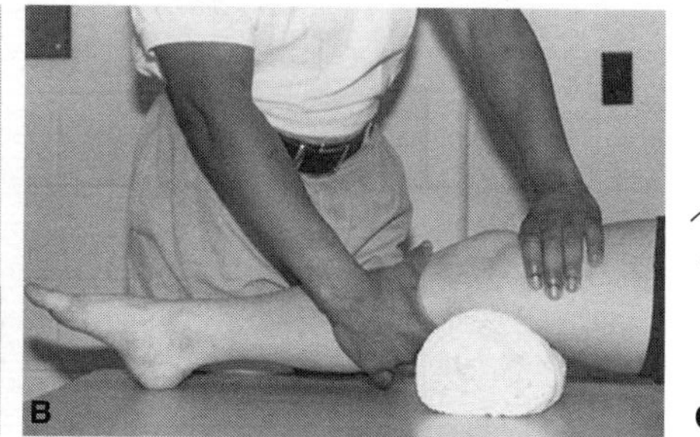

The Lachman's test **(A)** and modification of the Lachman's test **(B)**. Schematic representation of tibiofemoral translation in the presence of ACL deficiency **(C)**.

Patient Position	Lying supine The knee passively flexed to 20°–25°
Position of Examiner	One hand grasps the tibia around the level of the tibial tuberosity and the other hand grasps the femur just above the level of the condyles.
Evaluative Procedure	While the examiner supports the weight of the leg and the knee is flexed to 20°–25°, the tibia is drawn anteriorly while a posterior pressure is applied to stabilize the femur.
Positive Test	An increased amount of anterior tibial translation compared with the opposite (uninvolved) limb or the lack of a firm end-point
Implications	Sprain of the ACL, sprain of the posterolateral bundle of the ACL

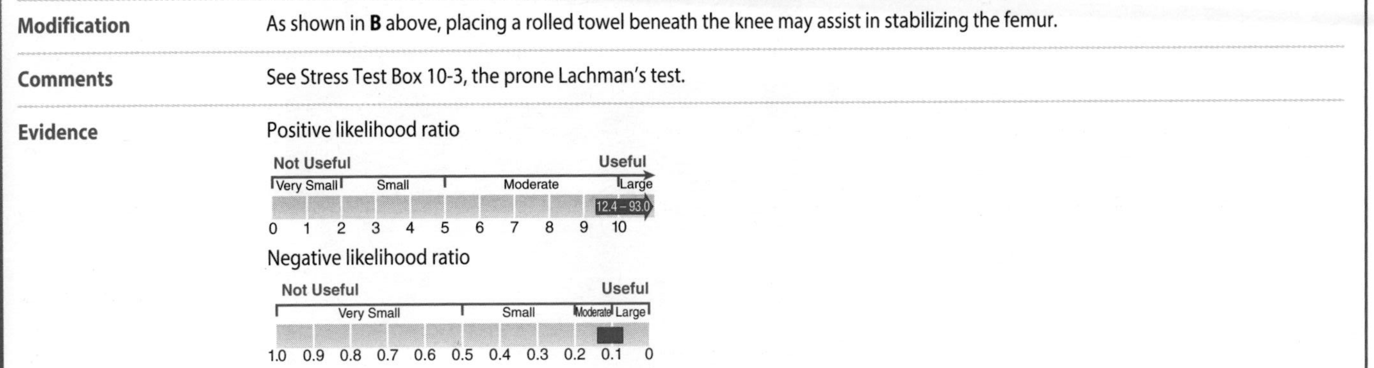

Modification	As shown in **B** above, placing a rolled towel beneath the knee may assist in stabilizing the femur.
Comments	See Stress Test Box 10-3, the prone Lachman's test.
Evidence	Positive likelihood ratio Negative likelihood ratio

ACL = anterior cruciate ligament.

Biomechanics of the Anterior Drawer and Lachman's Tests

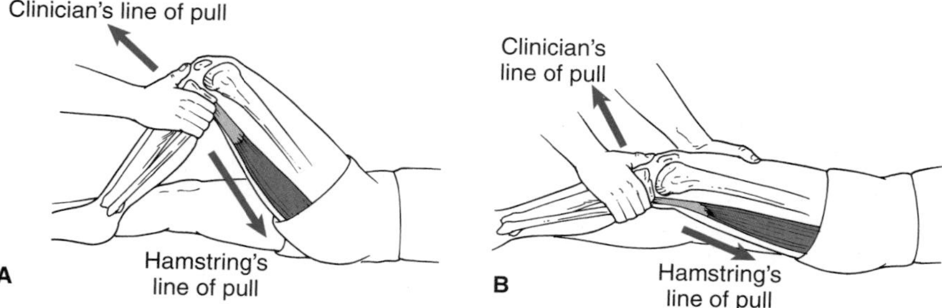

FIGURE 10-3 ■ Biomechanics of the **(A)** anterior drawer test and **(B)** Lachman's test for anterior cruciate laxity. **(A)** During the drawer test contraction of the hamstring group pulls the tibia posteriorly, the direction opposite the line of pull, potentially masking a positive result. **(B)** The joint position used during the Lachman's test (20° of flexion) alters the hamstring's force vector, thereby reducing the possibility of a false-negative result.

Modifications of the Lachman's Test

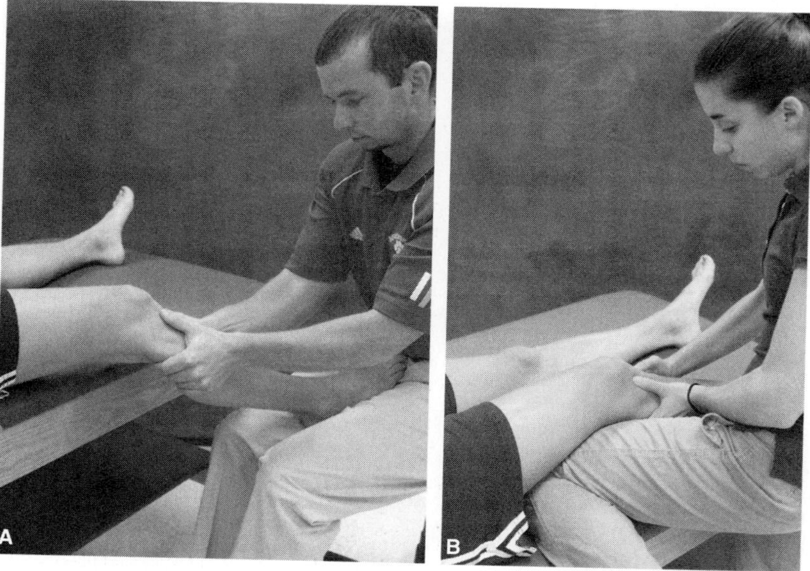

FIGURE 10-4 ■ **(A, B)** Modifications of the Lachman's test.

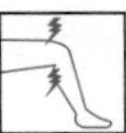

Stress Test 10-3
Prone Lachman's Test

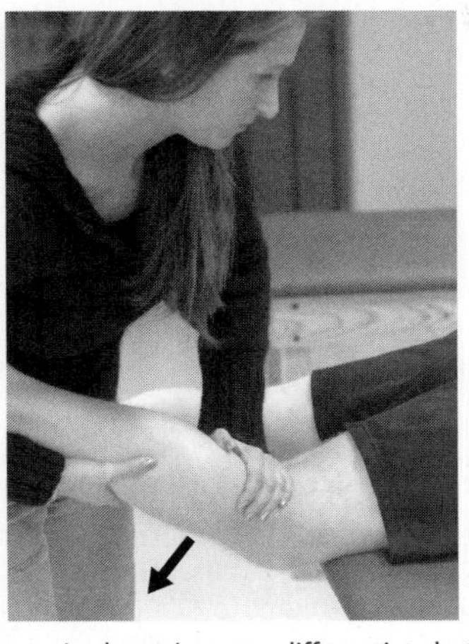

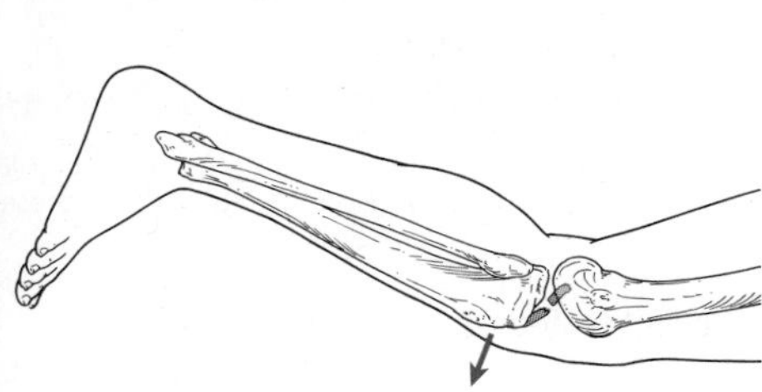

Prone Lachman's test to differentiate between anterior tibial glide caused by ACL versus PCL laxity and may be easier to perform than the Lachman's test for individuals with small hands or patients with large legs.

Patient Position	Prone, with the leg hanging off the end of the table. The knee passively flexed to 30°
Position of Examiner	One hand is placed over the posterior aspect of the proximal leg. The opposite hand supports the leg.
Evaluative Procedure	A downward pressure is placed on the proximal portion of the posterior tibia as the examiner notes any anterior tibial displacement.
Positive Test	Excessive anterior translation relative to the uninvolved knee indicates a sprain of the ACL.
Implications	Positive test results found in the anterior drawer and/or Lachman's test and in the alternate Lachman's test indicate a sprain of the ACL. A positive anterior drawer test and/or Lachman's test result and a negative alternate Lachman's test result implicate a sprain in the PCL.
Evidence	Inconclusive or absent in the literature

ACL = anterior cruciate ligament; PCL = posterior cruciate ligament.

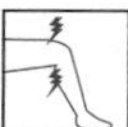

Stress Test 10-4
Posterior Drawer Test for Posterior Cruciate Ligament Laxity

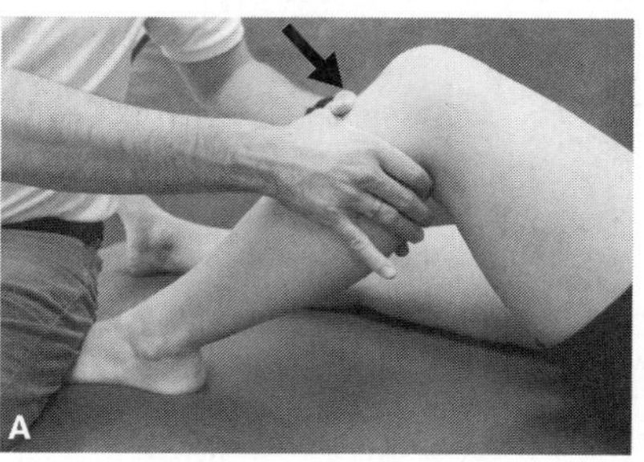

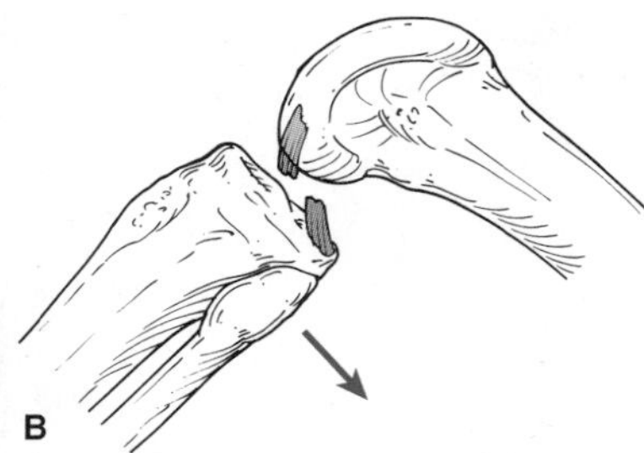

Posterior drawer test for PCL instability. **(A)** The tibia is moved posteriorly relative to the femur. **(B)** Translation of the tibia on the femur in the presence of a PCL tear. The posterior drawer test is also used to assess posterior joint play.

Patient Position	Lying supine The hip flexed to 45° and the knee flexed to 90°
Position of Examiner	Sitting on the examination table in front of the involved knee The patient's tibia stabilized in the neutral position
Evaluative Procedure	The examiner grasps the tibia just below the joint line of the knee with the fingers placed along the joint line on either side of the patellar tendon. The proximal tibia is pushed posteriorly.
Positive Test	An increased amount of posterior tibial translation compared with the opposite (uninvolved) limb or the lack of a firm end-point
Implications	A sprain of the PCL
Modification	To identify injury to the posterolateral corner of the knee, perform the posterior drawer test at 30° of flexion. The drawer test may also be performed with the tibia internally and externally rotated. In isolated PCL tears there will be decreased tibial translation with the tibia internally rotated.[53]
Comments	Increased posterior translation relative to the uninvolved knee at 30° but not at 90° implicates injury to the posterolateral corner. Increased posterior translation relative to the uninvolved knee at 30° and at 90° indicates injury to the PCL.[54]
Evidence	Inconclusive or absent in the literature

PCL = posterior cruciate ligament.

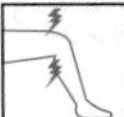

Stress Test 10-5
Godfrey's Test for Posterior Cruciate Ligament Laxity

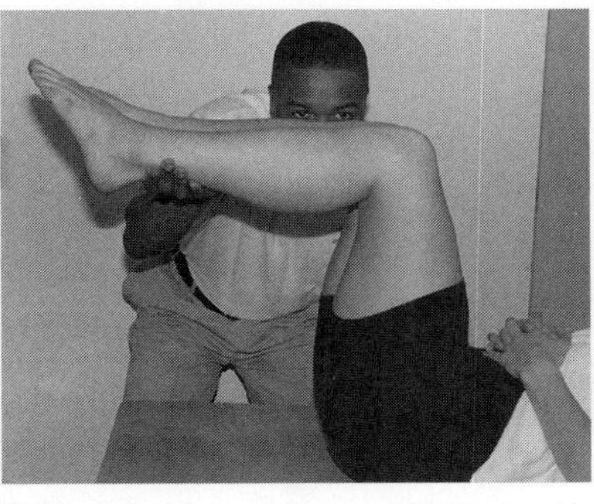

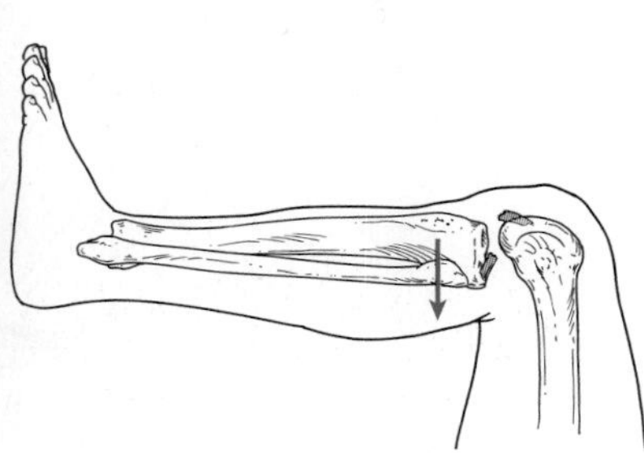

Godfrey's test for posterior cruciate ligament laxity. Note the downward displacement of the left (facing) tibia.

Patient Position	Lying supine with the knees extended and legs together
Position of Examiner	Standing next to the patient
Evaluative Procedure	Lift the patient's lower legs and hold them parallel to the table so that the knees are flexed to 90°. Observe the level of the tibial tuberosities.
Positive Test	A unilateral posterior (downward) displacement of the tibial tuberosity
Implications	A sprain of the PCL
Modification	A straight-edge (such as a ruler) can be placed between the patella and tibia to better visualize the posterior sag.
Comments	The lower leg must be stabilized as distally as possible; supporting the tibia proximally prevents it from sagging posteriorly. An assistant may be used to hold the distal legs.
Evidence	Inconclusive or absent in the literature

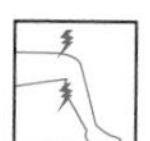

Stress Test 10-6
Valgus Stress Test for Medial Collateral Ligament Laxity

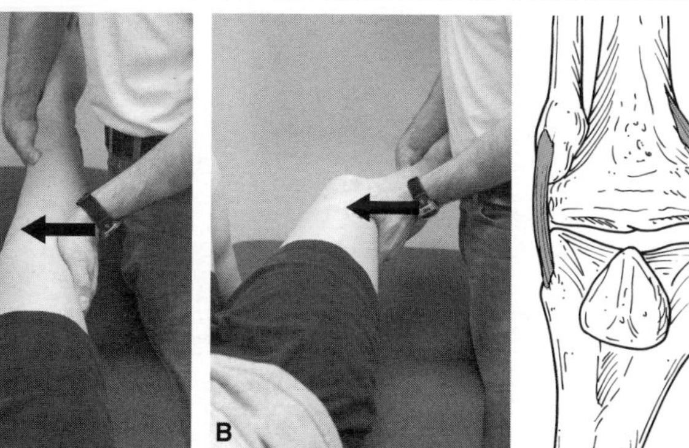

Valgus stress test **(A)** in full extension to determine the integrity of medial capsular restraints and cruciate ligaments, **(B)** with the knee flexed to 25° to isolate the medial collateral ligament, and **(C)** schematic representation of the opening of the medial joint line.

Patient Position	Lying supine with the involved leg close to the edge of the table
Position of Examiner	Standing lateral to the involved limb One hand supports the medial portion of the distal tibia while the other hand grasps the knee along the lateral joint line. To test the entire medial joint capsule and other medial restraining structures, the knee is kept in complete extension. To isolate the MCL, the knee is flexed to 25°.
Evaluative Procedure	A medial (valgus) force is applied to the knee while the distal tibia is moved laterally.

Positive Test	Increased laxity, decreased quality of the end-point, and/or pain compared with the uninvolved limb
Implications	In complete extension: A sprain of the MCL, medial joint capsule, and possibly the cruciate ligaments, distal femoral epiphyseal fracture In 25° flexion: A sprain of the MCL
Modification	To promote relaxation of the patient's musculature, the thigh may rest on the table with the knee flexed over the side edge of the table.[55] The patient's leg may be held against the clinician's torso to improve the amount of stress applied to the MCL.
Comments	When testing the knee in full extension, it is recommended that the thigh be left on the table, preventing shortening of the hamstring muscle group. The apprehension test (see Chapter 11) should be performed before valgus stress testing in patients who have a history of patellar dislocations or subluxations.
Evidence	Inconclusive or absent in the literature

MCL = medial collateral ligament.

Stress Test 10-7
Varus Stress Test for Lateral Collateral Ligament Laxity

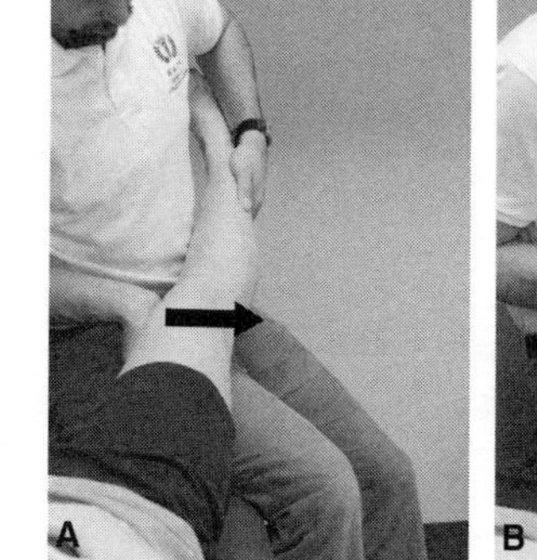
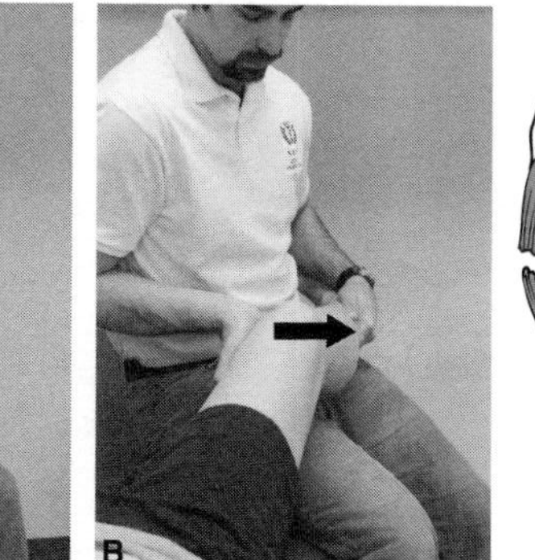

Varus stress test **(A)** in full extension to determine the integrity of lateral capsular restraints, **(B)** with the knee flexed to 25°–30° to isolate the lateral collateral ligament, and **(C)** schematic representation of the opening of the medial joint line.

Patient Position	Lying supine with the involved leg close to the edge of the table
Position of Examiner	Sitting on the table One hand supports the lateral portion of the distal tibia, while the other hand grasps the knee along the medial joint line. To test the entire lateral joint capsule and other lateral restraining structures, the knee is kept in complete extension. To isolate the LCL, the knee is flexed to 25°.
Evaluative Procedure	A lateral (varus) force is applied to the knee while the distal tibia is moved inward.

Positive Test	Increased laxity, decreased quality of the end-point, and/or pain compared with the uninvolved limb
Implications	In complete extension: A sprain of the LCL, lateral joint capsule, cruciate ligaments, and related structures, indicating possible rotatory instability of the joint, distal femoral epiphyseal fracture In 25° of flexion: A sprain of the LCL
Modification	The patient is supine. The examiner is standing to allow the patient's abducted thigh to rest on the table for improved stabilization and relaxation during the varus stress.
Comments	Avoid hip external rotation during the maneuver. The varus force must be applied perpendicular to the ligament in both testing positions.
Evidence	Inconclusive or absent in the literature

LCL = lateral collateral ligament.

Special Test 10-2
Sweep Test for Intracapsular Swelling/Effusion

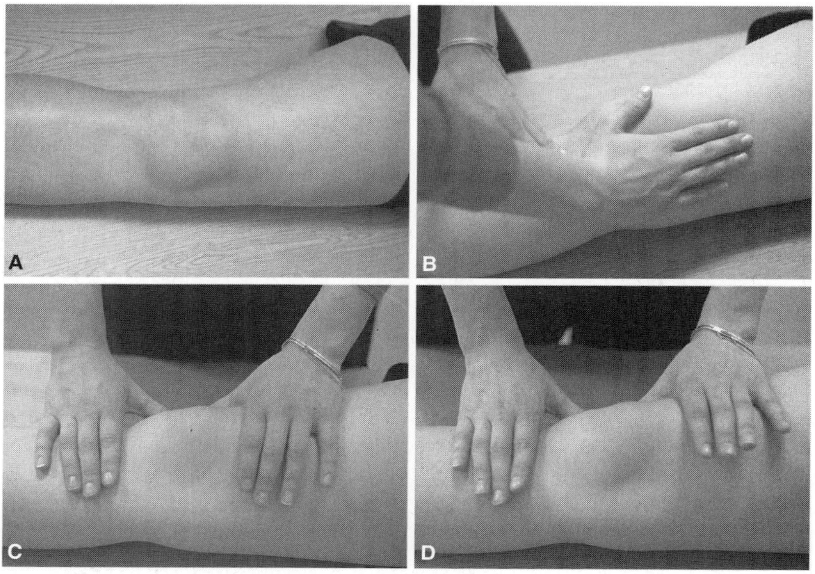

A B C D

Sweep test to determine the presence of intracapsular swelling.

Patient Position	Lying supine with the knee extended
Position of Examiner	Standing lateral to the patient
Evaluative Procedure	Assuming that the fluid is on the medial side of the knee **(A):** **(B)** The edema is stroked ("milked") proximally and laterally. **(C)** The normal contour of the knee is restored. **(D)** When pressure is applied on the lateral aspect of the knee, a fluid bulge immediately appears on the medial aspect.
Positive Test	Reformation of edema on the medial side of the knee when pressure is applied to the lateral aspect
Implications	Swelling within the joint capsule, indicating possible anterior cruciate ligament trauma, osteochondral fracture, synovitis, meniscal lesion, or patellar dislocation
Modification	If swelling is more prevalent on the lateral aspect of the knee, the steps are performed on the lateral side of the knee joint.
Evidence	Inconclusive or absent in the literature

Special Test 10-3
Ballotable Patella

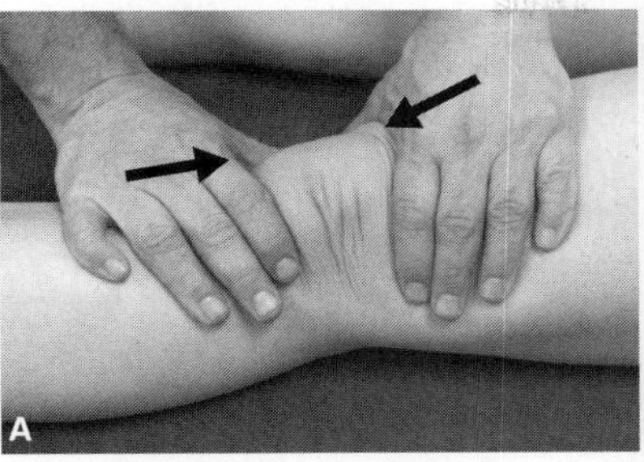

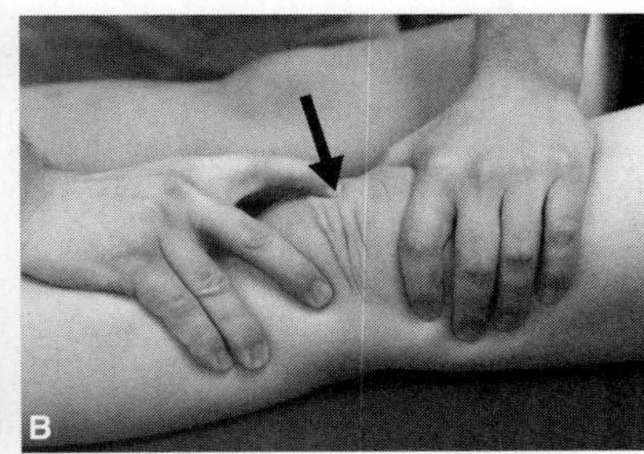

Excess fluid is manually moved inferior to the patella. In the presence of knee effusion, the patella will "float" over the femoral trochlea when the knee is extended.

Patient Position	Supine The knee is extended and the quadriceps are relaxed.
Position of Examiner	Standing to the side being tested
Evaluative Procedure	**(A)** The superior hand pushes any fluid in the superior portion of the knee inferiorly toward the patella. The opposite hand pushes any fluid in the inferior portion of the knee superiorly toward the patella. **(B)** A finger is used to press the patella down towards the patellar groove.
Positive Test	The patella fails to "bounce back" after being depressed.
Implications	Effusion within the joint capsule
Comments	Knee effusions, especially those of rapid onset, are associated with fractures or cruciate ligament sprains.
Evidence	Inconclusive or absent in the literature

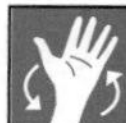

Special Test 10-4
Quadriceps Active Test

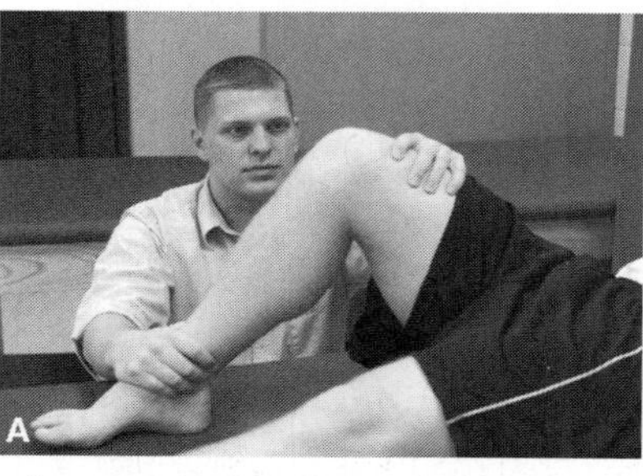

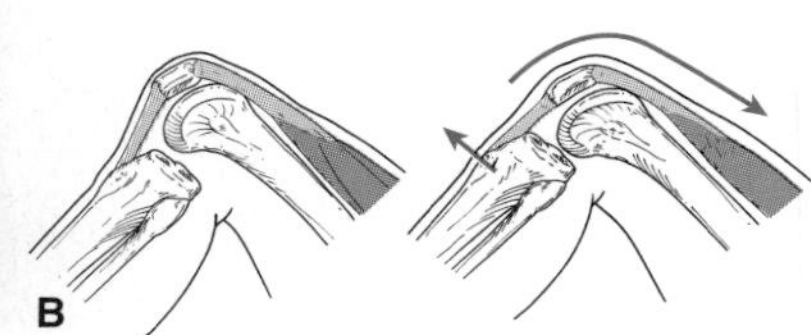

In the presence of a posterior tibial sag, contraction of the quadriceps muscle group will cause the tibia to shift back to its normal resting position.

Patient Position	Lying supine with the knee flexed to 90°
Position of Examiner	At the side of the patient One hand stabilizes the distal tibia and the opposite hand stabilizes the distal femur.
Evaluative Procedure	**(A)** While resisting knee extension the patient is asked to slide the foot forward by contracting the quadriceps. The examiner observes for anterior translation of the tibia.
Positive Test	Anterior translation of the tibia on the femur **(B)**
Implications	Grade II or III PCL sprain[56]
Comments	Interpretation of the results of this test is more accurate in the presence of higher-grade or chronic PCL lesions.[56]
Evidence	Inconclusive or absent in the literature

PCL = posterior cruciate ligament.

Special Test 10-5
Slocum Drawer Test for Rotational Knee Instability

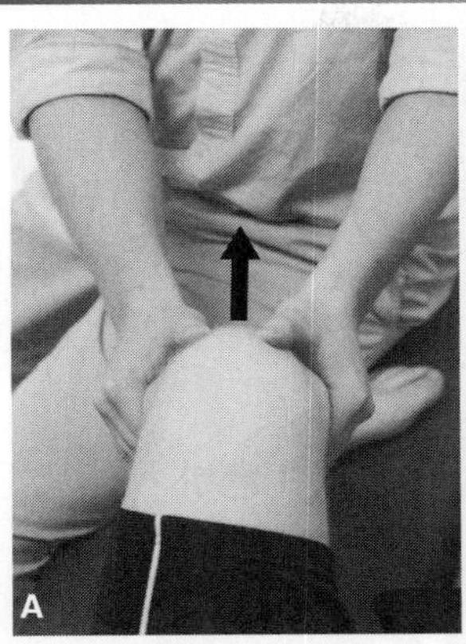

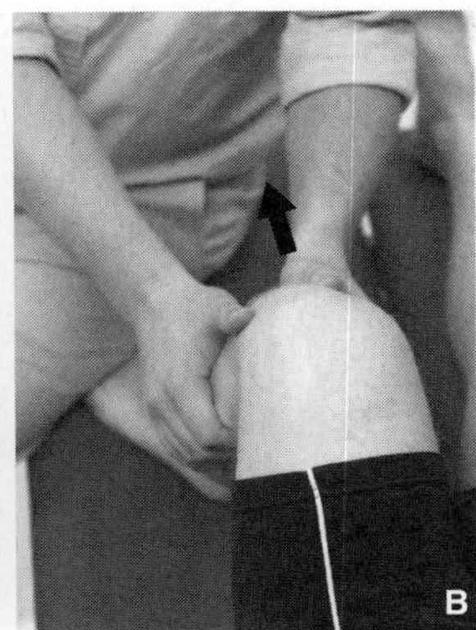

Slocum drawer test with the tibia internally rotated to isolate the lateral capsular structures **(A)** and with the tibia externally rotated to isolate the medial capsule **(B)**.

Patient Position	Lying supine with the knee flexed to 90°
Position of Examiner	Sitting on the patient's foot: **(A)** The tibia is internally rotated to 25° to test for anterolateral capsular instability. **(B)** The tibia is externally rotated to 15° to test for anteromedial capsular instability.
Evaluative Procedure	The tibia is drawn anteriorly.
Positive Test	An increased amount of anterior tibial translation compared with the opposite (uninvolved) limb or the lack of a firm end-point
Implications	**(A)** Test for anterolateral instability: Damage to the ACL, anterolateral capsule, LCL, IT band, popliteus tendon, posterolateral complex, lateral meniscus **(B)** Test for anteromedial instability: Damage to the MCL, anteromedial capsule, ACL, posteromedial capsule, pes anserine, medial meniscus
Comments	Excessive tibial rotation can cause a false-negative test due to wedging of the menisci in the joint space.
Evidence	Inconclusive or absent in the literature

ACL = anterior cruciate ligament; IT = iliotibial; LCL = lateral collateral ligament; MCL = medial collateral ligament.

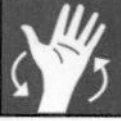

Special Test 10-6
Crossover Test for Rotational Knee Instability

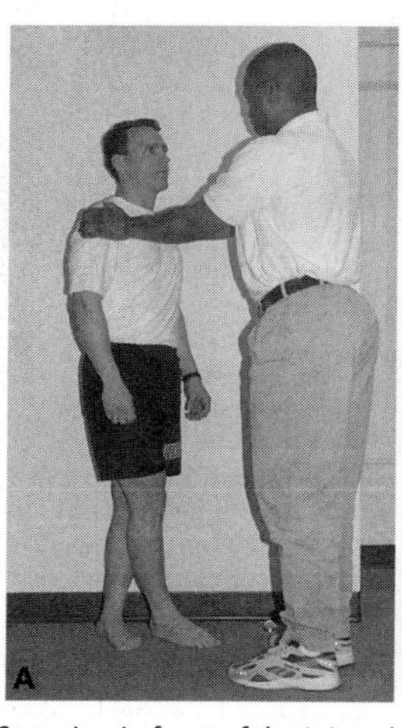

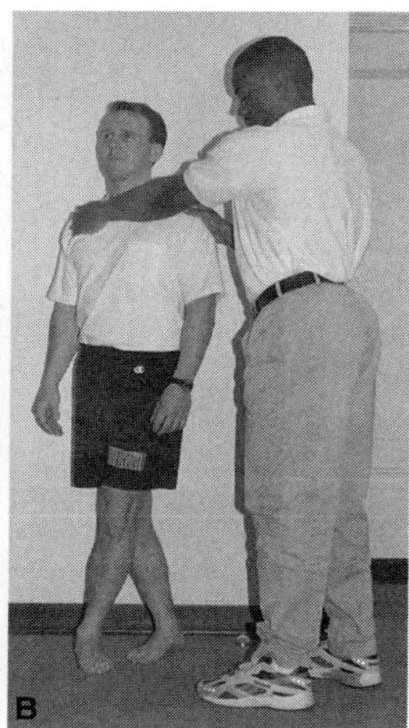

Crossover test: Stepping in front of the injured leg determines the presence of anterolateral rotatory instability **(A)**. Stepping behind the injured leg determines anteromedial rotatory instability **(B)**. Note that patient's left leg is being tested.

Patient Position	Standing with the weight on the involved limb
Position of Examiner	Standing in front of the patient
Evaluative Procedure	**(A) ALRI:** The patient steps across and in front with the uninvolved leg, rotating the torso in the direction of movement. The weight-bearing foot remains fixated. **(B) AMRI:** The patient steps across and behind with the uninvolved leg rotating the torso in the direction of movement. The weight-bearing foot remains fixated.
Positive Test	Patient reports pain, instability, or apprehension.
Implications	**(A) ALRI:** Instability of the lateral capsular restraints **(B) AMRI:** Instability of the medial capsular restraints
Comments	This test can be used as a prelude to assessing the patient's ability to perform a more functional cutting maneuver.
Evidence	Inconclusive or absent in the literature

ALRI = anterolateral rotatory instability; AMRI = anteromedial rotatory instability.

Special Test 10-7
Pivot Shift Test for Anterolateral Knee Instability Jerk Test

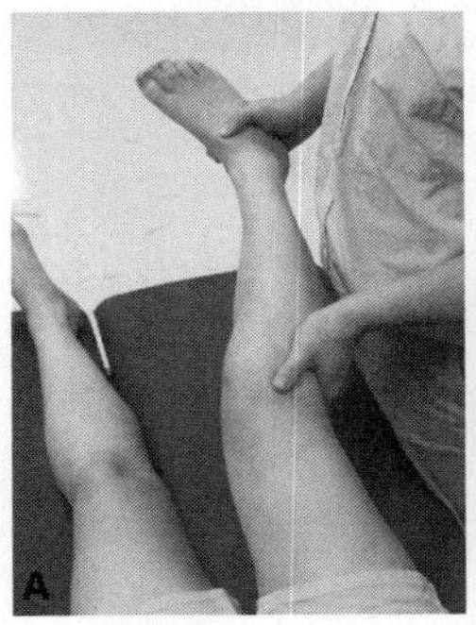

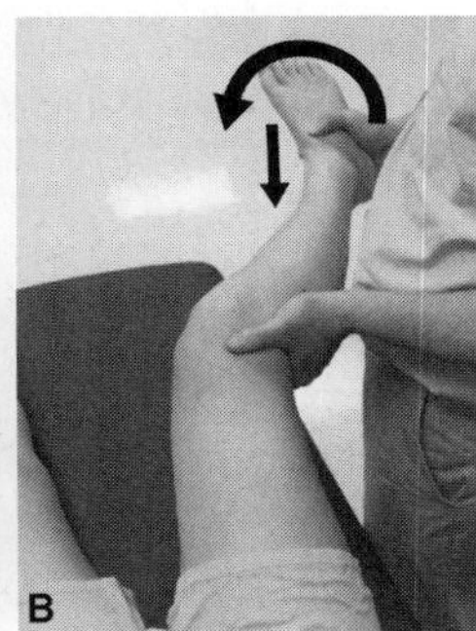

When positive, the pivot shift test (lateral pivot shift) reproduces the subluxation/reduction of the tibia on the femur experienced during gait.

Patient Position	Lying supine with the hip passively flexed to 30°
Position of Examiner	Standing lateral to the patient, the distal lower leg and/or ankle is grasped, maintaining 20° of internal tibial rotation. The knee is allowed to sag into complete extension **(A)**. The opposite hand grasps the lateral portion of the leg at the level of the superior tibiofibular joint, increasing the force of internal rotation.
Evaluative Procedure	While maintaining internal rotation, a valgus force is applied to the knee while it is slowly flexed **(B)**. To avoid masking any positive test results, the patient must remain relaxed throughout this test.
Positive Test	The tibia's position on the femur reduces as the leg is flexed in the range of 30°–40°. During extension in the jerk test, the anterior subluxation is felt in the same range.
Implications	ACL, anterolateral capsule, LCL, biceps femoris, lateral meniscus, popliteus, posterolateral capsule
Modification	The jerk test is a modification of the lateral pivot shift test: The patient's hip is flexed to 45° and the knee flexed to 90°. A valgus and internal rotation force is applied as the knee is extended.
Comments	Meniscal involvement may limit ROM to produce a false-negative test result. Muscle guarding can produce a false-negative result. This test is most reliable when performed while the patient is under anesthesia.
Evidence	Positive likelihood ratio Not Useful — Useful Very Small / Small / Moderate / Large 93.0 0 1 2 3 4 5 6 7 8 9 10 Negative likelihood ratio Not Useful — Useful Very Small / Small / Moderate / Large 1.0 0.9 0.8 0.7 0.6 0.5 0.4 0.3 0.2 0.1 0

ACL = anterior cruciate ligament; LCL = lateral collateral ligament; ROM = range of motion.

Special Test 10-8
Slocum Anterolateral Rotatory Instability (ALRI) Test

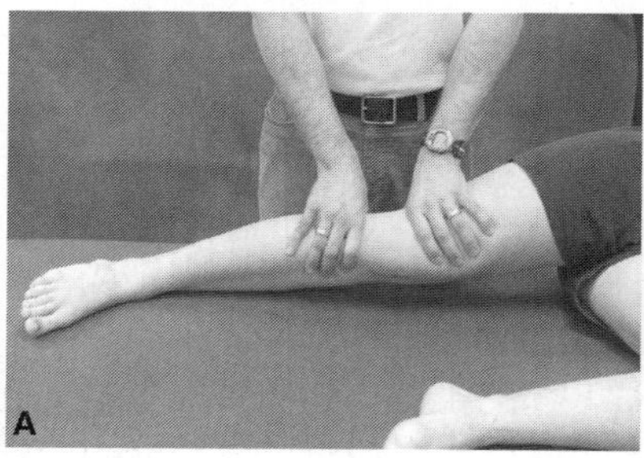

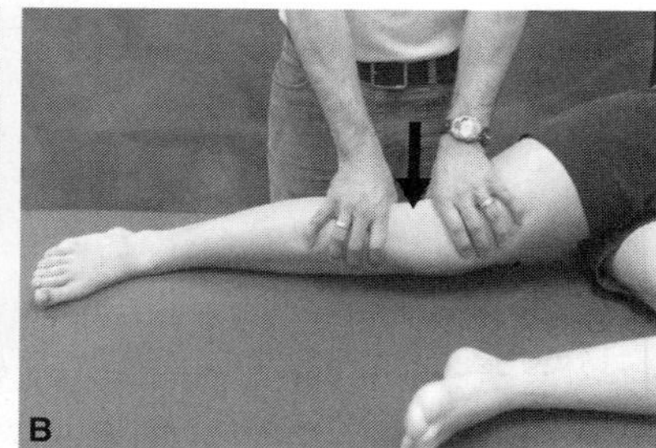

A modification of the valgus stress test, the Slocum ALRI accentuates the amount of internal tibial rotation, causing the tibial plateau to subluxate.

Patient Position	**(A)** Lying on the uninvolved side The uninvolved leg is flexed at the hip and knee, positioning it anterior to the involved extremity. The involved hip is externally rotated. The involved leg is extended with the medial aspect of the foot resting against the table to provide stability.
Position of Examiner	Standing behind the patient, grasping the knee on the distal aspect of the femur and the proximal fibula
Evaluative Procedure	A valgus force is placed on the knee, causing it to move into 30°–50° of flexion **(B)**.
Positive Test	An appreciable "clunk" or instability as the lateral tibial plateau subluxates or pain or instability is reported.
Implications	Tear of the ACL, LCL, anterolateral capsule, arcuate ligament complex, biceps femoris tendon and/or IT band
Comments	Muscle guarding can produce false-negative results. This test should be performed with caution and, if performed, should be done so only at the end of the examination.
Evidence	Inconclusive or absent in the literature

ACL = anterior cruciate ligament; IT = iliotibial; LCL = lateral cruciate ligament.

Special Test 10-9
Flexion–Rotation Drawer Test for Anterolateral Rotatory Instability

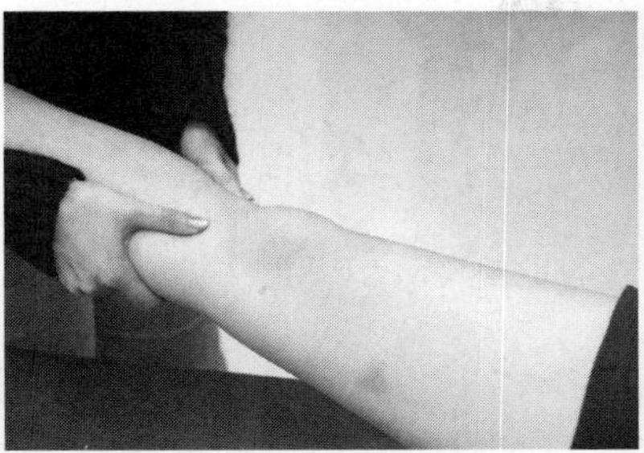

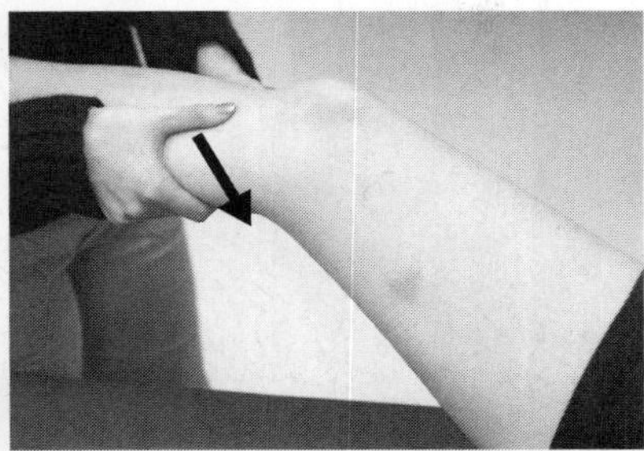

The flexion–rotation drawer replicates the femur relocating itself on the tibia as seen in a closed kinetic chain.

Patient Position	Lying supine The clinician lifts the calf and ankle so that the knee is flexed to approximately 25°. Heavier patients may require that the tibia be supported between the examiner's arm and torso.
Position of Examiner	Standing lateral and distal to the involved knee
Evaluative Procedure	The tibia is depressed posteriorly to the femur.
Positive Test	The femur is relocating itself on the tibia by moving anteriorly and internally, rotating on the tibia.
Implications	Tears of the ACL, LCL, anterolateral capsule, arcuate ligament complex, and/or biceps femoris tendon.
Modification	A valgus stress and axial compression along the tibial shaft can be applied as the knee is slowly flexed.
Evidence	Inconclusive or absent in the literature

ACL = anterior cruciate ligament; LCL = lateral cruciate ligament.

Special Test 10-10
External Rotation Test (Dial Test) for Posterolateral Knee Instability

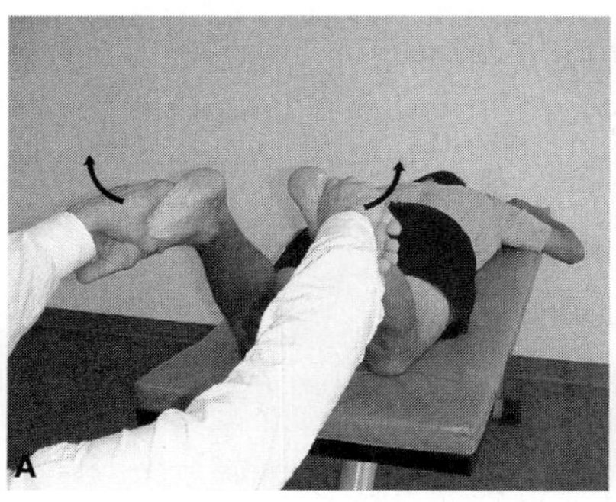

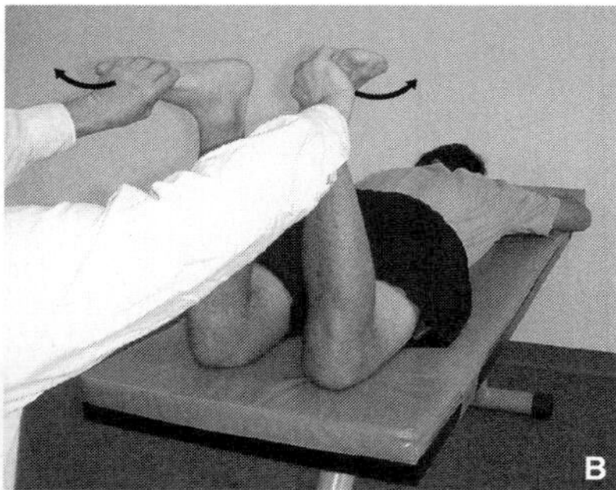

The external rotation test (Dial test) for posterolateral knee instability at 30° of the knee flexion **(A)** and at 90° of knee flexion **(B)**.

Patient Position	Prone or supine
Position of Examiner	Standing at the patient's feet
Evaluative Procedure	The knee is flexed to 30°. Using the medial border of the foot as a point of reference, the examiner forcefully externally rotates the patient's lower leg. The position of external rotation of the foot relative to the femur is assessed and compared with the opposite extremity. The knee is then flexed to 90° and the test repeated. Care must be taken to keep the knees together during the examination.[57]
Positive Test	An increase of external rotation greater than 10° compared with the opposite side[58,59]
Implications	Difference at 30° of knee flexion but not at 90°: Injury isolated to the posterolateral corner of the knee Difference at 30° and 90° of knee flexion: Trauma to the PCL, posterolateral knee structures, and the posterolateral corner Difference at 90° of knee flexion but not at 30°: Isolated PCL sprain
Modification	This test can also be performed with the patient in the supine position. A goniometer can be used to quantify the amount of external rotation.[54]
Comments	Normal variations for rotation are expected. The results of one extremity must be compared with those of the opposite leg.
Evidence	Inconclusive or absent in the literature

PCL = posterior cruciate ligament.

Special Test 10-11
External Rotation Recurvatum Test

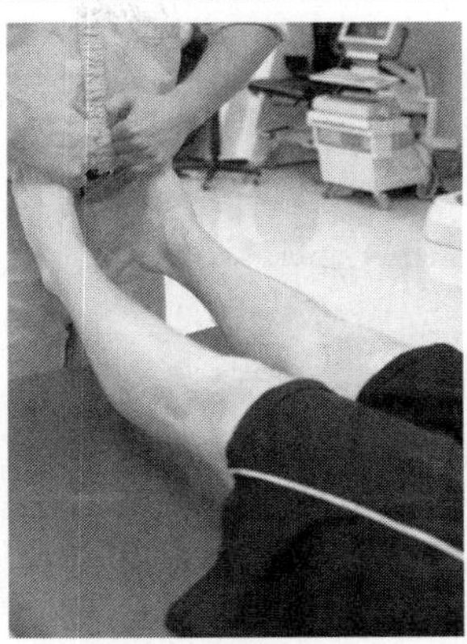

This test is a gross evaluation of the amount of external femoral rotation that occurs when the knees are hyperextended.[60]

Patient Position	Lying supine.
Position of Examiner	Standing at the patient's feet grasping the great toes/distal midfeet.
Evaluative Procedure	The examiner lifts the patient's legs approximately 12 inches off the table. Observe the bilateral alignment of the two knees.
Positive Test	A marked difference in hyperextension, external femoral rotation, and varus alignment between the two knees
Implications	Posterolateral corner trauma PCL sprain Posterolateral rotatory instability
Modification	While holding the heel, the examiner flexes the knee 40°. The opposite hand grasps the posterolateral aspect of the knee. The examiner passively extends the knee while noting external rotation and hyperextension relative to the opposite extremity.
Evidence	Positive likelihood ratio Not Useful — Useful Very Small, Small, Moderate, Large 30 0 1 2 3 4 5 6 7 8 9 10 Negative likelihood ratio Not Useful — Useful Very Small, Small, Moderate, Large 1.0 0.9 0.8 0.7 0.6 0.5 0.4 0.3 0.2 0.1 0

PCL = posterior cruciate ligament.

Special Test 10-12
Posterolateral/Posteromedial Drawer Test

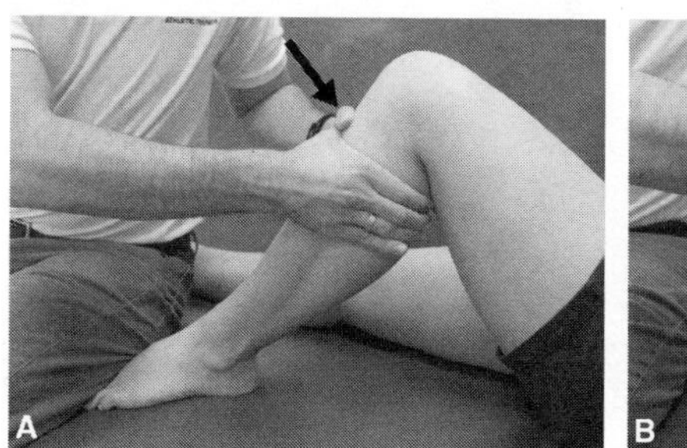

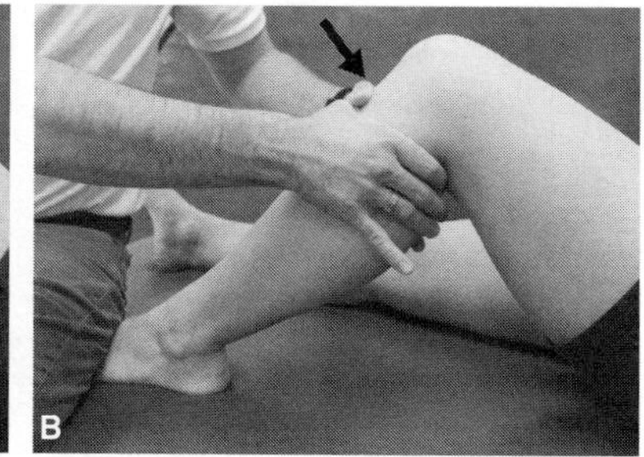

A modification of the posterior drawer test to identify lesions to the posterolateral corner of the knee.[60]

Patient Position	Supine with the hip flexed to 45° and the knee flexed to 80° **(A)** The tibia is externally rotated 15° (posterolateral test). **(B)** The tibia is internally rotated 15° (posteromedial test).
Position of Examiner	Sitting on the foot of the limb being tested. The hands grasp the proximal tibia.
Evaluative Procedure	A posterior force is applied to the proximal tibia.
Positive Test	Increased external rotation of the lateral (posterolateral) or medial (posteromedial) tibial condyle relative to the lateral femoral condyle relative to the uninvolved side

Implications	**(A)** Tibia externally rotated 15° (posterolateral test) Trauma to the posterolateral corner and PCL Possible posterolateral rotatory instability **(B)** Tibia internally rotated 15° (posteromedial test) PCL tear, oblique ligament, MCL, posteromedial capsule, semimembranosus
Modification	The posterolateral drawer test is sometimes performed with the knee flexed to 90°. This test can be performed with the patient sitting with the knees off the edge of the table.
Comments	Excessive tibial rotation can produce false-negative results, especially in the presence of a meniscal tear.
Evidence	***Posterolateral drawer test:*** Inconclusive or absent in the literature ***Posteromedial drawer test:*** Inconclusive or absent in the literature

MCL = medial collateral ligament; PCL = posterior cruciate ligament.

Special Test 10-13
Reverse Pivot-Shift Test

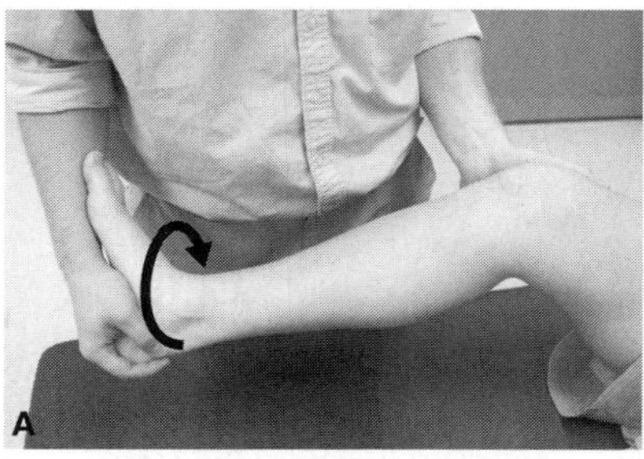

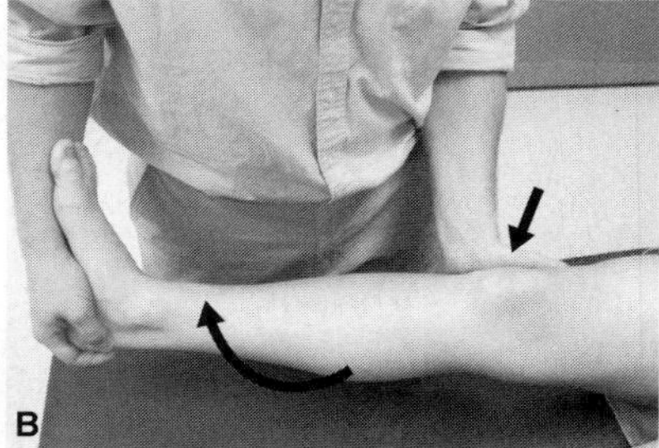

The reverse pivot-shift test is used to identify trauma to the PCL or posterolateral corner of the knee.[58]

Patient Position	Supine
Position of Examiner	Standing to the side of the involved leg
Evaluative Procedure	**(A)** The examiner flexes the knee and externally rotates the tibia of the involved leg. **(B)** The patient's knee is passively extended while a valgus stress is applied to the knee.
Positive Test	Appreciable reduction ("clunk") of the tibia on the femur
Implications	Posterolateral rotatory instability and/or trauma to the posterolateral corner
Comments	This test may be positive in 35% of knees examined under anesthesia.[58,61]
Evidence	Inconclusive or absent in the literature

PCL = posterior cruciate ligament.

Special Test 10-14
Dynamic Posterior Shift Test

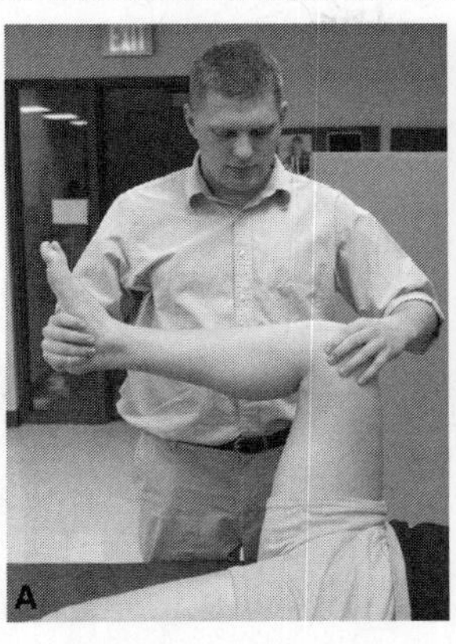

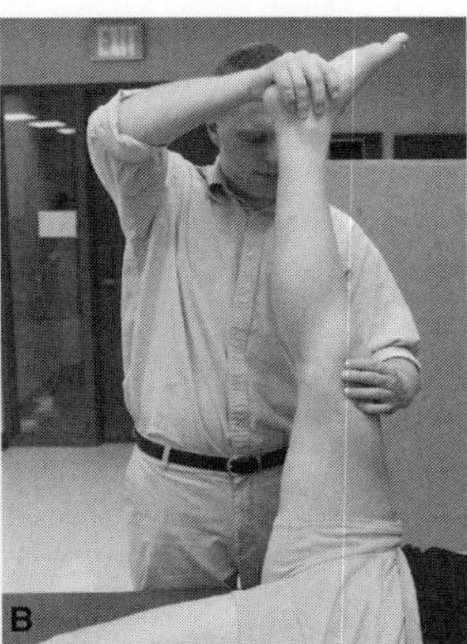

In the presence of posterolateral instability, the lateral tibial plateau is subluxed during knee flexion and reduces during knee extension.[58]

Patient Position	Supine
Position of Examiner	Standing on the side being tested
Evaluative Procedure	**(A)** The examiner passively flexes the patient's hip and knee to 90°. **(B)** The knee is then passively extended.
Positive Test	A "clunk" or "jerk" as the knee nears full extension, representing the subluxated tibia reducing on the femur
Implications	Posterolateral instability
Comments	During knee flexion, the tibia is posteriorly subluxated on the femur. Relocation is noted by an appreciable clunk during extension.[56]
Evidence	Inconclusive or absent in the literature

Special Test 10-15
McMurray's Test for Meniscal Lesions

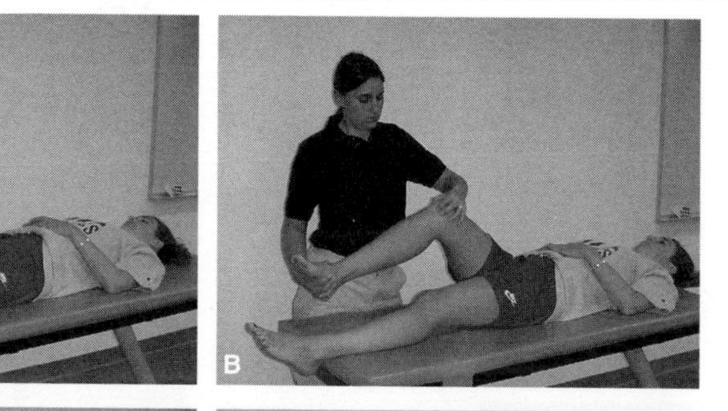
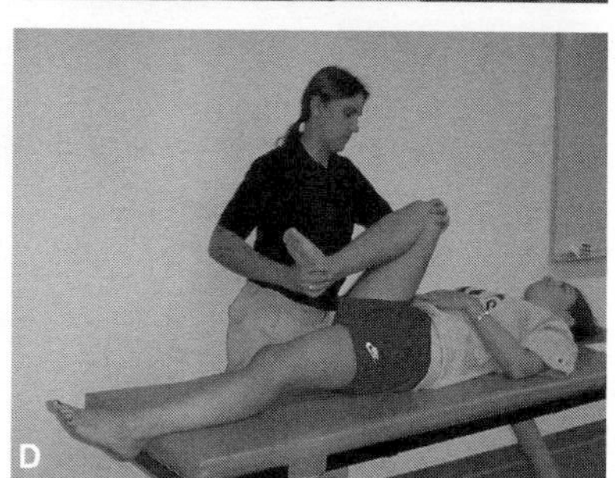
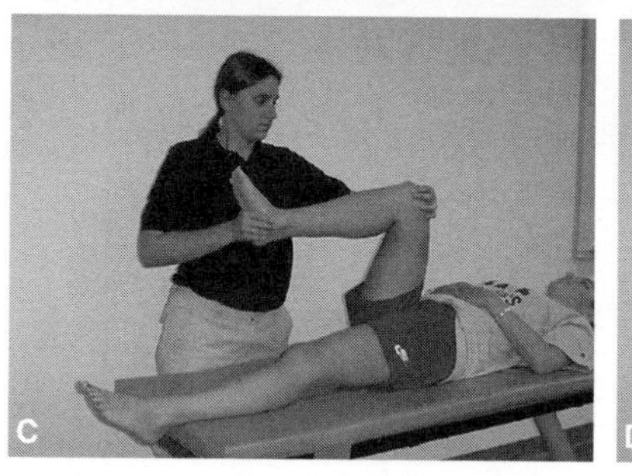
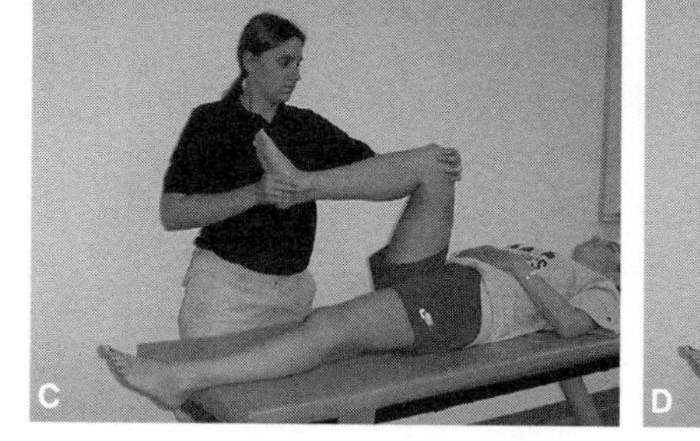

The McMurray's test aims to impinge the meniscus, especially the posterior and anterior horns, between the tibia and femur.

Patient Position	Lying supine
Position of Examiner	Standing lateral and distal to the involved knee One hand supports the lower leg while the thumb and index finger of the opposite hand is positioned in the anteromedial and anterolateral joint line on either side of the patellar tendon **(A)**.

Evaluative Procedure	**(B) Pass one:** With the tibia maintained in its neutral position, a valgus stress is applied while the knee is flexed through its available ROM. A varus stress is then applied as the knee is returned to full extension. **(C) Pass two:** The examiner internally rotates the tibia and applies a valgus stress while the knee is flexed through its available ROM. A varus stress is then applied as the knee is returned to full extension. **(D) Pass three:** With the tibia externally rotated, the examiner applies a valgus stress while the knee is flexed through its available ROM. A varus stress is then applied as the knee is returned to full extension.
Positive Test	A popping, clicking, or locking of the knee; pain emanating from the menisci; or a sensation similar to that experienced during ambulation
Implications	A meniscal tear on the side of the reported symptoms
Modification	Multiple modifications have been derived from the original test, including variations of additional varus and valgus stress and internally and externally rotating the tibia.
Comments	In acute injuries, the available ROM may not be sufficient to perform this test. Full flexion is required to isolate the posterior horns of the meniscus. Chondromalacia patellae or improper tracking of the patella may produce a click resembling that is associated with a meniscal tear, leading to false-positive results. Sensitivity is greater for lateral meniscus tears than the medial meniscus.[61] Different interpretations and methods of performing the test lead to widely varied opinions about the diagnostic usefulness of this test.
Evidence	Positive likelihood ratio Not Useful — Useful Very Small, Small, Moderate, Large 17.3 0 1 2 3 4 5 6 7 8 9 10 Negative likelihood ratio Not Useful — Useful Very Small, Small, Moderate, Large 1.0 0.9 0.8 0.7 0.6 0.5 0.4 0.3 0.2 0.1 0

ROM = range of motion.

Special Test 10-16
Apley's Compression and Distraction Tests for Meniscal Lesions

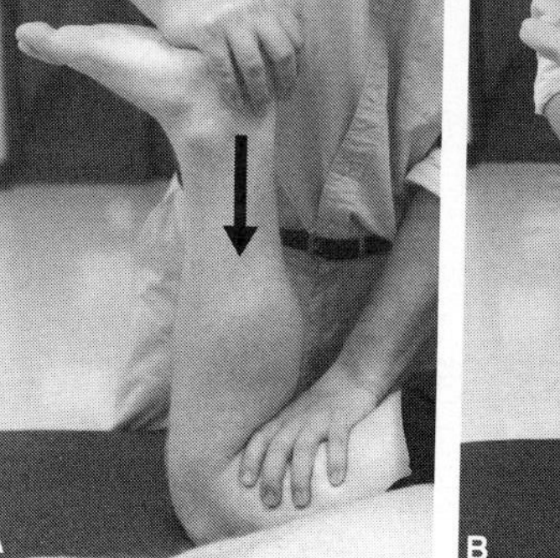

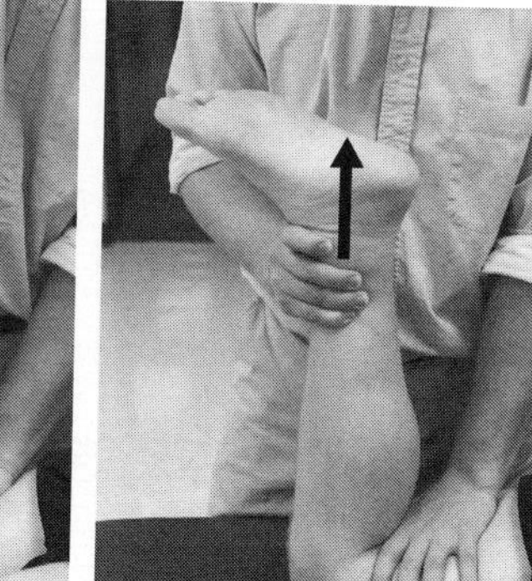

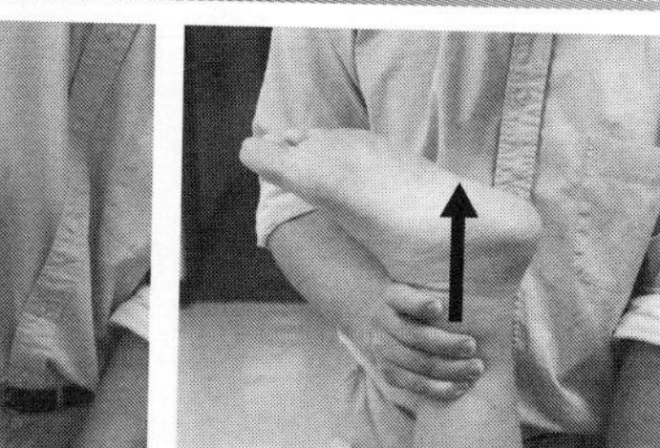

During the compression segment, pain may be caused by the menisci being caught between the tibia and femur **(A)**. During the distraction segment, the joint's ligaments are stressed **(B)**. Also, pain exhibited during compression should be reduced as the tibia is distracted from the femur.

Patient Position	Lying prone with knee flexed to 90°
Position of Examiner	Standing lateral to the involved side
Evaluative Procedure	**(A)** Compression test: The clinician applies pressure to the plantar aspect of the heel, applying an axial load to the tibia while simultaneously internally and externally rotating the tibia. **(B)** Distraction test: The clinician grasps the lower leg and stabilizes the knee proximal to the femoral condyles. The tibia is distracted away from the femur while internally and externally rotating the tibia.

Positive Test	Pain experienced during compression that is reduced or eliminated during distraction
Implications	Meniscal tear
Comments	90° of knee flexion is required to perform this test. Pain that is experienced only during distraction or during both compression and distraction may indicate trauma to the collateral ligaments, joint capsule, or cruciate ligaments.
Evidence	Positive likelihood ratio Not Useful — Useful Very Small · Small · Moderate · Large 58 0 1 2 3 4 5 6 7 8 9 10 Negative likelihood ratio Not Useful — Useful Very Small · Small · Moderate · Large 1.0 0.9 0.8 0.7 0.6 0.5 0.4 0.3 0.2 0.1 0

Special Test 10-17
Thessaly Test for Meniscal Tears

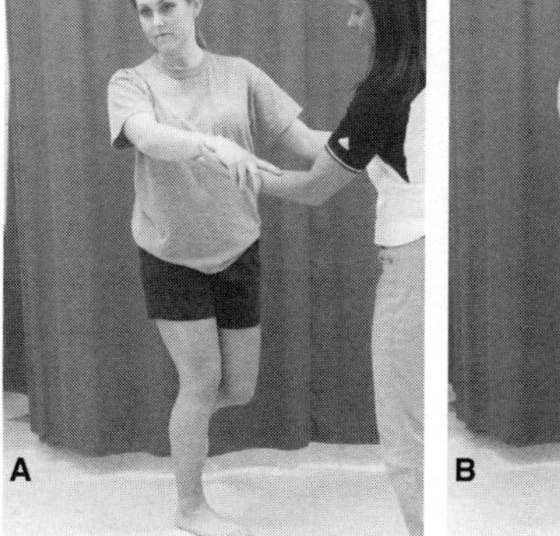

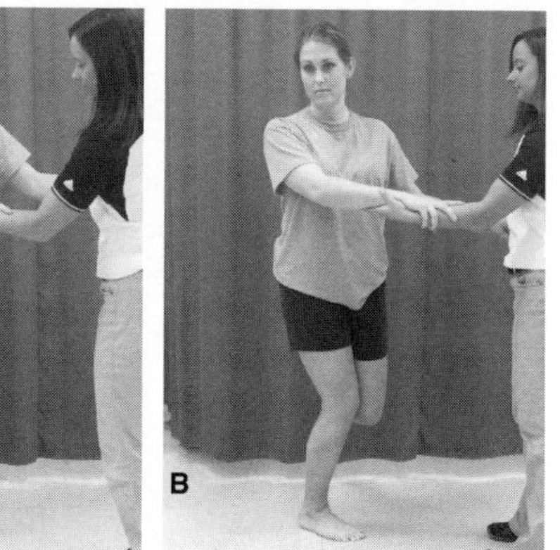

Performed weight-bearing and with femoral internal and external rotation, the Thessaly test is used to identify meniscal lesions. **(A)** The patient rotates on a fixed leg with the knee flexed to 5° and again **(B)** with the knee flexed to 20°.

Patient Position	Standing flatfooted on the involved leg The knee of the opposite leg is flexed to approximately 45°.
Position of Examiner	Standing in front of the patient, supporting the patient's arms

Evaluative Procedure	The uninvolved limb is tested first, allowing the patient to practice the maneuver. **Bout 1** The patient flexes the knee to 5°. The patient rotates the body to internally and externally rotate the femur on the tibia. Repeat three times. **Bout 2** The patient flexes the knee to 20°. The patient rotates the body to internally and externally rotate the femur on the tibia. Repeat three times.
Positive Test	Joint-line discomfort Complaints of "locking" or "catching"
Implications	A lesion of the medial or lateral meniscus, depending on the source of the pain and/or catching sensation
Evidence	Positive likelihood ratio* 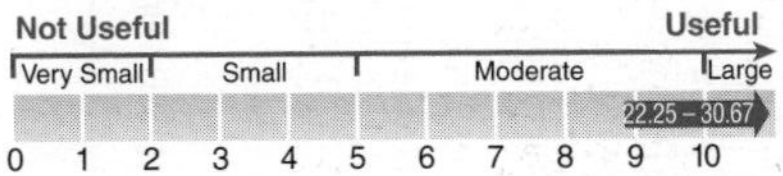 Not Useful — Useful Very Small / Small / Moderate / Large 22.25 – 30.67 0 1 2 3 4 5 6 7 8 9 10 Negative likelihood ratio* 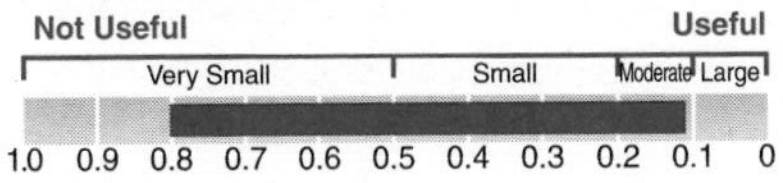 Not Useful — Useful Very Small / Small / Moderate / Large 1.0 0.9 0.8 0.7 0.6 0.5 0.4 0.3 0.2 0.1 0 *20° of flexion

Special Test 10-18
Wilson's Test for Osteochondral Defects of the Knee

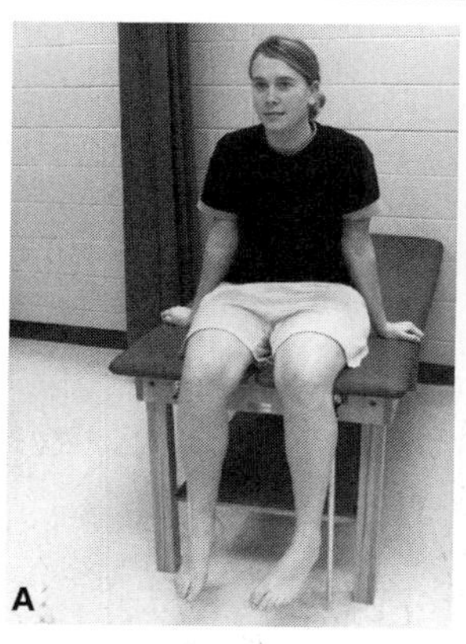

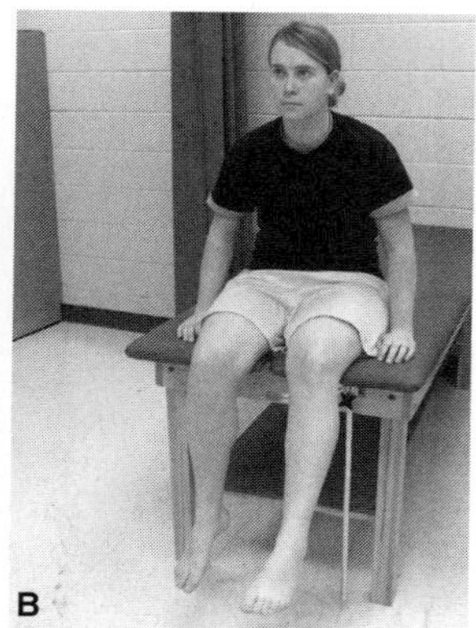

While the tibia is internally rotated, the patient extends the knee **(A)**. When pain is experienced, the patient externally rotates the tibia **(B)**. In the presence of some OCDs, pain is relieved during the external rotation.

Patient Position	Sitting with the knee flexed to 90°
Position of Examiner	In front of the patient to observe any reactions secondary to pain
Evaluative Procedure	**(A)** The patient actively extends the knee while maintaining the tibia in internal rotation. The patient is told to stop the motion and hold the knee in the position in which pain is experienced. **(B)** If pain is experienced, the patient is instructed to externally rotate the tibia while the knee is held at its present point of flexion.
Positive Test	Pain experienced during extension with internal tibial rotation that is relieved by externally rotating the tibia
Implications	OCD or osteochondritis dissecans on the intercondylar area of the medial femoral condyle
Evidence	Inconclusive or absent in the literature

OCD = osteochondral defect.

Special Test 10-19
Noble's Compression Test for Iliotibial Band Friction Syndrome Renne's Test

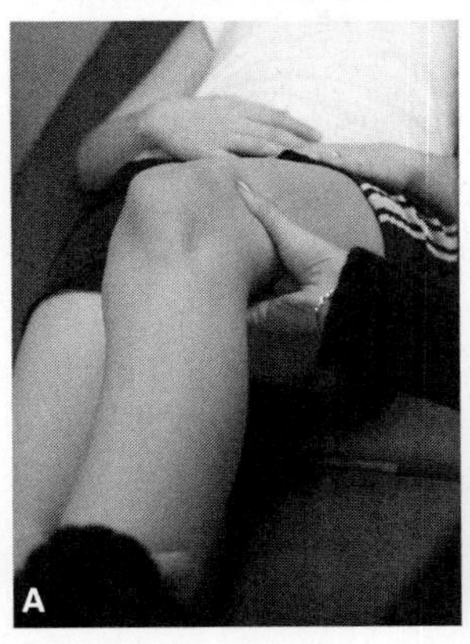

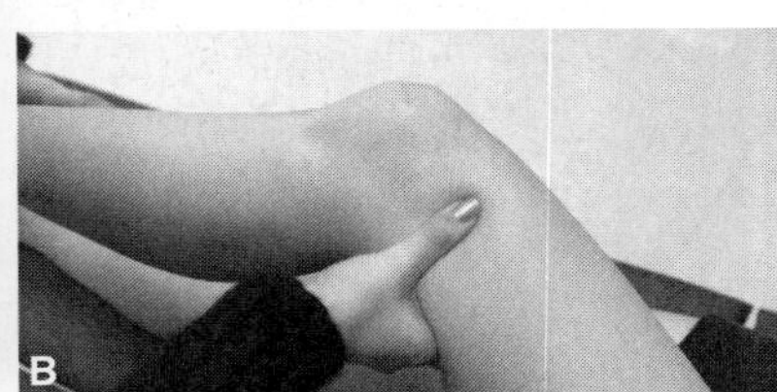

The examiner attempts to compress the distal portion of the IT band against the lateral femoral condyle during passive motion of the knee. In the presence of IT band inflammation, pain will be elicited.

Patient Position	Lying supine with the knee flexed
Position of Examiner	Standing lateral to the side being tested The knee is supported above the joint line with the thumb over or just superior to the lateral femoral condyle **(A)**. The opposite hand controls the lower leg.
Evaluative Procedure	While applying pressure over the lateral femoral condyle, the knee is passively extended and flexed **(B)**.
Positive Test	Pain under the thumb, most commonly as the knee approaches 30°
Implications	Inflammation of the IT band, its associated bursa, or inflammation of the lateral femoral condyle
Modification	Renne's test replicates the mechanics of the Noble compression test, but is performed with the patient standing on the involved leg and flexing the knee. No pressure is applied to the lateral femoral epicondyle.
Evidence	Inconclusive or absent in the literature

IT = iliotibial.

Special Test 10-20
Ober's Test for Iliotibial Band Tightness

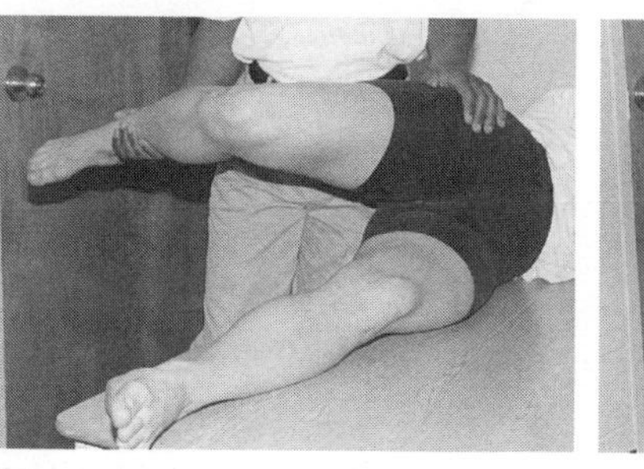

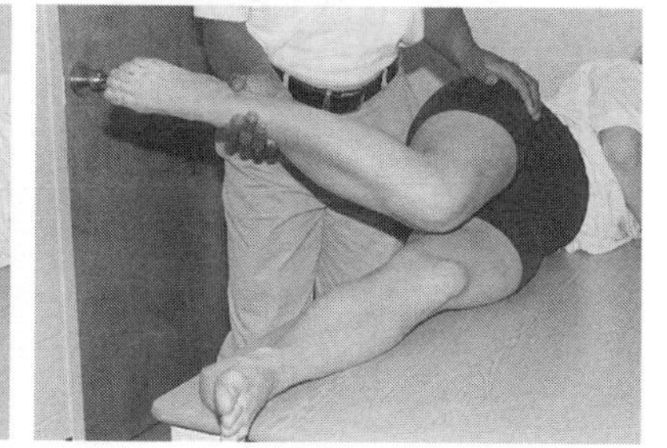

The original Ober's test. To eliminate false-positive test results, the tensor fasciae latae must first clear the greater trochanter. A positive test result occurs when the knee does not adduct past horizontal.

Patient Position	Lying on the side opposite that being tested The opposite hip (the bottom leg) is flexed to 45° and the knee flexed to 90° to stabilize the torso and pelvis. ***Ober's Test:*** The knee of the involved leg is flexed to 90°. ***Modified Ober's Test:*** The knee of the involved leg is extended.
Position of Examiner	Standing behind the patient One hand stabilizes the patient's pelvis. The opposite hand supports the leg being tested along the medial aspect of the distal tibia.
Evaluative Procedure	Passively abduct and extend the patient's hip to allow the tensor fasciae latae to clear the greater trochanter. The hip is then allowed to passively adduct to the table.
Positive Test	Normal: The femur adducts past horizontal. Minimal tightness: The femur adducts to horizontal. Maximal tightness: The leg is unable to adduct to horizontal.

Implications	Tightness of the IT band, predisposing the individual to IT band friction syndrome and/or lateral patellar malalignment
Modification	A goniometer can be used to quantify the results. The proximal arm is aligned with both ASIS and the distal arm is aligned with the midline of the thigh. An inclinometer can be placed over the lateral femoral condyle. If the leg remaining in abduction relative to 0° it is recorded as a negative value. If the leg adducts past 0° it is recorded as a positive value.[62]
Comments	Flexing the knee to 90° can place tension on the femoral nerve (see Femoral Nerve Stretch Test in Chapter 13) and on the medial structures of the knee. Adequate pelvic stabilization (limiting trunk lateral flexion) is important to avoid false-negative results. The modified Ober's test produces less adduction; therefore both tests should be performed.[63]
Evidence	***Ober's test*** Intra-rater reliability: Not Reliable — Very Reliable; Poor / Moderate / Good; 0 0.1 0.2 0.3 0.4 0.5 0.6 0.7 0.8 0.9 1.0 ***Modified Ober's test*** Intra-rater reliability: Not Reliable — Very Reliable; Poor / Moderate / Good; 0 0.1 0.2 0.3 0.4 0.5 0.6 0.7 0.8 0.9 1.0

ASIS = anterior superior iliac spine; IT = iliotibial.

Neurologic Assessment

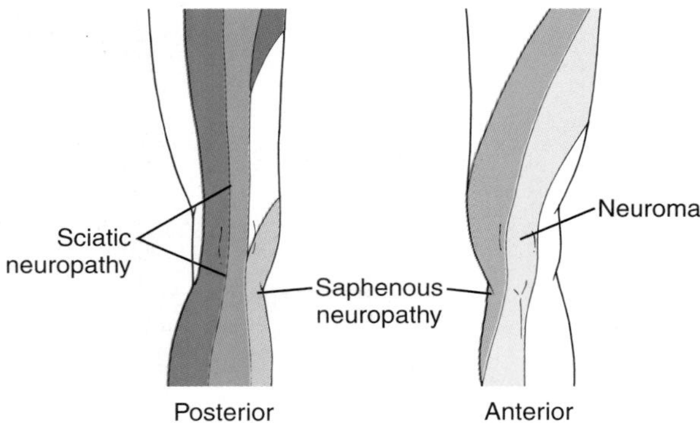

FIGURE 10-5 ■ Local neuropathies of the knee. These findings should also be correlated with a lower quarter neurologic screen.

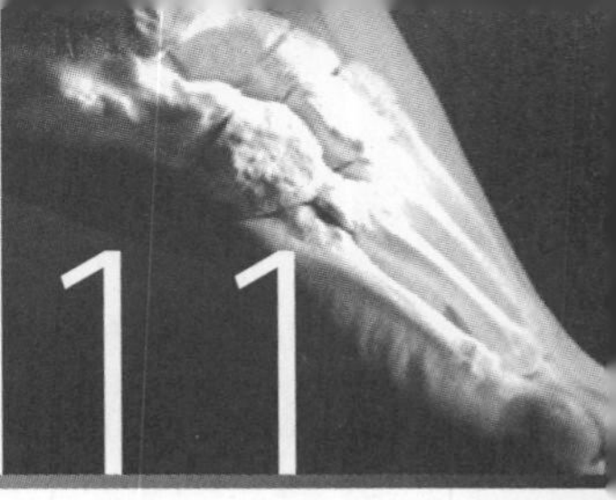

CHAPTER 11

Patellofemoral Articulation Pathologies

Examination Map

HISTORY

Past Medical History

History of the Present Condition

INSPECTION

Functional Assessment

Patella Alignment

Normal

Patella alta

Patella baja

Squinting

"Frog eyed"

Patellar Orientation

Medial/lateral glide

Spin

Anterior/posterior tilt

Medial/lateral tilt

Lower Extremity Posture

Genu varum

Genu valgum

Genu recurvatum

Q-Angle

Patellar Tendon

Tubercle Sulcus Angle

Leg Length Difference

Foot Posture

PALPATION

Palpation of the Anterior Structures

Tibial tuberosity

Patellar tendon

Patellar bursae

- Subcutaneous infrapatellar
- Deep infrapatellar

Fat pads

Patellar articulating surface

Femoral trochlea

Suprapatellar bursa

Medial patellofemoral ligament

Medial patellar retinaculum

Synovial plica

Lateral patellar retinaculum

Pes anserine insertion

Iliotibial band

JOINT AND MUSCLE FUNCTION ASSESSMENT

Goniometry

Knee flexion

Knee extension

Active Range of Motion

Knee flexion

Knee extension

Patellar tracking

Manual Muscle Tests

Knee extension

Knee flexion

Isolating the sartorius

Passive Range of Motion

Flexion

Extension

Continued

Evaluation Map—cont'd

JOINT STABILITY TESTS

Stress Testing

Testing of the major knee ligaments may be indicated

Joint Play Assessment

Medial patellar glide

Lateral patellar glide

Patellar tilt

Patellar spin

NEUROLOGIC EXAMINATION

Lower Quarter Screen

Common Peroneal Nerve

VASCULAR EXAMINATION

Distal Capillary Refill

Distal Pulse

Posterior tibial artery

Dorsal pedal artery

PATHOLOGIES AND SPECIAL TESTS

Patellofemoral Pain with Malalignment

Patellofemoral instability

- Apprehension test

Acute Patellar Dislocation

Patellofemoral Pain without Malalignment

Patellofemoral tendinopathy

Apophysitis

Osgood–Schlatter's disease

Sinding–Larsen–Johansson disease

Patellofemoral bursitis

Synovial plica

Traumatic Conditions

Patellar fracture

Patellar tendon rupture

Table 11-1 Subjective Findings in the Differentiation of Meniscal and Patellar Pain

History	Meniscus	Patella
Onset	Usually acute twisting injury	Occasionally direct anterior knee blow but usually insidious related to overuse and training errors
Symptom Site	Localized medial or lateral joint line	Diffuse, most commonly anterior
Locking	Frank transient locking episodes with the knee unable to fully terminally extend	Catching without locking, stiffness after immobility, but not true locking
Weight Bearing	Pain sharp and simultaneous with loaded weight bearing	Pain possibly coming on during weight bearing but often continuing into the evening and night
Cutting Sports	Pain with loaded twisting maneuvers	Some pain possible, but not sharp and clearly related to cutting
Squatting	Pain at full squat; inability to "duck walk"	Pain when extensors used to descend or rise from a squat
Kneeling	Not painful because meniscus is not weight loaded	Pain from patellar compression
Jumping	Weight loaded without torque or twist tolerated	Extensors heavily stressed, causing pain on descent impact
Stairs or Hills	Pain often going upstairs with loaded knee flexion, causing squatlike meniscal compression	More patellar loading and pain going downstairs because gravity-assisted impact increases patellofemoral stress
Sitting	No pain	Stiffness and pain from lack of the distraction–compression effect on abnormal articular cartilage

Inspection Findings 11-1
Patellar Alignment

Patella Alta	Patella Baja	Squinting Patellae	"Frog Eyed" Patella
Patella alta	Patella baja	Squinting patella	"Frog Eyed" patella
Description			
High-riding patellae; the camel sign may be present.	Low-riding patellae	Patellae positioned medially	Patellae high riding and laterally
Potential Causes			
Congenitally long patellar tendon	Congenitally short patellar tendon Arthrofibrosis after surgery or injury	Femoral anteversion, internal tibial rotation Arthrofibrosis after surgery or injury	Femoral retroversion, external tibial rotation
Consequences			
Increased patellar mobility, decreased quadriceps strength, increased patellofemoral compressive forces when the knee is flexed	Decreased patellar glide, decreased tibiofemoral range of motion, decreased quadriceps strength, increased compressive patellofemoral forces when the knee is flexed	Increased Q-angle, tight medial retinaculum, maltracking of the patella, altered patellofemoral compressive forces Compensations include external tibial torsion.	Increased lateral patellar glide, tight lateral retinaculum, patellar maltracking, decreased quadriceps strength, increased patellofemoral compressive forces when the knee is flexed

Inspection Findings 11-2
Patellar Orientatiopn

Medial/Lateral Patellar Glide	Patellar Rotation (Spin)	Anterior/Posterior Patellar Tilt	Medial/Lateral Patellar Tilt
Medial/lateral patellar glide	Patellar rotation (spin)	Anterior/posterior patellar tilt	Medial/lateral patellar tilt
Description			
Position of the patella in the frontal plane.	The longitudinal (superior to inferior pole) orientation in the frontal plane	Rotation in the sagittal plane	Rotation in the transverse plane
Evaluation of Alignment			
The patella should be centered between the medial and lateral patellar condyles. Displacement is described in the direction to which the patella is shifted. See Joint Play 11-1	The long axis of the patella should be directed toward the ASIS. If the long axis is directed lateral to the ASIS then the patella is laterally rotated and vice versa.	The inferior patellar pole should be palpable when the knee is extended and the quadriceps are relaxed. The patella is anteriorly rotated if the superior pole of the patella must be depressed to make the inferior pole palpable.	See Joint Play 11-2.

ASIS = anterior superior iliac spine.

Table 11-2 Structural Abnormalities and Their Resultant Forces and Biomechanical Changes

Alignment	Resulting Forces and Biomechanical Changes
Genu Varum	Increased compressive forces on the medial tibiofemoral articulating surfaces Tensile forces on the lateral tibiofemoral soft tissue structures and LCL Quadriceps exerting medially directed forces on the patella Compressive forces on the lateral facet Stretching of the lateral patellar restraints
Genu Valgum	Increased compressive forces on the lateral tibiofemoral articulating surfaces Tensile forces on the medial tibiofemoral ligaments Quadriceps exerting laterally directed forces on the patella Compressive forces on the odd and medial facets Stretching of the medial patellar restraints
Increased Q-angle or Lax Medial Restraints	Lateral tracking of the patella Compressive forces on the lateral facet Stretching of the medial patellar restraints
Decreased Q-angle or Lax Lateral Restraints	Medial tracking of the patella Compressive forces on odd and medial facets Stretching of the lateral patellar restraints
Genu Recurvatum	Decreased compressive forces in terminal knee extension

LCL = lateral collateral ligament.

Dislocated Patella

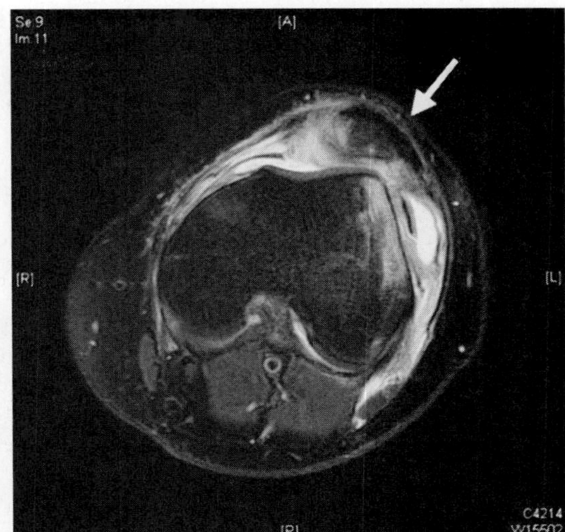

FIGURE 11-1 ■ Radiograph of a laterally dislocated patella. This view, taken from the left knee's posterior aspect, shows the patella resting on the lateral femoral condyle.

PALPATION

Palpation of the Patellofemoral Region

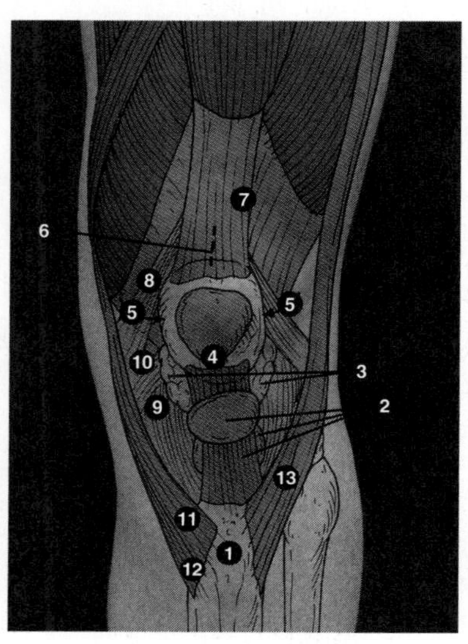

1 Tibial tuberosity

2 Patellar tendon and bursae

Subcutaneous infrapatellar bursa

Deep infrapatellar bursa

3 Fat pads

4 Patella and bursae

Prepatellar bursa

5 Patellar articulating surface

6 Femoral trochlea

7 Suprapatellar bursa

8 Medial patellofemoral ligament

9 Retinacular and capsular structures

10 Pes anserine bursa

11 Pes anserine tendon

12 Saphenous nerve

13 Iliotibial band

Tubercle Sulcus Angle

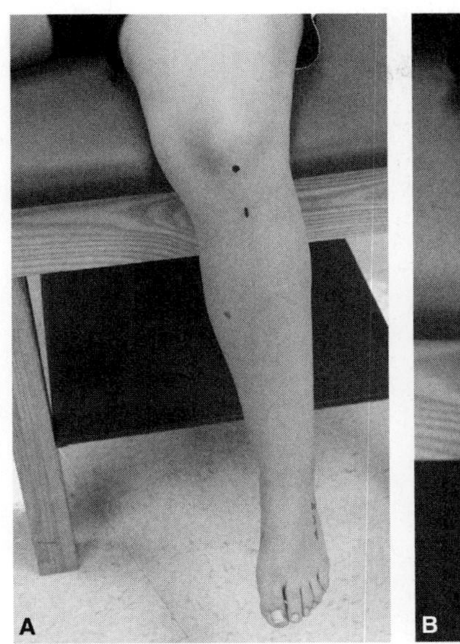

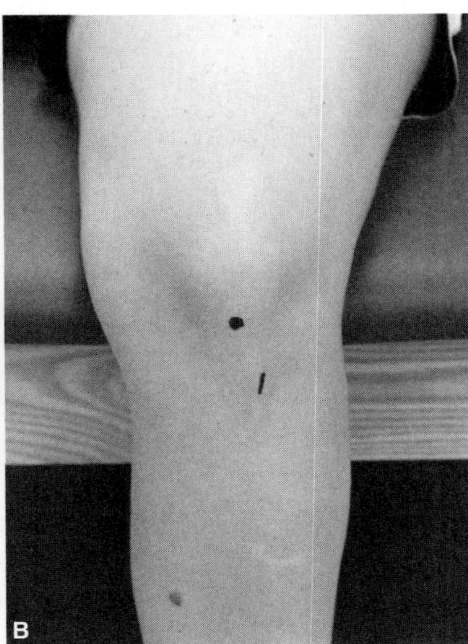

FIGURE 11-2 ■ Tubercle sulcus angle. **(A)** The tibial tuberosity is positioned inferior to the inferior pole of the patella, demonstrating normal alignment. **(B)** Laterally positioned tibial tuberosity, increasing lateral tracking of the patella.

Joint Play 11-1
Medial and Lateral Patellar Glide Test

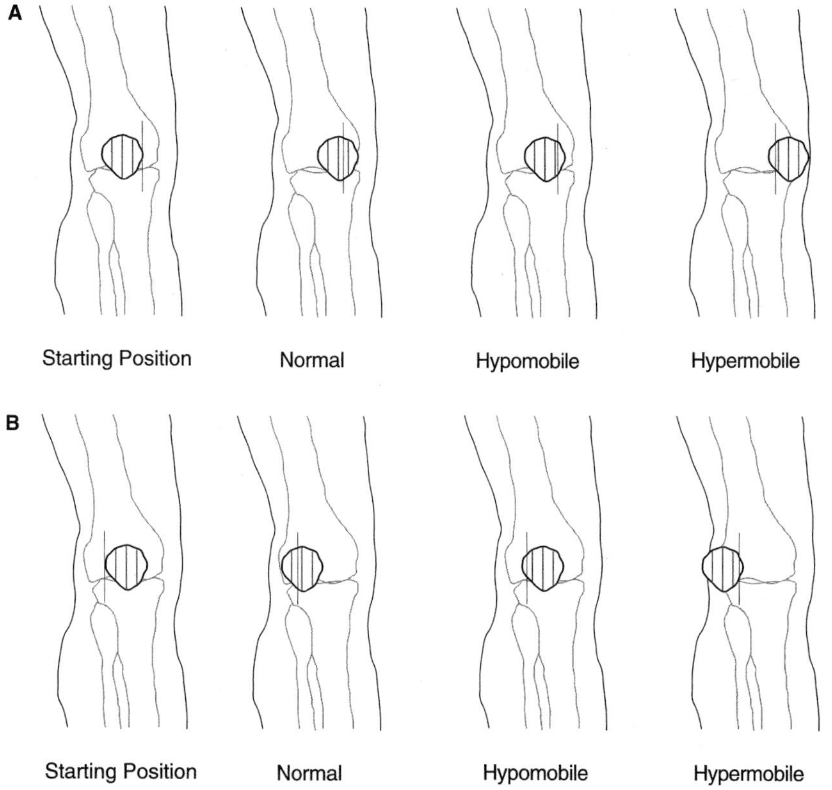

During medial **(A)** and lateral **(B)** patellar glide tests, the patella is viewed as having four quadrants. The amount of glide is based on the movement relative to the quadrants.

Patient Position	Supine with a bolster placed under the knee so that it is flexed to 30°
Position of Examiner	Standing lateral to the patient
Evaluative Procedure	**(A)** Medial glide: Move the patella medially, placing stress on the lateral retinaculum and other soft tissue restraints. **(B)** Lateral glide: Move the patella laterally, placing stress on the medial retinaculum, VMO, and medial capsule.
Positive Test	***Medial glide:*** The patella should glide one to two quadrants (approximately half its width) medially. Movement of less than one quadrant is considered hypomobile. Movement of more than two quadrants is hypermobile medial glide. ***Lateral glide:*** Normal lateral motion is 0.5–2.0 quadrants of glide. Less than that is hypomobile lateral glide; greater than two quadrants is hypermobile lateral glide.
Implications	***Medial glide:*** Hypomobile glide: Tightness of the lateral retinaculum or IT band. Hypermobile glide: Laxity of the lateral restraints. ***Lateral glide:*** Hypomobile glide: Tightness of the medial restraints, specifically the medial patellofemoral ligament.[64] Hypermobile glide: Laxity of the medial restraints
Comments	The patient may be apprehensive during lateral glide tests, fearful that the motion could result in a patella dislocation or subluxation. Hypermobile lateral glide creates a predisposition to patellar dislocations. Hypomobile medial glide is more common than hypermobile medial glide.
Evidence	Absent or inconclusive in the literature

IT = iliotibial; VMO = oblique fibers of the vastus medialis.

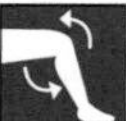

Joint Play 11-2
Patellar Tilt Assessment

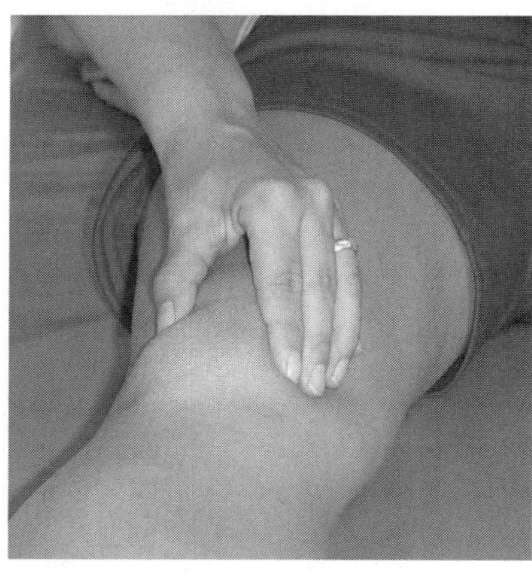

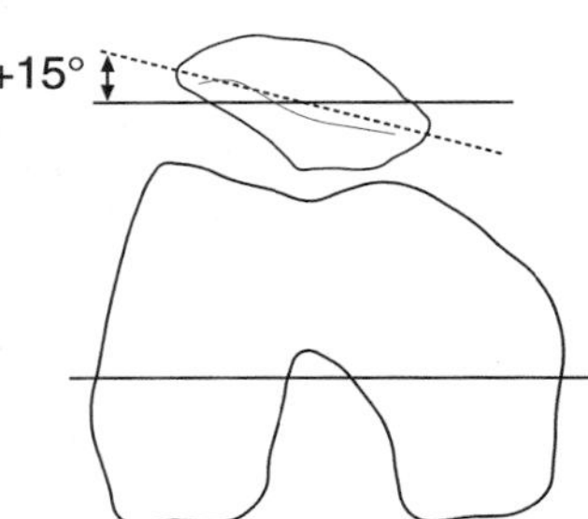

The patellar tilt test evaluates rotation of the patella around its midsagittal axis.

Patient Position	Supine with the knee extended and the femoral condyles parallel to the table
Position of Examiner	Standing lateral to the patient
Evaluative Procedure	Grasp the patella with the forefinger and thumb, elevating the lateral border and depressing the medial border.
Positive Test	A normal result is the lateral border raising between 0° and 15°. More than 15° is hypermobile lateral tilt; less than 0° is a hypomobile lateral tilt.
Implications	A tilt of less than 0° indicates tightness of the lateral restraints and often occurs in the presence of a hypomobile medial glide.[65] A tilt of more than 15° may predispose the individual to anterior knee pain
Evidence	Inter-rater reliability

Not Reliable — Very Reliable

Poor | Moderate | Good

0 0.1 0.2 0.3 0.4 0.5 0.6 0.7 0.8 0.9 1.0

Special Test 11-1
Q-Angle Measurement

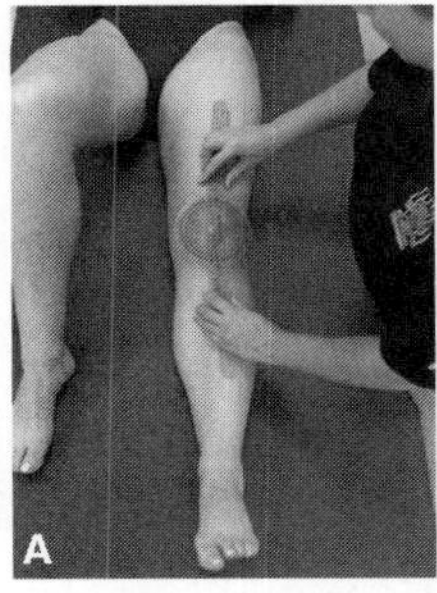

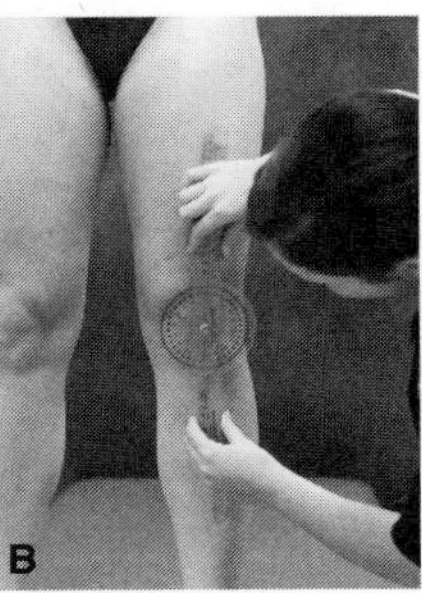

Measurement of the Q-angle with the knee extended in **(A)** a non–weight-bearing position and **(B)** weight-bearing; the anatomic landmarks of the ASIS, center of the patella, and the tibial tuberosity are used to align the goniometer.

Patient Position	**(A)** Lying supine with the knee fully extended with the ankle in neutral and the toes pointing up, replicating the standing position. Standardized foot position improves the reliability of this assessment.[66] **(B)** Standing with the feet shoulder-width apart.
Position of Examiner	Standing on the side of the limb to be measured
Evaluative Procedure	The examiner identifies and marks the ASIS, the midpoint of the patella, and the tibial tuberosity. A goniometer is placed so that the axis is located over the patellar midpoint, the center of the stationary arm is over the line from the ASIS to the patella, and the moving arm is placed over the line from the patella to the tibial tuberosity.
Positive Test	A Q-angle greater than 13° in men or 18° in women
Implications	Increased lateral forces leading to a laterally tracking patella
Modification	Re-measure the Q-angle with the quadriceps isometrically contracted. Differences between the two measures may provide insight to patellar tracking abnormalities.[67]
Comments	Measurement of the Q-angle in standing better replicates the functional alignment of the lower extremity. If the Q-angle is measured with the patient supine, this stance position should be replicated as indicated above. Q-angle measured with the patient short-sitting should be smaller than measures obtained with the patient standing or long-sitting. When correlated with radiographic Q-angle measurements, clinical measurements routinely overestimate the angle.[68]
Evidence	Inter-rater reliability Not Reliable — Very Reliable Poor / Moderate / Good 0 0.1 0.2 0.3 0.4 0.5 0.6 0.7 0.8 0.9 1.0 Intra-rater reliability Not Reliable — Very Reliable Poor / Moderate / Good 0 0.1 0.2 0.3 0.4 0.5 0.6 0.7 0.8 0.9 1.0

ASIS = anterior superior iliac spine.

Patellar Angles

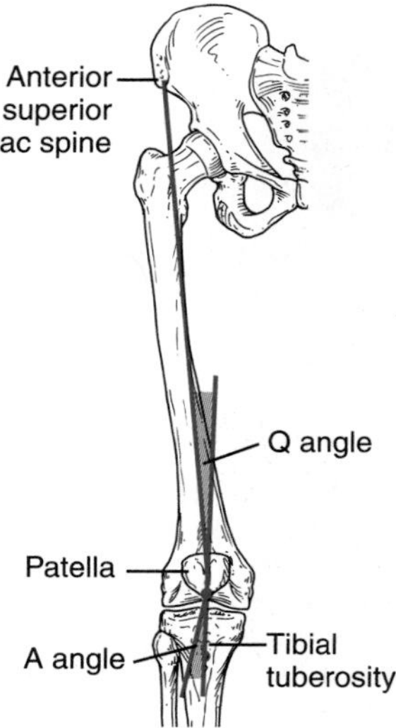

FIGURE 11-3 ■ The Q-angle describes the relationship between the long axis of the femur, measured from the anterior superior iliac spine to the center of the patella, to the long axis of the patella tendon, measured from the midpoint of the patella to the center of the tibial tuberosity. The A-angle is the relationship between the long axis of the patella and the tibial tuberosity.

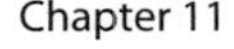

Special Test 11-2
Clarke's Sign for Chondromalacia Patella

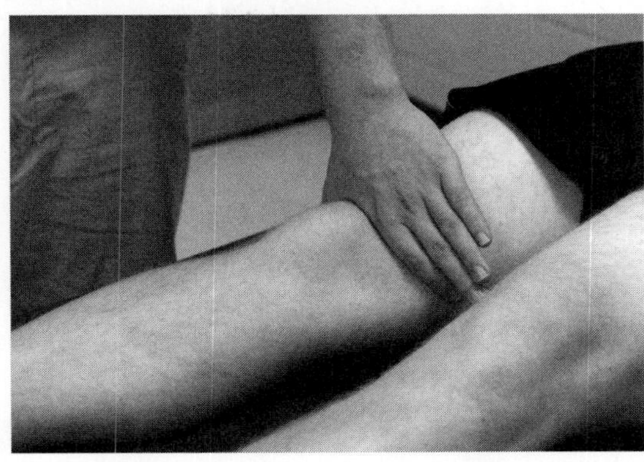

Clarke's sign for chondromalacia patella; this test elicits a great deal of pain and elicits a positive result in otherwise asymptomatic knees.

Patient Position	Lying supine with the knee extended
Position of Examiner	Standing lateral to the limb being evaluated; one hand is placed proximal to the superior patellar pole, applying a gentle downward pressure.
Evaluative Procedure	The patient is asked to contract the quadriceps muscle while pressure is maintained on the patella, pushing it into the femoral trochlea.
Positive Test	The patient experiences patellofemoral pain and the inability to hold the contraction.
Implications	Possible chondromalacia patella
Modification	The test may be performed with the knee flexed to various angles to assess different areas of patellofemoral contact.
Comments	The Clarke's sign is an unreliable test, producing false-positive results in otherwise asymptomatic knees.

Evidence

Positive likelihood ratio

Not Useful — Useful
Very Small | Small | Moderate | Large
0 1 2 3 4 5 6 7 8 9 10

Negative likelihood ratio

Not Useful — Useful
Very Small | Small | Moderate | Large
1.0 0.9 0.8 0.7 0.6 0.5 0.4 0.3 0.2 0.1 0

Special Test 11-3
Apprehension Test for a Subluxating/Dislocating Patella Fairbanks Test

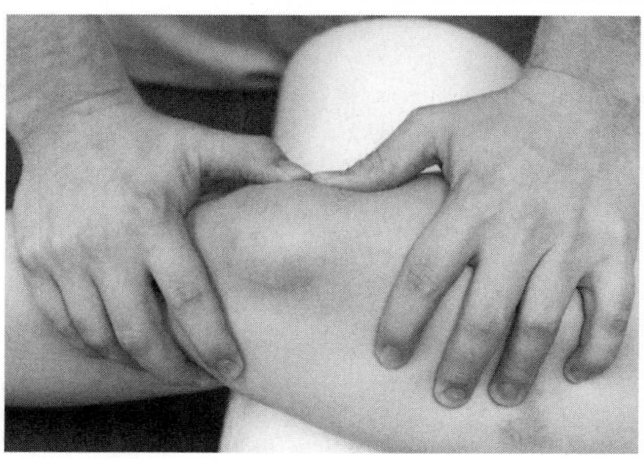

The apprehension test for patellar dislocation on a left knee. The examiner glides the patella laterally. A positive test is indicated by the patient's contracting the muscle or showing apprehension (anticipation) of an impending dislocation.

Patient Position	Lying supine with the knee extended
Position of Examiner	Standing to the patient's side
Evaluative Procedure	The examiner attempts to move the patella as far laterally as possible, taking care not to cause it to actually dislocate.
Positive Test	Forcible contraction of the quadriceps by the patient to guard against dislocation of the patella. The patient may also demonstrate apprehension verbally or through facial expression.
Implications	Laxity of the medial patellar retinaculum, predisposing the patient to patellar subluxations or dislocations
Modification	To improve the specificity of the test by isolating the medial patellofemoral ligament, move the patella distally and laterally.[69] The **Fairbanks Apprehension test** is performed with the patient's knee passively flexed to 30°. A lateral gliding force is placed on the patella while the knee is passively extended to the point where pain or apprehension is experienced.[70]
Evidence	Positive likelihood ratio Not Useful — Useful Very Small, Small, Moderate, Large 0 1 2 3 4 5 6 7 8 9 10 Negative likelihood ratio Not Useful — Useful Very Small, Small, Moderate, Large 1.0 0.9 0.8 0.7 0.6 0.5 0.4 0.3 0.2 0.1 0

Special Test 11-4
Test for Medial Synovial Plica

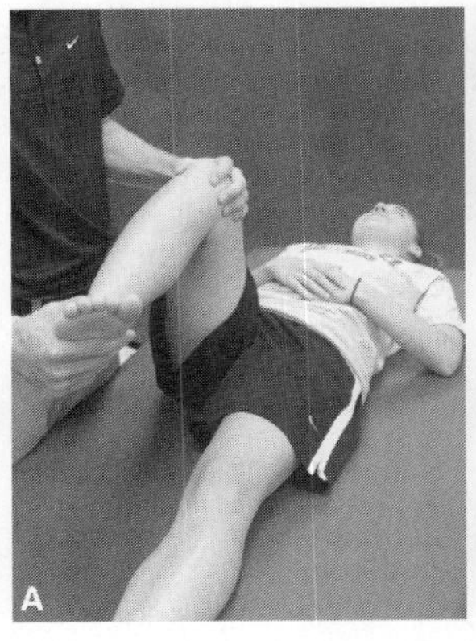

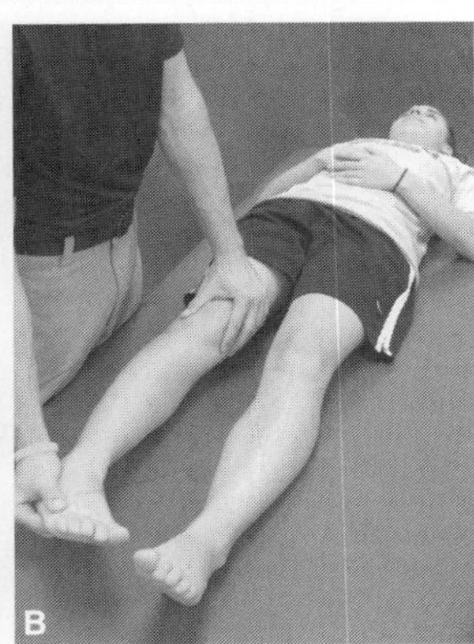

A positive test reproduces the patient's symptoms; the examiner may feel the plica as it crosses the medial femoral condyle.

Patient Position	Lying supine with the knee flexed or with the patient seated.
Position of Examiner	Standing on the side being tested.
Evaluative Procedure	**(A)** With the knee flexed to 90° and the tibia internally rotated, the examiner passively moves the patella medially while palpating the anteromedial capsule. **(B)** The knee is then extended and flexed from 90° to 0° while the tibia is internally rotated.
Positive Test	Reproduction of the symptoms is described by the patient. The clinician may feel the plica as it crosses the medial femoral condyle, especially in the range of 60°–45° of flexion.
Implications	Symptomatic medial synovial plica
Evidence	Absent or inconclusive in the literature

Special Test 11-5
Stutter Test for Medial Synovial Plica

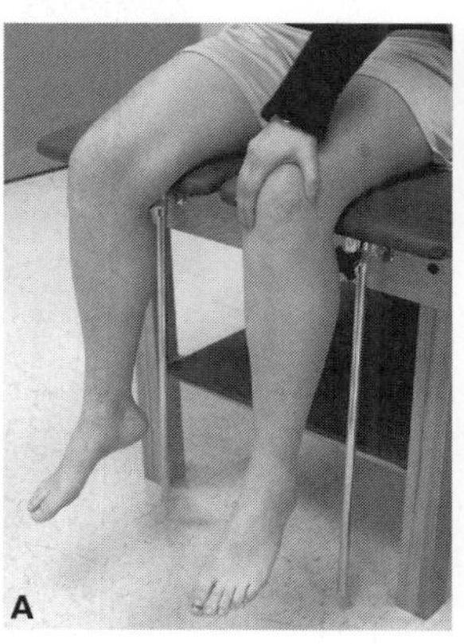

A

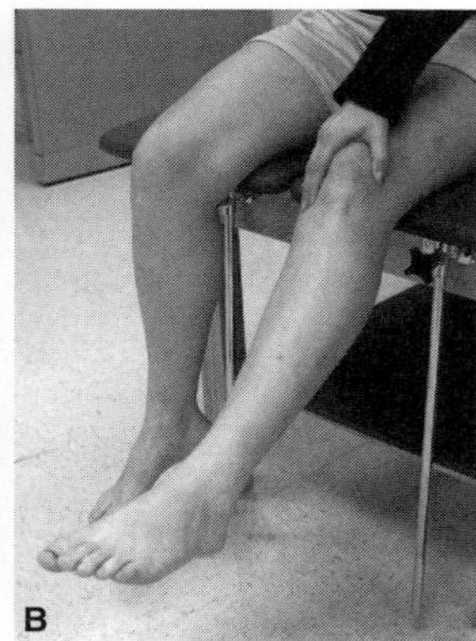

B

The examiner palpates the patella for irregular movement (stutter) as the patient extends the knee. When a plica snags against the medial femoral condyle, it may cause a momentary disruption in patellar motion.

Patient Position	**(A)** Sitting with the knee flexed over the edge of the table.
Position of Examiner	Standing lateral to the involved side, lightly cupping one hand over the patella, being careful not to compress the articular surfaces.
Evaluative Procedure	**(B)** The patient slowly extends the knee.
Positive Test	Irregular motion or stuttering between 40° and 60° as the plica passes over the medial condyle.
Implications	Medial synovial plica
Evidence	Absent or inconclusive in the literature.

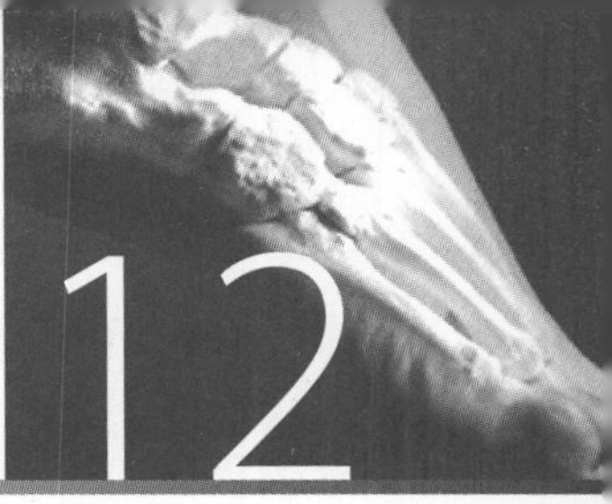

CHAPTER 12

Pelvis and Thigh Pathologies

Examination Map

HISTORY

Past Medical History

History of the Present Condition

Mechanism of injury

INSPECTION

Functional Assessment

Hip Angulations

Angle of inclination

Angle of torsion

Inspection of the Anterior Structures

Hip flexors

Inspection of the Medial Structures

Adductor group

Inspection of the Lateral Structures

Iliac crest

Nélaton's line

Inspection of the Posterior Structures

Posterior superior iliac spine

Gluteus maximus

Hamstring muscle group

Median sacral crests

Leg Length Discrepancy

PALPATION

Palpation of the Medial Structures

Gracilis

Adductor longus

Adductor magnus

Adductor brevis

Palpation of the Anterior Structures

Pubic bone/pubic symphysis

Inguinal ligament

Anterior superior iliac spine

Anterior inferior iliac spine

Sartorius

Rectus femoris

Palpation of the Lateral Structures

Iliac crest

Tensor fasciae latae

Gluteus medius

Iliotibial band

Greater trochanter

Trochanteric bursa

Palpation of the Posterior Structures

Median sacral crests

Posterior superior iliac spine

Gluteus maximus

Ischial tuberosity

Ischial bursa

Sciatic nerve

Hamstring muscles

JOINT AND MUSCLE FUNCTION ASSESSMENT

Goniometry

Flexion

Extension

Abduction

Adduction

Internal rotation

External rotation

Active Range of Motion

Flexion

Extension

Abduction

Adduction

Internal rotation

External rotation

Continued

Examination Map—cont'd

Manual Muscle Tests
Hip flexion (iliopsoas)
Knee extension (rectus femoris)
Hip extension
Abduction
Adduction
Internal rotation
External rotation

Passive Range of Motion
Flexion
- Thomas test
- Hip flexion contracture test
- Ely's test

Extension
Abduction
Adduction
Internal rotation
External rotation

JOINT STABILITY TESTS

Stress Testing
Not applicable

Joint Play Assessment
Passive range of motion

NEUROLOGIC EXAMINATION

Lower Quarter Screen

Sciatic Nerve

Femoral Nerve

VASCULAR EXAMINATION

Distal Capillary Refill

Distal Pulse
Posterior tibial artery
Dorsal pedal artery

PATHOLOGIES AND SPECIAL TESTS

Iliac Crest Contusions

Muscle Strains
Hamstring strain

Quadriceps Contusion

Slipped Capital Femoral Epiphysis

Iliotibial Band Friction Syndrome

Legg–Calvé–Perthes Disease

Femoral Neck Stress Fracture

Degenerative Hip Changes

Labral Tears
Hip subluxation

Athletic Pubalgia

Osteitis Pubis

Piriformis Syndrome

Snapping Hip Syndrome
Internal cause
External cause
Intra-articular cause

Bursitis
Trochanteric bursitis
Ischial bursitis
Iliopsoas bursitis

Table 12-1 Possible Pathology Based on the Location of Pain*

	Location of Pain			
	Medial	**Anterior**	**Lateral**	**Posterior**
Soft Tissue	Adductor strain Gracilis strain	Rectus femoris strain Iliopsoas strain Sartorius strain Symphysis pubis sprain Rectus femoris or iliopsoas tendinopathy Hip sprain Labral tear Iliofemoral bursitis Lymphatic edema/infection	Trochanteric bursitis Gluteus medius strain Gluteus minimus strain Nerve compression	Ischial bursitis Hamstring strain Gluteus maximus strain Nerve compression
Bony	Adductor avulsion fracture Stress fracture	Pubic bone fracture Osteoarthritis Stress fracture	Iliac crest contusion Hip joint dysfunction Stress fracture	Sacroiliac pathology Stress fracture

*Excluding gross injury.

PALPATION

Palpation of the Medial Structures

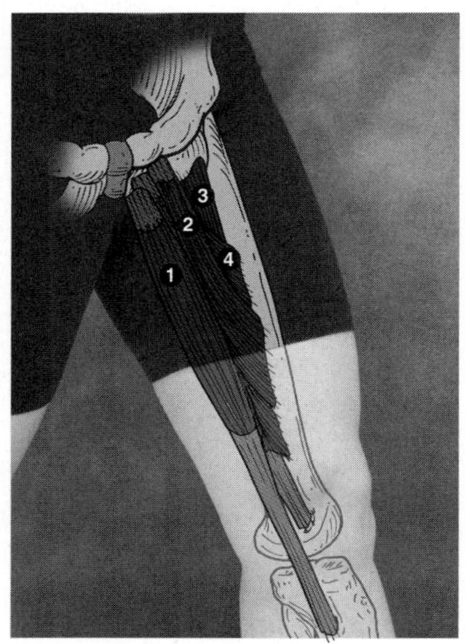

1 Gracilis

2 Adductor longus

3 Adductor magnus

4 Adductor brevis

Palpation of the Anterior Structures

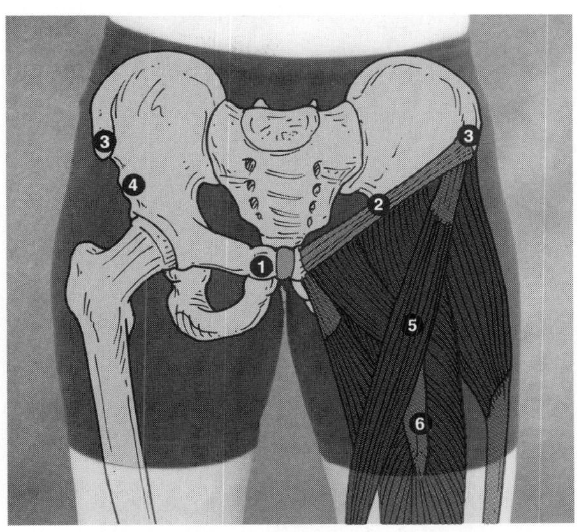

1 Pubic bone

2 Inguinal ligament

3 Anterior superior iliac spine

4 Anterior inferior iliac spine

5 Sartorius

6 Rectus femoris

Palpation of the Lateral Structures

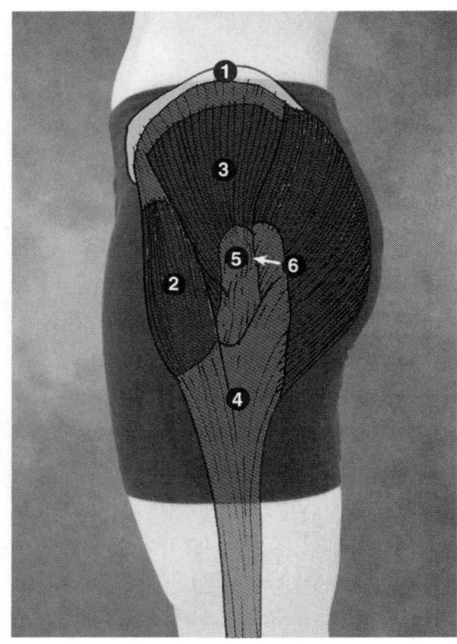

1	Iliac crest	4	IT band
2	Tensor fasciae latae	5	Greater trochanter
3	Gluteus medius	6	Trochanteric bursa

Isolating the Gluteus Medius

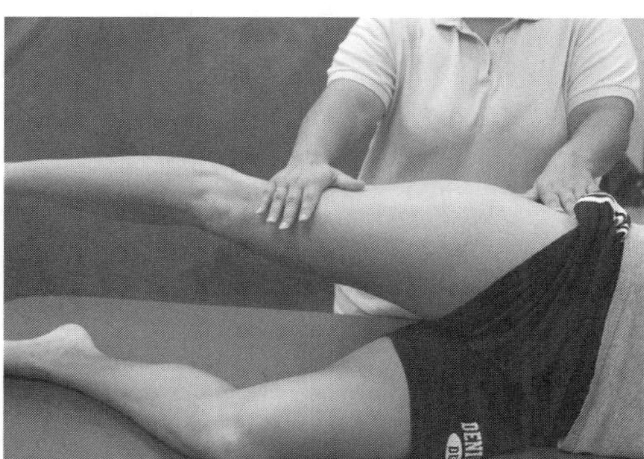

FIGURE 12-1 ■ Positioning of the patient to isolate the gluteus medius during palpation. Slightly abducting the hip makes the gluteus medius palpable.

Palpation of the Posterior Structures

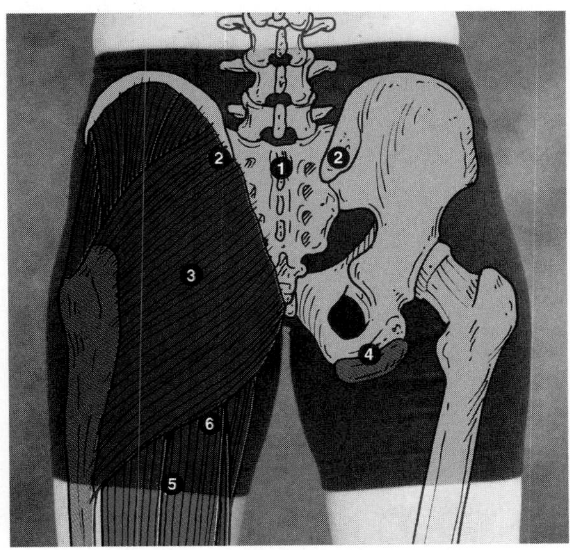

1 Median sacral crests

2 Posterior superior iliac spine

3 Gluteus maximus

4 Ischial tuberosity and bursa

5 Sciatic nerve

6 Hamstring muscle origin

Active Range of Motion

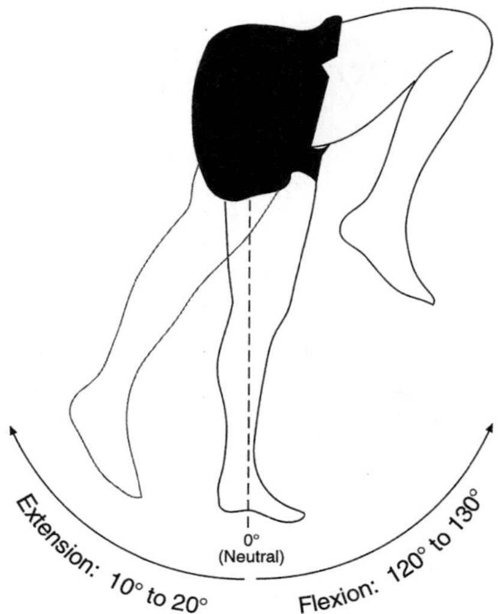

FIGURE 12-2 ■ Active range of motion available to the hip during flexion and extension. The range for hip flexion is decreased when the knee is extended secondary to tightness of the hamstring muscles and is limited during extension when the knee is flexed because of tightness of the rectus femoris.

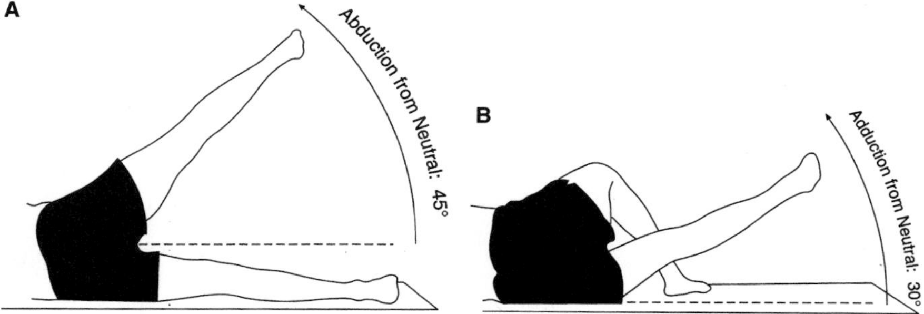

FIGURE 12-3 ■ Active hip abduction **(A)** and adduction **(B)**.

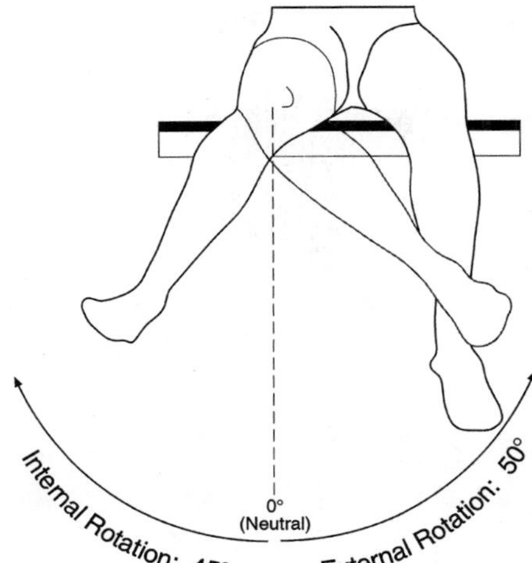

FIGURE 12-4 ■ Active hip internal and external rotation. Note that, in the seated position, the lower leg moves in a direction opposite that of the femur (i.e., during internal femoral rotation the lower leg rotates outwardly).

Passive Range of Motion

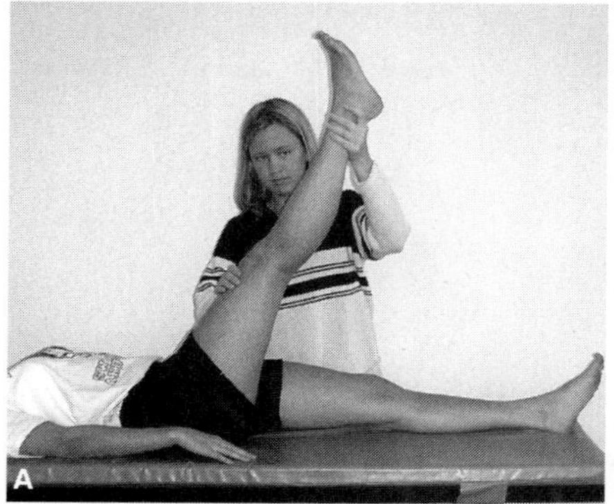

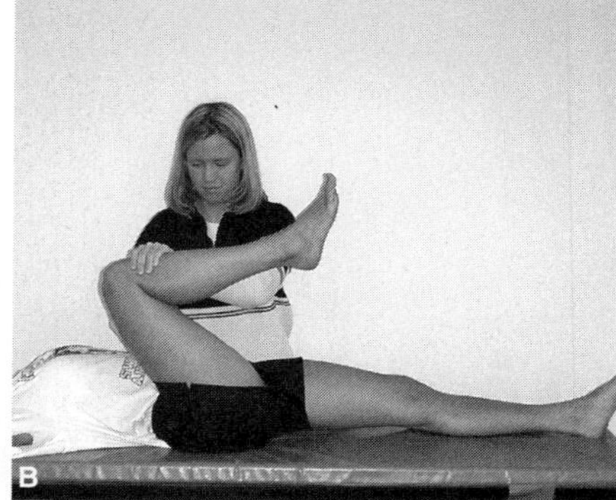

FIGURE 12-5 ■ Passive hip flexion: **(A)** knee extended; **(B)** knee flexed. The motion should also be replicated by adding pressure to the posterior distal femur. Note that hip flexion with the knee extended (shown in **A**) is the provocative phase of the straight-leg raise test and may produce sciatic nerve symptoms (see Chapter 13).

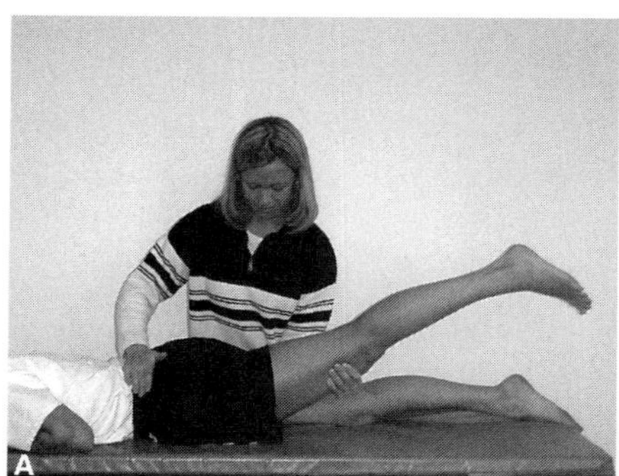

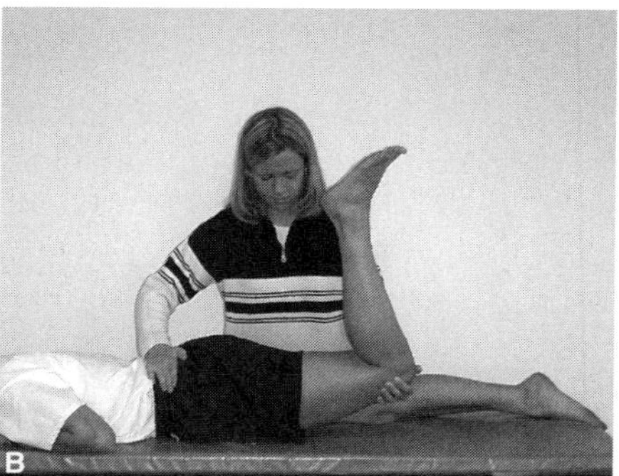

FIGURE 12-6 ■ Passive hip extension: **(A)** knee extended; **(B)** knee flexed.

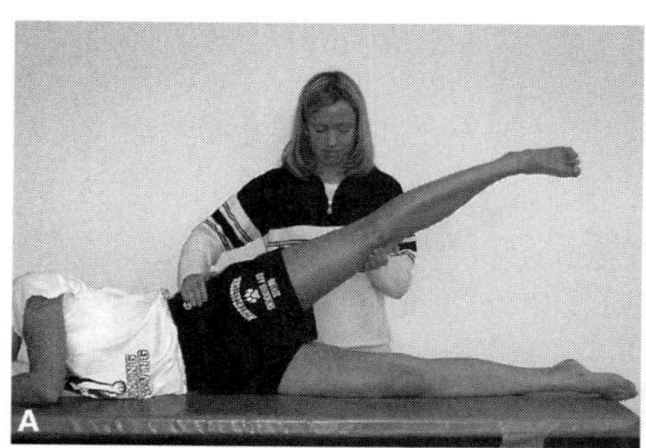

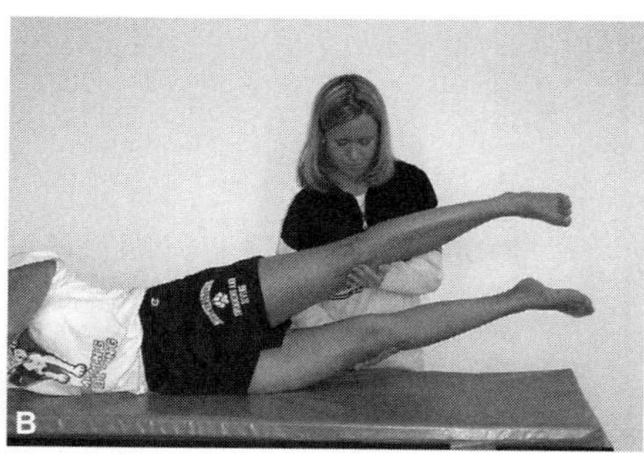

FIGURE 12-7 ■ **(A)** Passive hip abduction. **(B)** Passive hip adduction.

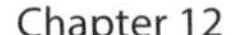

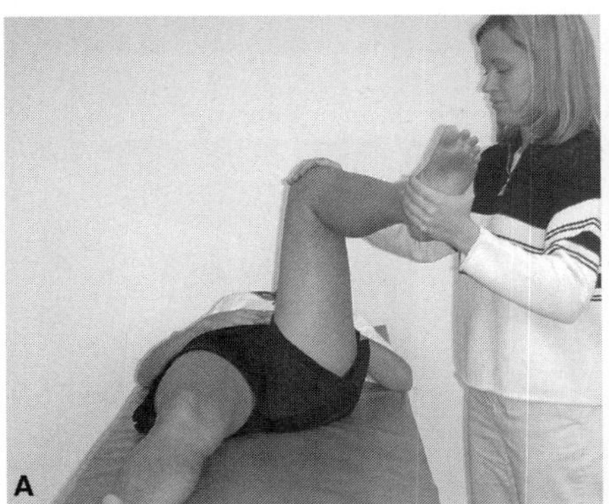

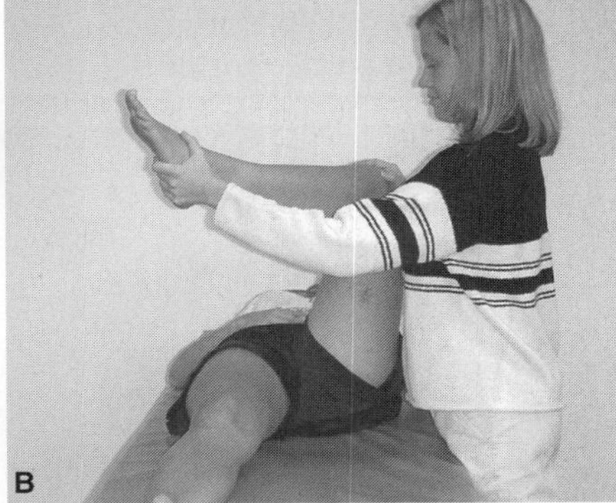

FIGURE 12-8 ■ **(A)** Passive hip internal rotation, and **(B)** passive hip external rotation.

Table 12-2 Hip Capsular Pattern and End-Feels

Capsular Pattern: Internal rotation, abduction, flexion, extension	
End-Feels:	
Flexion	Firm or soft: Soft tissue approximation or hamstring tension
Abduction	Firm: Stretch of the adductors
Adduction	Firm: Stretch of the abductors and joint capsule
Internal rotation	Firm: Stretch of the external rotators
External rotation	Firm: Stretch of the internal rotators
Extension	Firm: Stretch of the iliopsoas and joint capsule

Goniometry Box 12-1
Flexion and Extension

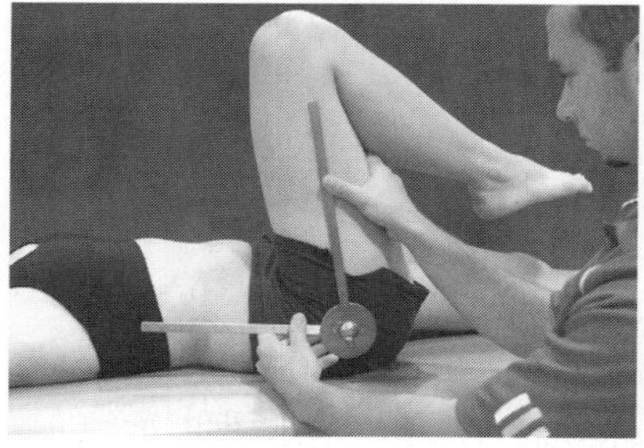

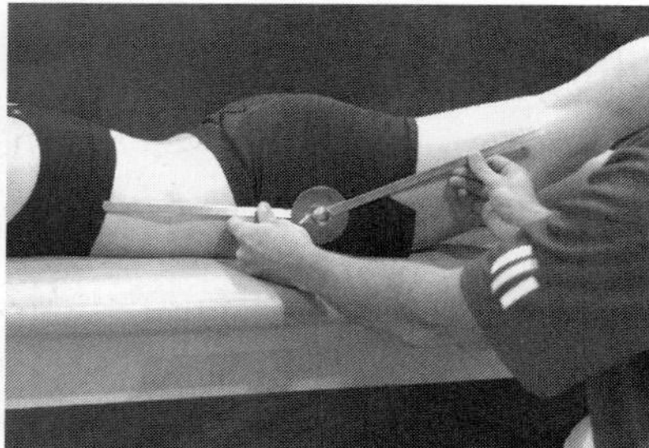

	Flexion 0°–120°	Extension 0°–30°
Patient Position	Supine	Prone
Goniometer Alignment		
Fulcrum	The axis is aligned over the greater trochanter.	
Proximal Arm	The stationary arm is aligned over the midline of the pelvis.	
Distal Arm	The movement arm is aligned over the long axis of the femur, using the lateral epicondyle as the distal reference point.	
Comments	Allow the knee to flex during the hip flexion measurement. The hip flexion measurement can also be taken with the knee extended to determine the influence of the hamstrings length. When measuring hip extension, stabilize the pelvis to avoid trunk extension. This may require help from someone. The hip extension measurement can also be taken with the knee flexed to determine the influence of the rectus femoris length.	

Goniometry Box 12-2
Hip Abduction and Adduction

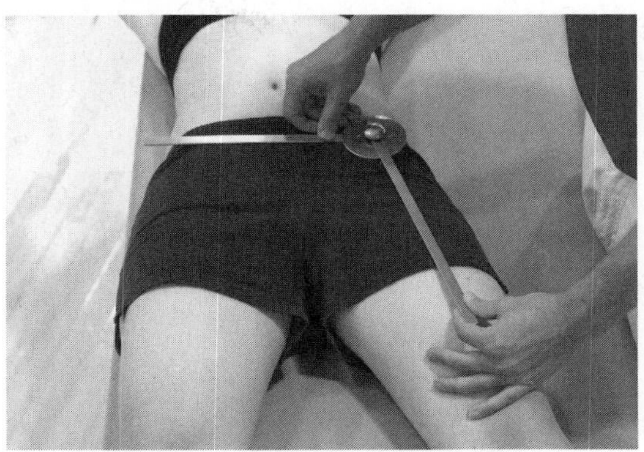

	Abduction 0°–45°	Adduction 0°–30°
Patient Position	Supine	Supine; the opposite leg is abducted.
Goniometer Alignment		
Fulcrum	The axis is aligned over the ASIS.	
Proximal Arm	The stationary arm is placed over the opposite ASIS.	
Distal Arm	The movement arm is positioned over the long axis of the femur, using the middle of the patella as the distal reference.	
Comments	Note that the start position of the goniometer is 90°, which is the baseline. Measurements are made relative to that position. The end of hip adduction is reached when the pelvis begins to laterally tilt.	

ASIS = anterior superior iliac spine.

Goniometry Box 12-3
Hip Internal and External Rotation

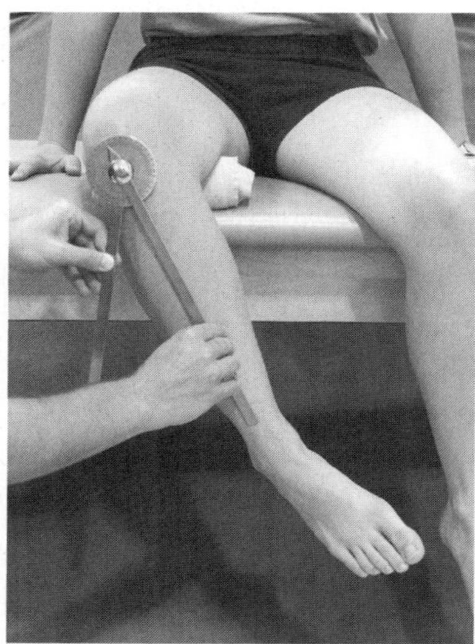

Internal Rotation 0°–45° **External Rotation 0°–45°**

Patient Position	Seated Place a bolster under the distal femur to keep it parallel with the tabletop.
Goniometer Alignment	
Fulcrum	The axis is aligned over the center of the patella.
Proximal Arm	The stationary arm is held perpendicular to the floor.
Distal Arm	The movement arm is positioned over the long axis of the femur, using the center of the talocrural joint as the distal reference.

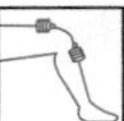

Manual Muscle Test 12-1
Iliopsoas (Hip Flexion)

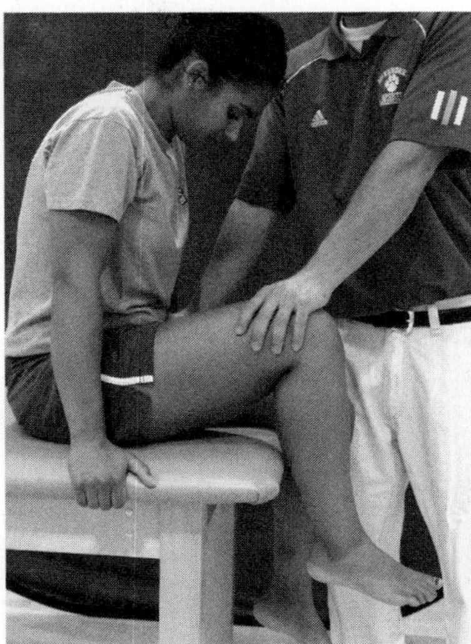

Iliopsoas

Patient Position	Seated, leaning slightly forward The patient should lightly grip the table.
Starting Position	The knee is flexed over the edge of the table.
Stabilization	Over the ASIS
Palpation	The insertion of the iliopsoas can be palpated in the inguinal crease, medial to the origin of the rectus femoris.
Resistance	Anterior aspect of the distal femur just proximal to the knee
Primary Mover(s) (Innervation)	Iliopsoas (L1, L2, L3, L4)
Secondary Mover(s) (Innervation)	Rectus femoris (L2, L3, L4) Sartorius (L2, L3)
Substitution	The patient may attempt to lean backwards to maximize the contribution of the rectus femoris.
Comments	There is no agreement on the optimal position for testing the hip flexors.

ASIS = anterior superior iliac spine.

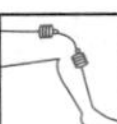

Manual Muscle Test 12-2
Hip Extension

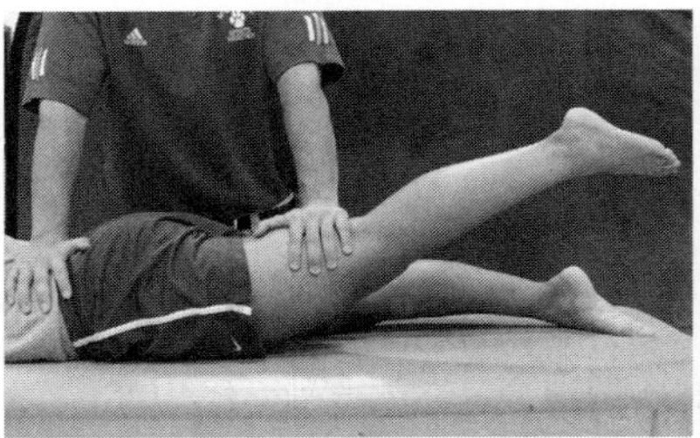

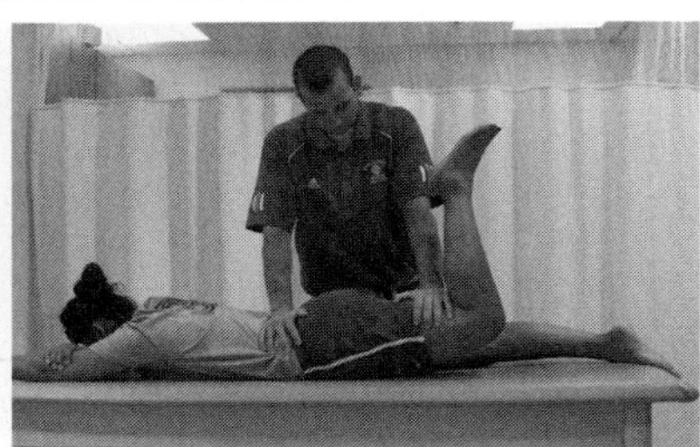

	Hamstrings and Gluteus Maximus	Gluteus Maximus
Patient Position	Prone	Prone
Starting Position	The knee is extended.	The knee is flexed to 90°.
Stabilization	Posterior pelvis	Posterior pelvis
Palpation	Posterior thigh	Buttock
Resistance	Proximal to the popliteal fossa	Posterior aspect of the distal femur
Primary Mover(s) (Innervation)	Hamstrings (L4, L5, S1, S2, S3) Gluteus maximus (L5, S1, S2)	Gluteus maximus (L5, S1, S2)
Secondary Mover(s) (Innervation)	Not applicable	Hamstrings (L4, L5, S1, S2, S3)
Substitution	Trunk rotation	Trunk extension
Comments	Pain with the knee extended decreases with knee flexed that implicates the hamstrings. This can be confirmed by resisting knee flexion.	Not applicable

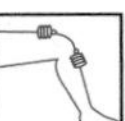

Manual Muscle Test 12-3
Hip Adduction and Abduction

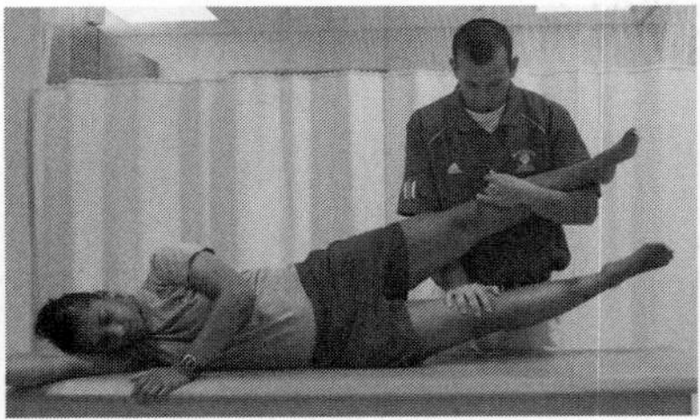

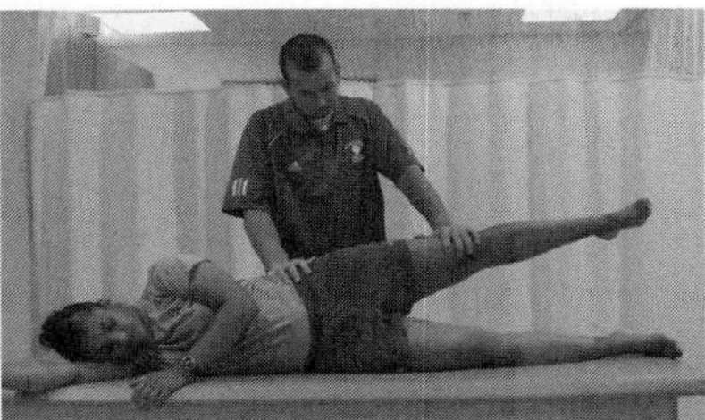

	Adduction	Abduction
Patient Position	Side-lying on the side being tested	Side-lying on the opposite side being tested
Starting Position	The knee is extended. The opposite (nontested) leg is supported by the examiner.	The knee is flexed slightly.
Stabilization	The pelvis and torso are actively stabilized by the patient.	The pelvis and torso are actively stabilized by the patient.
Palpation	Medial thigh	Proximal to greater trochanter
Resistance	Over the medial femur, proximal to the knee	Over the lateral femoral condyle
Primary Mover(s) (Innervation)	Adductor magnus (L2, L3, L4, L5, S1) Adductor longus (L2, L3, L4) Adductor brevis (L2, L3, L4) Gracilis	Gluteus medius (L4, L5, S1) Gluteus minimus (L4, L5, S1)
Secondary Mover(s) (Innervation)	Gluteus maximus (lower fibers) (L5, S1, S2) Pectineus (L3, L4)	Tensor fasciae latae (L4, L5, S1) Sartorius (L2, L3)
Substitution	Not applicable	Hip flexion
Comments	The test can also be performed with the patient prone.	The tensor fasciae latae is more active with slight hip flexion. The gluteus medius is more active more straight abduction.

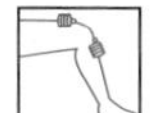

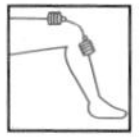

Manual Muscle Test 12-4
Hip Internal and External Rotation

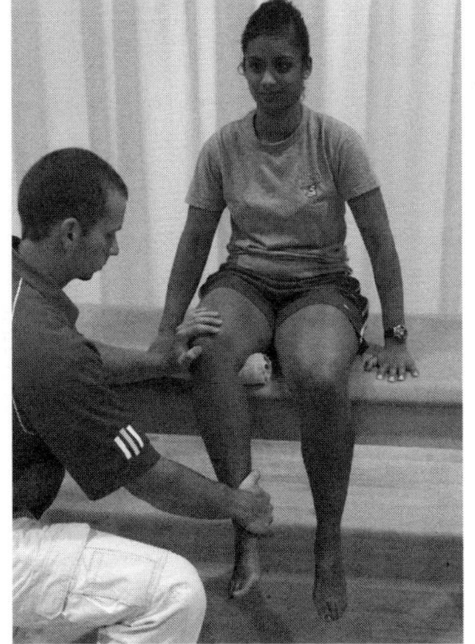

Internal Rotation and External Rotation

	Internal Rotation	External Rotation
Patient Position	Seated with the knees flexed over the edge of the table A bolster is placed under the distal femur to keep it parallel with the tabletop.	Seated with the knees flexed over the edge of the table A bolster is placed under the distal femur to keep it parallel with the tabletop.
Starting Position	Leg perpendicular to the ground	Leg perpendicular to the ground

Stabilization	The patient's arms are extended and support the torso on the table.	The patient's arms are extended and support the torso on the table.
Resistance	On the lateral aspect of the distal lower leg	On the medial aspect of the distal lower leg
Primary Mover(s) (Innervation)	Gluteus minimus (L4, L5, S1) Tensor fasciae latae (L4, L5, S1) Gluteus medius (anterior fibers) (L4, L5, S1)	Obturator internus (L5, S1, S2) Obturator externus (L3, L4) Quadratus femoris (L4, L5, S1) Piriformis (S1, S2) Gemellus inferior and superior (L4, L5, S1) Gluteus maximus (L5, S1, S2)
Secondary Mover(s) (Innervation)	Adductor longus (L2, L3, L4) Adductor magnus (L2, L3, L4, L5, S1) Adductor brevis (L2, L3, L4) Semimembranosus (L5, S1) Semitendinosus (L5, S1, S2)	Sartorius (L2, L3) Biceps femoris (long head) (S1, S2, S3) Psoas major (L1, L2, L3, L4)
Substitution	Trunk lateral flexion	Knee flexion

Table 12-3 Muscles Acting on the Hip

Muscle	Action	Origin	Insertion	Innervation	Root
Adductor Brevis	Hip adduction Hip internal rotation	Pubic ramus	Pectineal line Medial lip of linea aspera	Obturator	L2, L3, L4
Adductor Longus	Hip adduction Hip internal rotation	Pubic symphysis	Middle one third of medial linea aspera	Obturator	L2, L3, L4
Adductor Magnus	Hip adduction Hip internal rotation	Inferior pubic ramus Ramus of ischium Ischial tuberosity	Line spanning from the gluteal tuberosity to the adductor tubercle of the medial femoral condyle	Obturator Sciatic	L2, L3, L4 L5, S1
Biceps Femoris	Hip extension Hip external rotation Knee flexion External rotation of the tibia	Long head • Ischial tuberosity • Sacrotuberous ligament Short head • Lateral lip of the linea aspera • Upper two thirds of the supracondylar line	Lateral fibular head Lateral tibial condyle	Long head • Tibial Short head • Common peroneal	Long head • S1, S2, S3 Short head • L4, L5, S1
Gemellus Inferior	Hip external rotation	Tuberosity of ischium	Greater trochanter of femur via the obturator internus tendon	Sacral plexus	L4, L5, S1
Gemellus Superior	Hip external rotation	Spine of ischium	Greater trochanter of femur via the obturator internus tendon	Sacral plexus	L4, L5, S1

Gluteus Maximus	Hip extension Hip external rotation Hip adduction (lower fibers) Hip adduction (upper fibers)	Posterior gluteal line of ilium Posterior sacrum Posterior coccyx	Gluteal tuberosity of femur Through a fibrous band to the iliotibial tract	Inferior gluteal	L5, S1, S2
Gluteus Medius	Hip abduction **Anterior fibers** Hip flexion Hip internal rotation **Posterior fibers** Hip extension Hip external rotation	External surface of superior ilium Anterior gluteal line Gluteal aponeurosis	Greater trochanter of femur	Superior gluteal	L4, L5, S1
Gluteus Minimus	Hip abduction Hip internal rotation Hip flexion	Lower portion of ilium Margin of greater sciatic notch	Greater trochanter of femur	Superior gluteal	L4, L5, S1
Gracilis	Hip adduction Knee flexion	Symphysis pubis Inferior pubic ramus	Medial tibial flare	Obturator	L3, L4
Iliacus	Hip flexion	Superior surface of the iliac fossa Internal iliac crest Sacral ala	Lateral to the psoas major, distal to the lesser trochanter	Lumbar plexus	L1, L2, L3, L4

Continued

Table 12-3 Muscles Acting on the Hip—cont'd

Muscle	Action	Origin	Insertion	Innervation	Root
Obturator Externus	Hip external rotation	Pubic ramus	Trochanteric fossa of femur	Obturator	L3, L4
Obturator Internus	Hip external rotation	Obturator membrane Margin of obturator foramen Pelvic surface of ischium	Greater trochanter of femur	Sacral plexus	L5, S1, S2
Pectineus	Hip adduction	Superior symphysis pubis	Pectineal line of femur	Obturator	L3, L4
Piriformis	Hip external rotation	Pelvic surface of sacrum Rim of greater sciatic foramen	Greater trochanter of femur	Sacral plexus	S1, S2
Psoas Major and Minor	Hip flexion	Transverse process of T12 and all lumbar vertebrae	Lesser trochanter of femur	Lumbar plexus	L1, L2, L3, L4
Quadratus Femoris	Hip external rotation	Tuberosity of ischium	Intertrochanteric crest of femur	Sacral plexus	L4, L5, S1
Rectus Femoris	Hip flexion Knee extension	Anterior inferior iliac spine Groove located superior to the acetabulum	To the tibial tuberosity via the patella and patellar ligament	Femoral	L2, L3, L4
Sartorius	Hip flexion Hip abduction Hip external rotation Knee flexion Internal tibial rotation	Anterior superior iliac spine	Proximal portion of the anteromedial tibial flare	Femoral	L2, L3

Semimembranosus	Hip extension Hip internal rotation Knee flexion Internal tibial rotation	Ischial tuberosity	Posteromedial portion of the medial condyle of the tibia	Tibial	L5, S1
Semitendinosus	Hip extension Hip internal rotation Knee flexion Internal tibial rotation	Ischial tuberosity	Medial portion of the tibial flare	Tibial	L5, S1, S2
Tensor Fasciae Latae	Hip flexion Hip internal rotation Hip abduction	Anterior superior iliac spine External lip of the iliac crest	Iliotibial tract	Superior gluteal	L4, L5, S1

Special Test 12-1
Clinical Determination of the Angle of Torsion

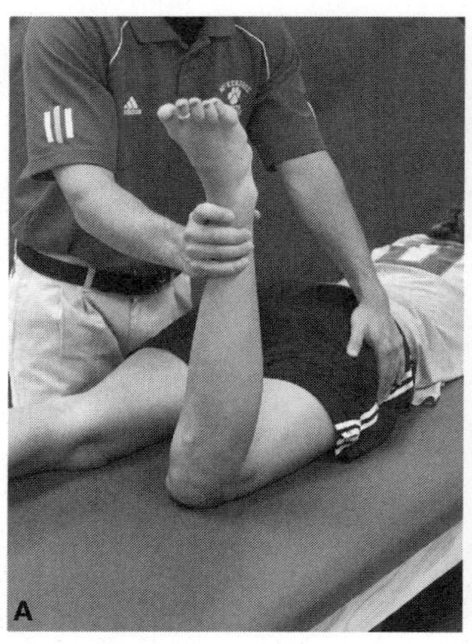

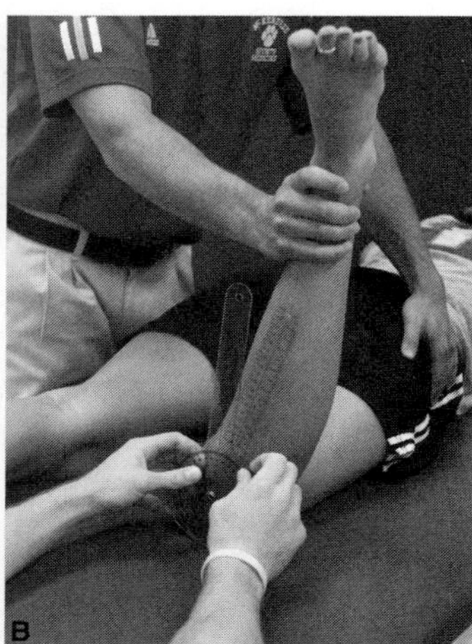

This procedure is most easily performed by two clinicians, one to manipulate the leg and the other to goniometrically measure the angle of the lower leg perpendicular to the table.

Patient Position

Prone with the knee of the leg being evaluated flexed to 90°

Position of Examiner

The use of two examiners is recommended.

Examiner 1: On the contralateral side to that being tested; one hand palpates the greater trochanter and the other hand manipulates the lower extremity.

Examiner 2: Holding a goniometer distal to the flexed knee with the stationary arm perpendicular to the tabletop.

Evaluative Procedure

(A) Examiner 1 internally rotates the femur by moving the lower leg inward and outward until the greater trochanter is maximally prominent. This represents the point at which the femoral head is parallel with the tabletop.

(B) Examiner 2 then measures the angle formed by the lower leg while the knee remains flexed to 90°.

Positive Test

Angles less than 15° represent femoral retroversion; angles greater than 20° represent anteversion.[71]

Implications

As described in Positive Test above

Evidence

Inter-rater reliability

Not Reliable — Very Reliable

Poor | Moderate | Good

0 0.1 0.2 0.3 0.4 0.5 0.6 0.7 0.8 0.9 1.0

Intra-rater reliability

Not Reliable — Very Reliable

Poor | Moderate | Good

0 0.1 0.2 0.3 0.4 0.5 0.6 0.7 0.8 0.9 1.0

Special Test 12-2
Trendelenburg Test for Gluteus Medius Weakness

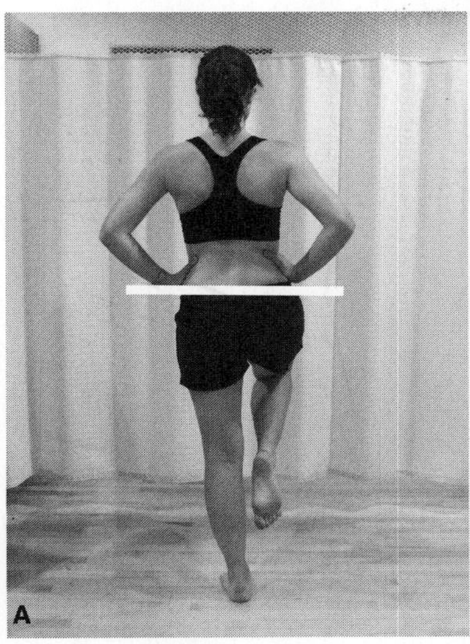

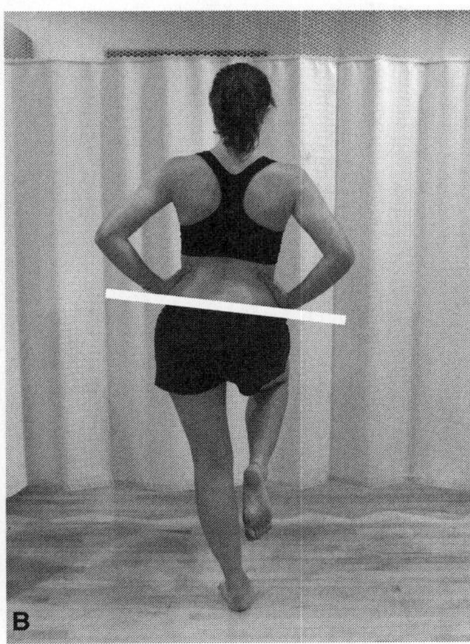

The patient is asked to stand on the affected leg **(A)**. In the presence of gluteus medius weakness, the pelvis lowers on the opposite side of the affected leg **(B)**.

Patient Position	Standing with the weight evenly distributed between both feet The patient's shorts are lowered to the point at which the iliac crests or posterior superior iliac spines are visible.
Position of Examiner	Behind the patient
Evaluative Procedure	The patient lifts the leg opposite the side being tested.
Positive Test	The pelvis lowers on the non–weight-bearing side.
Implications	Insufficiency of the gluteus medius to support the torso in an erect position, indicating weakness in the muscle
Modification	Repeated testing may be necessary, as fatigue can magnify this weakness.
Comments	Muscle weakness can result from nerve root impingement or damage to the superior gluteal nerve.
Evidence	Absent or inconclusive in the literature

Special Test 12-3
Thomas Test for Hip Flexor Tightness/Rectus Femoris Contracture Test

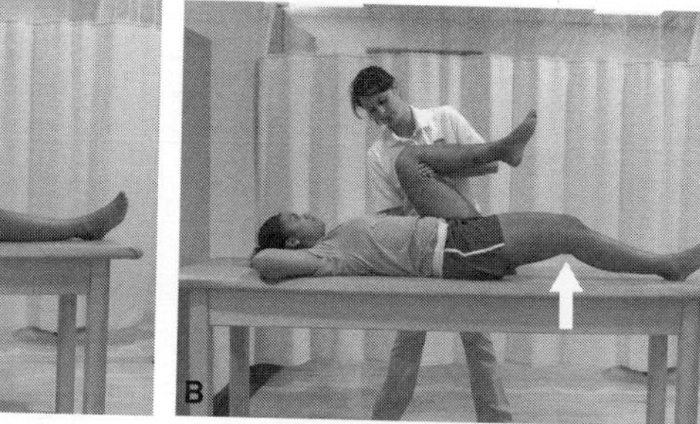

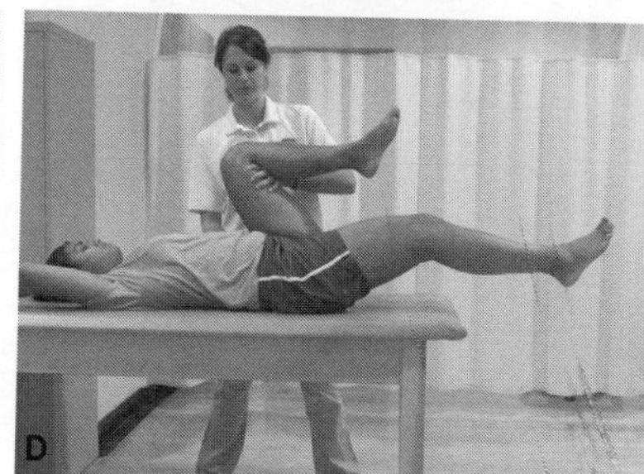

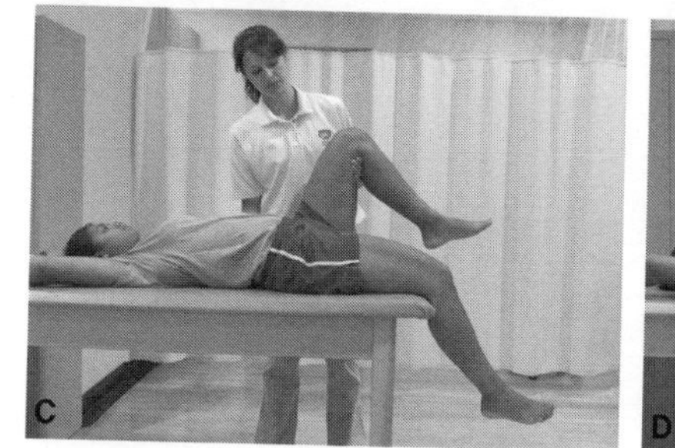

Thomas test for hip flexor tightness. The patient's left (forward) leg is tested. **(A)** Tightness of the left rectus femoris muscle; **(B)** tightness of the left iliopsoas group. Rectus femoris contracture test (a modification of the Thomas test). **(C)** A modification of the Thomas test, the patient is positioned so that the knee of the test leg is off the table. **(D)** Tightness of the hip flexors results in the opposite knee and hip flexing.

Patient Position	TT: Lying prone on the table RFCT: Lying supine with the knees bent at the end of the table
Position of Examiner	Standing beside the patient

Evaluative Procedure	The examiner places one hand between the lumbar lordotic curve and the tabletop. One leg is passively flexed to the patient's chest, allowing the knee to flex during the movement. The opposite leg (the leg being tested) rests flat on the table.
Positive Test	**(A)** The lower leg moves into extension. **(B)** The involved leg rises off the table.
Implications	**(A)** Tightness of the rectus femoris. **(B)** Tightness of the iliopsoas muscle group.
Modification	The patient can use the arms to passively flex the hip. The hip position may be measured goniometrically.
Comments	The patient may passively flex the hip and knee by using the arms to pull the leg to the chest.[72] The amount of lumbar flattening can be determined by placing a hand under the lumbar spine.
Evidence	***Modification*** Inter-rater reliability Not Reliable — Very Reliable; Poor, Moderate, Good; 0 0.1 0.2 0.3 0.4 0.5 0.6 0.7 0.8 0.9 1.0 Intra-rater reliability Not Reliable — Very Reliable; Poor, Moderate, Good; 0 0.1 0.2 0.3 0.4 0.5 0.6 0.7 0.8 0.9 1.0

RFCT = rectus femoris contracture test; TT = Thomas test.

Special Test 12-4
Ely's Test

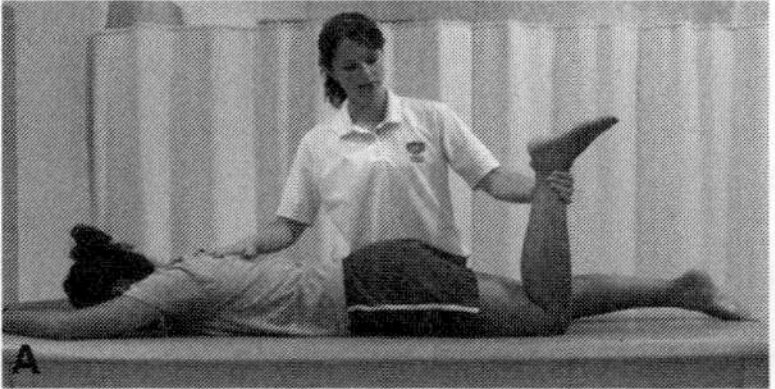

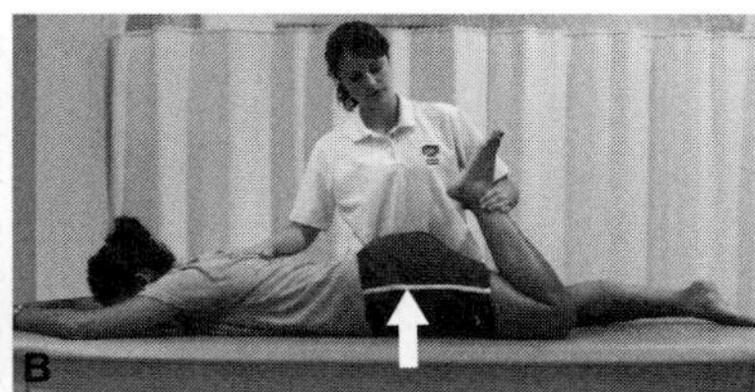

Ely's test for hip flexor tightness **(A)**. Passive flexion of the knee results in hip flexion, causing it to rise off the table **(B)**.

Patient Position	Lying prone
Position of Examiner	Standing beside the patient
Evaluative Procedure	The knee is passively flexed toward the patient's buttock.
Positive Test	The hip on the side being tested flexes, causing it to rise from the table.
Implications	Tightness of the rectus femoris
Evidence	Absent or inconclusive in the literature

Special Test 12-5
Hip Scouring Test (Hip Quadrant Test)

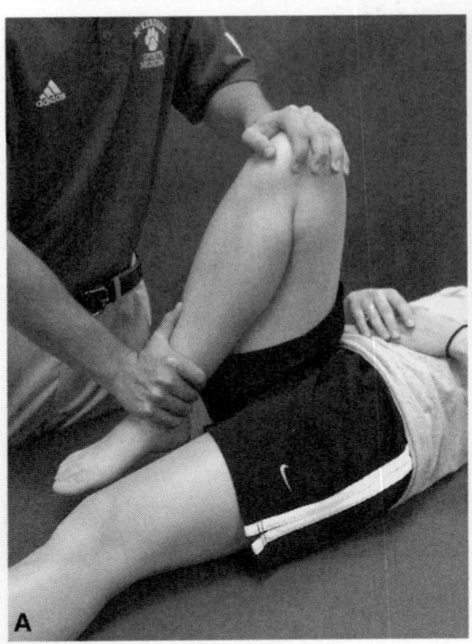

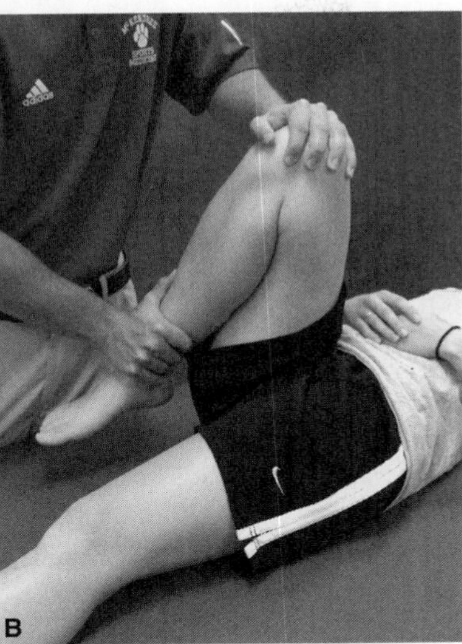

This procedure moves the hip through its range of motion while an axial load is placed on the femur. Pain within a specific location may indicate a defect of the articular surface or labral tear.

Patient Position	Supine
Position of Examiner	At the side of the patient, fully flexing the patient's hip and knee
Evaluative Procedure	The examiner applies pressure downward along the shaft of the femur to compress the joint surfaces. The femur is **(A)** internally and **(B)** externally rotated with the hip in multiple angles of flexion.
Positive Test	Pain described or symptoms in the hip are reproduced
Implications	A possible defect in the articular cartilage of the femur or acetabulum (e.g., osteochondral defects, arthritis) This test may also produce pain in the presence of a labral tear.
Evidence	Absent or inconclusive in the literature

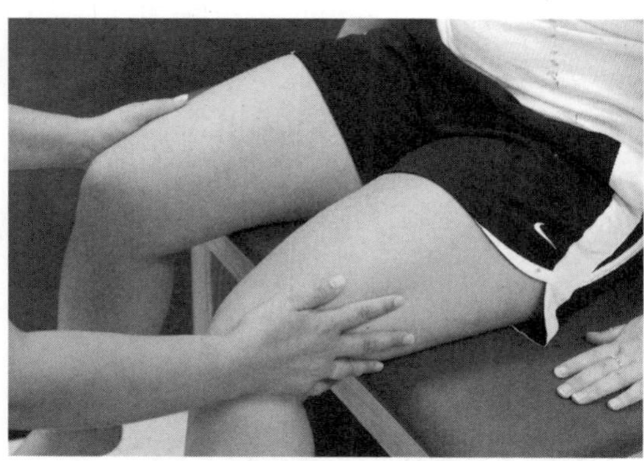

FIGURE 12-9 ■ Resisted hip abduction with the patient seated to duplicate pain caused by piriformis syndrome.

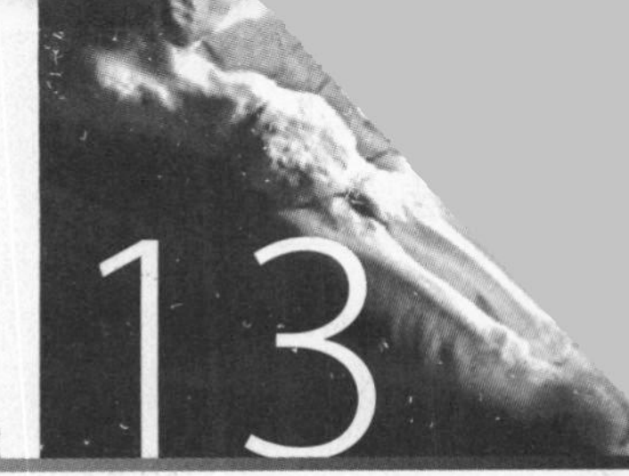

CHAPTER 13

Thoracic and Lumbar Spine Pathologies

Examination Map

HISTORY

Past Medical History
Mental health status

History of the Present Condition
Location of pain
Radicular symptoms
Onset and severity of symptoms

INSPECTION

Functional Assessment
Gait
Movement and posture

General Inspection
Frontal curvature
Sagittal curvature
Skin markings

Inspection of the Thoracic Spine
Breathing patterns
Skin folds
Chest shape

Inspection of the Lumbar Spine
Lordotic curve
Standing posture
Erector muscle tone
Faun's beard

PALPATION

Palpation of the Thoracic Spine
Spinous processes
Supraspinous ligaments
Costovertebral junction
Trapezius
Paravertebral muscles
Scapular muscles

Palpation of the Lumbar Spine
Spinous processes
- Step-off deformity

Paravertebral muscles

Palpation of the Sacrum and Pelvis
Median sacral crests
Iliac crests
Posterior superior iliac spine
Gluteals
Ischial tuberosity
Greater trochanter
Sciatic nerve
Pubic symphysis

JOINT AND MUSCLE FUNCTION ASSESSMENT

Goniometry
Flexion
Extension
Lateral bending
Rotation

Active Range of Motion
Flexion
Extension
Lateral bending
Rotation

Manual Muscle Tests
Flexion
Extension
Rotation
Pelvic elevation

Continued

tion Map—cont'd

Passive Range of Motion
Flexion
Extension
Rotation
Side gliding

JOINT STABILITY TESTS

Joint Play Assessment
Spring test

SPECIAL TESTS

Test for Nerve Root Impingement
Valsalva
Milgram
Kernig
Straight leg raise
Well straight leg raise
Slump test
Quadrant test

NEUROLOGIC EXAMINATION

Lower quarter screen

PATHOLOGIES AND SPECIAL TESTS

Spinal Stenosis

Intervertebral Disk Lesions
Femoral nerve stretch test
Tension sign

Segmental Instability
Erector spinae strain
Facet joint dysfunction

Spondylopathies
Spondylolysis
Spondylolisthesis
- Single leg stance test

Sacroiliac dysfunction
- Fabere sign
- Patrick's test
- Gaenslen's test
- Long sit test

Table 13-1 Ramifications of Spinal Pain Exhibited During the Activities of Daily Living

Activity	Ramifications
Bending	Pain may be initially worsened with flexion exercises.
Sitting	Pain may be initially worsened with flexion exercises.
Rising from Sitting	This motion causes changes in the interdiscal forces. Sharp pain suggests derangement of the disk.
Standing	The spine is placed in extension. Pain may be initially experienced with extension exercises.
Walking	The amount of spinal extension increases as the speed of gait increases.
Lying Prone	The spine is placed in or near full extension.
Lying Supine	When lying supine on a hard surface, the amount of extension is maintained. When lying on a soft surface, the spine falls into flexion.

PALPATION

Palpation of the Thoracic Spine

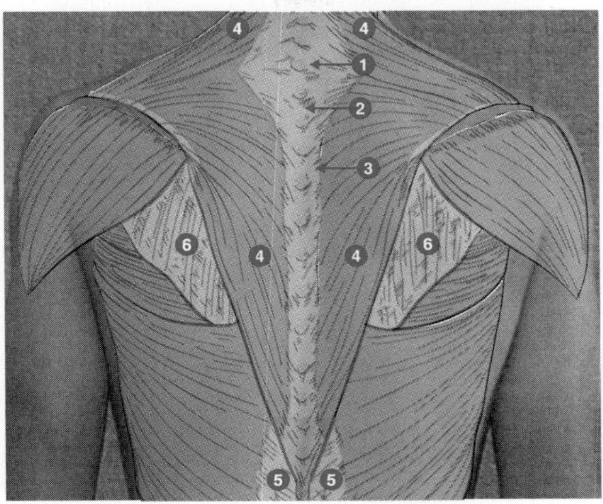

1 Spinous processes

2 Supraspinous ligaments

3 Costovertebral junction

4 Trapezius

5 Paravertebral muscles

6 Scapular muscles

Palpation of the Lumbar Spine

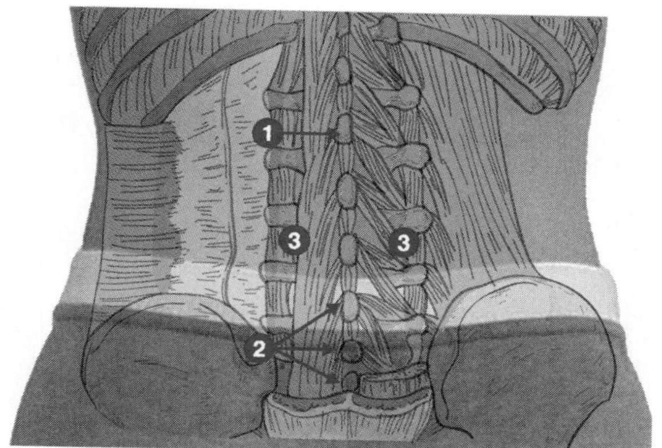

1 Spinous processes

2 Step-off deformity

3 Paravertebral muscles

Palpation of the Sacrum and Pelvis

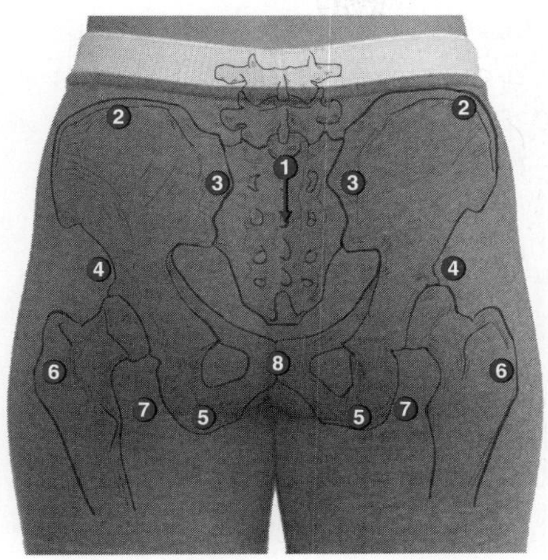

1 Median sacral crests

2 Iliac crests

3 Posterior superior iliac spine

4 Gluteals

5 Ischial tuberosity

6 Greater trochanter

7 Sciatic nerve

8 Pubic symphysis

Table 13-2 Bony Landmarks During Palpation

Structure	Landmark
Cervical Vertebral Bodies	On the same level as the spinous processes
C1 Transverse Process	One finger's breadth inferior to the mastoid process
C3–C4 Vertebrae	Posterior to the hyoid bone
C4–C5 Vertebrae	Posterior to the thyroid cartilage
C6 Vertebra	Posterior to the cricoid cartilage; moves during flexion and extension of the cervical spine
C7 Vertebra	Prominent posterior spinous process
Thoracic Spinal Bodies	Underlying the spinous processes of the superior vertebra
T1 Vertebra	Prominent protrusion inferior to the cervical spine; does not disappear during extension
T2 Vertebra	Posterior from the jugular notch of the sternum
T3 Vertebra	Even with the medial border of the scapular spine
T7 Vertebra	Even with the inferior angle of scapula
Lumbar Spinal Bodies	Upper portion of the spinous processes overlying the inferior half of the same vertebra
L3 Vertebra	In normal body build, posterior from the umbilicus
L4 Vertebra	Level with the iliac crest
L5 Vertebra	Typically demarcated by bilateral dimples, but variable from person to person
S2	At the level of the posterior superior iliac spine

Table 13-3 Spinal Ligaments Stressed During the End-Range of Passive Range of Motion Assessment

Motion	Ligaments Stressed
Flexion	Posterior longitudinal ligament Supraspinous ligament (thoracic and lumbar spine) Interspinous ligament Ligamentum flavum
Extension	Anterior longitudinal ligament
Rotation	Interspinous ligament Ligamentum flavum
*Lateral Bending**	Interspinous ligament Ligamentum flavum

*Testing these motions is usually inconclusive.

Goniometry Box 13-1
Trunk Flexion and Extension (Tape Measure)

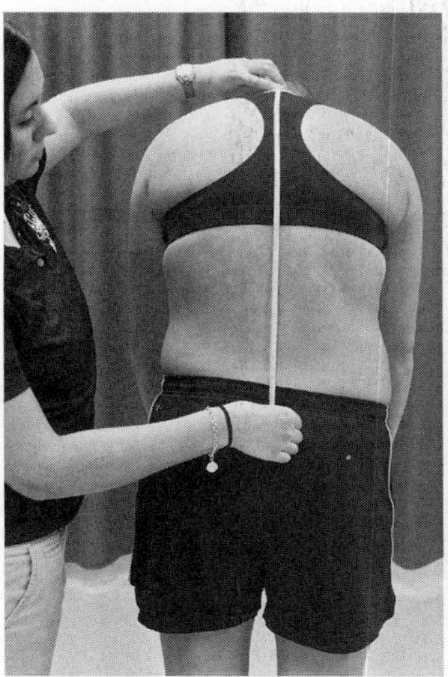

Flexion

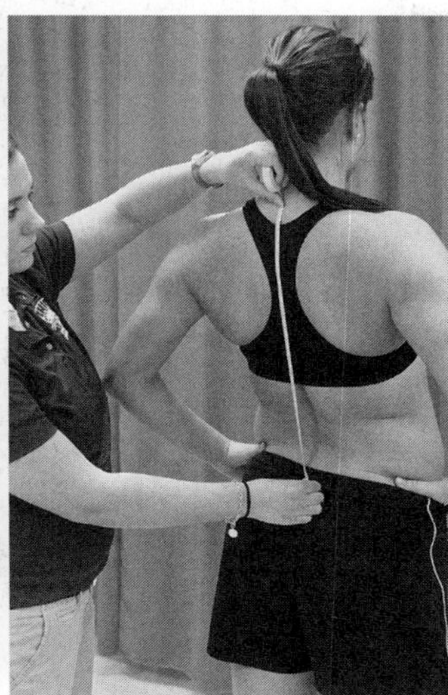

Extension

Patient Position	Standing with the knees extended, feet shoulder-width apart, and the spine in the neutral position
Procedure	
Initial Measurement	Using a tape measure, the distance (in cm) between the C7 and S1 spinous processes is determined.
Motion	The patient fully flexes or extends the trunk. Observe for pelvic rotation that is indicative of compensatory spinal motion.
Final Measurement	The distance between the C7 and S1 spinous processes is determined. The difference between the initial and final measurement is calculated and the value is recorded.

Goniometry Box 13-2
Lateral Bending and Rotation

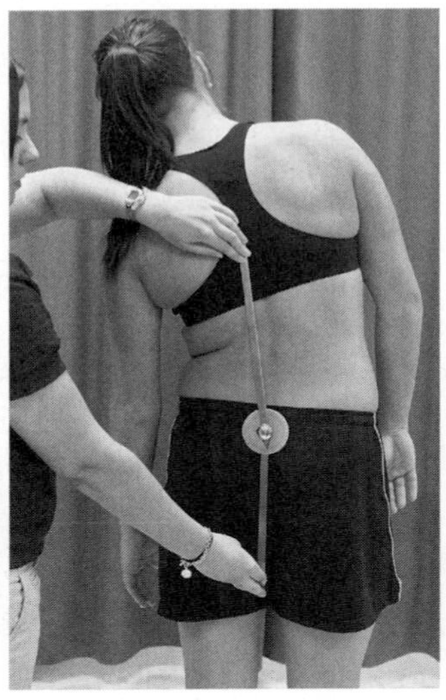

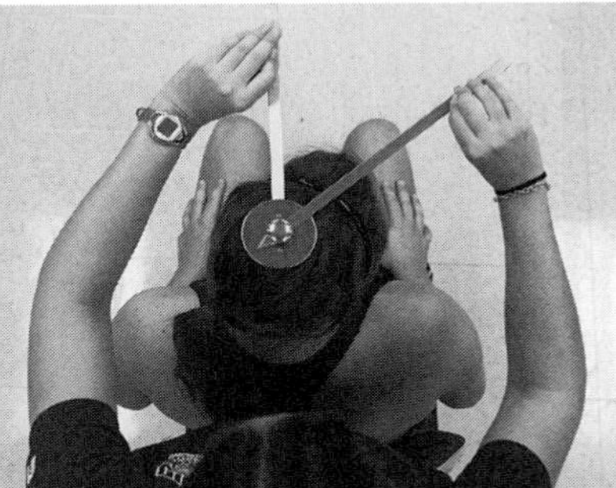

	Lateral Bending	Rotation
Patient Position	Standing with the knees extended and the spine in the neutral position	Seated The feet are placed firmly on the floor
Goniometer Alignment		
Fulcrum	The axis is aligned over the S1 spinous process	Aligned over the center of the patient's head
Proximal Arm	Aligned over the median sacral crest	Parallel to a line formed by the iliac crests
Distal Arm	Aligned with the C7 vertebrae	Parallel to a line formed by the two acromion processes.

Goniometry Box 13-3
Trunk Flexion and Extension (Inclinometer)

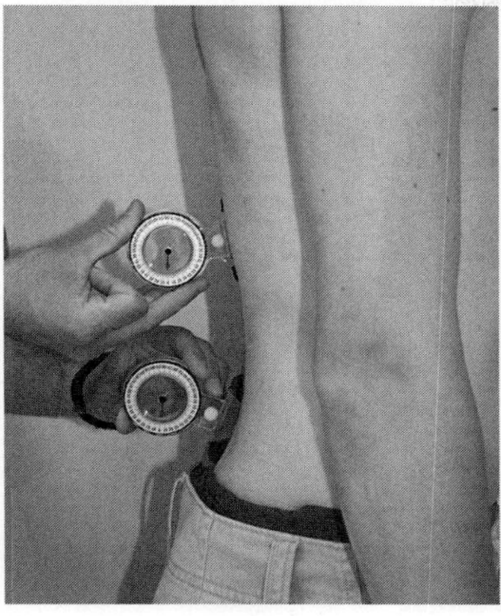

Flexion

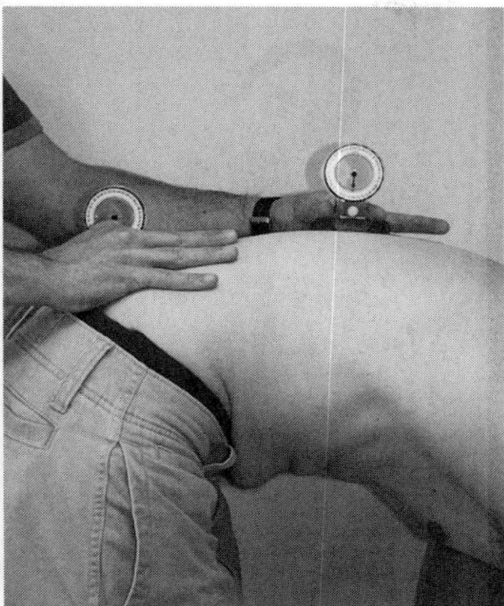

Extension

Patient Position	Standing with the feet shoulder-width apart
Procedure	Place one inclinometer at midline of spine in line with PSIS. The second inclinometer is placed 15 cm above first. Both inclinometers are set at 0°.
Measurement	
Motion	The patient forward flexes while the clinician holds the inclinometers.
Final Measurement	Flexion ROM is recorded as superior inclinometer reading minus the reading obtained from the inferior inclinometer. The reading at the superior inclinometer represents hip and spine motion; reading at the inferior inclinometer represents hip motion only.
Comments	This technique can be performed using a single inclinometer: Have the patient forward flex. Position and read the inferior goniometer, moving the inferior goniometer proximally and taking a reading. Motion measurements taken using inclinometers demonstrate a high correlation with measurements taken on MRI images.[73]

MRI = magnetic resonance imaging; PSIS = posterior superior iliac spine; ROM = range of motion.

Active Range of Motion

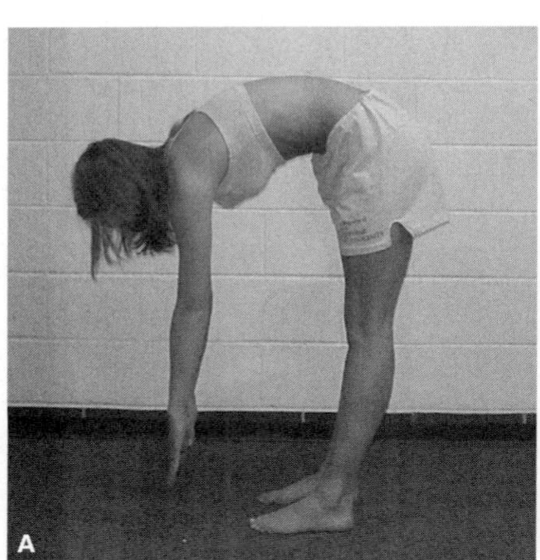

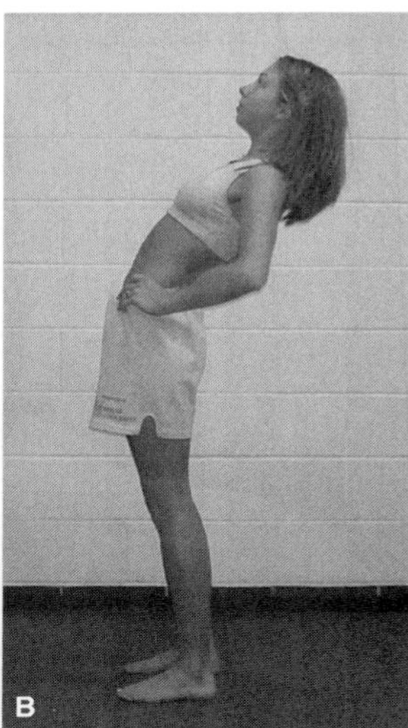

FIGURE 13-1 ■ Active trunk **(A)** flexion and **(B)** extension.

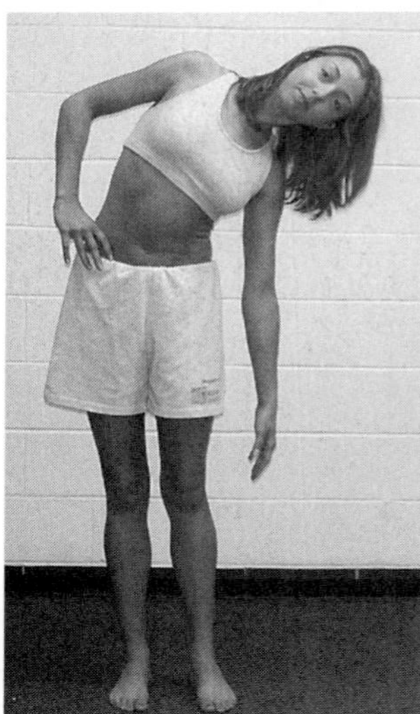

FIGURE 13-2 ■ Active lateral bending with gravity. The patient attempts to touch the fingers to the floor. Observe for normal segmental motion.

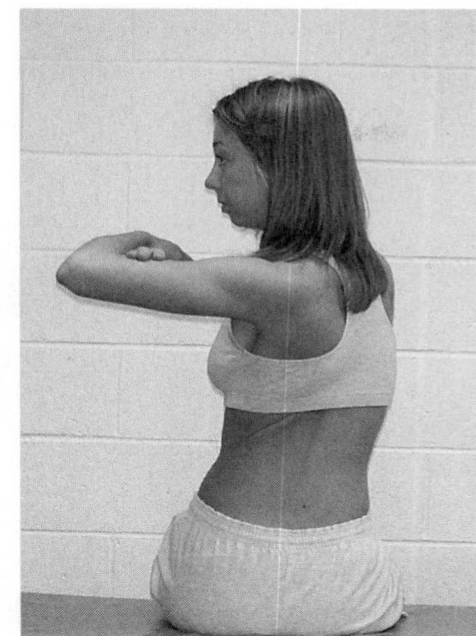

FIGURE 13-3 ■ Active trunk rotation. This motion occurs primarily in the thoracic spine.

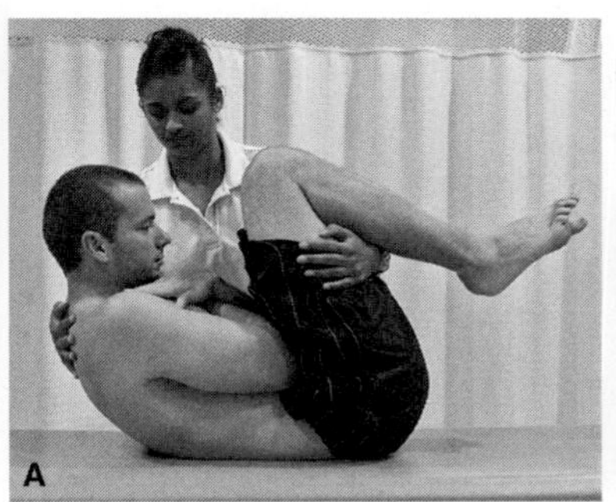

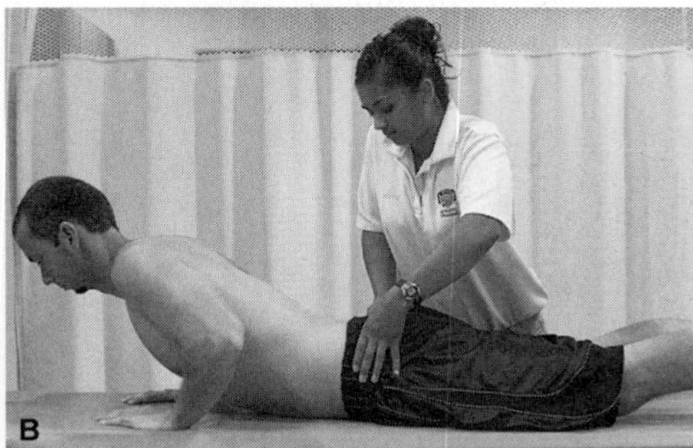

FIGURE 13-4 ■ Passive trunk **(A)** flexion and **(B)** extension.

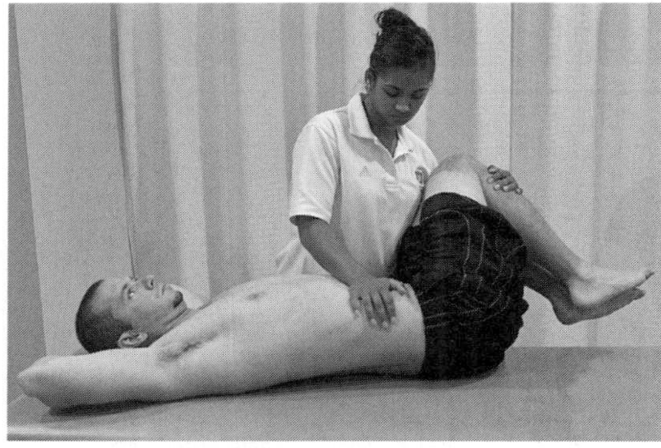

FIGURE 13-5 ■ Passive trunk rotation.

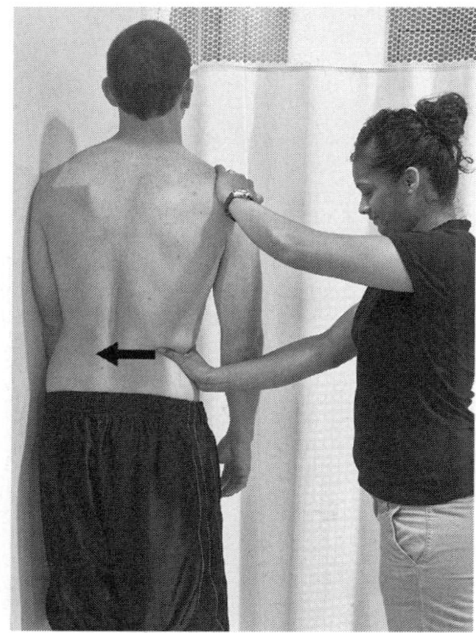

FIGURE 13-6 ■ Passive lateral glide of the trunk. The patient's shoulder is stabilized against the wall while the examiner forces the pelvis laterally.

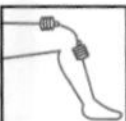

Manual Muscle Test 13-1
Trunk Flexion and Extension

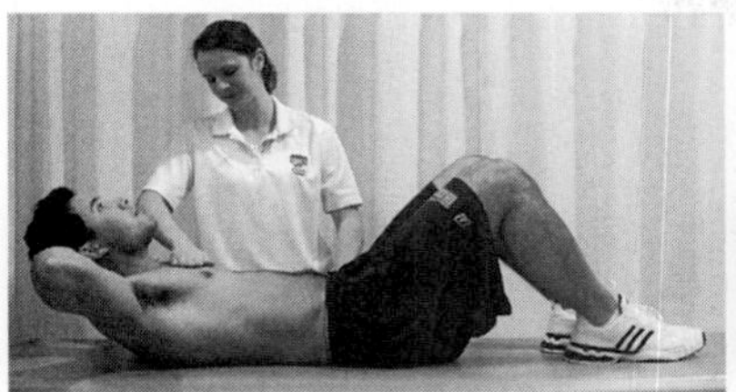

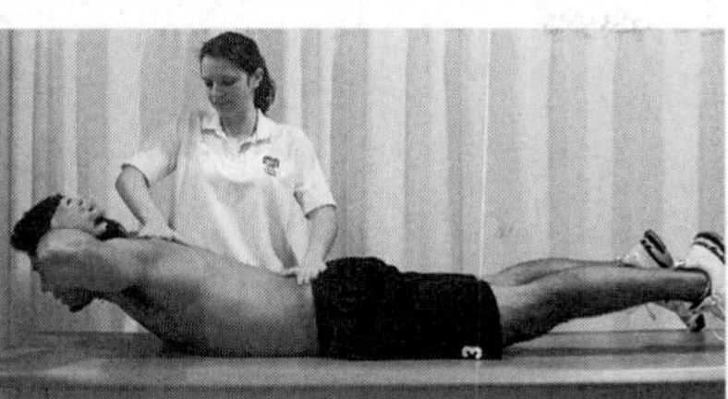

	Flexion	Extension
Patient Position	Supine	Prone
Starting Position	The knees are flexed and the feet flat on the table The patient's hands are interlocked behind the head with the elbow in line with the ears.	The elbows flexed with the hands interlocked behind the head
Stabilization	Pelvis	Pelvis
Palpation	Lateral to the abdominal midline	Lateral to the spine
Resistance	Resistance is applied to the superior sternum as the patient lifts the scapulae off the table.	Resistance is applied to the upper thoracic spine as the patient lifts the head, chest, and arms off the table.
Primary Mover(s) (Innervation)	Rectus abdominis	Iliocostalis lumborum, iliocostalis thoracis, longissimus thoracis, spinalis thoracis, semispinalis thoracis, multifidus
Secondary Mover(s) (Innervation)	Iliopsoas, rectus femoris, internal oblique and external oblique	Rotatores, latissimus dorsi, quadratus lumborum
Substitution	Reaching with shoulders/ elbows, hip flexion	Hip extension
Comments	The ability to sit up with the elbow by the head constitutes a grade of 5/5. If the patient cannot do this, try again with the arms folded across the chest.	The ability to extend the trunk with the elbows by the hand constitutes a grade of 5/5. If the patient cannot do this, try again with the arms at the side and the hands behind the back.

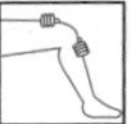

Manual Muscle Test 13-2
Trunk Rotation

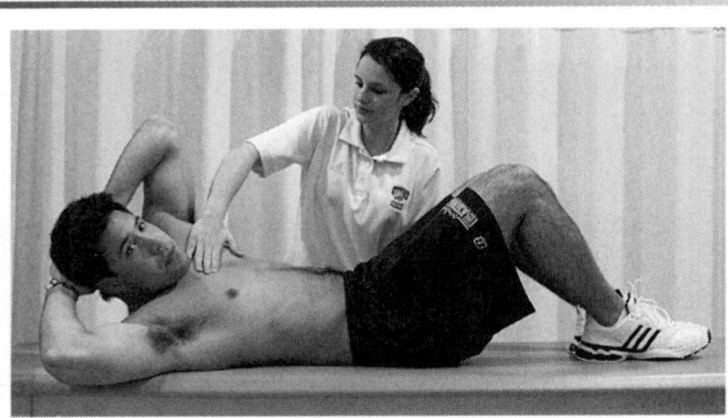

Patient Position	Supine
Starting Position	The knees are flexed and the feet flat on the table. The patient's hands are interlocked behind the head, with the elbows in line with the ears.
Stabilization	Opposite ASIS
Palpation	External oblique: Just below rib cage Internal oblique: Medial and just above anterior superior iliac spine
Resistance	Resistance is applied over the anterior aspect of the shoulder as it is rotated off the table. This procedure is repeated for the opposite side.
Primary Mover(s) (Innervation)	Internal oblique, external oblique (opposite side)
Secondary Mover(s) (Innervation)	Rotatores, multifidii (opposite side), latissimus dorsi
Substitution	Cervical flexion
Comments	The ability to sit up with the elbow by the head constitutes a grade of 5/5, even with no resistance. If the patient cannot do this, try again with the arms folded across the chest.

ASIS = anterior superior iliac spine.

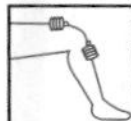

Manual Muscle Test 13-3
Pelvic Elevation

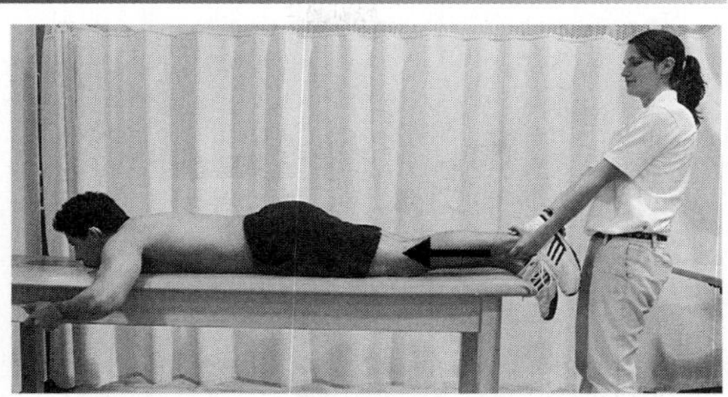

Patient Position	Supine or prone
Starting Position	The examiner grasps the patient's leg just proximal to the ankle.
Stabilization	The patient holds the edges of the table to maintain stabilization.
Palpation	Lateral lumbar spine
Resistance	The examiner distracts the leg by applying longitudinal resistance. The patient is then instructed to "hike" the pelvis, attempting to move the pelvis on the side being tested toward the rib cage.
Primary Mover(s) (Innervation)	Quadratus lumborum External oblique Internal oblique
Secondary Mover(s) (Innervation)	Latissimus dorsi (with the patient's arm's flexed) Iliocostalis lumborum
Substitution	Trunk lateral flexion (abdominals)
Comments	The test may also be performed with the patient standing on a lift and hiking the opposite leg.

Table 13-4 Extrinsic Muscles Acting on the Spinal Column

Muscle	Action	Origin	Insertion	Innervation	Root
Rectus Abdominis	Flexion of the lumbar spine against gravity Posterior rotation of the pelvis	Pubic crest Pubic symphysis	Costal cartilage of the 5th–7th ribs Xiphoid process of sternum	Ventral rami	T5–T12
External Oblique	Bilateral contraction: Flexion of the lumbar spine Posterior rotation of the pelvis Unilateral contraction: Rotation of the lumbar spine to the opposite side Lateral bending of the lumbar spine to the same side	5th– 8th ribs (anterior fibers) 9th–12th ribs (lateral fibers)	Via an aponeurosis to the linea alba (anterior fibers) Anterior superior iliac spine, pubic tubercle, and the anterior portion of the iliac crest (lateral fibers)	Iliohypogastric Ilioinguinal Ventral rami	T1–T12
Internal Oblique	Bilateral contraction: Support of the abdominal viscera Posterior rotation of the pelvis Flexion of the lumbar spine Unilateral contraction: Rotation of the lumbar spine to the same side Lateral bending of the lumbar spine to the same side	Lateral two thirds of the inguinal ligament (lower fibers) • Anterior one third of the iliac crest (upper fibers) • Middle one third of the iliac crest (lateral fibers)	Crest of pubis, pectineal line (lower fibers) 10th–12th ribs (lateral fibers) • Linea alba (all portions)	Iliohypogastric Ilioinguinal Ventral rami	T7–T12

Latissimus Dorsi	Extension of the spine Anterior rotation of the pelvis (also see shoulder function) Stabilization of the lumbar spine via the thoracodorsal fascia	Spinous processes of T6–T12 and the lumbar vertebrae via the thoracodorsal fascia Posterior iliac crest	Intertubercular groove of the humerus	Thoracodorsal	C6, C7, C8
Trapezius (middle one third)	Retraction of scapula Fixation of thoracic spine	Lower portion of the ligamentum nuchae Spinous processes of the 7th cervical vertebra and T1–T5	Acromion process Spine of the scapula (superior, lateral border)	Accessory	Cranial nerve XI
Trapezius (lower one third)	Depression of scapula Retraction of scapula Upward rotation of the scapula Fixation of thoracic spine	Spinous processes and supraspinal ligaments of T8–T12	Spine of the scapula (medial portion)	Accessory	Cranial nerve XI
Rhomboid Major	Retraction of scapula Elevation of scapula Downward rotation of scapula Fixation of thoracic spine	Spinous processes of T2, T3, T4, and T5	Vertebral border of scapula (lower two thirds)	Dorsal scapular	C5
Rhomboid Minor	Retraction of scapula Elevation of scapula Downward rotation of scapula Fixation of thoracic spine	Inferior portion of the ligamentum nuchae Spinous processes C7 and T1	Vertebral border of scapula (upper one third and superior angle)	Dorsal scapular	C5

Table 13-5 Intrinsic Muscles Acting on the Spinal Column

Muscle	Action	Origin	Insertion	Innervation	Root
Iliocostalis Lumborum	Bilateral contraction: Extension of spinal column Unilateral contraction: Lateral bending of spinal column to the same side	Posterior aspect of the iliac crest	Inferior angles of ribs 6–12	Posterior primary divisions of the spinal nerves	Multiple roots, segmentally along the length of the muscle
Iliocostalis Thoracis	Bilateral contraction: Extension of spinal column Unilateral contraction: Lateral bending of spinal column to the same side	Ribs 6–12	Ribs 1–6 Transverse process of C7	Posterior primary divisions of the spinal nerves	Multiple roots, segmentally along the length of the muscle
Longissimus Thoracis	Bilateral contraction: Extension of spinal column Unilateral contraction: Lateral bending of spinal column	Common erector spinae tendon	Transverse process of T3–T21 Ribs 3–12	Posterior primary divisions of the spinal nerves	Multiple roots, segmentally along the length of the muscle
Spinalis Thoracis	Bilateral contraction: Extension of the spine Unilateral contraction: Lateral bending of the spine to the same side	Common erector spinae tendon	Spinous processes of upper thoracic spine	Posterior primary divisions of the spinal nerves	Multiple roots, segmentally along the length of the muscle
Semispinalis Thoracis	Bilateral contraction: Extension of thoracic and cervical spine Unilateral contraction: Rotation to the opposite side	Transverse process	Travel upwardly and medially to attach to a spinous process 5 or 8 vertebrae above the origin	Posterior primary divisions of the spinal nerves	Multiple roots, segmentally along the length of the muscle

Multifidus* *(or multifidi)	Bilateral contraction: Stabilization of vertebral column Unilateral contraction: Rotation of spine to the opposite side	Lumbar region • Superior aspect of sacrum Thoracic region • Transverse processes Cervical region • Articular processes	Spinous process	Posterior primary divisions of the spinal nerves	Multiple roots, segmentally along the length of the muscle
Rotatores	Bilateral contraction: Extension of spine Stabilization of vertebral column Unilateral contraction: Rotation of spine	Transverse process	Spinous process of the vertebra immediately above the origin	Posterior primary divisions of the spinal nerves	Multiple roots, segmentally along the length of the muscle

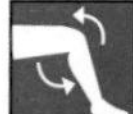

Joint Play 13-1
Posterior–Anterior Vertebral Joint Play (Spring Test)

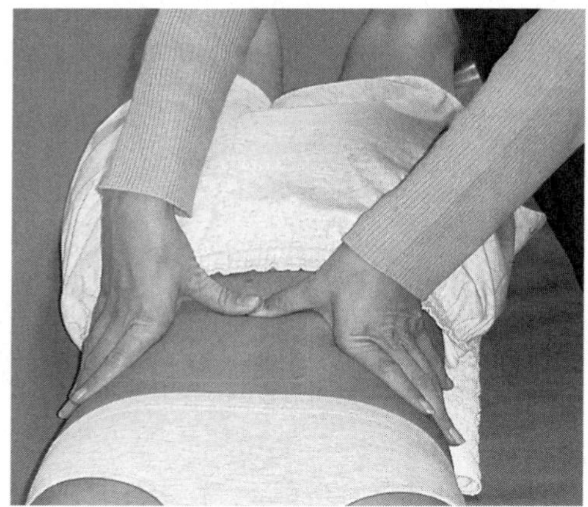

Posterior–anterior joint play is used to determine normal vertebral movement (spring).

Patient Position	Prone
Position of Examiner	Standing over the patient with the thumbs placed over the spinous process to be tested
Evaluative Procedure	The examiner carefully pushes the spinous process anteriorly, feeling for the springing of the vertebrae.
Positive Test	The vertebra does not move ("spring"), moves excessively, or pain is elicited.
Implications	Hypomobility or hypermobility of the vertebral segment
Evidence	Inter-rater reliability (pain)

Inter-rater reliability (pain)

Not Reliable — Very Reliable
Poor | Moderate | Good
0 0.1 0.2 0.3 0.4 0.5 0.6 0.7 0.8 0.9 1.0

Inter-rater reliability (stiffness)

Not Reliable — Very Reliable
Poor | Moderate | Good
0 0.1 0.2 0.3 0.4 0.5 0.6 0.7 0.8 0.9 1.0

Positive likelihood ratio

Not Useful — Useful
Very Small | Small | Moderate | Large
0 1 2 3 4 5 6 7 8 9 10

Negative likelihood ratio

Not Useful — Useful
Very Small | Small | Moderate | Large
1.0 0.9 0.8 0.7 0.6 0.5 0.4 0.3 0.2 0.1 0

Special Test 13-1
Hoover Test

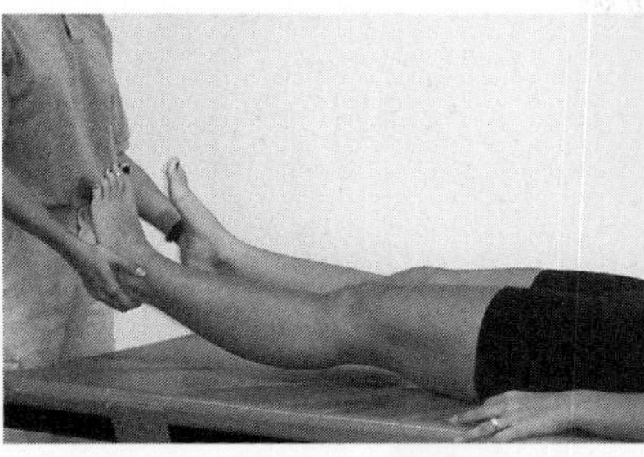

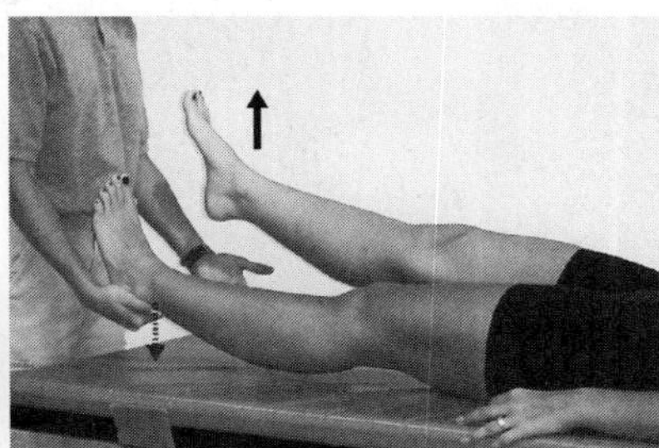

The Hoover Test is used to identify if a patient is actually exerting effort during the testing procedure. A positive test suggests that the patient is malingering.

Patient Position	Supine
Position of Examiner	At the feet of the patient with the evaluator's hands cupping the calcaneus of each leg
Evaluative Procedure	The patient attempts an active straight leg raise on the involved side
Positive Test	The patient does not attempt to lift the leg and the examiner does not sense pressure from the uninvolved leg pressing down on the hand as should instinctively happen.
Implications	The patient is not attempting to perform the test (i.e., malingering).
Evidence	Absent or inconclusive in the literature

Special Test 13-2
Test for Scoliosis (Adams Forward Bend Test)

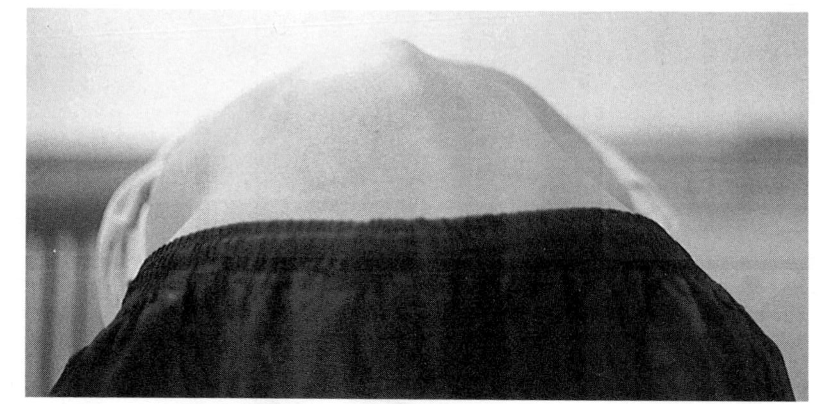

Posterior view of the spinal column while the patient flexes the spine; note the presence of a hump over the left thoracic spine, suggesting scoliosis.

Patient Position	Standing with hands held in front with the arms straight
Position of Examiner	Seated in front of or behind the patient
Evaluative Procedure	The patient bends forward, sliding the hands down the front of each leg.
Positive Test	An asymmetrical hump is observed along the lateral aspect of the thoracolumbar spine and rib cage.
Implications	If scoliosis is present but disappears during flexion, then functional scoliosis is suggested. Scoliosis that is present while the patient is standing upright and while forwardly flexed indicates structural scoliosis.

Evidence

Inter-rater reliability

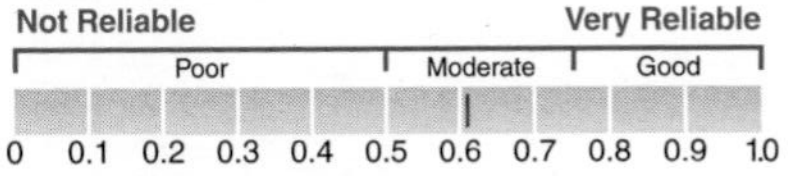

Not Reliable **Very Reliable**

Poor | Moderate | Good

0 0.1 0.2 0.3 0.4 0.5 0.6 0.7 0.8 0.9 1.0

Thoracic curvature

Positive likelihood ratio

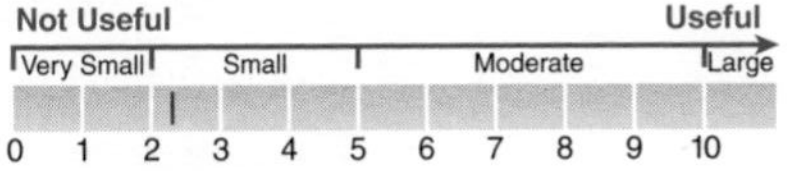

Not Useful **Useful**

Very Small | Small | Moderate | Large

0 1 2 3 4 5 6 7 8 9 10

Negative likelihood ratio

Not Useful **Useful**

Very Small | Small | Moderate | Large

1.0 0.9 0.8 0.7 0.6 0.5 0.4 0.3 0.2 0.1 0

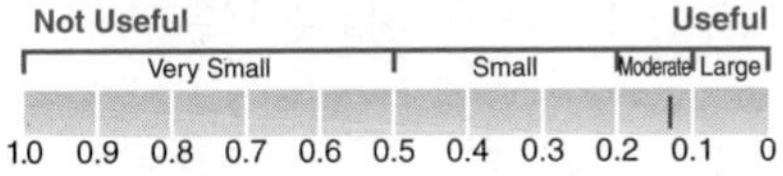

Lumbar curvature

Positive likelihood ratio

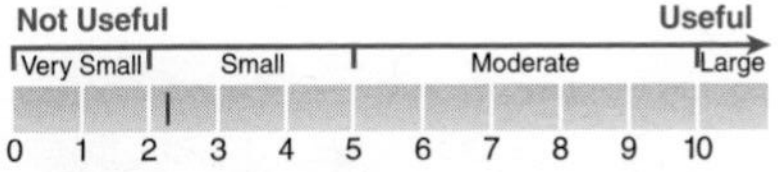

Not Useful **Useful**

Very Small | Small | Moderate | Large

0 1 2 3 4 5 6 7 8 9 10

Negative likelihood ratio

Not Useful **Useful**

Very Small | Small | Moderate | Large

1.0 0.9 0.8 0.7 0.6 0.5 0.4 0.3 0.2 0.1 0

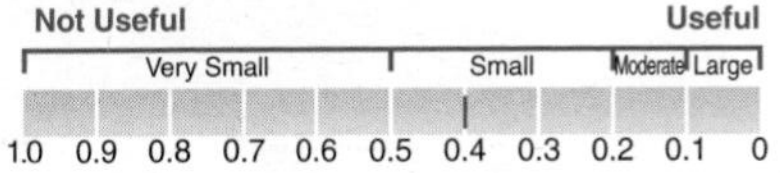

Special Test 13-3
Beevor's Sign for Thoracic Nerve Inhibition

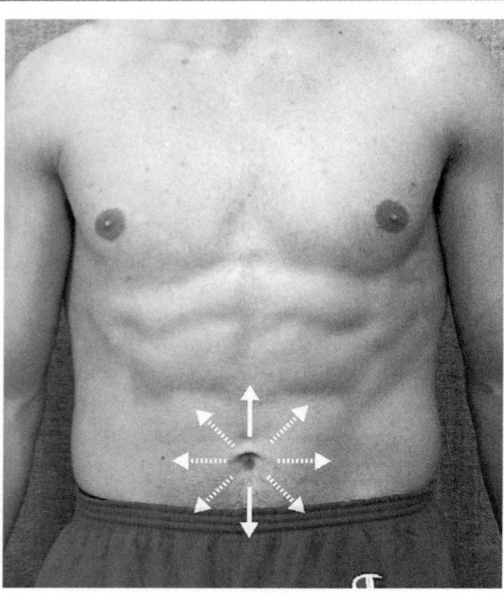

Lateral movement of the umbilicus can indicate inhibition of the thoracic nerves innervating the abdominal muscles.

Patient Position	Hook-lying
Position of Examiner	At the side of the patient
Evaluative Procedure	The patient performs an abdominal curl (partial sit-up).
Positive Test	The umbilicus moves up, down, or to one side.
Implications	Segmental involvement of the nerves innervating the rectus abdominis (T5–T12); this should draw suspicion to the paraspinal muscles innervated by the same nerve roots.
Comments	Normally the umbilicus should not move at all during this test, but will move toward the stronger muscle group in the presence of pathology.
Evidence	Absent or inconclusive in the literature

Special Test 13-4
Valsalva Test

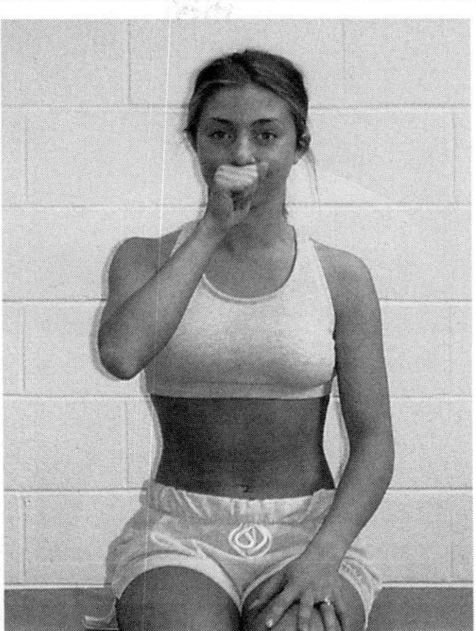

The Valsalva test attempts to increase intrathecal pressure, duplicating nerve-root pain that may be elicited while coughing or with bowel movements.

Patient Position	Sitting
Position of Examiner	Standing within arms' reach in front of the patient
Evaluative Procedure	The patient takes and holds a deep breath while bearing down similar to performing a bowel movement.
Positive Test	Increased spinal or radicular pain
Implications	Increase in intrathecal pressure causes pain secondary to a space-occupying lesion such as a herniated disk, tumor, or osteophyte anywhere along the spinal column Athletic pubalgia
Modification	If the patient is embarrassed or apprehensive about simulating a bowel movement, he or she may be instructed to blow into a closed fist as if inflating a balloon.
Comments	This can be performed for any level of the spine. The test increases intrathecal pressure, resulting in a slowing of the pulse, decreased venous return, and increased venous pressure, all of which may cause fainting.
Evidence	Inter-rater reliability Not Reliable — Very Reliable Poor — Moderate — Good 0 0.1 0.2 0.3 0.4 0.5 0.6 0.7 0.8 0.9 1.0

Special Test 13-5
Milgram Test

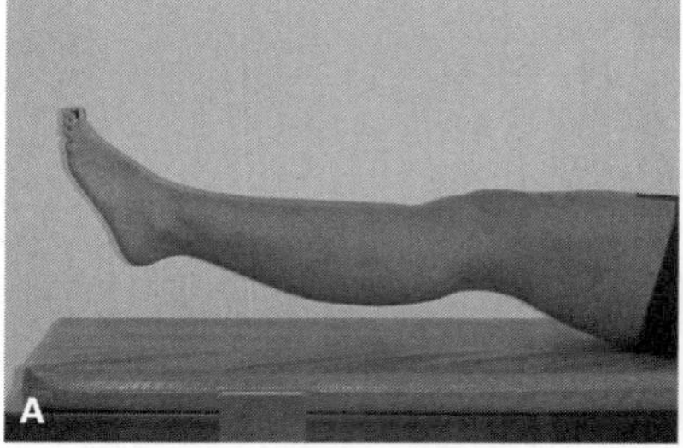

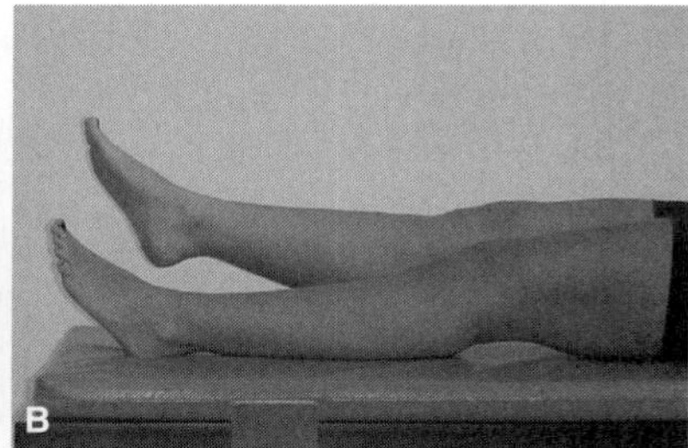

A bilateral straight leg raise is used to increase pressure on the lumbar nerve roots. In the presence of a disk lesion one or both legs will drop.

Patient Position	Supine
Position of Examiner	At the feet of the patient
Evaluative Procedure	The patient performs a bilateral straight leg raise to the height of 2–6 inches and is asked to hold the position for 30 seconds **(A)**.
Positive Test	The patient is unable to hold the position, cannot lift the leg, or experiences pain with the test **(B)**.
Implications	Intrathecal or extrathecal pressure causing an intervertebral disk to place pressure on a lumbar nerve root
Evidence	Absent or inconclusive in the literature

Special Test 13-6
Kernig's Test/Brudzinski Test

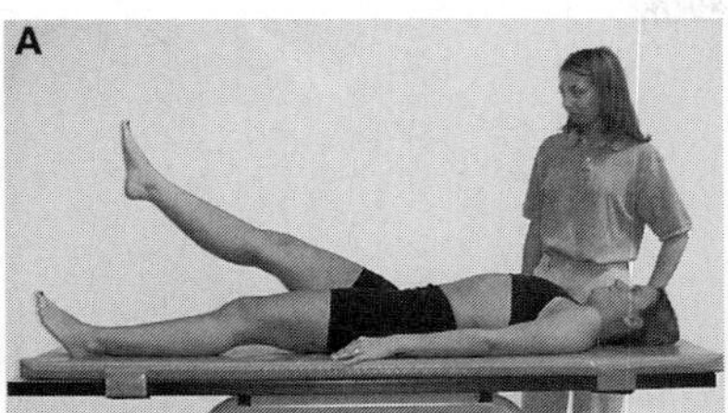

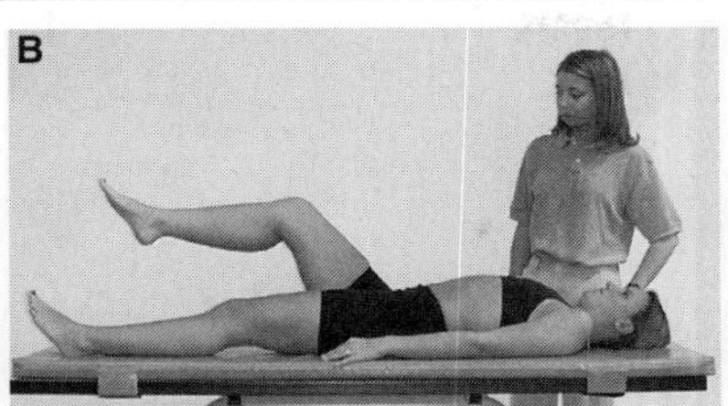

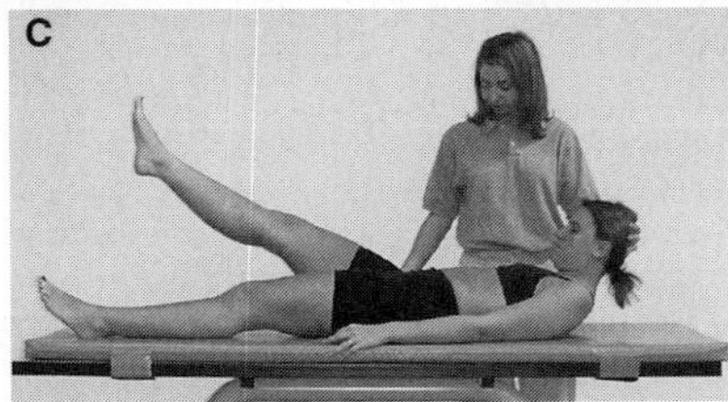

The Kernig test identifies nerve root entrapment caused by a bulging of an intervertebral disk or narrowing of the intervertebral foramen. The Brudzinski test **(C)** identifies symptoms caused by a stretching of the dural sheath.

Patient Position	Supine
Position of Examiner	At the side of the patient
Evaluative Procedure	The patient performs a unilateral active straight leg raise with the knee extended until pain occurs **(A)**. After pain occurs, the patient flexes the knee **(B)**.
Positive Test	Pain is experienced in the spine and possibly radiating into the lower extremity. This pain is relieved when the patient flexes the knee.
Implications	Nerve root impingement secondary to a bulging of the intervertebral disk or bony entrapment; irritation of the dural sheath; or irritation of the meninges.
Modification	In the absence of pain during the active straight leg raise, the examiner may further elongate the spinal cord and increase the tension on the dural sheath by passively flexing the patient's cervical spine (**Brudzinski's test**) and repeating the test **(C)**.
Evidence	Absent or inconclusive in the literature

Special Test 13-7
Straight Leg Raise Test (Test of Lasègue)

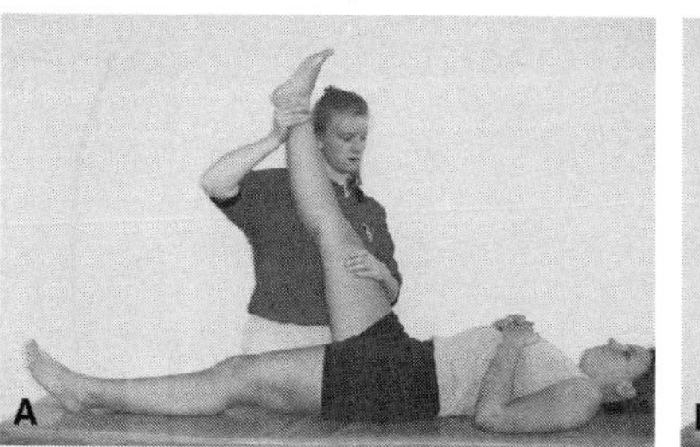

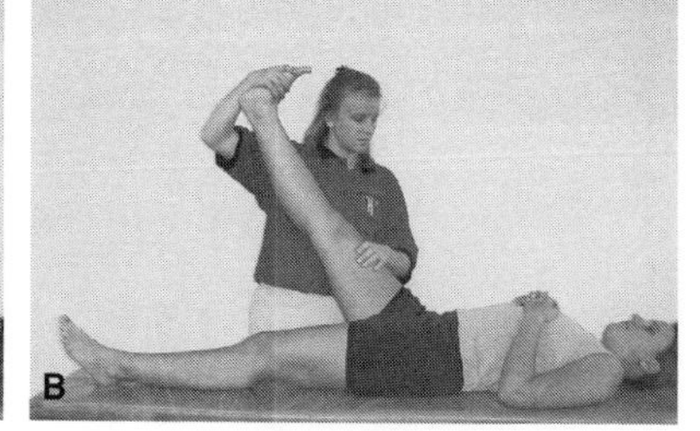

(A) The involved leg is flexed at the hip until symptoms are experienced. **(B)** The involved leg is extended approximately 10° (until symptoms subside) and the ankle is then passively dorsiflexed. A return of the symptoms indicates a stretching of the dural sheath.

Patient Position	Supine
Position of Examiner	At the side to be tested; one hand grasps under the heel while the other is placed on the anterior knee to keep it in full extension during the examination.
Evaluative Procedure	While keeping the knee in extension, the examiner raises the leg by flexing the hip until discomfort is experienced or the full ROM is obtained.
Positive Test	The patient complains of pain before the end of the normal ROM (70°). The pain may be described as radiating distally along the tested leg, usually in the posterior thigh, radiating into the calf and perhaps the foot. The findings are highly significant if they are elicited at 30° or less of hip flexion.[74]
Implications	Sciatic nerve irritation/compression Pain described before the hip reaches 70° of hip flexion may indicate disk involvement.[75]
Modification	After pain is experienced, the leg is lowered to the point at which the pain stops. The examiner passively dorsiflexes the ankle and/or has the patient flex the cervical spine. Serving to stretch the dural sheath, this flexion recreates the symptoms. If the patient's prior pain was caused by tight hamstrings, this modification does not elicit pain.

Comments	The SLR may be helpful in differentiating between tarsal tunnel syndrome and plantar fasciitis. Beginning with the foot dorsiflexed and everted additionally stresses the tibial nerve. The SLR is then performed. An increase in symptoms points to tibial nerve entrapment because strain on the plantar fascia would not further increase.[76]
Evidence	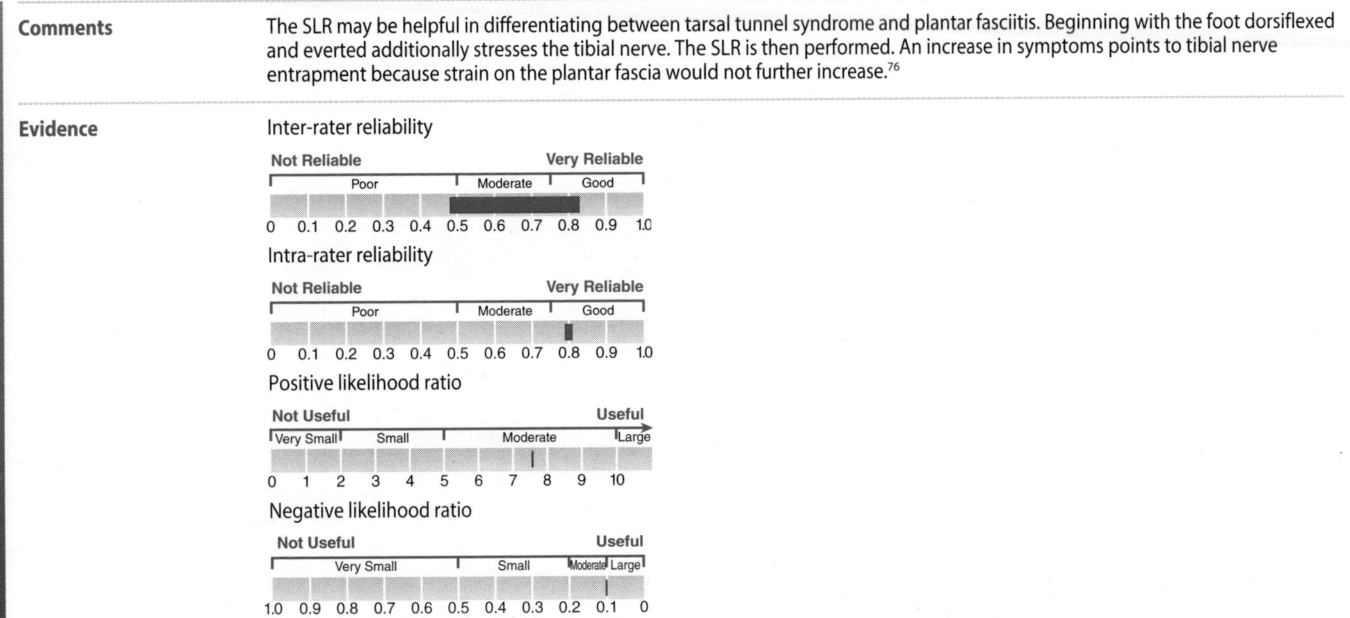

ROM = range of motion.

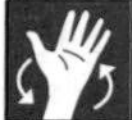

Special Test 13-8
Well (Cross) Straight Leg Raising Test

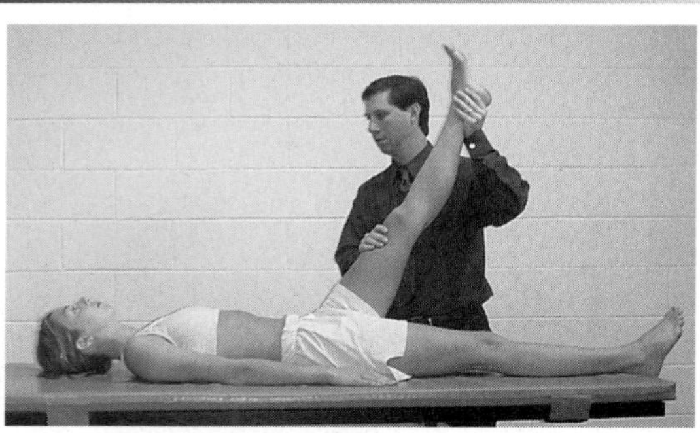

The well straight leg raise test differs from the straight leg raise test in that the unaffected leg is elevated.

Patient Position	Supine
Position of Examiner	At the side to be tested (the side not suffering the symptoms); one hand grasps under the heel while the other is placed on the anterior thigh just superior to the knee to maintain the leg in extension.
Evaluative Procedure	Keeping the knee in extension, the examiner raises the leg by flexing the hip until discomfort is reported.
Positive Test	Pain is experienced on the side opposite that being raised.
Implications	A large space-occupying lesion such as a herniated intervertebral disk
Evidence	Positive likelihood ratio Not Useful — Useful Very Small, Small, Moderate, Large 0 1 2 3 4 5 6 7 8 9 10 Negative likelihood ratio Not Useful — Useful Very Small, Small, Moderate, Large 1.0 0.9 0.8 0.7 0.6 0.5 0.4 0.3 0.2 0.1 0

Special Test 13-9
Slump Test

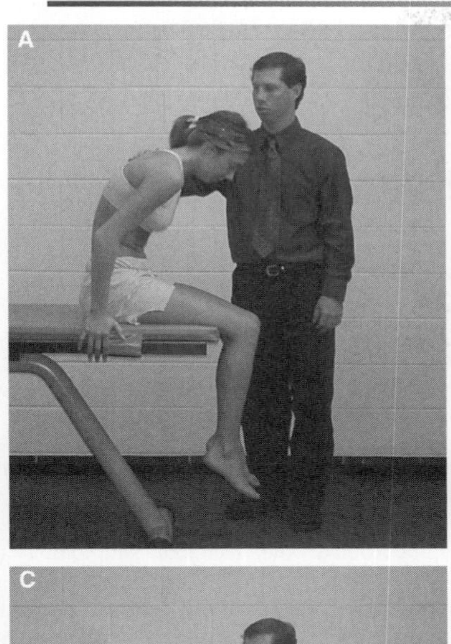

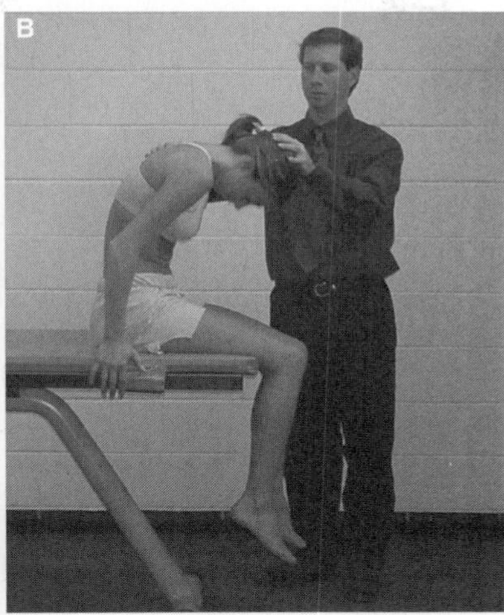

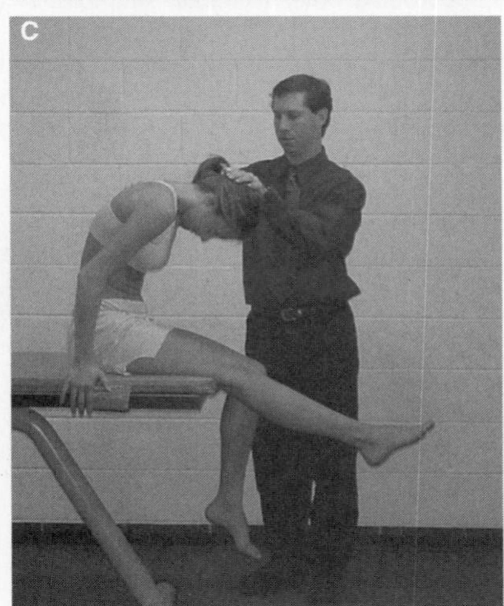

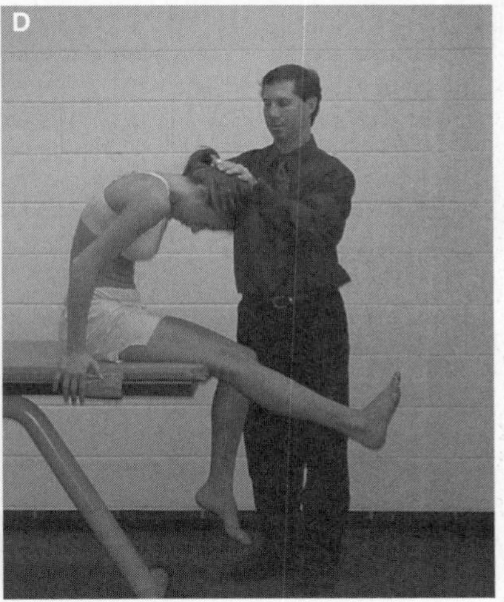

The slump test is designed to place progressively more tension on the nerve and nerve roots by changing positions and then systematically positioning the patient to provoke or alleviate symptoms.

Patient Position	Sitting over the edge of the table
Position of Examiner	At the side of the patient

Continued

Special Test 13-9—cont'd
Slump Test

Evaluative Procedure	The following sequence is followed until symptoms are provoked: **1.** The patient slumps forward along the thoracolumbar spine, rounding the shoulders while keeping the cervical spine in neutral **(A)**. Overpressure to trunk flexion is then applied. **2.** The patient flexes the cervical spine by bringing the chin to the chest. The clinician then holds the patient in this position **(B)**. **3.** The knee is actively extended **(C)**. **4.** The ankle is actively dorsiflexed **(D)**. **5.** Repeat steps 2–4 on the opposite side. **6. Alleviation maneuver**: At any step that symptoms are elicited, the provoking position is slightly relieved and tension is reduced at the other end of the nervous system. For example, if knee extension reproduces symptoms, slightly flex the patient's knee and extend the cervical spine. Extend the patient's knee again. In this example if the symptoms reappear the cause is nerve tension as opposed to hamstring pathology.
Positive Test	Sciatic pain or reproduction of other neurologic symptoms
Implications	Impingement of the dural lining, spinal cord, or nerve roots
Modification	Many modifications have been proposed, most of which describe different sequences of motions.
Evidence	Absent or inconclusive in the literature

Special Test 13-10
Quadrant Test

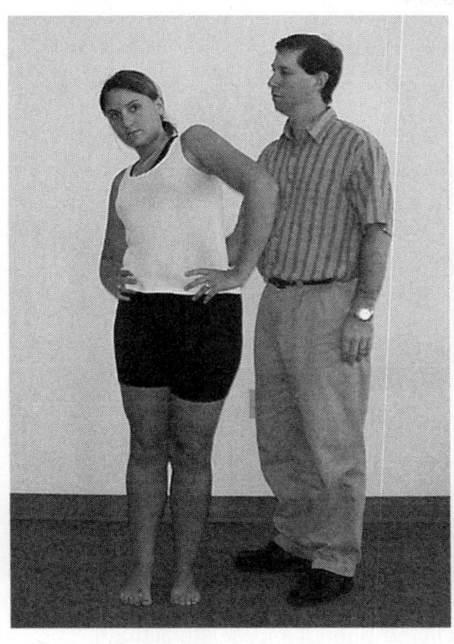

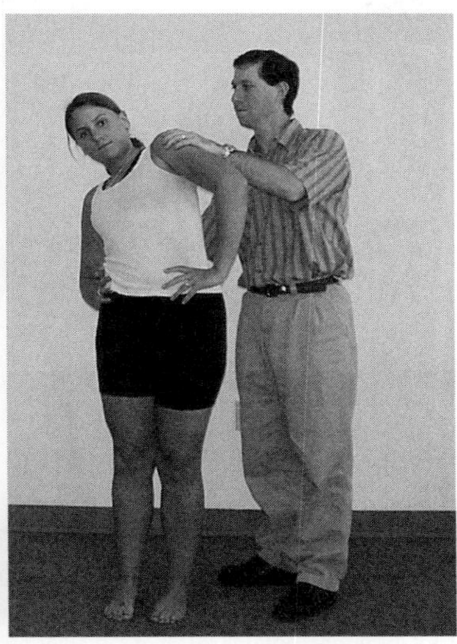

The patient moves into extension, followed by sidebending and rotation to the same side. The examiner provides overpressure to emphasize the position.

Patient Position	Standing with the feet shoulder-width apart
Position of Examiner	Standing behind the patient, grasping the patient's shoulders
Evaluative Procedure	The patient extends the spine as far as possible, then sidebends and rotates to the affected side. The examiner provides overpressure through the shoulders, supporting the patient as needed.
Positive Test	Reproduction of the patient's symptoms
Implications	Radicular pain indicates compression of the intervertebral foramina that impinges on the lumbar nerve roots. Local (nonradiating) pain indicates facet joint pathology. Symptoms isolated to the area of the PSIS; may also indicate SI joint dysfunction
Evidence	Inter-rater reliability Not Reliable — Very Reliable Poor — Moderate — Good 0 0.1 0.2 0.3 0.4 0.5 0.6 0.7 0.8 0.9 1.0

PSIS = posterior superior iliac spine; SI = sacroiliac.

Special Test 13-11
Femoral Nerve Stretch Test

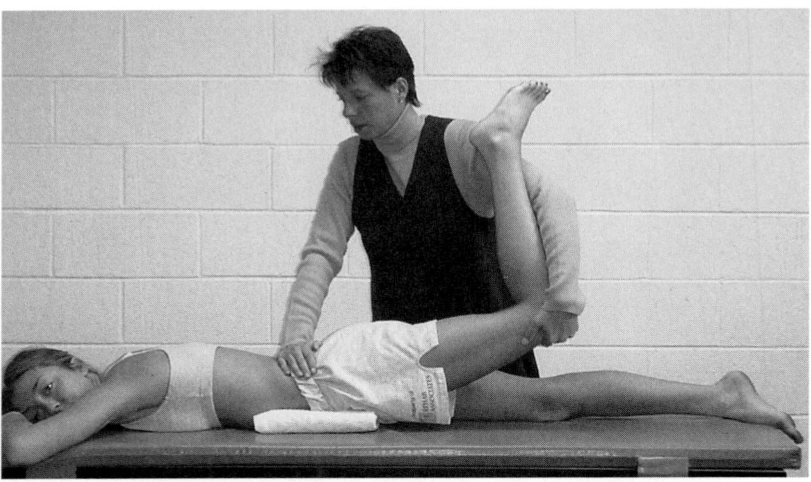

The femoral nerve (L2, L3, L4) is placed on stretch by passively flexing the patient's knee. Nerve root impingement will result in radicular pain in the anterior and/or lateral thigh.

Patient Position	Prone with a pillow under the abdomen
Position of Examiner	At the side of the patient
Evaluative Procedure	The examiner passively flexes the patient's knee.
Positive Test	Pain is elicited in the anterior and lateral thigh.
Implications	Nerve root impingement at the L2, L3, or L4 level
Modification	The femoral nerve may be further stressed by passively extending the patient's hip while maintaining knee flexion. If the patient cannot lie prone, the test can be performed in side-lying with the pelvis stabilized.
Comments	The examiner should attempt to fully flex the knee with the hip in the neutral position to determine any strain of the quadriceps muscle that may also cause pain. This test is associated with a high number of false positives due to tight or injured quadriceps.
Evidence	Absent or inconclusive in the literature

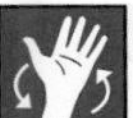

Special Test 13-12
Tension Sign

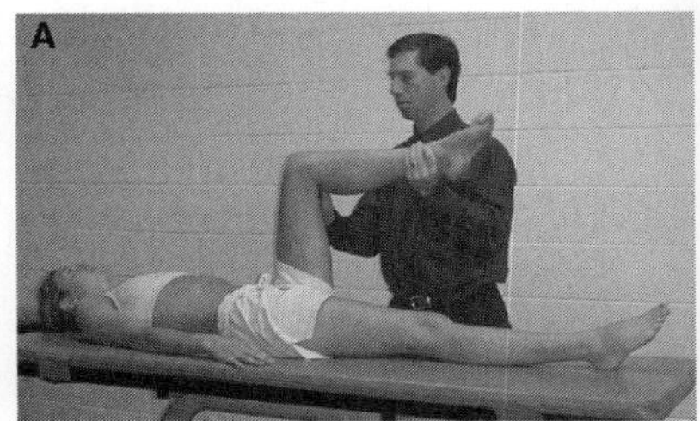

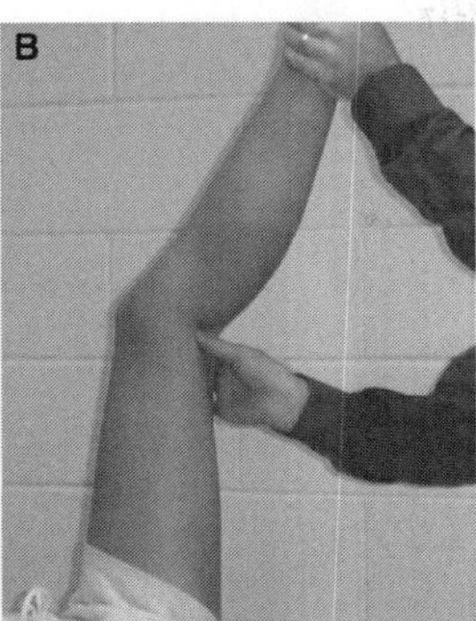

The sciatic nerve is stretched by extending the patient's knee with the hip flexed to 90° while palpating the nerve as it passes through the popliteal fossa.

Patient Position	Supine
Position of Examiner	At the patient's side that is to be tested; one hand grasps the heel while the other grasps the thigh.
Evaluative Procedure	The hip is flexed to 90°, with the knee flexed to 90°. The knee is then extended as far as possible with the examiner palpating the tibial portion of the sciatic nerve as it passes through the popliteal space **(A)**.
Positive Test	Exquisite tenderness with possible duplication of sciatic symptoms, as compared with the opposite side.
Implications	Sciatic nerve irritation
Modification	The Bowstring test is a variation of this technique **(B)**. The examiner extends the patient's knee until radiating symptoms are experienced. The knee is then flexed approximately 20° or until the symptoms are relieved. The examiner then pushes on the tibial portion of the sciatic nerve to reestablish the symptoms.
Evidence	Absent or inconclusive in the literature

Special Test 13-13
Single Leg Stance Test

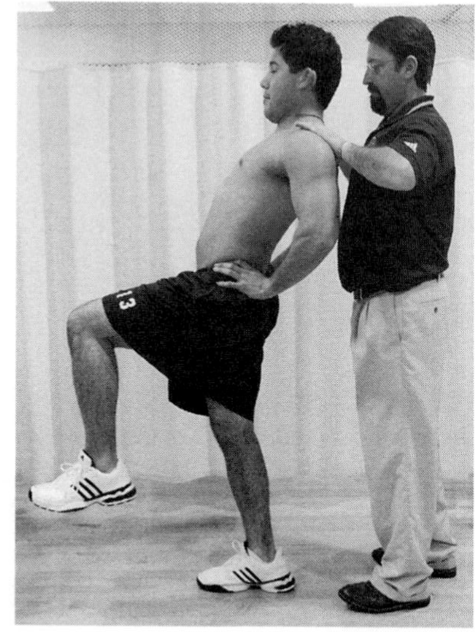

This test reproduces the positions that maximally stress the pars interarticularis by positioning the patient in extension and rotation.

Patient Position	Standing with the body weight evenly distributed between the two feet
Position of Examiner	Standing behind the patient, ready to provide support if the patient begins to fall

Evaluative Procedure	The patient lifts one leg, then places the trunk in hyperextension. The examiner may assist the patient during this motion. The procedure is then repeated for the opposite leg.
Positive Test	Pain is noted in the lumbar spine or SI area.
Implications	Shear forces are placed on the pars interarticularis by the iliopsoas pulling the vertebra anteriorly, resulting in pain.
Comments	When the lesion to the pars interarticularis is unilateral, pain is evoked when the opposite leg is raised. Bilateral pars fractures result in pain when either leg is lifted. This test may also result in pain specifically at the area of the PSIS secondary to SI joint irritation.
Evidence	Absent or inconclusive in the literature

PSIS = posterior superior iliac spine; SI = sacroiliac.

Special Test 13-14
Sacroiliac Joint Compression and Distraction Tests

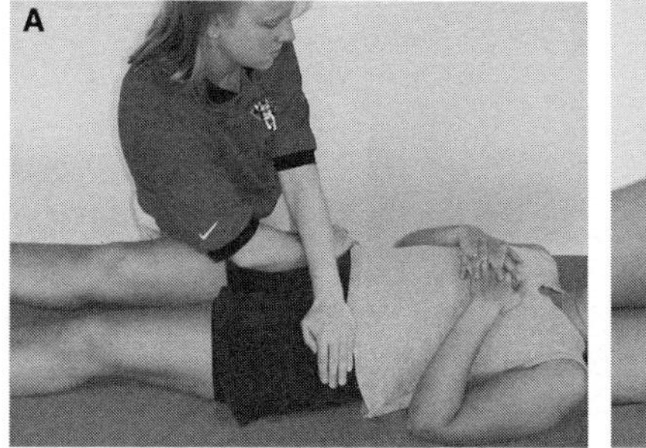

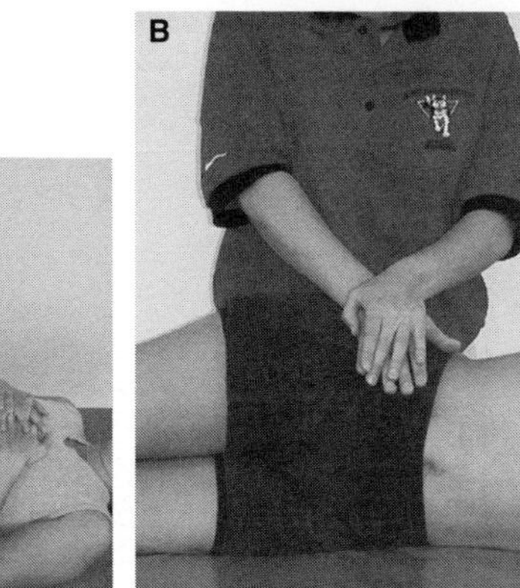

(A) Sacroiliac joint compression test. Spreading the ASIS compresses the SI joint. **(B)** Sacroiliac joint distraction test. Compressing the ASIS distracts the SI joints. The distraction test should be performed on both sides.

Patient Position	***Compression:*** Sidelying ***Distraction:*** Supine
Position of Examiner	***Compression:*** At the side of the patient with the hands placed over the opposite ASIS bilaterally ***Distraction:*** Behind the patient with both hands over the lateral aspect of the pelvis.
Evaluative Procedure	***Compression:*** The examiner applies pressure to spread the ASIS, thus compressing the SI joints. ***Distraction:*** The examiner applies pressure down through the anterior portion of the ilium, spreading the SI joints.
Positive Test	Pain arising from the SI joint
Implications	Sacroiliac pathology

Evidence

Compression inter-rater reliability

Not Reliable — Very Reliable
Poor | Moderate | Good
0 0.1 0.2 0.3 0.4 0.5 0.6 0.7 0.8 0.9 1.0

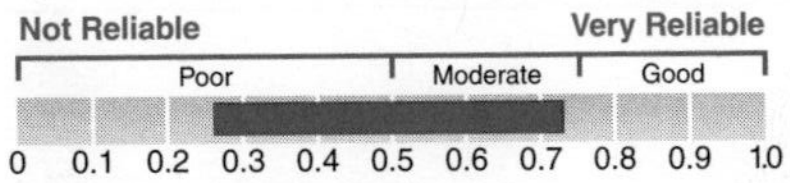

Distraction inter-rater reliability

Not Reliable — Very Reliable
Poor | Moderate | Good
0 0.1 0.2 0.3 0.4 0.5 0.6 0.7 0.8 0.9 1.0

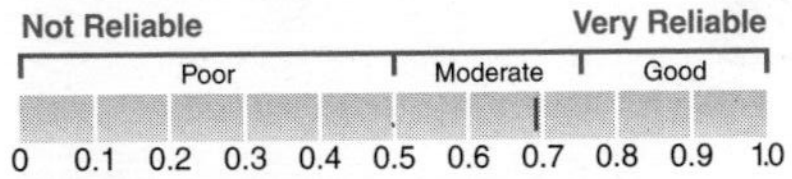

Compression positive likelihood ratio

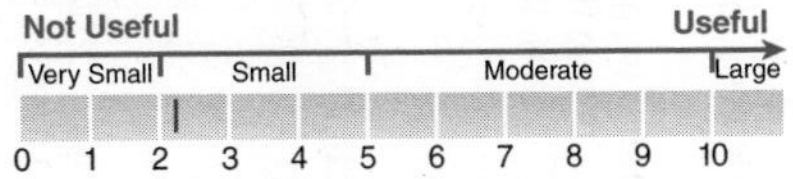

Not Useful — Useful
Very Small | Small | Moderate | Large
0 1 2 3 4 5 6 7 8 9 10

Compression negative likelihood ratio

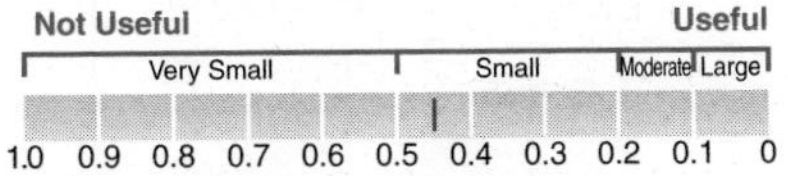

Not Useful — Useful
Very Small | Small | Moderate | Large
1.0 0.9 0.8 0.7 0.6 0.5 0.4 0.3 0.2 0.1 0

ASIS = anterior superior iliac spine; SI = sacroiliac.

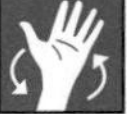

Special Test 13-15
Fabere (Patrick's) Test

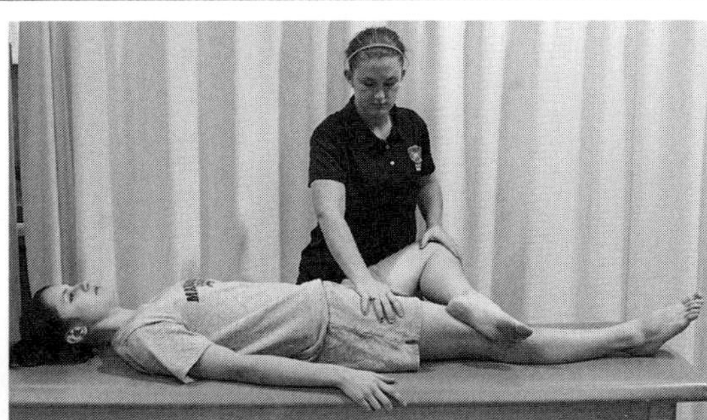

Fabere (flexion, abduction, external rotation, and extension) test for hip or sacroiliac pathology.

Patient Position	Supine, with the foot of the involved side crossed over the opposite thigh
Position of Examiner	At the side of the patient to be tested with one hand on the opposite ASIS and the other on the medial aspect of the flexed knee
Evaluative Procedure	The extremity is allowed to rest into full external rotation followed by the examiner's applying overpressure at the knee and ASIS.
Positive Test	Reproduction of symptoms in the sacroiliac joint or hip
Implications	Pain in the inguinal area anterior to the hip may indicate hip pathology. Pain in the SI area during the application of overpressure may indicate SI joint pathology.
Evidence	Positive likelihood ratio Not Useful — Useful Very Small — Small — Moderate — Large 0 1 2 3 4 5 6 7 8 9 10 Negative likelihood ratio Not Useful — Useful Very Small — Small — Moderate — Large 1.0 0.9 0.8 0.7 0.6 0.5 0.4 0.3 0.2 0.1 0

ASIS = anterior superior iliac spine; SI = sacroiliac.

Special Test 13-16
Gaenslen's Test

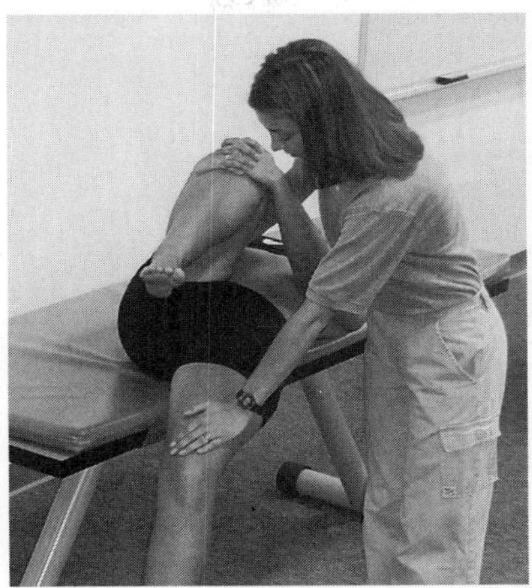

Gaensten's test places a rotational force on the SI joints.

Patient Position	Supine, lying close to the side of the table
Position of Examiner	Standing at the side of the patient
Evaluative Procedure	The examiner slides the patient close to the edge of the table. The patient pulls the far knee up to the chest. The near leg is allowed to hang over the edge of the table. While stabilizing the patient, the examiner applies pressure to the near leg, forcing the hip into extension.
Positive Test	Pain in the SI region
Implications	SI joint dysfunction
Comments	The lumbar spine should not go into extension during this test.
Evidence	Inter-rater reliability Not Reliable — Very Reliable Poor · Moderate · Good 0 0.1 0.2 0.3 0.4 0.5 0.6 0.7 0.8 0.9 1.0 Positive likelihood ratio Not Useful — Useful Very Small · Small · Moderate · Large 0 1 2 3 4 5 6 7 8 9 10 Negative likelihood ratio Not Useful — Useful Very Small · Small · Moderate · Large 1.0 0.9 0.8 0.7 0.6 0.5 0.4 0.3 0.2 0.1 0

SI = sacroiliac.

Special Test 13-17
Long Sit Test

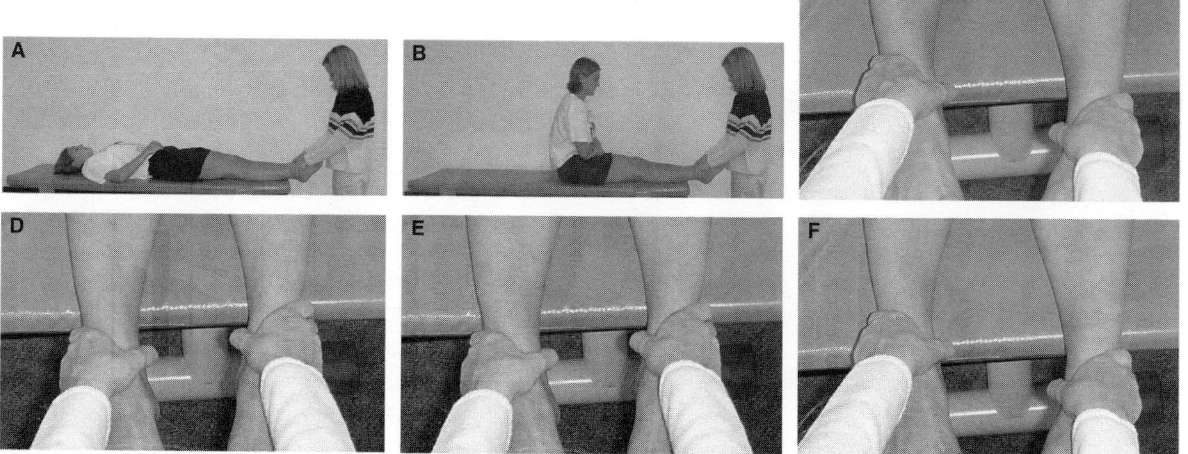

(A) Starting position. **(B)** Finishing position. **(C)** Left leg is longer when supine and becomes shorter when assuming a sitting position. **(D)** Signifying anterior rotation of the ilium. **(E)** Left leg is shorter when supine and becomes longer when assuming a sitting position. **(F)** Signifying posterior rotation of the ilium.

Patient Position	Supine with the heels off the table
Position of Examiner	Holding the feet with the thumbs placed over the medial malleoli
Evaluative Procedure	The examiner provides slight traction on the legs while the patient arches and lifts the buttocks off the table. The patient then rests supine on the table. The patient then moves from a supine to a long sit position. The examiner must pay close attention to the position of the malleoli at all times throughout the test. This test is done actively if possible, without assistance provided by the upper extremities.

Positive Test	The movement of the medial malleoli is observed. If the involved leg (painful side) goes from a longer to a shorter position, there is an anterior rotation of the ilium on that side. If the involved side goes from a shorter to a longer position, posterior rotation of the ilium on the sacrum is indicated.
Implications	Rotated ilium as noted above
Evidence	Inter-rater reliability Not Reliable / Very Reliable Poor / Moderate / Good 0 0.1 0.2 0.3 0.4 0.5 0.6 0.7 0.8 0.9 1.0 Positive likelihood ratio Not Useful / Useful Very Small / Small / Moderate / Large 0 1 2 3 4 5 6 7 8 9 10 Negative likelihood ratio Not Useful / Useful Very Small / Small / Moderate / Large 1.0 0.9 0.8 0.7 0.6 0.5 0.4 0.3 0.2 0.1 0

Lower Quarter Screen

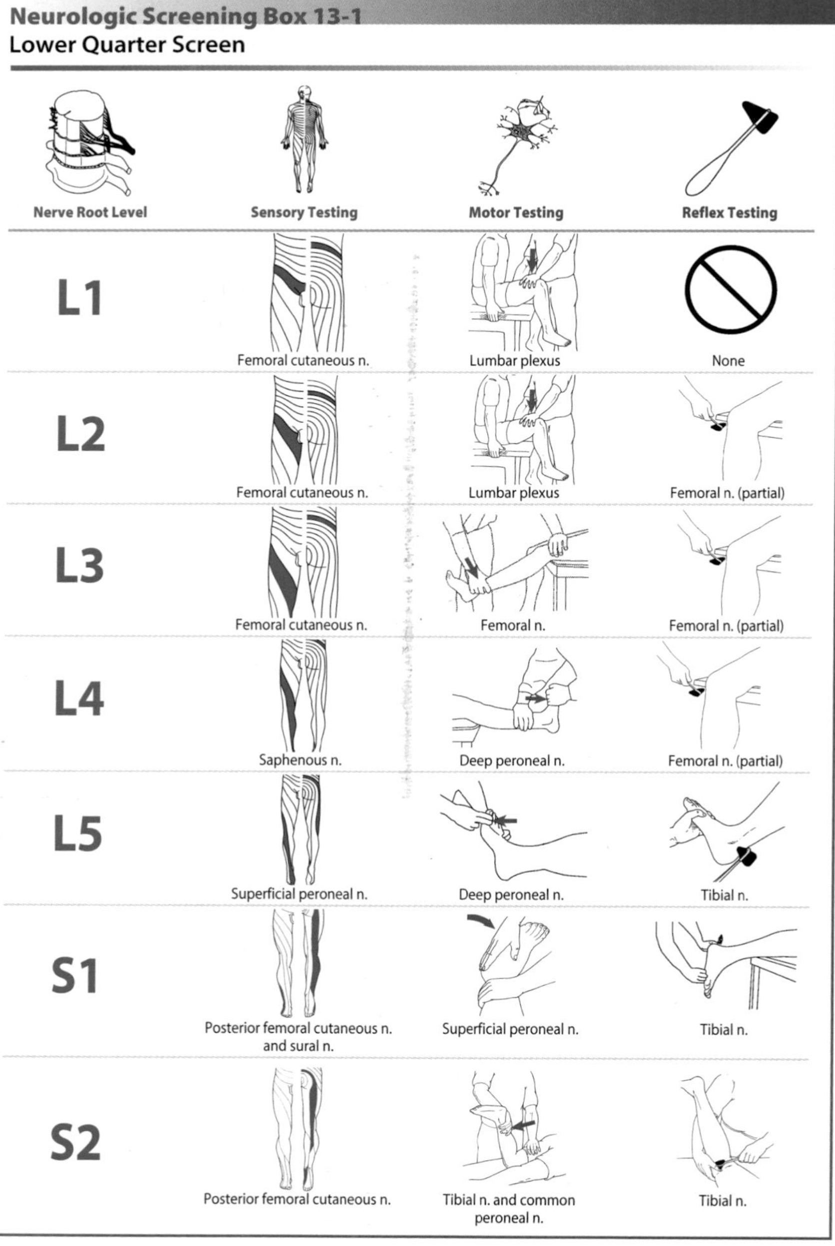

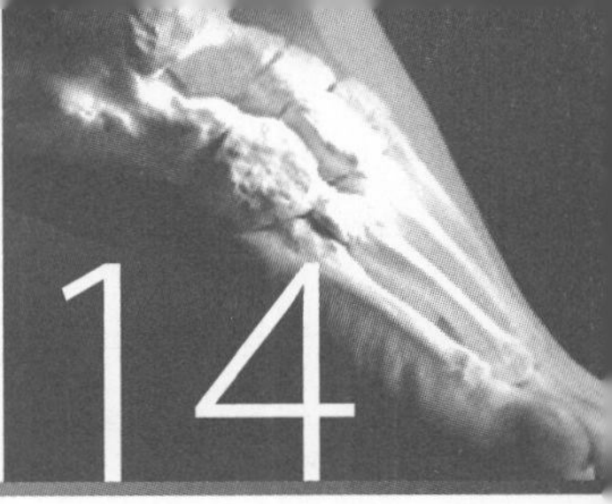

CHAPTER 14

Cervical Spine Pathologies

Examination Map

HISTORY

Past Medical History
Mental health status

History of the Present Condition
Location of pain
Radicular symptoms
Onset and severity of symptoms
Mechanism of injury
Postural influences

INSPECTION

Functional Assessment
Movement and posture

Inspection of the Lateral Structures
Cervical curvature
Forward head posture

Inspection of the Anterior Structures
Level of the shoulders
Position of the head

Inspection of the Posterior Structures
Bilateral soft tissue comparison

PALPATION

Palpation of the Anterior Structures
Hyoid
Thyroid cartilage
Cricoid cartilage
Sternocleidomastoid
Scalenes
Carotid artery
Lymph nodes

Palpation of the Posterior and Lateral Spine
Occiput and superior nuchal line
Transverse processes
Spinous processes
Trapezius
Levator scapulae

JOINT AND MUSCLE FUNCTION ASSESSMENT

Goniometry
Flexion
Extension
Lateral bending
Rotation

Active Range of Motion
Flexion
Extension
Lateral bending
Rotation

Manual Muscle Tests
Flexion
Extension
Lateral bending
Rotation

Passive Range of Motion
Flexion
Extension
Lateral bending
Rotation

JOINT STABILITY TESTS

Joint Play Assessment
Spring test
Mobility of the first rib

NEUROLOGIC EXAMINATION

Upper Quarter Screen

Upper Limb Nerve Tension Test

Continued

Examination Map—cont'd

Upper Motor Neuron Lesions
Babinski test
Oppenheim test

PATHOLOGIES AND SPECIAL TESTS

Cervical Radiculopathy
Cervical compression test
Spurling test
Cervical distraction test
Vertebral artery test

Intervertebral Disk Lesions
Shoulder abduction test
Valsalva maneuver

Degenerative Joint and Disk Disease

Cervical Instability

Facet Joint Dysfunction

Brachial Plexus Pathology
Brachial plexus traction test

Thoracic Outlet Syndrome
Adson's test
Allen test
Costoclavicular syndrome test
Roos test

Table 14-1 Key Signs and Symptoms Associated with Serious Pathological Cervical Spine Conditions

Cervical Myelopathy	Neoplastic Conditions	Upper Cervical Ligamentous Instability	Vertebral Artery Insufficiency	Inflammatory or Systemic Disease
Sensory disturbance of the hands	Age older than 50	Occipital headache and numbness	Drop attacks	Temperature > 37°C
Muscle wasting of hand intrinsic muscles	Previous history of cancer	Severe limitation during neck active range of motion in all directions	Dizziness or lightheadedness related to neck movement	BP > 160/95 mm Hg
Unsteady gait	Unexplained weight loss	Signs of cervical myelopathy	Dysphasia	Resting pulse >100 bpm
Hyperreflexia	Constant pain; no relief with bed rest		Dysarthria	Fatigue
Bowel/bladder disturbance	Night pain		Double vision	
Multisegmental weakness and/or sensory changes			Positive cranial nerve signs	

Table 14-2 Overview of Cervical Spinal Nerve Root Dysfunction

Cervical Nerve Root	Sensory Complaints	Motor/Functional Deficit
C2	Jaw Occipital headaches	None
C3	Headache Posterior cervical spine pain Occipital pain Ear	None
C4	Cervical spine pain Trapezius pain Superior/proximal shoulder	No skeletal muscle deficits Diaphragmatic dysfunction possible
C5	Superior aspect of the shoulder Lateral aspect of the upper arm	Deltoid muscle group weakness Biceps brachii weakness Impingement tests may be negative
C6	Cervical spine Area over the biceps brachii Dorsal hand between thumb and index fingers	Weak wrist extension Weak elbow extension Weak thumb extension
C7	Posterior aspect of arm Posterolateral forearm Middle finger	Triceps brachii weakness Wrist extensor weakness Finger extensor weakness Wrist pronator weakness
C8	Fourth or fifth finger	Weak interossei

Table 14-3 **Possible Pathology Based on the Mechanism of Injury**

Mechanism	Pathology
Flexion	Compression of the anterior vertebral body and intervertebral disk Sprain of the supraspinous, interspinous, and posterior longitudinal ligaments and ligamentum flavum Sprain of the facet joints Strain of the posterior cervical musculature
Extension	Sprain of the anterior longitudinal ligament Compression of the posterior vertebral body and intervertebral disk Compression of the facet joints Fracture of the spinous processes
Lateral Bending	On the side toward the bending: Compression of the cervical nerve roots Compression of the vertebral bodies and intervertebral disk Compression of the facet joints On the side opposite the bending: Stretching of the cervical nerve roots Sprain of the lateral ligaments Sprain of the facet joints Strain of the cervical musculature
Rotation	Disk trauma Ligament sprain Facet sprain or dislocation Vertebral dislocation
Axial Load	Compression fracture of the vertebral body Compression of the intervertebral disk
Whiplash	Cervical instability Cervical muscle strain Facet joint dysfunction

Referred Pain Patterns

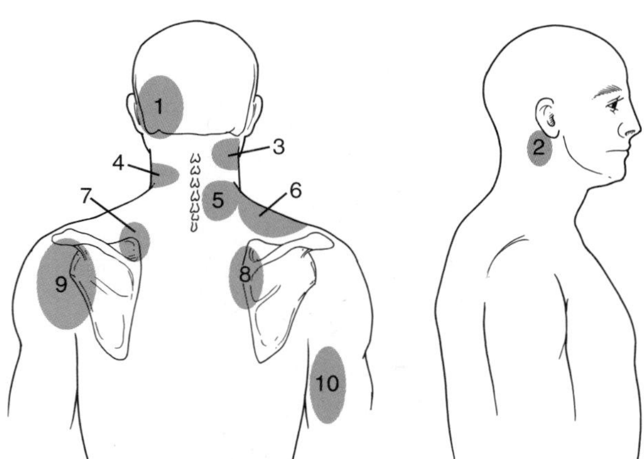

FIGURE 14-1 ■ Referred pain patterns from the cervical spine. *1*, Occipital region; *2*, upper posterolateral cervical region; *3*, upper posterior cervical region; *4*, middle posterior cervical region; *5*, lower posterior cervical region; *6*, suprascapular region; *7*, superior angle of the scapula; *8*, midscapular region; *9*, shoulder joint; *10*, upper arm.

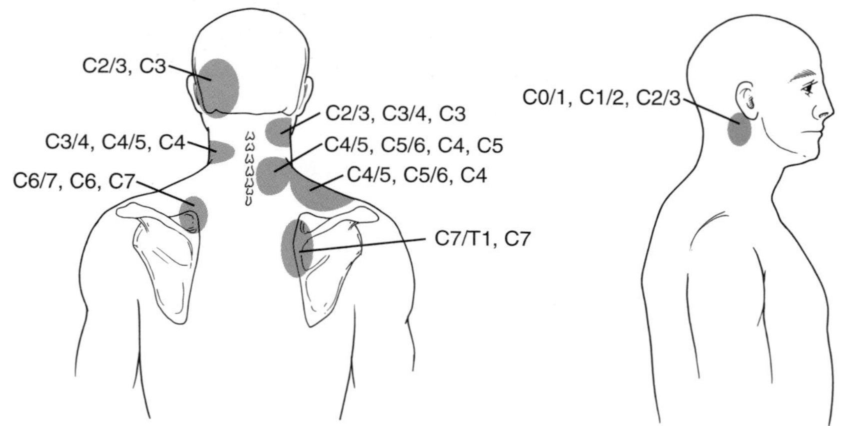

FIGURE 14-2 ■ Referred pain patterns from cervical facet joints.

PALPATION

Palpation of the Anterior Cervical Spine Structures

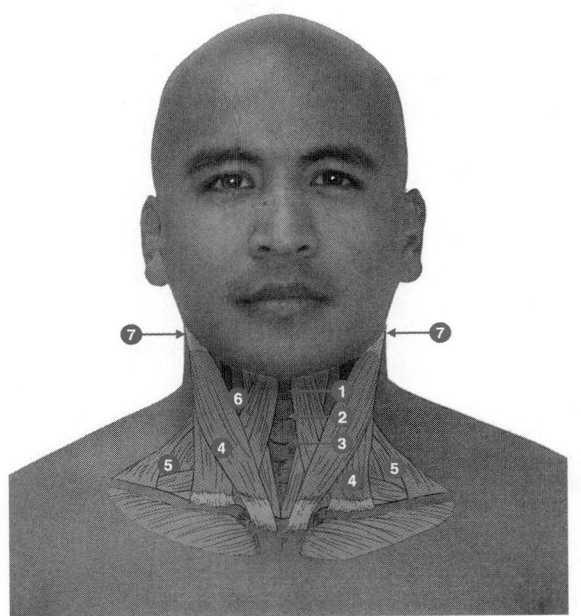

1 Hyoid bone

2 Thyroid cartilage

3 Cricoid cartilage

4 Sternocleidomastoid

5 Scalenus

6 Carotid artery

7 Lymph nodes

Palpation of the Posterior and Lateral Spine Structures

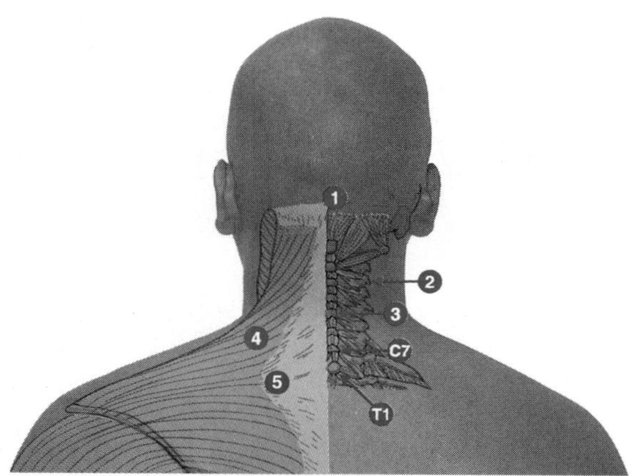

1 Occiput and superior nuchal line

2 Transverse processes

3 Spinous processes

4 Trapezius

5 Levator scapulae

Table 14-4 Bony Landmarks for Palpation

Structure	Landmark
Cervical Vertebral Bodies	On the same level as the spinous processes
C1 Transverse Process	One finger breadth inferior to the mastoid process
C3–C4 Vertebrae	Posterior to the hyoid bone
C4–C5 Vertebrae	Posterior to the thyroid cartilage
C6 Vertebra	Posterior to the cricoid cartilage; movement during flexion and extension of the cervical spine
C7 Vertebra	Prominent posterior spinous process

Active Range of Motion

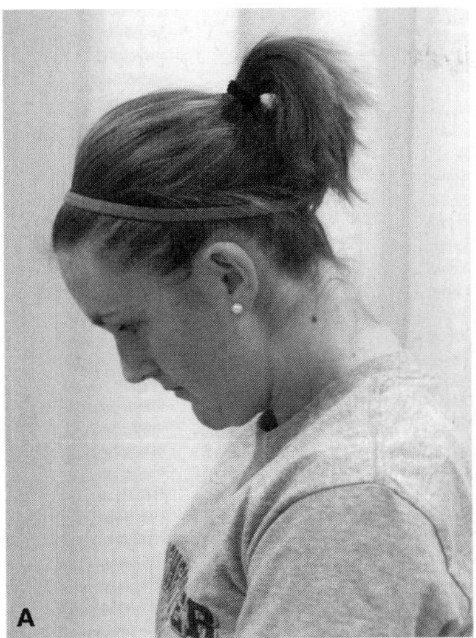

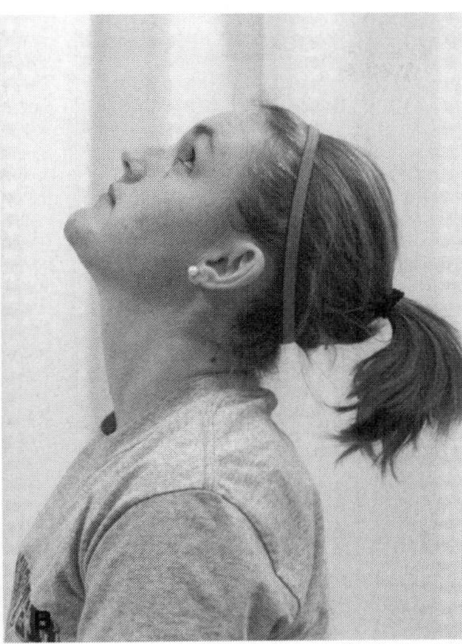

FIGURE 14-3 ■ Active **(A)** flexion and **(B)** extension of the cervical spine. The patient may attempt to compensate for a lack of cervical flexion by rounding the shoulders and compensate for a lack of extension by retracting the scapulae.

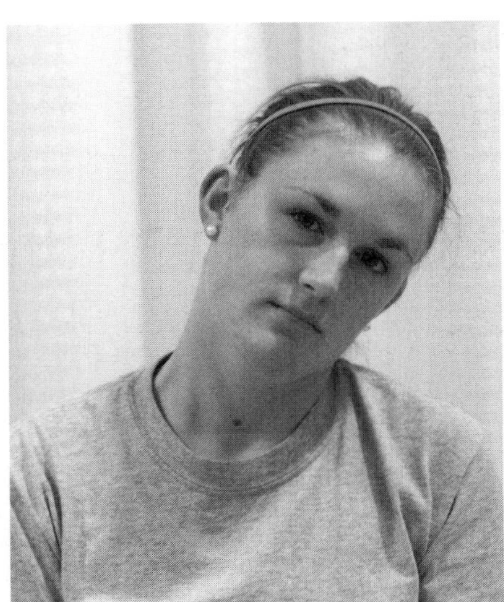

FIGURE 14-4 ■ Active left lateral bending of the cervical spine. The patient may attempt to compensate for decreased cervical ROM by elevating the shoulder girdle.

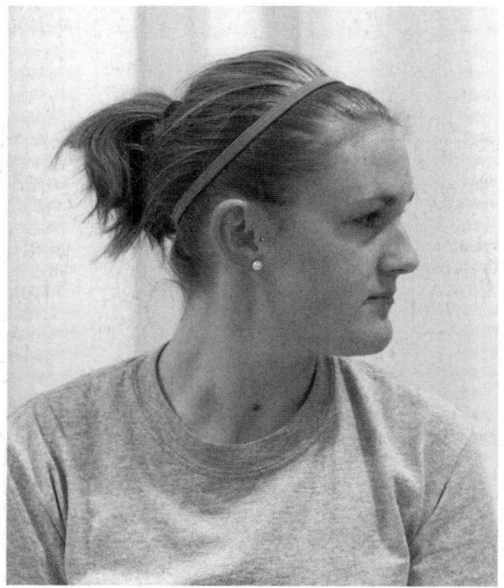

FIGURE 14-5 ■ Active left rotation of the cervical spine. The patient may compensate for a lack of cervical rotation by rotating the torso in the direction opposite that of the cervical movement.

Goniometry Box 14-1
Cervical Flexion and Extension

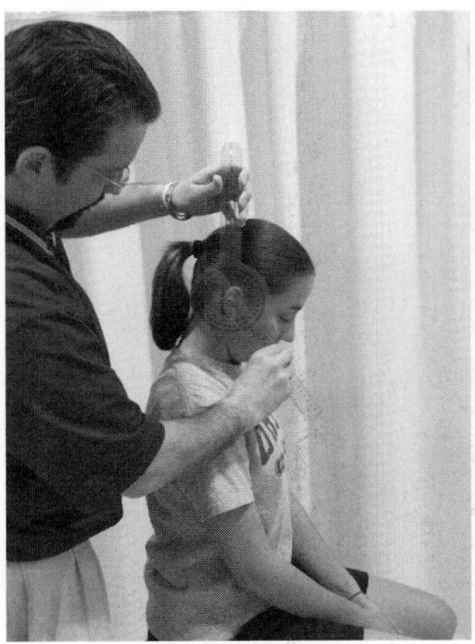

Flexion: 0 to 40–70°

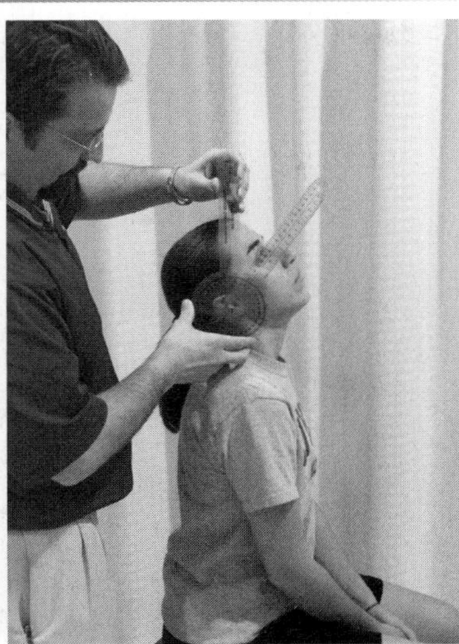

Extension: 0 to 60–80°

Patient Position	Seated
Goniometer Alignment	
Fulcrum	The axis is positioned over the external auditory meatus.
Proximal Arm	The stationary arm is positioned parallel with base of nasal openings.
Distal Arm	The movement arm is held perpendicular to the floor.
Comments	Start and end positions should be noted. Cervical flexion and extension can also be assessed using a tape measure to measure the distance between the chin and the suprasternal notch. Avoid trunk flexion/extension during testing

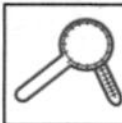

Goniometry Box 14-2
Cervical Rotation

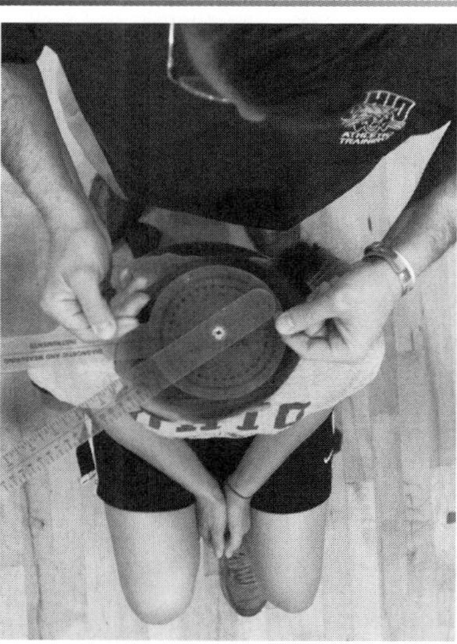

Rotation: 0 to 70–90° (each direction)

Patient Position	Seated with trunk supported
Goniometer Alignment	
Fulcrum	The axis is positioned over the center of patient's head.
Proximal Arm	The stationary arm is aligned with imaginary line between patient's acromion processes.
Distal Arm	The movement arm is positioned so that it bisects the patient's nose.
Comments	Inter-rater reliability

Not Reliable — Very Reliable

Poor | Moderate | Good

0 0.1 0.2 0.3 0.4 0.5 0.6 0.7 0.8 0.9 1.0

Goniometry Box 14-3
Cervical Lateral Flexion (Side-bending)

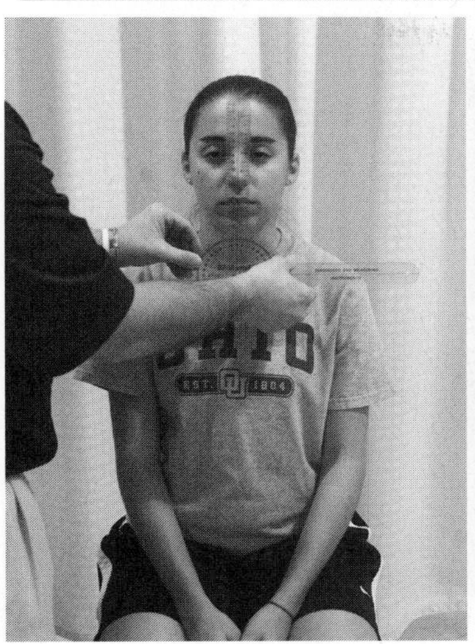

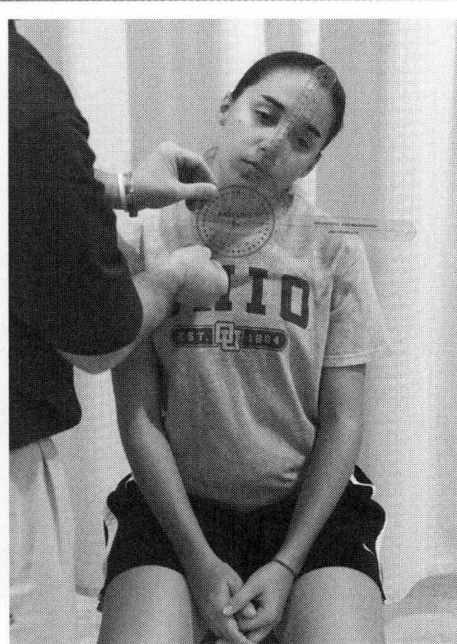

Lateral Flexion 40–50° (each direction)

Patient Position	Seated with the trunk supported
Goniometer Alignment	
Fulcrum	The axis is centered on the patient's sternal notch.
Proximal Arm	The stationary arm is aligned parallel to an imaginary line between patient's acromion processes.
Distal Arm	The movement arm is positioned so that it bisects the patient's nose.

Cervical Range of Motion

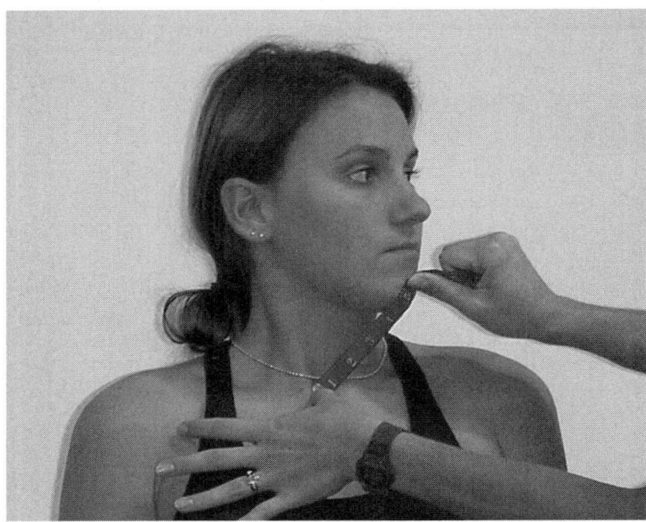

FIGURE 14-6 ■ Measuring cervical range of motion with a tape measure. The distance from the jugular notch on the sternum to the point of the chin is measured and recorded for each motion. Cervical rotation is demonstrated in this photograph.

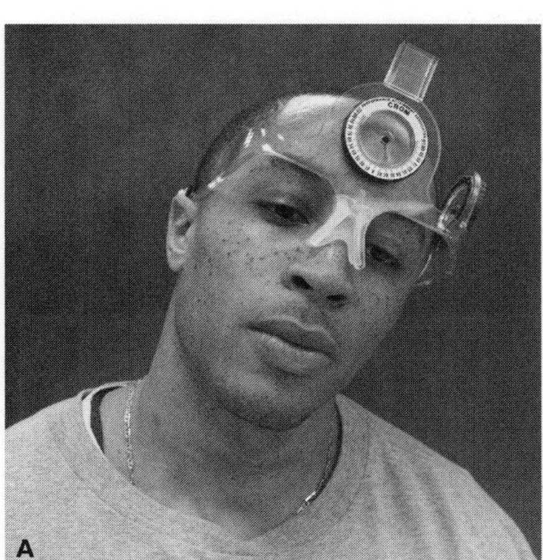

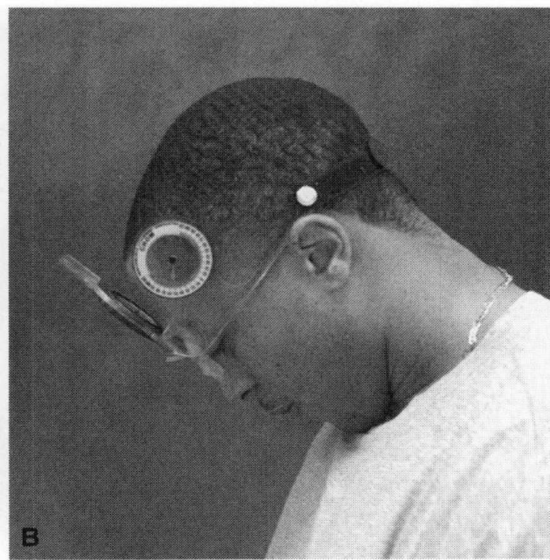

FIGURE 14-7 ■ (A, B) Inclinometer. The use of an inclinometer provides improved interrater reliability for determining cervical range of motion than traditional goniometric measurements.

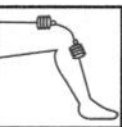

Manual Muscle Test 14-1
Flexion

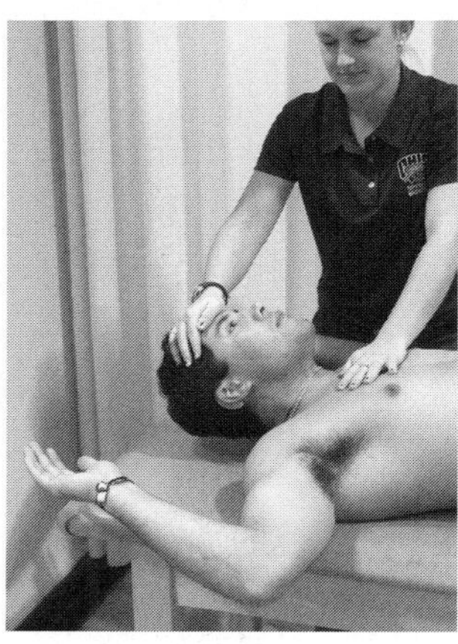

Patient Position	Supine. The shoulders are abducted to 90° with the elbows flexed to 90°.
Starting Position	The cervical spine and head are in the neutral position.
Stabilization	Over the superior aspect of the sternum if patient is unable to self-stabilize trunk
Palpation	Sternocleidomastoid at anterolateral neck and anterior scalene just posterior to sternocleidomastoid. Others are too deep to palpate.
Resistance	To the forehead
Prime Mover(s) (Innervation)	Sternocleidomastoid (spinal accessory: CN XI, C2, C3) Anterior scalene (dorsal rami: C4, C5, C6) Longus capitis (branches of CN C4, C5, C6, C7, C8) Longus colli (anterior rami, C2, C3, C4, C5, C6) Rectus capitis anterior (suboccipital nerve: C1) Anterior scalene (C4, C5, C6)
Secondary Mover(s) (Innervation)	Middle scalene (C3, C4, C5, C6, C7, C8) Posterior scalene (C7, C8) Suprahyoid Infrahyoid Rectus capitis lateralis (C1, C2)
Substitutions	Inability to keep the chin tucked during the movement signals weakness of the deep cervical flexors and overreliance on the sternocleidomastoid.[77]
Comments	Instruct the patient to first tuck the chin and then continue flexing the neck. Weakness with upper cervical motion (tucking the chin) is a common impairment associated with chronic, nonspecific cervical pain.[78]

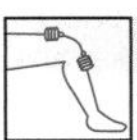

Manual Muscle Test 14-2
Extension

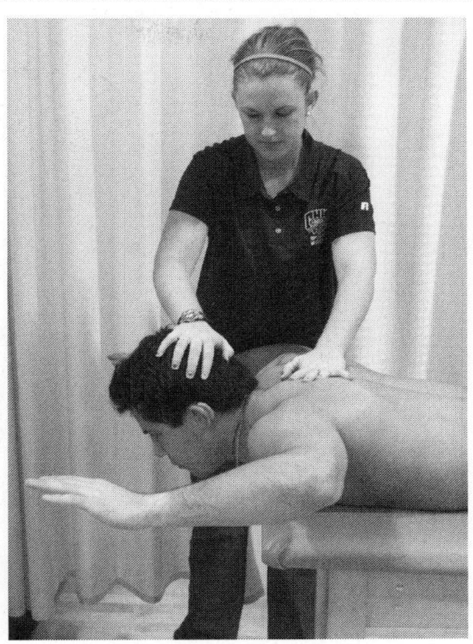

Patient Position	Prone. The shoulders are abducted to 90° and the elbows flexed to 90°.
Starting Position	The cervical spine and head are in the neutral position.
Stabilization	Superior aspect of the thoracic spine (e.g., T2–T9)
Palpation	Posterior cervical region
Resistance	To the skull over the occiput
Prime Mover(s) (Innervation)	Trapezius (upper one third) (spinal accessory: CN XI) Levator scapulae (dorsal subscapular: C3, C4, C5) Cervical extensor muscles (see Table 14-5)
Secondary Mover(s) (Innervation)	None
Substitutions	Lumbar and thoracic paraspinals

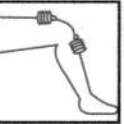

Manual Muscle Test 14-3
Lateral Flexion

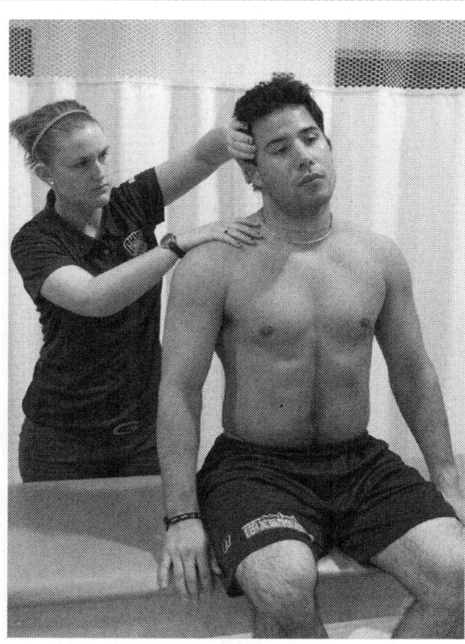

Starting Position	Seated with the cervical spine and head in the neutral position
Stabilization	Over the acromioclavicular joint on the side toward the motion
Resistance	Over the temporal and parietal bones on the side toward the motion
Prime Movers (Innervation)	Sternocleidomastoid (spinal accessory: CN XI, C2, C3) Scalenes (dorsal rami: C3–C8) Paraspinal muscles on the side being tested
Secondary Mover(s) (Innervation)	None
Substitutions	Cervical flexors
Comments	The muscles tested during lateral flexion are redundant with those tested for cervical rotation, flexion, and extension.

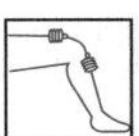

Manual Muscle Test 14-4
Rotation and Flexion

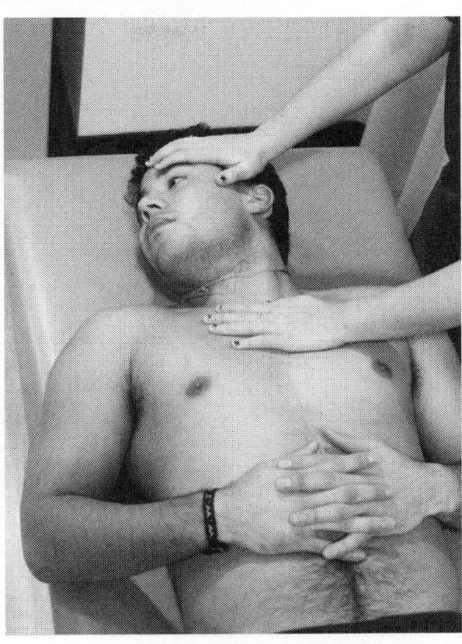

Patient Position	Supine. The shoulders are abducted to 90° and the elbows flexed to 90°.
Starting Position	The head is rotated to the side opposite that being tested.
Stabilization	Over the sternum
Resistance	Over the temporal bone on the side toward the motion
Prime Movers (Innervation)	Sternocleidomastoid (accessory nerve CN XI, C2, C3)
Secondary Mover(s) (Innervation)	Cervical flexors on same side
Substitutions	Uniplanar cervical flexion

Table 14-5 Intrinsic Muscles that Extend the Cervical Spine and Head

Muscle	Action	Origin	Insertion	Innervation	Root
Iliocostalis Cervicis	Extension of spinal column Lateral bending of spinal column	Ribs 3–6	Transverse processes of C4–C6	Posterior rami of spinal nerves	C4–C8
Longissimus Capitis	Extension of skull and cervical spine Rotation of the face toward the same side	Articular processes of C5–C7	Mastoid process of skull	Posterior rami of spinal nerves	C4–C8
Longissimus Cervicis	Extension of spinal column Lateral bending of spinal column	Transverse processes of T1–T5	Transverse processes of C2–C6	Posterior rami of spinal nerves	C4–C8
Longissimus Thoracis	Extension of spinal column Lateral bending of spinal column	Common erector spinae tendon	Transverse process of T3–T12 Ribs 3–12	Posterior rami of spinal nerves	C4–C8
Multifidus (or Multifidi)	Rotation of spine to the opposite side Stabilization of vertebral column	Articular processes	Spinous process	Posterior rami of spinal nerves	C4–C8
Semispinalis Capitis	Extension of neck and head Rotation to the opposite side	Transverse process	Travel upwardly and medially to attach to a spinous process 5 or 8 vertebrae above the origin	Posterior rami of spinal nerves	C4–C8
Semispinalis Cervicis	Extension of thoracic and cervical spine	Transverse process	Travel upwardly and medially to attach to a spinous process 5 or 8 vertebrae above the origin	Posterior rami of spinal nerves	C4–C8
Semispinalis Thoracis	Extension of thoracic and cervical spine Rotation to the opposite side	Transverse process	Travel upwardly and medially to attach to a spinous process 5 or 8 vertebrae above the origin	Posterior rami of spinal nerves	C4–C8
Spinalis Capitis	Extension of the spine Lateral bending of the spine	Upper thoracic and lower cervical spinous processes	Ligamentum nuchae	Posterior rami of spinal nerves	C4–C8
Spinalis Cervicis	Extension of the spine Lateral bending of the spine	Upper thoracic and lower cervical spinous processes	Ligamentum nuchae	Posterior rami of spinal nerves	C4–C8
Splenius Capitis	Lateral bending of the cervical spine	Lower half of the ligamentum nuchae	Mastoid process of the temporal bone and adjacent occipital bone (capitis portion)	Posterior rami of middle cervical spinal nerves.	C4–C8
Splenius Cervicis	Rotation of the head toward the same side Extension of the cervical spine	Spinous processes of C7–T6 vertebrae	Transverse processes of C2–C4 vertebrae (cervicis portion)	Posterior rami of spinal nerves	C4–C8

Table 14-6 Intrinsic Muscles Acting on the Head (atlanto-occipital flexion and extension)

Muscle	Action	Origin	Insertion	Innervation	Root
Longus Capitis	Flex head (atlanto–occipital motion)	Base of occiput	Anterior tubercles of C3–C6 transverse processes	Anterior rami of C1–C3 spinal nerves	C1, C2, C3
Longus Colli	Cervical flexion with rotation to opposite if unilateral.	Anterior tubercle of C1; bodies of C1–C3 and transverse processes of C3–C6	Bodies of C5–T3 vertebrae; transverse processes of C3–C5 vertebrae	Anterior rami of spinal nerves	C2, C3, C4, C5, C6
Obliquus Capitis Inferior	Unilateral: ipsilateral rotation	Lateral surface of spinous process of axis	Inferior surface of transverse process of C1 (atlas)	Suboccipital nerve	C1
Obliquus Capitis Superior	Bilateral: Extension of head on atlas. Unilateral: Ipsilateral rotation	Transverse process of atlas	Occipital bone	Suboccipital nerve	C1
Rectus Capitis Anterior	Flex head (atlanto–occipital motion)	Base of skull, anterior to occipital condyle	Anterior surface of lateral portion of C1 (atlas)	Branches from C1 and C2 spinal nerves	C1, C2
Rectus Capitis Lateralis	Flex (atlanto-occipital motion) and stabilize head.	Jugular process of occiput.	Transverse process of C1 (atlas)	Branches from C1 and C2 spinal nerves	C1, C2
Rectus Capitis Posterior Major	Bilateral: Extension of head on atlas. Unilateral: Ipsilateral rotation	Posterior edge of spinous process of axis	Inferior nuchal line on occipital bone	Suboccipital nerve	C1
Rectus Capitis Posterior Minor	Bilateral: Extension of head on atlas. Unilateral: ipsilateral rotation	Posterior tubercle of axis	Inferior nuchal line on occipital bone (medial aspect)	Suboccipital nerve	C1

Table 14-7 Extrinsic Muscles Acting on the Cervical Spinal Column

Muscle	Action	Origin	Insertion	Innervation	Root
Trapezius (upper one-third)	Cervical extension Cervical side bending Elevation of scapula Upward rotation of scapula Rotation of the cervical spine to the opposite side	Occipital protuberance Nuchal line of the occipital bone Upper portion of the ligamentum nuchae	Lateral one third of clavicle Acromion process	Spinal accessory	CN XI
Levator Scapulae	Elevation of the scapula Downward rotation of the scapula Extension of cervical spine	Spinous process of C7 Transverse processes of cervical vertebrae C1 through C4	Superior medial border of scapula	Dorsal subscapular	C3, C4, C5
Sternocleidomastoid	Flexion of the cervical spine Rotation of the skull to the opposite side Lateral bending of the cervical spine Elevation of the clavicle and sternum	Medial clavicular head Superior sternum	Mastoid process of the skull	Spinal accessory	CN XI C2, C3
Scalene, Anterior	Lateral bending of the cervical spine Elevation of the rib cage	Anterior portion of the transverse processes of C3 to C6	Sternal attachment of the 1st rib	Cervical spinal nerves	C4, C5, C6
Scalene, Middle	Lateral bending of the cervical spine Elevation of the rib cage	Anterior portion of the transverse processes of C2–C7	Lateral to the insertion of the anterior scalene on the 1st rib	Anterior rami of cervical spinal nerves	C3, C4, C5, C6, C7, C8
Scalene, Posterior	Lateral bending of the cervical spine Elevation of the rib cage	Anterior portion of the transverse processes C5 and C6	Medial portion of the 2nd rib	Anterior rami of cervical spinal nerves	C7, C8

Passive Range of Motion

Table 14-8 Cervical Spine Ligaments Stressed During Passive Range of Motion Testing

Motion	Ligaments Stressed
Flexion	Posterior longitudinal ligament Ligamentum nuchae Interspinous ligament Ligamentum flavum
Extension	Anterior longitudinal ligament
Rotation	Interspinous ligament Ligamentum flavum
Lateral Bending*	Interspinous ligament Ligamentum flavum

*These tests are usually inconclusive.

Joint Play 14-1
Cervical Vertebral Joint Play

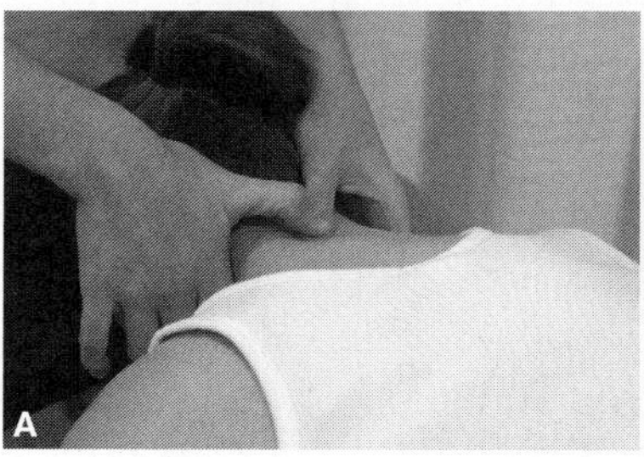

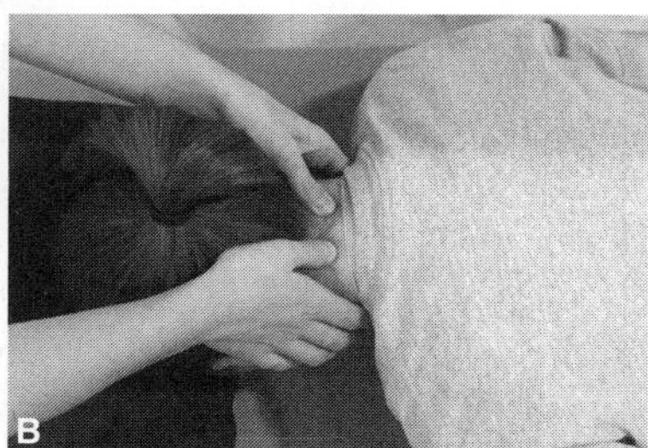

Joint play of the cervical spine. **(A)** Central posterior–anterior (CPA) and **(B)** unilateral posterior anterior (UPA).

Patient Position	Supine; the head is in a neutral position.
Position of Examiner	Standing at the head of the patient
Evaluative Procedure	**CPA:** Palpate the target spinous process using the tips of the thumbs. Apply a gradual anteriorly directed force until an end-feel is determined. Repeat at each level, noting any differences. **UPA:** Palpate the target spinous process and move laterally approximately one thumb breadth to the raised area, the articular pillar. Apply an anteriorly directed force. Repeat at each level, and then assess the opposite side.
Positive Test	Hyper- or hypomobility compared to the segment above and below
Implications	**Hypermobility:** Insufficiency of the passive supporting structures (e.g., ligaments). **Hypomobility:** Restriction of the passive supporting structures
Evidence	Inter-rater reliability Not Reliable — Very Reliable Poor — Moderate — Good 0 0.1 0.2 0.3 0.4 0.5 0.6 0.7 0.8 0.9 1.0

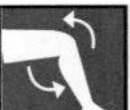

Joint Play 14-2
Mobility of the First Rib

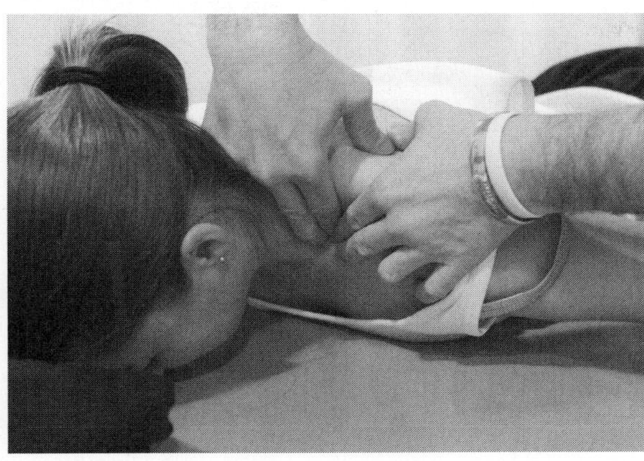

The first rib is manipulated to determine the amount of motion at the costovertebral junction.

Patient Position	Prone
Position of Examiner	Standing at the head of the patient
Evaluative Procedure	Palpate the posterior aspect of the first rib just anterior to the upper trapezius just above the vertebral border of the scapula. Provide an inferior gliding force to the rib.
Positive Test	Hypomobility and/or pain
Implications	Restricted mobility of the first costovertebral joint
Modification	There are several techniques for evaluating the mobility of the first rib.
Evidence	Absent or inconclusive in the literature

Special Test 14-1
Upper Limb Tension Test (ULTT)

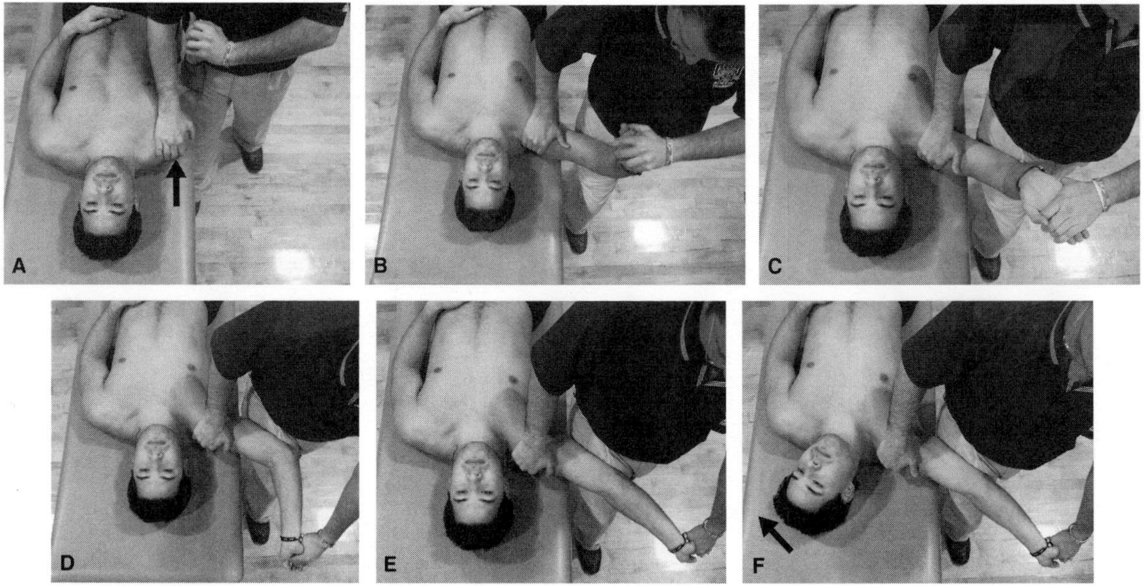

A B C D E F

The patient's limb is sequentially positioned, pausing after each step to elicit symptoms.

Patient Position	Supine The glenohumeral joint is adducted to the side, the wrist and fingers are relaxed, the forearm is pronated, and the elbow is flexed.
Position of Examiner	On the test side

Evaluative Procedure	Hold each position for 6 seconds after the addition of each sequential position: **(A)** Depress the shoulder girdle on the same side. Maintain this force throughout the remaining steps. **(B)** Abduct the glenohumeral joint to 110°. **(C)** Supinate the forearm and extend the wrist and fingers. **(D)** Externally rotate the glenohumeral joint. Note: Avoid over-rotating the glenohumeral joint if the patient has a history of glenohumeral instability. **(E)** Extend the elbow. **(F)** Add neck lateral flexion. Lateral flexion to the opposite side will increase symptoms, while lateral flexion to the same side will decrease symptoms. The test is discontinued at whatever position evokes positive findings.
Positive Test	Provocation of stated symptoms and restricted range of motion
Implications	Hyperirritability of the peripheral nerve due to adaptive shortening, entrapment or impingement (e.g., cervical disk herniation)[79]
Evidence	Inter-rater reliability **Not Reliable** **Very Reliable** Poor Moderate Good 0 0.1 0.2 0.3 0.4 0.5 0.6 0.7 0.8 0.9 1.0 Positive likelihood ratio **Not Useful** **Useful** Very Small Small Moderate Large 0 1 2 3 4 5 6 7 8 9 10 Negative likelihood ratio **Not Useful** **Useful** Very Small Small Moderate Large 1.0 0.9 0.8 0.7 0.6 0.5 0.4 0.3 0.2 0.1 0

Special Test 14-2
Cervical Compression Test

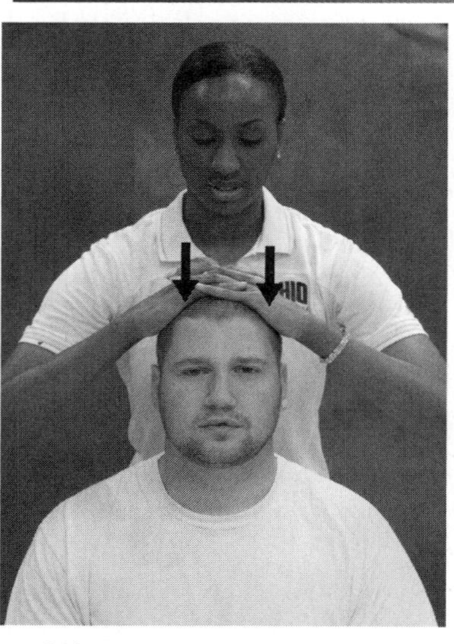

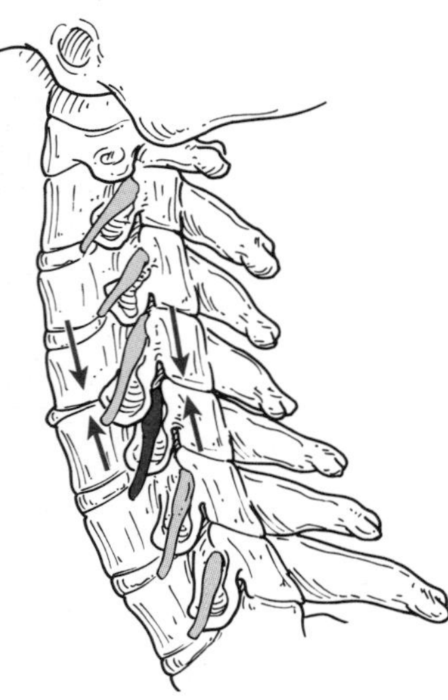

The cervical compression test attempts to duplicate the patient's symptoms by increasing pressure on the cervical nerve roots.

Patient Position	Sitting
Position of Examiner	Standing behind the patient with hands interlocked over the top of the patient's head
Evaluative Procedure	The examiner presses down on the crown of the patient's head.
Positive Test	The patient experiences pain or reproduction of symptoms in the upper cervical spine, upper extremity, or both.
Implications	Compression of the facet joints and narrowing of the intervertebral foramen resulting in pain
Comments	This test should not be performed until the possibility of a cervical fracture or instability has been ruled out.
Evidence	Absent or inconclusive in the literature

Special Test 14-3
Spurling Test

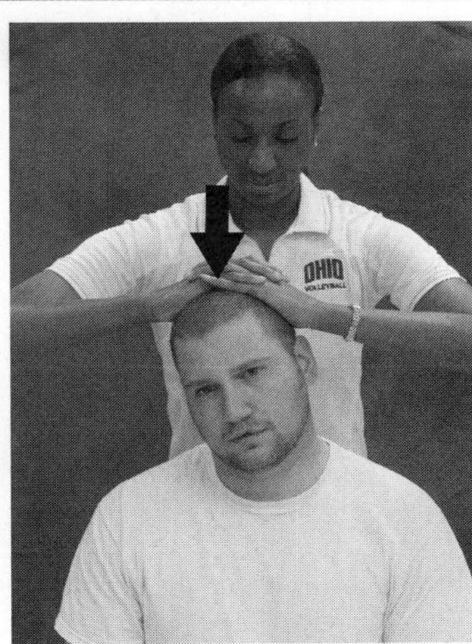

Similar to the cervical compression test, Spurling's test attempts to compress one of the cervical nerve roots.

Patient Position	Seated
Position of Examiner	Standing behind the patient with the hands interlocked over the crown of the patient's head
Evaluative Procedure	The patient laterally flexes the cervical spine. A compressive force is then placed along the cervical spine.
Positive Test	Pain or reproduction of symptoms radiating down the patient's arm
Implications	Nerve root impingement by narrowing of the neural foramina
Modification	The cervical spine may be extended and/or rotated.[80,81]
Comments	This test should not be performed until the possibility of a cervical fracture or dislocation has been ruled out.
Evidence	Inter-rater reliability

Not Reliable — Very Reliable
Poor | Moderate | Good
0 0.1 0.2 0.3 0.4 0.5 0.6 0.7 0.8 0.9 1.0

Positive likelihood ratio

Not Useful — Useful
Very Small | Small | Moderate | Large
0 1 2 3 4 5 6 7 8 9 10

Negative likelihood ratio

Not Useful — Useful
Very Small | Small | Moderate | Large
1.0 0.9 0.8 0.7 0.6 0.5 0.4 0.3 0.2 0.1 0

Special Test 14-4
Cervical Distraction Test

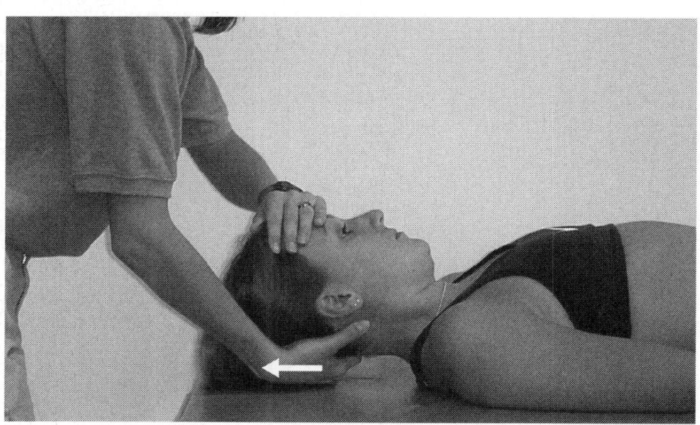

The cervical distraction test attempts to relieve the patient's symptoms by decreasing pressure on the cervical nerve roots.

Patient Position	Supine to relax the cervical spine postural muscles
Position of Examiner	At the head of the patient with one hand under the occiput and the other on top of the forehead, stabilizing the head
Evaluative Procedure	The examiner flexes the patient's cervical spine to a position of comfort.[80] A traction force is applied to the skull, producing distraction of the cervical spine.
Positive Test	The patient's symptoms are relieved or reduced.
Implications	Compression of the cervical facet joints and/or stenosis of the neural foramina
Modification	Not applicable
Comments	This test should not be performed until the possibility of a cervical fracture or dislocation has been ruled out.
Evidence	Inter-rater reliability **Not Reliable** — **Very Reliable** Poor / Moderate / Good 0 0.1 0.2 0.3 0.4 0.5 0.6 0.7 0.8 0.9 1.0 Positive likelihood ratio **Not Useful** — **Useful** Very Small / Small / Moderate / Large 0 1 2 3 4 5 6 7 8 9 10 Negative likelihood ratio **Not Useful** — **Useful** Very Small / Small / Moderate / Large 1.0 0.9 0.8 0.7 0.6 0.5 0.4 0.3 0.2 0.1 0

Special Test 14-5
Vertebral Artery Test

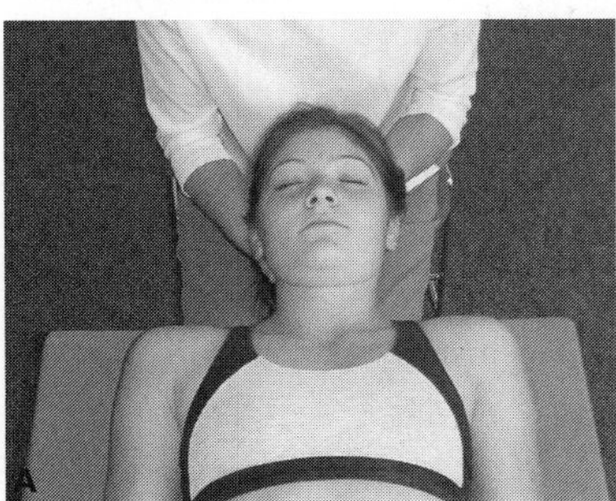

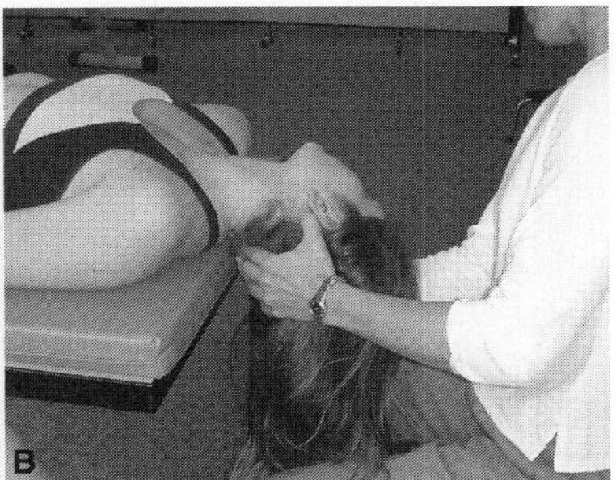

The vertebral artery test is performed to assess the competency of the vertebral artery before initiating treatment or rehabilitation techniques that may compromise a partially occluded artery. This test should not be performed until the presence of a cervical fracture, dislocation, or instability has been ruled out.

Patient Position	Supine
Position of Examiner	Seated at the head of the patient with the hands placed under the occiput to stabilize the head
Evaluative Procedure	The examiner passively extends the cervical spine **(A)**. The head is then rotated to one side and held for 30 s **(B)**. Repeat the procedure for the opposite side. During this procedure, the examiner must monitor the patient's pupillary activity.
Positive Test	Dizziness, confusion, nystagmus, unilateral pupil changes, nausea
Implications	Occlusion of the cervical vertebral arteries.
Comments	Patients with a positive test result should be referred to a physician before any other evaluative tests are performed or a rehabilitation plan is implemented and before being allowed to return to competition.
Evidence	Positive likelihood ratio Not Useful — Useful Very Small / Small / Moderate / Large 0 1 2 3 4 5 6 7 8 9 10 Negative likelihood ratio Not Useful — Useful Very Small / Small / Moderate / Large 1.0 0.9 0.8 0.7 0.6 0.5 0.4 0.3 0.2 0.1 0

Special Test 14-6
Shoulder Abduction Test

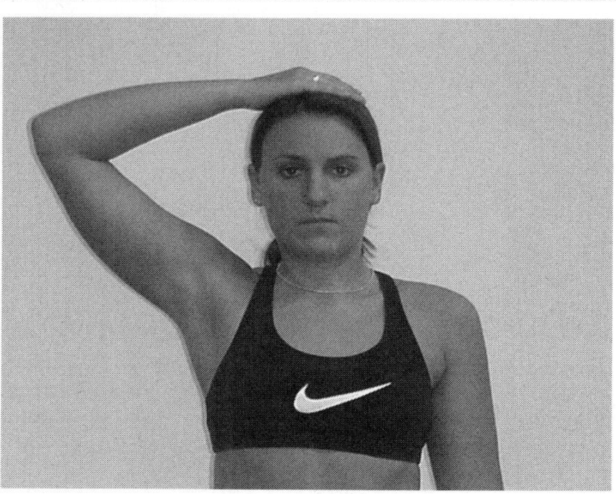

Because of its pain relieving qualities, the patient may assume this posture on his or her own.

Patient Position	Seated or standing
Position of Examiner	Standing in front of the patient
Evaluative Procedure	The patient actively abducts the arm so that the hand is resting on top of the head and maintains this position for 30 seconds.
Positive Test	Decrease in the patient's symptoms secondary to decreased tension on the involved nerve root
Implications	Herniated disk or nerve root compression
Evidence	Positive likelihood ratio

Not Useful — Useful

Very Small | Small | Moderate | Large

0 1 2 3 4 5 6 7 8 9 10

Negative likelihood ratio

Not Useful — Useful

Very Small | Small | Moderate | Large

1.0 0.9 0.8 0.7 0.6 0.5 0.4 0.3 0.2 0.1 0

Special Test 14-7
Brachial Plexus Traction Test

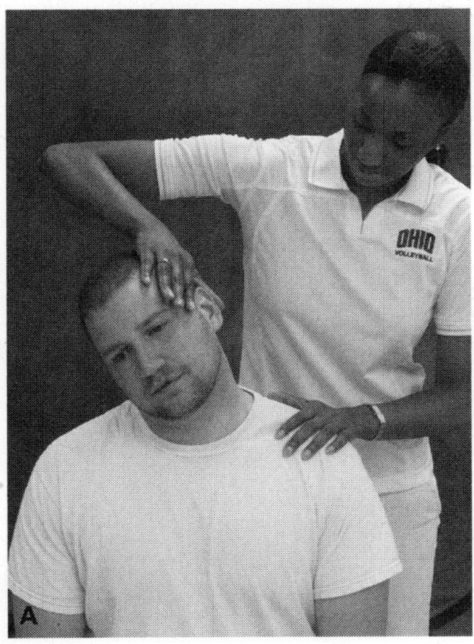

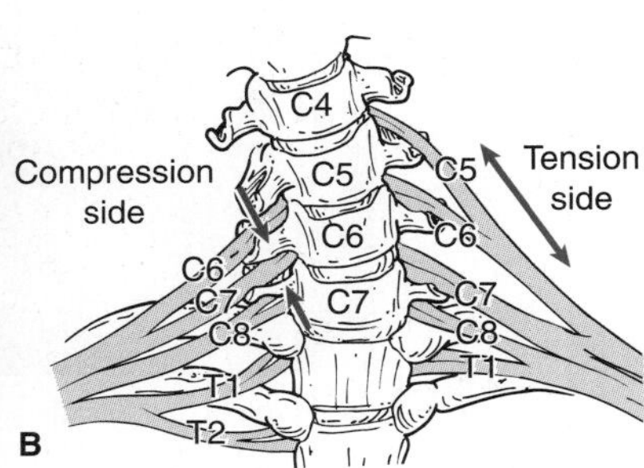

The examiner duplicates the mechanism of injury and replicate the patient's symptoms **(A)**. Pain radiates down the patient's left shoulder when a traction injury exists and down the patient's right shoulder when a compression injury exists **(B)**. This test should be duplicated in each direction.

Patient Position	Seated or standing
Position of Examiner	Standing behind the patient
Evaluative Procedure	One hand is placed on the side of the patient's head; the other hand is placed over the acromioclavicular joint, stabilizing the trunk. The cervical spine is laterally bent and the opposite shoulder depressed.
Positive Test	Reproduction of pain and/or paresthesia symptoms throughout the involved upper extremity.
Implications	Brachial plexus neurapraxia **Radiating pain on the side opposite the lateral bending:** Tension (stretching) of the brachial plexus **Radiating pain on the side toward the lateral bending:** Compression of the cervical nerve roots between two vertebrae
Comments	This test should not be performed until the possibility of a cervical fracture or dislocation has been ruled out.
Evidence	Absent or inconclusive in the literature

Special Test 14-8
Adson's Test for Thoracic Outlet Syndrome

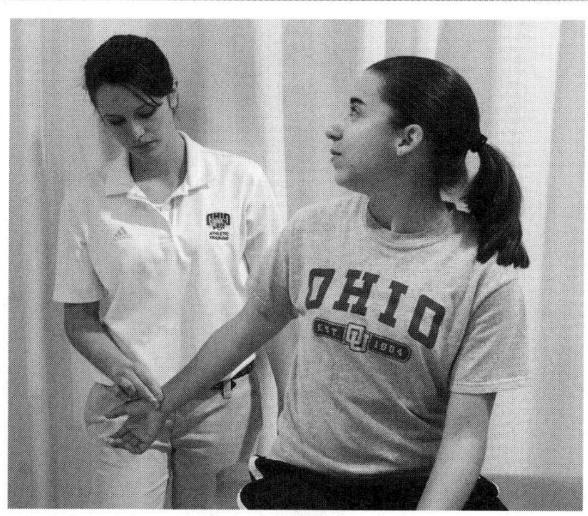

Identifies possible occlusion of the medial cord of the brachial plexus, subclavian artery, and subclavian vein secondary to entrapment of the anterior scalene.

Patient Position	Sitting The shoulder abducted to 30° The elbow extended with the thumb pointing upward The humerus externally rotated
Position of Examiner	Standing behind the patient One hand positioned so that the radial pulse is palpable
Evaluative Procedure	While still maintaining a feel for the radial pulse, the examiner externally rotates and extends the patient's shoulder while the face is rotated toward the involved side and extends the neck. The patient is instructed to inhale deeply and hold the breath.
Positive Test	The radial pulse disappears or markedly diminishes as compared to the opposite side.
Implications	The subclavian artery is being occluded between the anterior and middle scalene muscles and/or the pectoralis minor.
Evidence	Positive likelihood ratio Not Useful — Useful Very Small | Small | Moderate | Large 0 1 2 3 4 5 6 7 8 9 10 Negative likelihood ratio Not Useful — Useful Very Small | Small | Moderate | Large 1.0 0.9 0.8 0.7 0.6 0.5 0.4 0.3 0.2 0.1 0

Special Test 14-9
Allen Test for Thoracic Outlet Syndrome

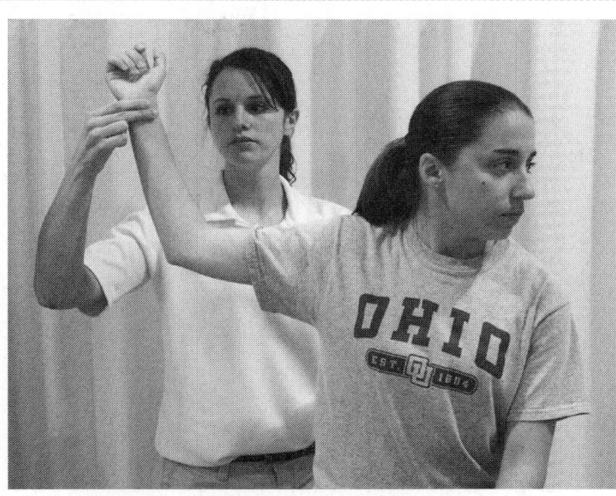

Identifies possible occlusion of the subclavian artery and vein caused by compression from the pectoralis minor.

Patient Position	Sitting The head facing forward
Position of Examiner	Standing behind the patient One hand positioned so that radial pulse is felt
Evaluative Procedure	The elbow is flexed to 90° while the clinician abducts the shoulder to 90°. The shoulder is then passively horizontally abducted and placed into external rotation. The patient then rotates the head toward the opposite shoulder.
Positive Test	The radial pulse disappears or reproduction of neurologic symptoms.
Implications	The pectoralis minor muscle is compressing the neurovascular bundle.
Evidence	Absent or inconclusive in the literature

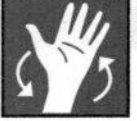

Special Test 14-10
Military Brace Position for Thoracic Outlet Syndrome

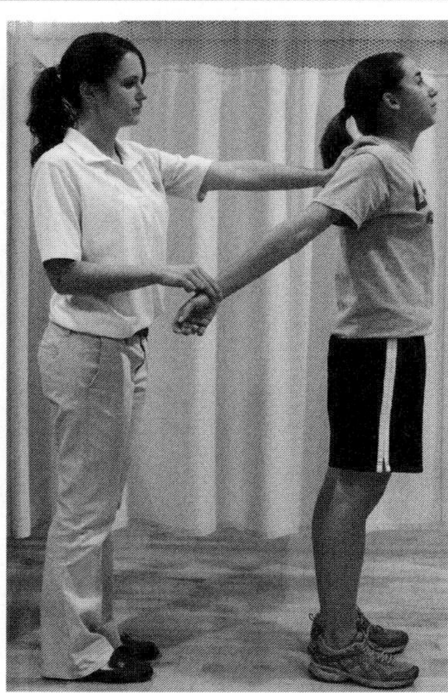

Identifies occlusion of the subclavian artery by the shoulder's costoclavicular structures.

Patient Position	Standing The shoulders in a relaxed posture The head looking forward
Position of Examiner	Standing behind the patient One hand positioned to locate the radial pulse on the involved extremity
Evaluative Procedure	The patient retracts and depresses the shoulders as if coming to military attention. The humerus is extended and abducted to 30°. The neck and head are hyperextended.
Positive Test	The radial pulse disappears.
Implications	The subclavian artery is being blocked by the costoclavicular structures of the shoulder.
Evidence	Absent or inconclusive in the literature

Special Test 14-11
Roos Test (or EAST–Elevated Arm Stress Test) for Thoracic Outlet Syndrome

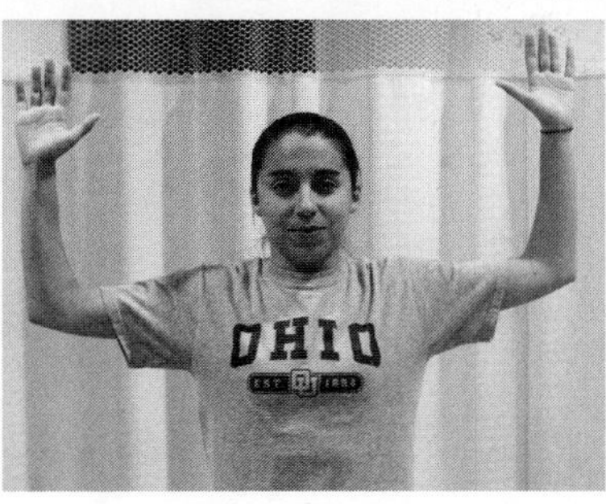

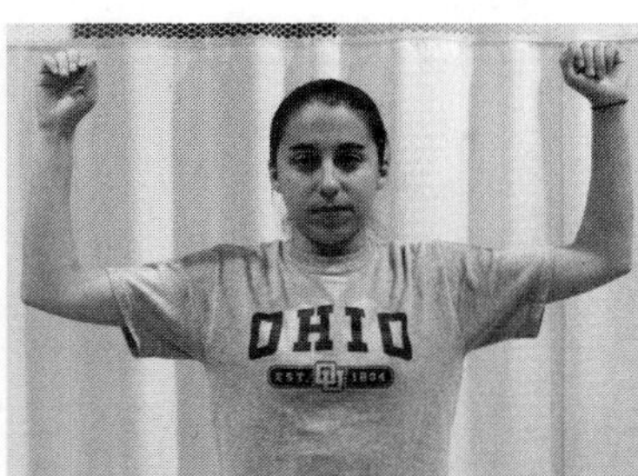

The Roos test identifies the presence of thoracic outlet syndrome of neurologic or vascular etiology.

Patient Position	Sitting or standing The shoulders are abducted to 90° and the humerus is externally rotated. The elbows are flexed to 90°.
Position of Examiner	Standing in front of the patient
Evaluative Procedure	The patient rapidly opens and closes both hands for 3 minutes.
Positive Test	Inability to maintain the testing position Replication of sensory and/or motor symptoms in the extremity.
Implications	Thoracic outlet syndrome of neurologic origin.
Evidence	Positive likelihood ratio Not Useful — Useful Very Small / Small / Moderate / Large 0 1 2 3 4 5 6 7 8 9 10 Negative likelihood ratio Not Useful — Useful Very Small / Small / Moderate / Large 1.0 0.9 0.8 0.7 0.6 0.5 0.4 0.3 0.2 0.1 0

Upper Quarter Screen

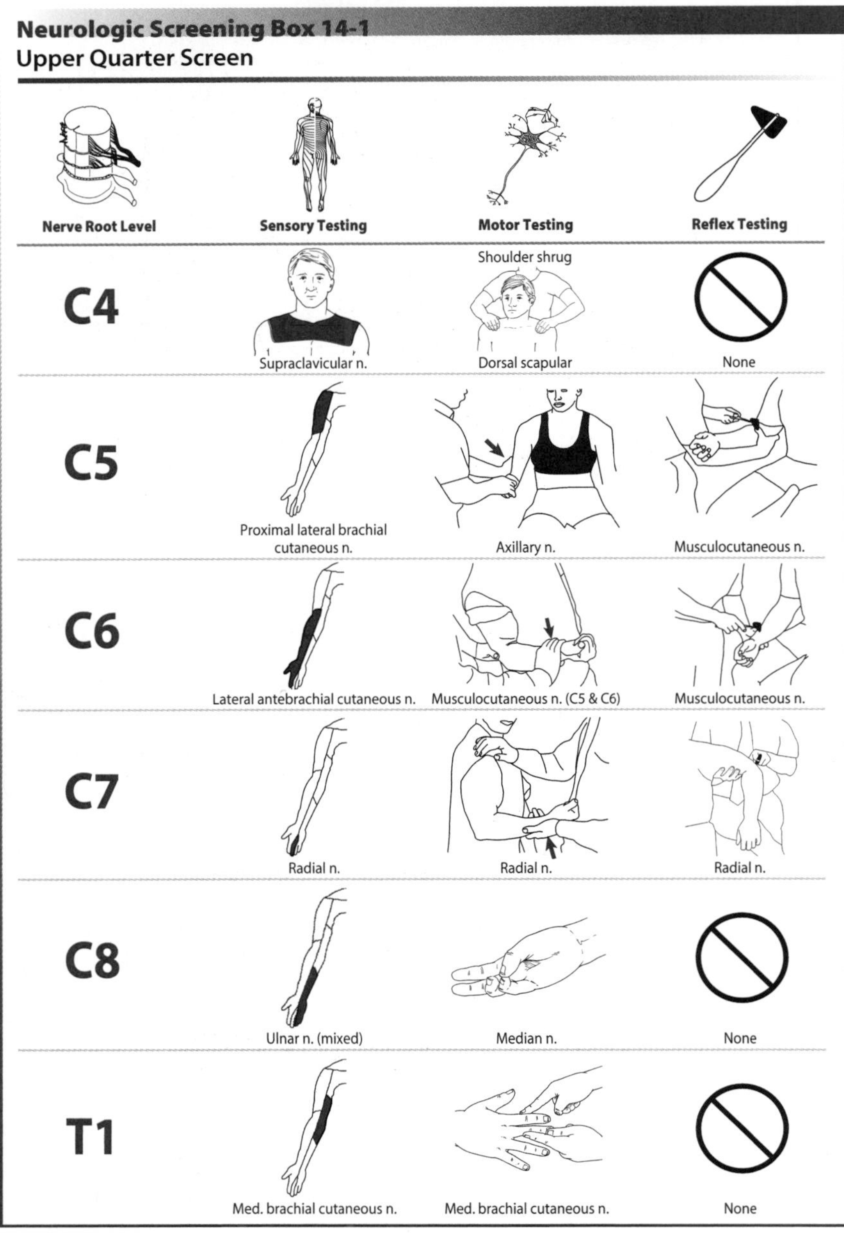

Special Test 14-12
Babinski Test for Upper Motor Neuron Lesions

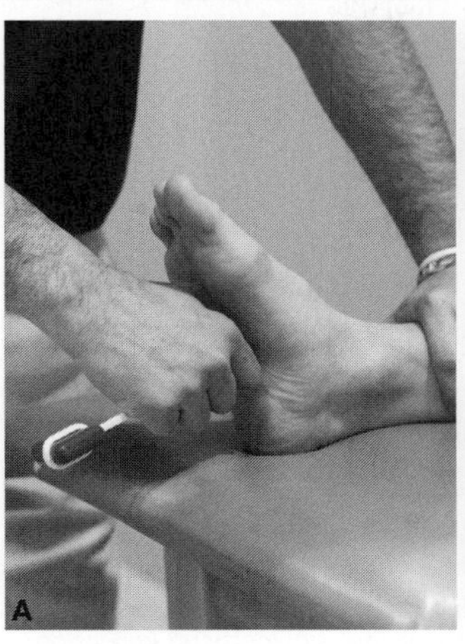

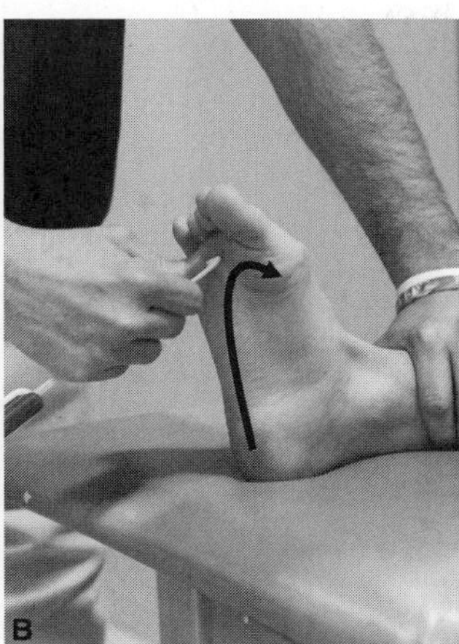

In adults, the Babinski test may be performed during the evaluation of an acute head or cervical spine injury to determine the presence of an upper motor neuron lesion.

Patient Position	Supine
Position of Examiner	At the foot of the patient; a blunt device, such as the handle of a reflex hammer or the handle of a pair of scissors, is needed.
Evaluative Procedure	The examiner runs the device up the plantar aspect of the foot, making an arc from the calcaneus medially to the ball of the great toe **(A)**. In the presence of normal innervation the toes should curl **(B)**.
Positive Test	The great toe extends and the other toes splay.
Implications	Upper motor neuron lesion, especially in the pyramidal tract, caused by brain or spinal cord trauma or pathology
Comments	The Babinski reflex occurs normally in newborns and should spontaneously disappear shortly after birth.
Evidence	Inter-rater reliability **Not Reliable** — **Very Reliable** Poor / Moderate / Good 0 0.1 0.2 0.3 0.4 0.5 0.6 0.7 0.8 0.9 1.0 Positive likelihood ratio **Not Useful** — **Useful** Very Small / Small / Moderate / Large 0 1 2 3 4 5 6 7 8 9 10 Negative likelihood ratio **Not Useful** — **Useful** Very Small / Small / Moderate / Large 1.0 0.9 0.8 0.7 0.6 0.5 0.4 0.3 0.2 0.1 0

Special Test 14-13
Oppenheim Test for Upper Motor Neuron Lesions

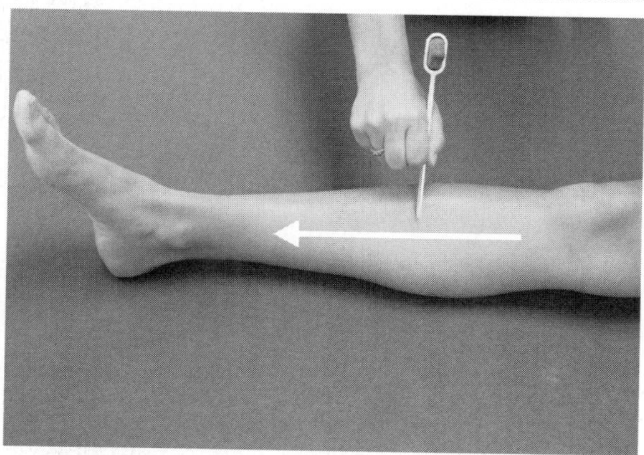

The Oppenheim test may be performed during the evaluation of a patient with acute head or cervical spine injury to determine the presence of an upper motor neuron lesion.

Patient Position	Supine
Position of Examiner	At the patient's side
Evaluative Procedure	A blunt object or the examiner's fingernail is run along the crest of the anteromedial tibia.
Positive Test	The great toe extends and the other toes splay or the patient reports hypersensitivity to the test.
Implications	Upper motor neuron lesion caused by brain or spinal cord trauma or pathology
Evidence	Absent or inconclusive in the literature

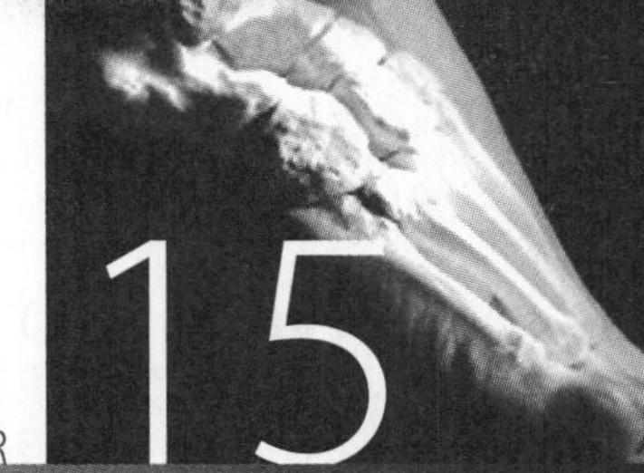

CHAPTER 15

Thoracic, Abdominal, and Cardiopulmonary Pathologies

Examination Map

HISTORY

Past Medical History
General medical history
Family history
History of drug/alcohol use
Mental health status

History of the Present Condition
Location of pain
Mechanism of injury
Onset and severity of symptoms

INSPECTION

General Assessment
Sweating
Throat
Muscle tone
Skin features

PALPATION

Palpation of the Thorax
Sternum
Costal cartilage and ribs
Spleen
Kidneys

Palpation of the Abdomen
McBurney's point
Quadrant analysis

REVIEW OF SYSTEMS

Cardiovascular
Heart rate
Blood pressure
Heart auscultation
Capillary refill

Respiratory
Breath sounds
Respiratory rate and pattern
Respiratory flow

Gastrointestinal
Vomiting
Abdominal auscultation

Genitourinary
Urinalysis

Neurologic

PATHOLOGIES AND SPECIAL TESTS

Thorax
Rib fractures
Rib compression test
Costochondral injury
Pneumothorax
Hemothorax

Abdominal and Urinary
Splenic injury
Kidney pathologies
Urinary tract infection
Appendicitis/appendix rupture
Hollow organ rupture

Reproductive Organs
Testicular contusion
Testicular torsion
Testicular dysfunction
Testicular cancer
Menstrual irregularities

Examination Map—cont'd

Female athlete triad
Pelvic inflammatory disease

Cardiopulmonary
Commotio cordis
Cardiac contusions
Syncope
Hypertrophic cardiomyopathy
Athlete's heart
Myocardial infarction
Arrhythmia
Tachycardia
Mitral valve prolapse
Hypertension
Asthma
Hyperventilation

Table 15-1 Signs and Symptoms of Cardiopulmonary Conditions

Cardiovascular	Both	Pulmonary
Panic	Chest pain	Congestion
Dizziness	Respiratory distress	Wheezing
Nausea	Pain in mid and upper posterior thorax	Fatigue
Vomiting		Anxiety
Sweating		Tingling in fingers and toes
Decreased blood pressure		Spasm in fingers and toes
Distended jugular vein		Periorbital numbness
Pallor		Deviated trachea
Clutching at chest		
Shoulder pain		
Epigastric pain		

Referred Pain Patterns

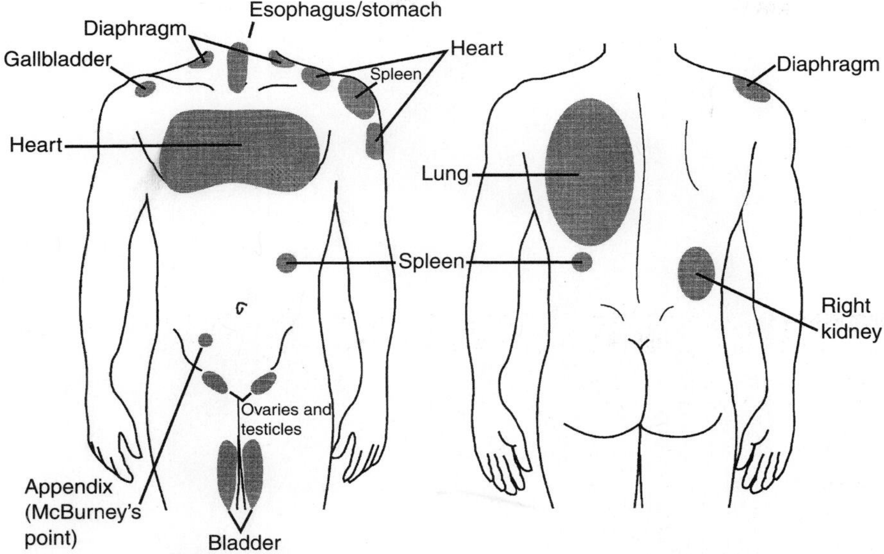

FIGURE 15-1 ■ Referred pain patterns from the viscera. Pain from the internal organs tends to radiate along the corresponding somatic sensory fibers.

PALPATION

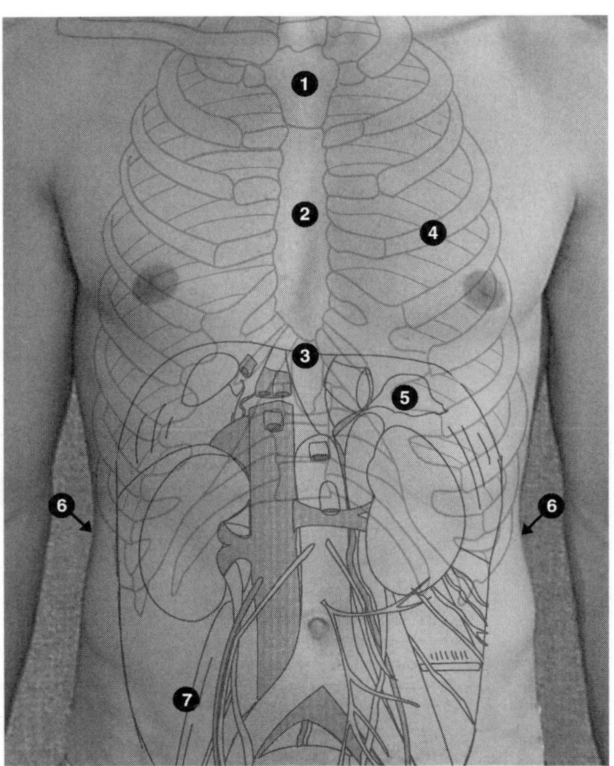

1 Manubrium

2 Sternal body

3 Xiphoid process

4 Costal cartilage and rib

5 Spleen

6 Kidneys

7 McBurney's point

Abdominal Palpation

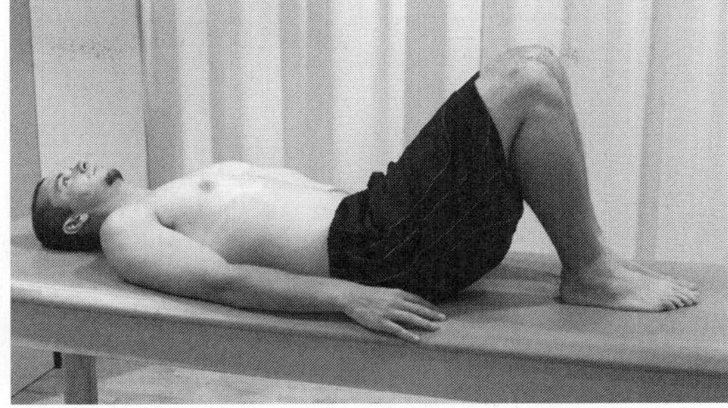

FIGURE 15-2 ■ Positioning of the patient during palpation of the abdomen. The hook-lying position relaxes the abdominal muscles, easing palpation of the underlying structures.

Abdominal Quadrants

	Right	Left
Upper	**Liver:** Pain is associated with cholecystitis or liver laceration. **Gallbladder:** Pain without the history of trauma indicates gallbladder disease.	**Spleen:** Rigidity under the last several ribs indicates trauma to the spleen.
Lower	**Appendix:** Rebound tenderness indicates appendicitis. **Colon:** Colitis or diverticulitis may cause pain. Pelvic inflammation results in diffuse tenderness.	**Colon:** Colitis or diverticulitis may cause pain. Pelvic inflammation results in diffuse tenderness.

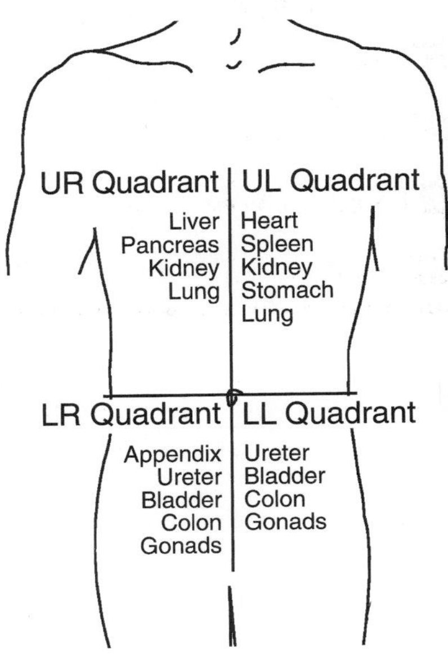

FIGURE 15-3 ■ Abdominal quadrant reference system. The sagittal quadrants are relative to the patient. Therefore, the right kidney is on the person's right-hand side.

Special Test 15-1
Abdominal Percussion

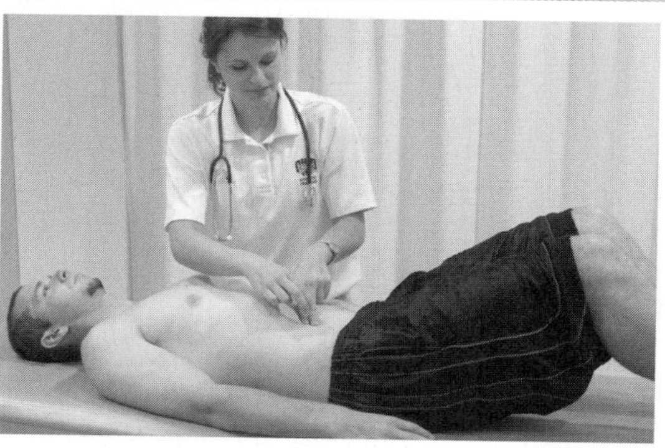

The abdominal quadrants are percussed by a quick tap of the finger tips lying gently on the abdomen. The resulting sound provides context to the density of the underlying tissues. Solid (or fluid-filled) areas produce a dull thud; hollow areas yield a more resonant sound.

Patient Position	Hook lying
Position of Examiner	Standing to the patient's side The examiner lightly places one hand palm down over the area to be assessed. The index and middle fingers of the opposite hand tap the DIP joints of the hand placed over the patient's abdomen.
Evaluative Procedure	The fingertips of the top hand quickly strike the middle phalanges of the bottom hand in a tapping motion. The sound of the echo within the abdomen is noted. Areas over solid organs have a dull thump associated with them. Hollow organs make a crisper, more resonant sound.
Positive Test	A hard, solid sounding echo over areas that should normally sound hollow.
Implications	Internal bleeding filling the abdominal cavity.
Evidence	Inter-rater reliability Not Reliable — Very Reliable Poor — Moderate — Good 0 0.1 0.2 0.3 0.4 0.5 0.6 0.7 0.8 0.9 1.0

DIP = distal interphalangeal.

Special Test 15-2
Determination of Heart Rate Using the Carotid Pulse

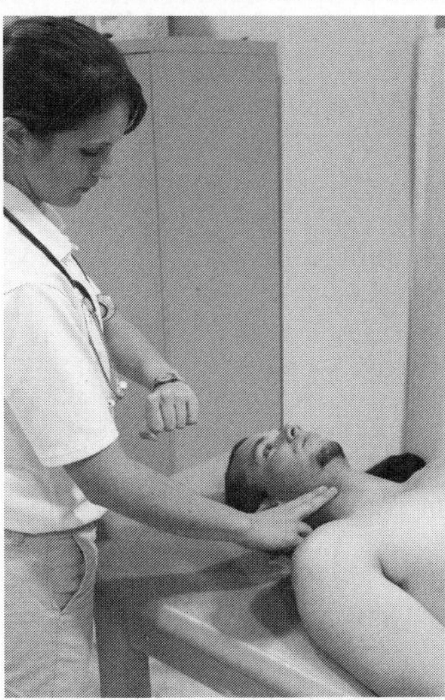

The carotid artery, palpated between the thyroid cartilage and sternocleidomastoid, is used to determine the frequency, quality, and rhythm of the pulse.

Patient Position	Seated or supine
Position of Examiner	Using the index and middle fingers to locate the thyroid cartilage, move the fingers laterally in either direction to find the common carotid artery between the thyroid cartilage and the sternocleidomastoid muscle.
Evaluative Procedure	Count the number of pulses in a 15-s interval and multiply that number by 4 to determine the number of beats per minute. The examiner also attempts to determine the quality of the pulse: strong (bounding) or weak.
Positive Test	Not applicable
Implications	The quality and quantity of the heart rate established. Normal (general population): 60–100 bpm Well-trained athletes: 40–60 bpm Tachycardia: Greater than 100 bpm Bradycardia: Less than 60 bpm
Comments	The baseline heart rate should be recorded and rechecked at regular intervals. Note the rhythm of the beats for symmetry and strength.
Evidence	Absent or inconclusive in the literature

Abnormal Pulses

Type	Characteristics	Implication
Accelerated	Pulse >150 beats per minute (bpm) (>170 bpm usually has fatal results).	Pressure on the base of the brain; shock
Bounding	Pulse that quickly reaches a higher intensity than normal, then quickly disappears	Ventricular systole and reduced peripheral pressure
Deficit	Pulse in which the number of beats counted at the radial pulse is less than that counted over the heart itself	Cardiac arrhythmia
High Tension	Pulse in which the force of the beat is increased; an increased amount of pressure is required to inhibit the radial pulse.	Cerebral trauma
Low Tension	Short, fast, faint pulse having a rapid decline	Heart failure; shock

Special Test 15-3
Blood Pressure Assessment

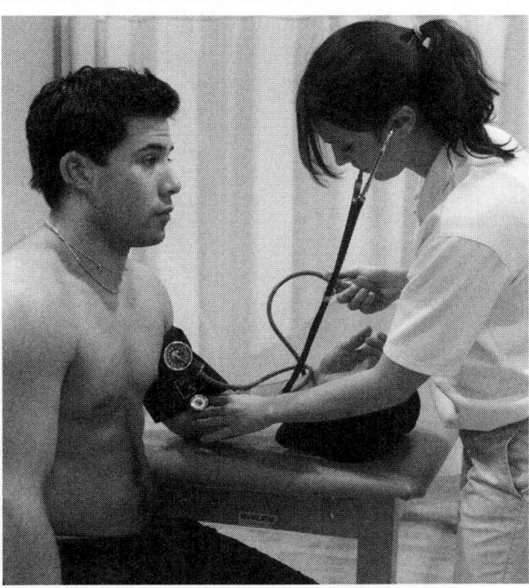

Blood pressure assessment at the brachial artery. Based on the findings of the systolic and diastolic pressures the patient's blood pressure is categorized as hypertensive, prehypertensive, normal, or hypotensive.

Patient Position	If possible, the patient should be seated; support the arm so that the middle section of the upper arm is at heart level.
Position of Examiner	In front of or beside the patient in a position to read the gauge on the BP cuff
Evaluative Procedure	The cuff is secured over the upper arm, with the lower edge of the bladder approximately 1 inch above the antecubital fossa. Many cuffs have an arrow that must be aligned with the brachial artery. The stethoscope is placed over the brachial artery. The cuff is inflated to 180 to 200 mm Hg. The air is slowly released from the cuff at a rate of 2 mm per second until the initial beat is heard.[82] While reading the gauge, note the point at which the first pulse sound, the systolic pressure, is heard. Continuing to slowly release the air from the cuff (approximately 2 mm Hg per second), note the value at which the last pulse, the diastolic value, is heard. Record to the nearest 2 mm Hg.
Positive Test	***Hypertension:*** Systolic pressure greater than 140 mm Hg Diastolic pressure greater than 90 mm Hg

Continued

Special Test 15-3—cont'd
Blood Pressure Assessment

	Prehypertension: Systolic pressure 120–139 mm Hg Diastolic pressure 80–89 mm Hg ***Normal:*** Systolic pressure 90–119 mm Hg Diastolic pressure 60–79 mm Hg ***Hypotension:*** Systolic pressure less than 90 mm Hg Diastolic pressure less than 60 mm Hg
Implications	Low BP may indicate shock or internal hemorrhage. High BP indicates hypertension.
Comments	Athlete's baseline BP should be obtained annually during the preparticipation physical examination and should be compared with the current readings. Larger patients may require the use of a larger BP cuff. A cuff that is too small erroneously increases the BP. The cuff's bladder should surround 80% of the arm.[82] Minimally, the blood pressure cuff must be 66% as wide as the upper arm from the top of the shoulder to the olecranon and encircle the arm completely.[83] The same arm should be used each time repeated measures are taken from the same patient. Multiple high readings on different days are needed for a diagnosis of hypertension.
Evidence	Inter-rater reliability

Not Reliable — Very Reliable

Poor | Moderate | Good

0 0.1 0.2 0.3 0.4 0.5 0.6 0.7 0.8 0.9 1.0

BP = blood pressure.

Heart Sounds

Special Test 15-4
Heart Auscultation

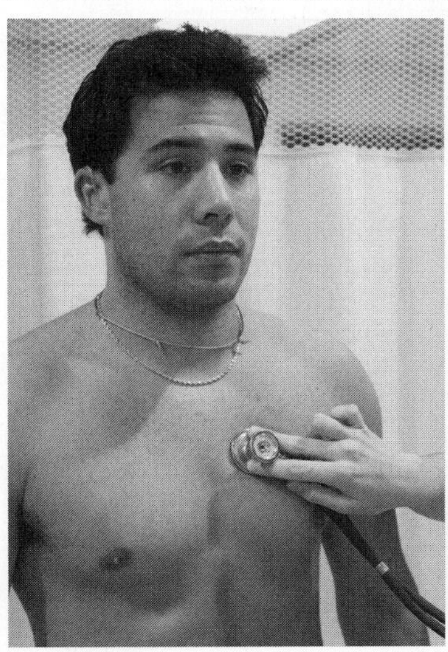

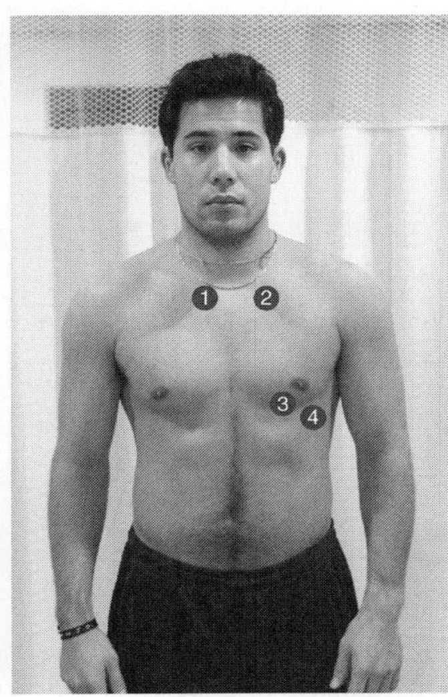

Heart auscultation identifies the presence or absence of abnormal heart sounds.

Patient Position	Supine and standing
Position of Examiner	Stand facing the patient's right side
Evaluative Procedure	Listen at four locations: **1.** Right sternal border between ribs 2 and 3: Aortic area **2.** Left sternal border between ribs 2 and 3: Pulmonary area **3.** Left sternal border between ribs 5 and 6: Tricuspid area **4.** Left mid clavicle line between ribs 5 and 6: Mitral area
Positive Test	Any deviation from typical "lub" "dub" warrants referral to a physician. For examples, see Table 15-2.
Implications	A range of cardiac conditions
Comments	Do not auscultate over clothing.
Evidence	Absent or inconclusive in the literature

Heart Sounds

Table 15-2 Heart Sounds

Sound	Status	Possible Interpretation
"Lub"	Normal systole	Closure of the mitral and mitral and tricuspid valves
"Dub"	Normal diastole	Closure of the aortic and pulmonary valves
Soft, blowing "lub"	Abnormal systole	Associated with anemia or other changes in blood constituents
Loud, booming "lub"	Abnormal systole	Aneurysm
Sloshing "dub"	Abnormal diastole	Incomplete closure of the valves; blood heard regurgitating backward
Friction sound	Abnormal	Inflammation of the heart's pericardial lining; pericarditis

Special Test 15-5
Lung Auscultation

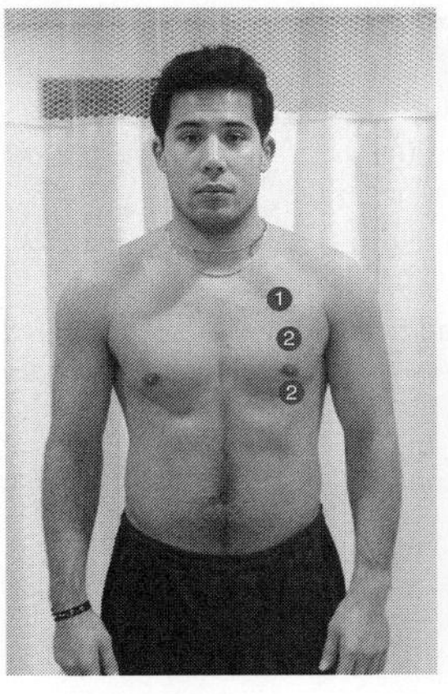

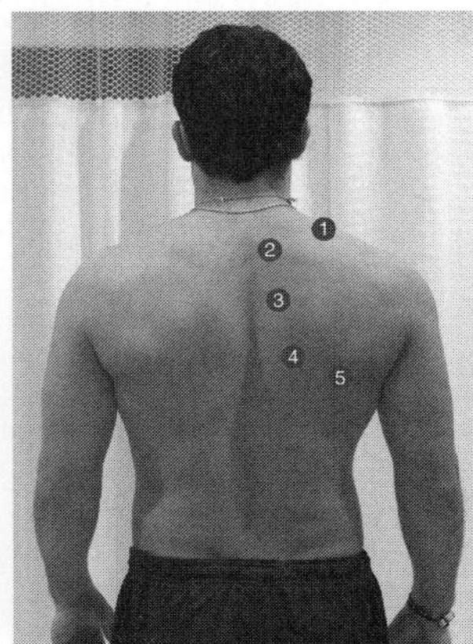

Lung sounds are obtained from the anterior and posterior thorax to determine the quality and quantity of respirations, noting for abnormal sounds.

Patient Position	Sitting
Position of Examiner	Standing on side of patient ideally with the ability to move behind
Evaluative Procedure	Instruct the patient to breathe slowly and deeply through the mouth. Listen left then right at each level ***Anterior:*** **1.** Midclavicle line just below clavicle **2.** Above and below the nipple line under breast tissue if present ***Posterior:*** Five spots each side, taking care not to listen over the scapula **1.** Above the spine of scapula **2.** At the level of scapula spine **3.** Midscapula **4.** Distal scapula **5.** Below the inferior angle
Positive Test	Absence of sound: Collapsed lung Hyper-resonance: Fluid in lung Crackles: Representing small airways "popping open" Wheeze: Narrowed airway (high pitch) Rhonchi: Secretions in larger airway (lower pitch); gurgling[84]
Comments	Do not auscultate over clothing.
Evidence	Inter-rater reliability Not Reliable — Very Reliable Poor — Moderate — Good 0 0.1 0.2 0.3 0.4 0.5 0.6 0.7 0.8 0.9 1.0

Abnormal Breathing Patterns

Type	Characteristics	Implications
Apneustic	Prolonged inspirations unrelieved by attempts to exhale	Trauma to the pons
Biot's	Periods of apnea followed by hyperapnea	Increased intracranial pressure
Cheyne-Stokes	Periods of apnea followed by breaths of increasing depth and frequency	Frontal lobe or brain stem trauma
Slow	Respiration consisting of fewer than 12 breaths per minute	CNS disruption
Thoracic	Respiration in which the diaphragm is inactive and breathing occurs only through expansion of the chest; normal abdominal movement is absent	Disruption of the phrenic nerve or its nerve roots

Special Test 15-6
Peak Flow Meter (Spirometer)

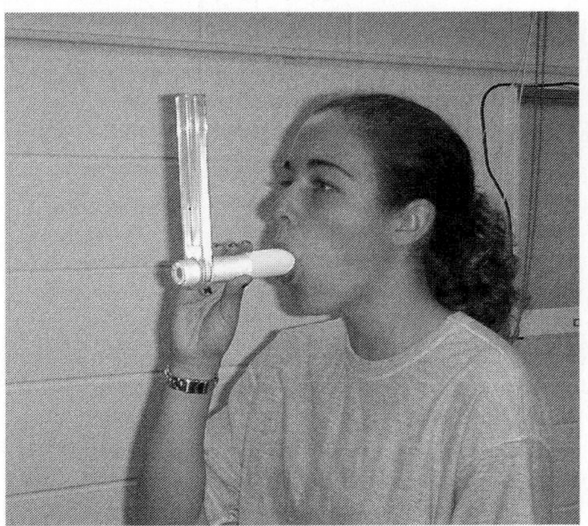

A spirometer measures the volume of air that can be displaced from the lungs.

Patient Position

Standing

Position of Examiner

Standing in front of the patient

Evaluative Procedure

The patient takes as deep a breath as possible.

The mouth is placed around the mouthpiece of the peak flow meter.

The patient blows as hard and as fast as possible into the device.

Positive Test

1. **Diagnostic**: Decreases greater or equal to a 15% decrease in peak expiratory flow rate from preexercise to postexercise
2. **Monitoring**: Daily percentage readings of 50%–80% of personal best or less than 50% of personal best

Implications

1. Exercise-induced asthma
2. Asthma attack requiring caution, possibly a temporary increase in bronchodilator dosage or immediate administration of bronchodilators and notification of the treating physician if levels do not return to at least 50% of personal best after medication administration

Comments

The patient must be careful not to block the mouthpiece opening with the tongue while performing the test.

Evidence

Positive likelihood ratio

Not Useful — Useful

Very Small | Small | Moderate | Large

0 1 2 3 4 5 6 7 8 9 10

Negative likelihood ratio

Not Useful — Useful

Very Small | Small | Moderate | Large

1.0 0.9 0.8 0.7 0.6 0.5 0.4 0.3 0.2 0.1 0

Gastrointestinal

Special Test 15-7
Abdomen Auscultation

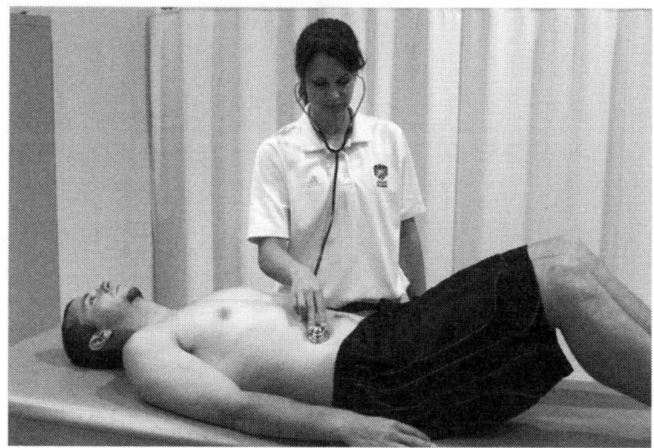

Auscultation of the abdomen. The integrity of the abdomen, the hollow organs, lungs, and descending blood vessels can be assessed through listening to the bowel sounds. Although the abdomen typically makes a gurgling sound, abdominal trauma reduces or eliminates this noise.

Patient Position	Supine; hook lying
Position of Examiner	Standing at the side of the patient
Evaluative Procedure	Examine the patient with empty bladder if possible. Bowel sounds: Place diaphragm of stethoscope gently over the lower right quadrant for 30 seconds. Medium pitched gurgles every 5–10 seconds are normal. If absent, listen in all other quadrants. Listen for bruits at the top border of the right and left upper quadrants and the lower border of the right and left lower quadrants.

Positive Test	Bowel sounds that are high pitched or tinkle indicate possible partial obstruction or early complete bowel obstruction. Absent sounds indicate bowel paralysis possibly secondary to complete obstruction or peritonitis. To be sure that bowel sounds are truly absent, must listen for 5 minutes. Bruits (sound of turbulent flow) at top border of upper quadrant indicates renal artery stenosis Lower border of lower quadrant iliac artery
Implications	Bowel obstruction, peritonitis
Comments	Auscultate before palpation. Palpation can stimulate the bowel and give false impression.
Evidence	Inter-rater reliability Not Reliable — Very Reliable Poor — Moderate — Good 0 0.1 0.2 0.3 0.4 0.5 0.6 0.7 0.8 0.9 1.0

Genitourinary

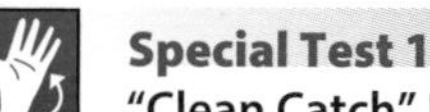

Special Test 15-8
"Clean Catch" Dipstick Urinalysis

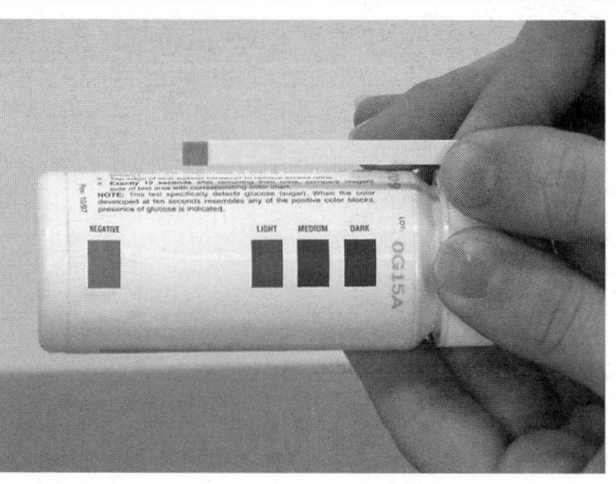

Dipstick urinalysis provides information regarding the patient's health and relative hydration level.

Evaluative Procedure

The external urethra and surrounding area is cleansed using soap and water and then rinsed.

To clear the urethra, the initial flow of urine is into a toilet bowl or "dirty" collection container.

One to 2 oz. of urine is then collected in a clean specimen cup.

The dipstick is then immersed into the specimen cup.

Follow the manufacturer's recommendations for immersion and interpretation times.

Test Results

The colors produced on the dipstick are matched to the values provided by the manufacturer.

Implications

Element	Normal	Interpretation
Specific Gravity:	1.006–1.030	Low reading: Diabetes mellitus, excessive hydration, renal failure High reading: Dehydration; heart or renal failure
pH:	4.6–8.0	Low reading: Chronic obstructive pulmonary disease, diabetic ketoacidosis High reading: Renal failure, urinary tract infection

	Glucose, dehydrogenase:	<0.5	Diabetes mellitus, stress
	Ketones:	0	Anorexia, poor nutrition, alcoholism, diabetes mellitus
	Protein:	0	Congestive heart failure, polycystic kidney disease
	Hemoglobin:	0	Urinary tract infection, kidney disease or trauma
	RBC:	0	Kidney disease or trauma, kidney stones, bladder infection, urinary tract infection
Comments	The above interpretations are partial lists. High or low readings should be interpreted by a physician. Factors such as diet and the level of exercise can alter the urinalysis readings.		

Evidence

Hematuria

Positive likelihood ratio

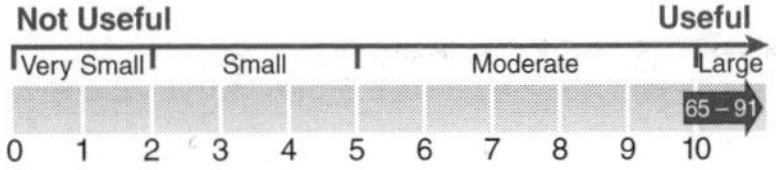

Not Useful — Useful
Very Small | Small | Moderate | Large
0 1 2 3 4 5 6 7 8 9 10
65 – 91

Negative likelihood ratio

Not Useful — Useful
Very Small | Small | Moderate | Large
1.0 0.9 0.8 0.7 0.6 0.5 0.4 0.3 0.2 0.1 0

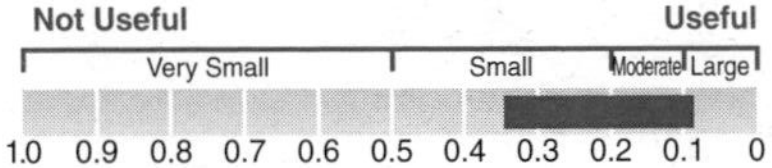

Proteinuria

Positive likelihood ratio

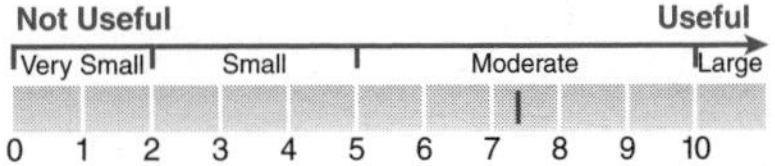

Not Useful — Useful
Very Small | Small | Moderate | Large
0 1 2 3 4 5 6 7 8 9 10

Negative likelihood ratio

Not Useful — Useful
Very Small | Small | Moderate | Large
1.0 0.9 0.8 0.7 0.6 0.5 0.4 0.3 0.2 0.1 0

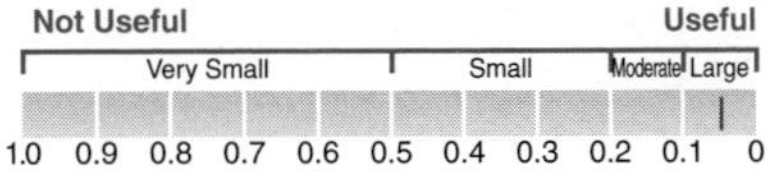

RBC = red blood cell.

Special Test 15-9
Compression Test for Rib Fractures

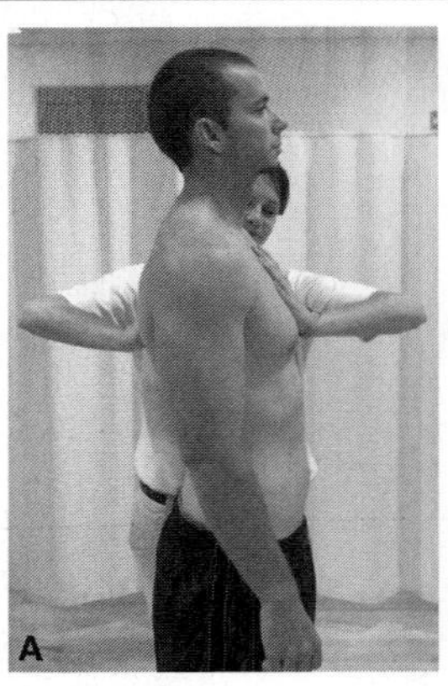

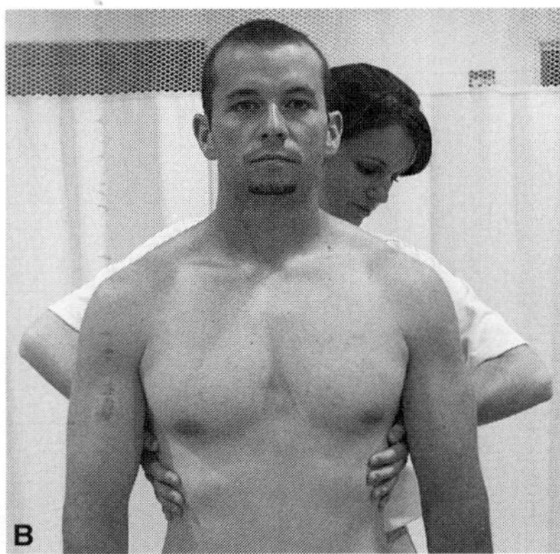

Manual compression causes deformation of the rib cage, causing pain in the presence of a rib fracture. **(A)** Anterior–posterior compression; **(B)** lateral compression. Costochondral injury may produce a false-positive result.

Patient Position	Seated or standing
Position of Examiner	Standing in front of the patient with the hands on opposite sides of the rib cage
Evaluative Procedure	The examiner compresses the rib cage in an anterior-posterior direction and quickly releases the pressure. The rib cage is then compressed from the patient's side and the pressure is quickly released.
Positive Test	Pain in the rib cage
Implications	Damage to the rib cage, including the possibility of a fracture, contusion, or costochondral separation
Comments	Do not perform this test in the presence of palpable rib deformity or crepitus.
Evidence	Absent or inconclusive in the literature

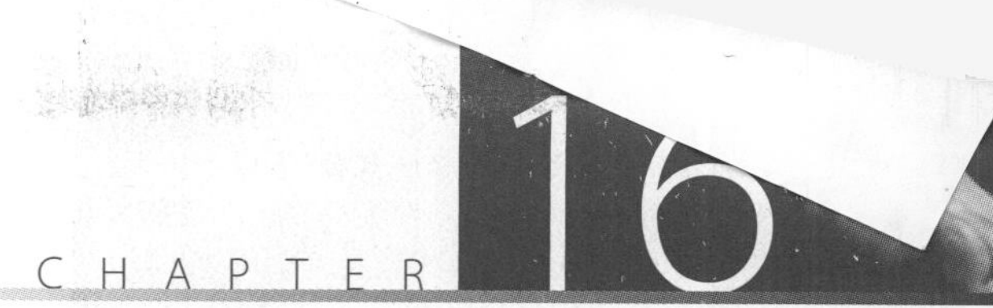

Shoulder and Upper Arm Pathologies

Examination Map

HISTORY

Past Medical History

History of Present Condition

Mechanism of injury

Onset of symptoms

Location of pain

INSPECTION

Functional Assessment

Inspection of the Anterior Structures

Level of the shoulders

Position of the head

Position of the arm

Contour of the clavicles

Deltoid muscle groups

Humerus

Inspection of the Lateral Structures

Deltoid muscle group

Acromion process

Position of the humerus

Inspection of the Posterior Structures

Vertebral column

Position of the scapula

Muscle development

Position of the humerus

PALPATION

Palpation of the Anterior Structures

Jugular notch

Sternoclavicular joint

Clavicular shaft

Acromion process

Acromioclavicular joint

Coracoid process

Humeral head

Greater tuberosity

Lesser tuberosity

Bicipital groove

Humeral shaft

Pectoralis major

Pectoralis minor

Coracobrachialis

Deltoid muscle group

Biceps brachii
- Long head
- Short head

Palpation of the Posterior Structures

Spine of the scapula

Superior angle

Inferior angle

Rotator cuff
- Infraspinatus
- Teres minor
- Supraspinatus

Teres major

Rhomboids

Levator scapulae

Trapezius

Latissimus dorsi

Posterior deltoid

Triceps brachii

Continued

Examination Map—cont'd

JOINT AND MUSCLE FUNCTION ASSESSMENT

Goniometry
Flexion

Extension

Abduction

Internal rotation

External rotation

Horizontal abduction

Horizontal adduction

Active Range of Motion
Apley's scratch test

Flexion/extension

Abduction/adduction
- Drop arm test

Internal and external rotation

Horizontal adduction/abduction

Manual Muscle Tests
Gerber lift-off test

Flexion/extension

Abduction/adduction

Internal/external rotation

Horizontal abduction/adduction

Scapular muscles
- Retraction and downward rotation
- Retraction
- Protraction and upward rotation
- Depression and retraction
- Elevation

Passive Range of Motion
Flexion

Extension

Abduction

Adduction

Internal rotation

External rotation

Horizontal abduction

Horizontal adduction

JOINT STABILITY TESTS

Joint Play Assessment
Sternoclavicular joint

Acromioclavicular joint

Glenohumeral joint

NEUROLOGIC EXAMINATION

Upper Quarter Screen

PATHOLOGIES AND SPECIAL TESTS

Sternoclavicular Joint

Acromioclavicular Joint
Acromioclavicular traction test

Acromioclavicular compression test

Glenohumeral Joint
Anterior instability
- Apprehension test
- Relocation test
- Anterior release test

Posterior instability
- Posterior apprehension test
- Jerk test

Inferior instability
- Sulcus sign

Multidirectional instability

Rotator Cuff Pathology
Impingement syndrome

Neer impingement test

Hawkins impingement test

Drop arm test

Rotator cuff tendinopathy
- Drop arm test
- Empty can test

Subacromial bursitis

Biceps Tendon Pathology
Bicipital tendinopathy
- Yergason's test
- Speed's test

SLAP lesions
- Active compression test
- Anterior slide test
- Compression–rotation test

Inspection of the Shoulder

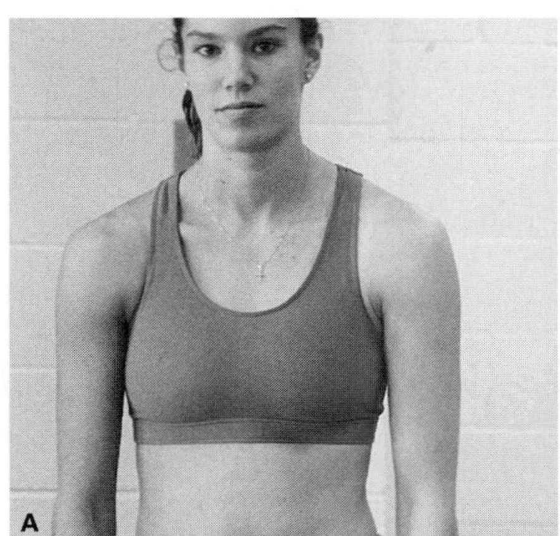

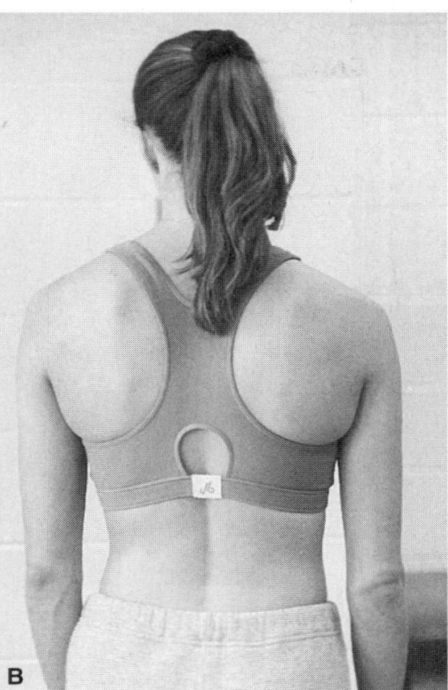

FIGURE 16-1 ■ **(A)** Anterior and **(B)** posterior view of the shoulders. Note that the shoulder of the dominant right arm hangs lower than the shoulder of the nondominant arm.

Clavicular Fracture

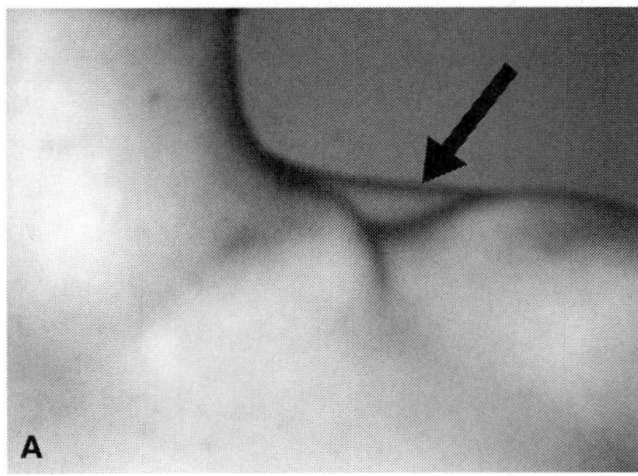

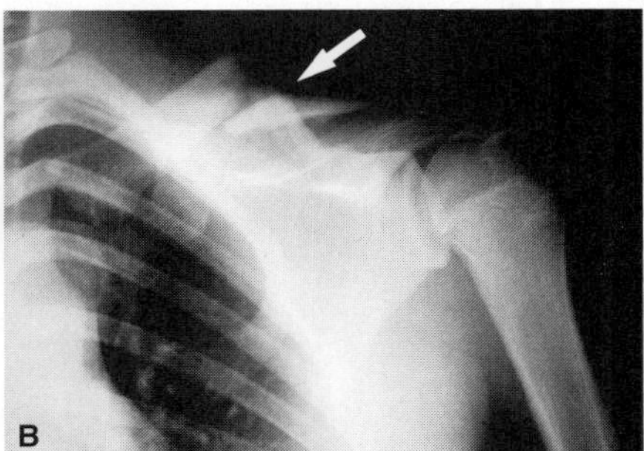

FIGURE 16-2 ■ Fracture of the left clavicle. **(A)** Inspection showing gross deformity. **(B)** Anterior–posterior radiograph demonstrating the fracture lines.

Biceps Tendon Rupture

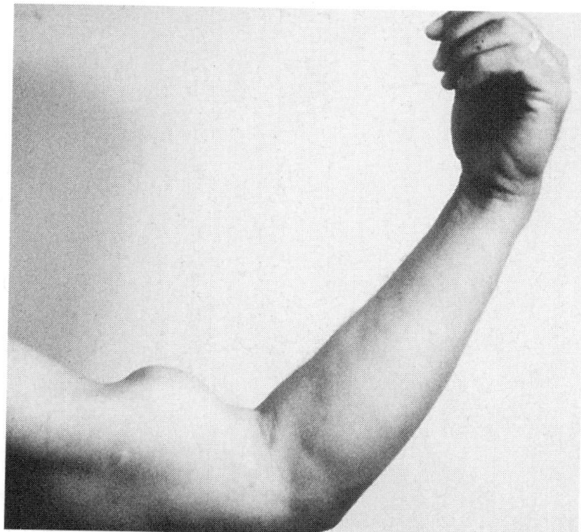

FIGURE 16-3 ■ Rupture of the long head of the biceps brachii tendon.

Acromioclavicular Joint Sprain

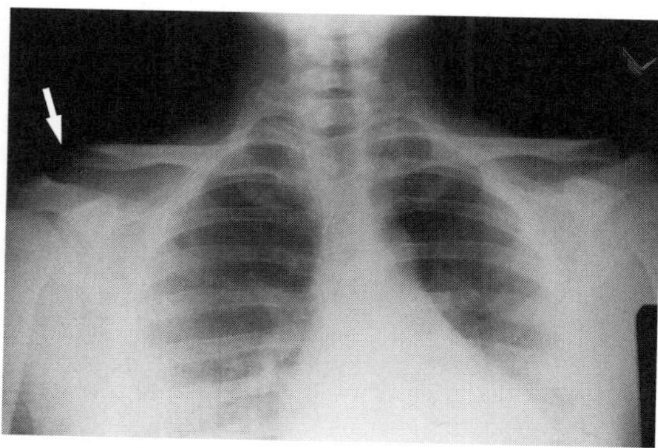

FIGURE 16-4 ■ Radiograph of a third-degree AC sprain. The superior displacement of the clavicle's distal aspect creates a characteristic "step deformity."

PALPATION

Palpation of the Anterior Shoulder

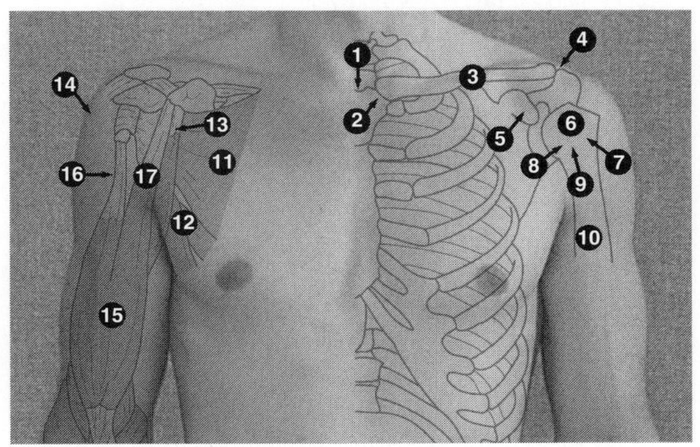

1 Jugular notch

2 Sternoclavicular joint

3 Clavicular shaft

4 Acromion process and AC joint

5 Coracoid process

6 Humeral head

7 Greater tuberosity

8 Lesser tuberosity

9 Bicipital groove

10 Humeral shaft

11 Pectoralis major

12 Pectoralis minor

13 Coracobrachialis

14 Deltoid group

15 Biceps brachii

16 Long head of the biceps brachii

17 Short head of the biceps brachii

Palpation of the Posterior Shoulder

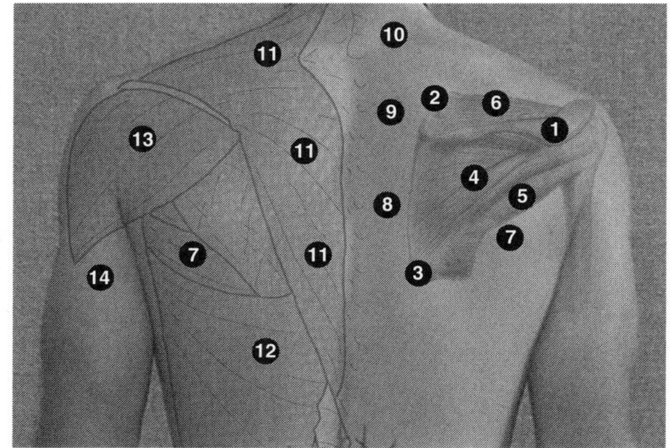

1 Spine of the scapula

2 Superior angle

3 Inferior angle

4 Infraspinatus

5 Teres minor

6 Supraspinatus

7 Teres major

8 Rhomboid major

9 Rhomboid minor

10 Levator scapulae

11 Trapezius

12 Latissimus dorsi

13 Posterior deltoid

14 Triceps brachii

Table 16-1 Glenohumeral Joint Capsular Patterns and End-Feels

End Feels: Capsular Pattern: External Rotation, Abduction, Internal Rotation	
Elevation	Firm or hard
Extension	Firm
Flexion	Firm
Abduction	Firm or hard
Horizontal Abduction	Firm
Horizontal Adduction	Firm or soft
Internal Rotation	Firm
External Rotation	Firm

Active Range of Motion Tests

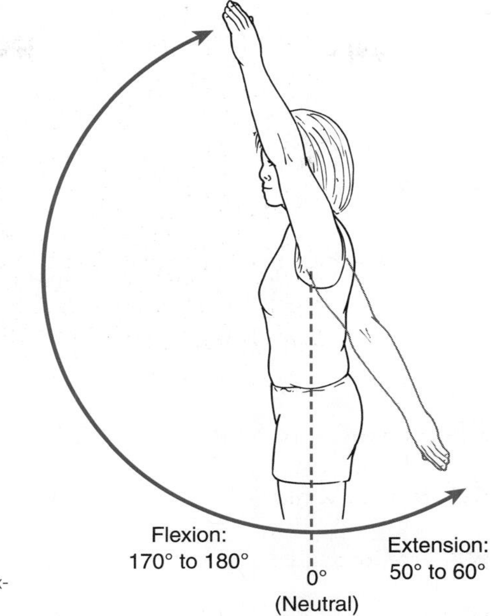

FIGURE 16-5 ■ Range of motion for shoulder flexion and extension.

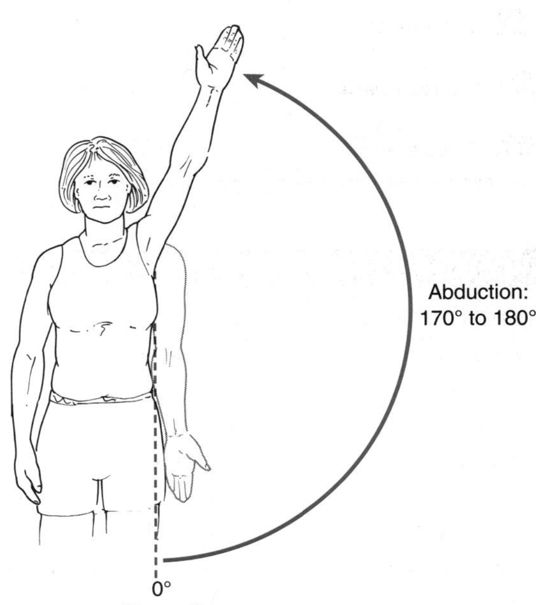

FIGURE 16-6 ■ Range of motion for shoulder abduction and adduction.

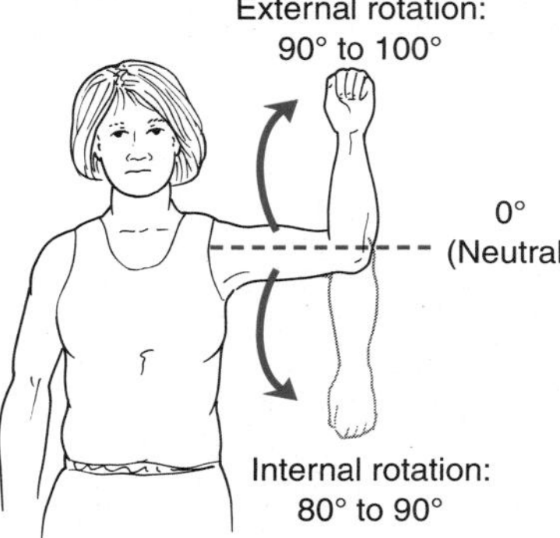

FIGURE 16-7 ■ Range of motion for shoulder internal rotation and external rotation.

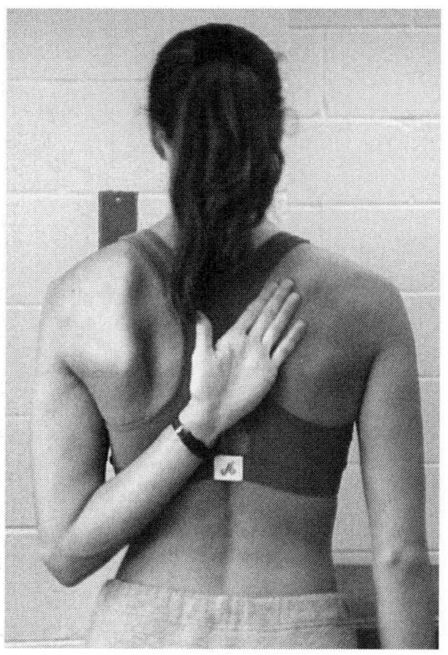

FIGURE 16-8 ■ Method of checking for shoulder internal rotation as recommended by the American Academy of Orthopaedic Surgeons. The amount of internal GH rotation is determined by measuring the distance up the spinal column the patient can reach and comparing this result to that of the opposite shoulder. This method is similar to part of the Apley's scratch test (see Box 16-1).

Box 16-1
Apley's Scratch Tests

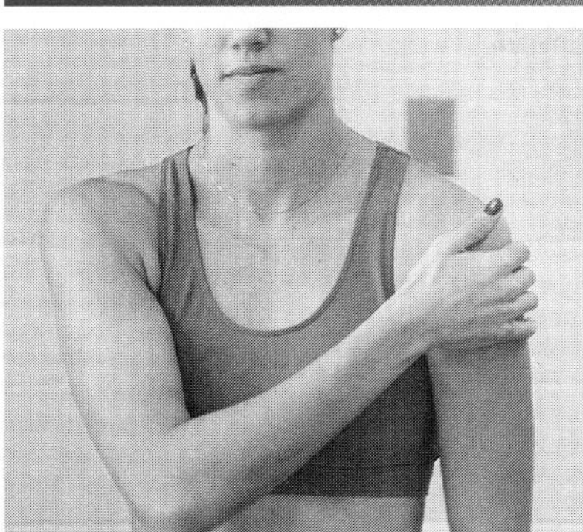

The patient touches the opposite shoulder by crossing the chest.

Motions produced: GH adduction, horizontal adduction, and internal rotation; scapular protraction

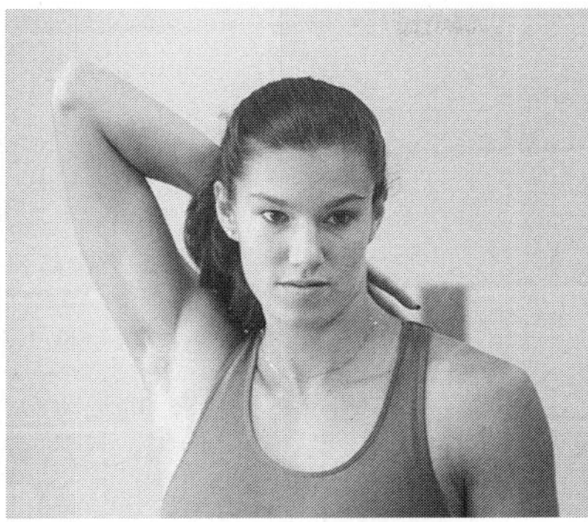

The patient reaches behind the head and touches the opposite shoulder from behind.

Motions produced: GH abduction and external rotation; scapular elevation, and upward rotation

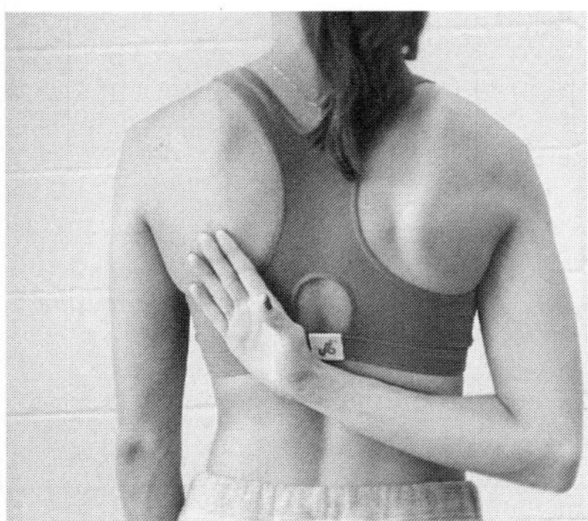

The patient reaches behind the back and touches the opposite scapula.

Motions produced: GH adduction and internal rotation; scapular retraction and downward rotation

GH = glenohumeral.

Goniometry Box 16-1
Shoulder Goniometry: Flexion and Extension

	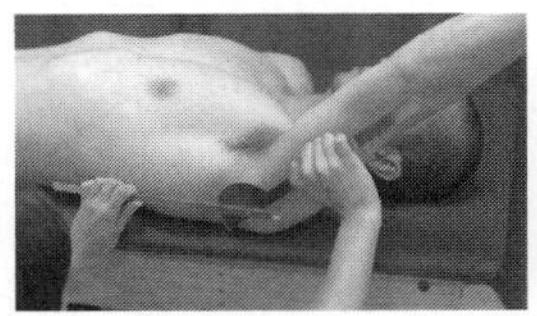 **GH Flexion 0° to 120° Elevation Through Flexion 0° to 180°**	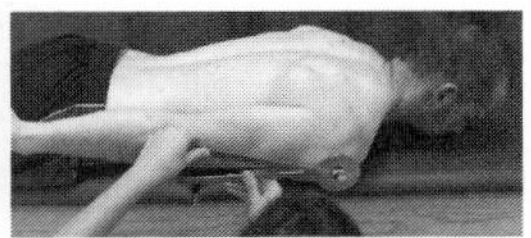 **GH Extension 0° to 60°**
Patient Position	Supine	Prone
Goniometer Alignment		
Fulcrum	Aligned lateral to the acromion process	Aligned lateral to the acromion process
Proximal Arm	The stationary arm is aligned parallel to the thorax.	The stationary arm is aligned parallel to the thorax.
Distal Arm	The movement arm is centered over the midline of the lateral humerus.	The movement arm is centered over the midline of the lateral humerus.
Comments	To isolate GH flexion, stabilize the scapula at its lateral border. Perform the measurement at the point where the scapula begins to move.	Stabilize the scapula on its posterior surface to isolate GH extension.

GH = glenohumeral.

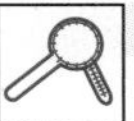

Goniometry Box 16-2
Shoulder Goniometry: Abduction

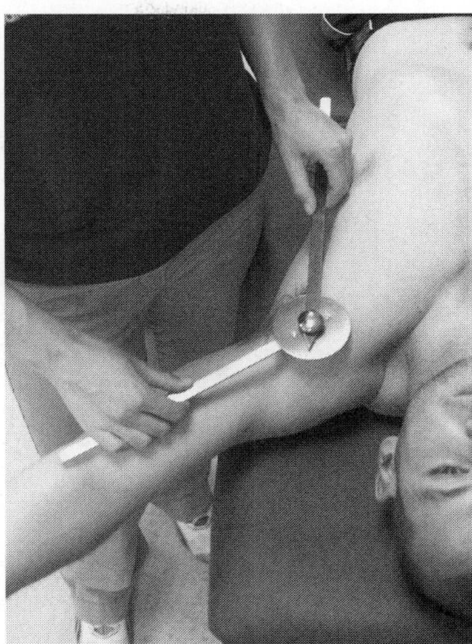

GH Abduction 0° to 120°
Elevation Through Abduction 0° to 180°

Patient Position	Supine or sitting
Goniometer Alignment	
Fulcrum	Anterior to the acromion process
Proximal Arm	The stationary arm is aligned parallel to the long axis of the torso.
Distal Arm	The movement arm is centered over the midline of the anterior humerus.
Comments	To isolate GH abduction, stabilize the scapula at its lateral border. Perform the measurement at the point where the scapula begins to move. Adduction is not normally measured.

GH = glenohumeral.

Goniometry Box 16-3
Shoulder Goniometry: Internal and External Rotation

	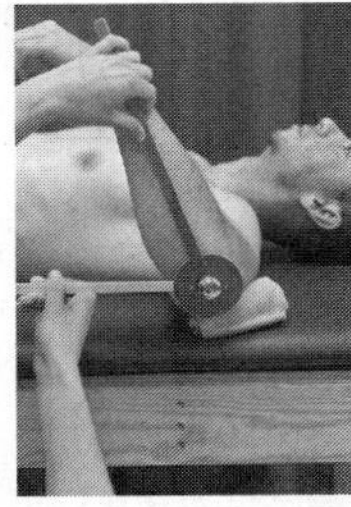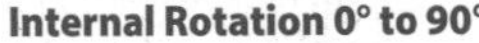 **Internal Rotation 0° to 90°**	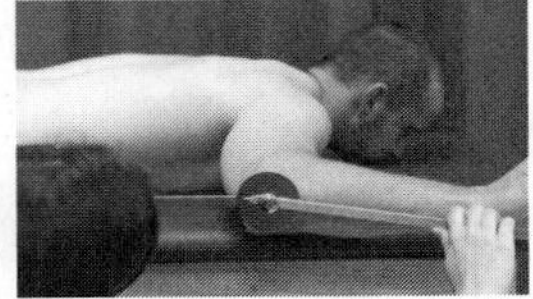 **External Rotation 0° to 100°**
Patient Position	Supine with the shoulder abducted to 90° and the elbow flexed to 90°	Prone with the shoulder abducted to 90° and the elbow flexed to 90°
Goniometer Alignment		
Fulcrum	Centered lateral to the olecranon process	
Proximal Arm	The stationary arm is aligned perpendicular to the floor or parallel to the tabletop.	
Distal Arm	The movement arm is centered over the long axis of the ulna.	
Comments	Anterior instability may result in pain and/or apprehension at the end range of external rotation (the apprehension test). To isolate GH motion, stabilize the scapula during external rotation. Perform the measurement at the point where the scapula begins to move. Scapular stabilization is provided by the body weight during internal rotation.	

GH = glenohumeral.

Goniometry Box 16-4
Shoulder Goniometry: Horizontal Abduction and Adduction

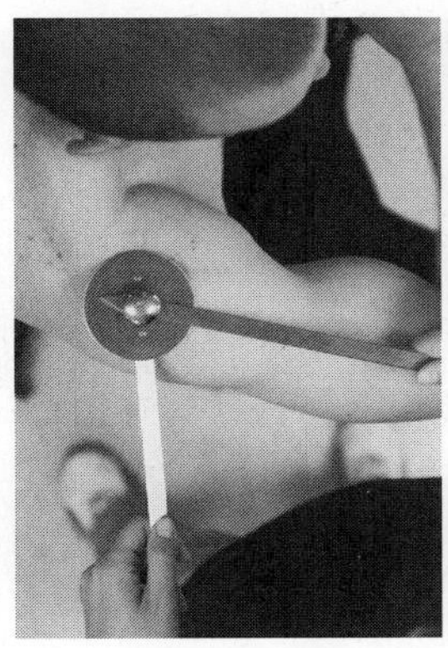

GH Horizontal Abduction 0° to 90°

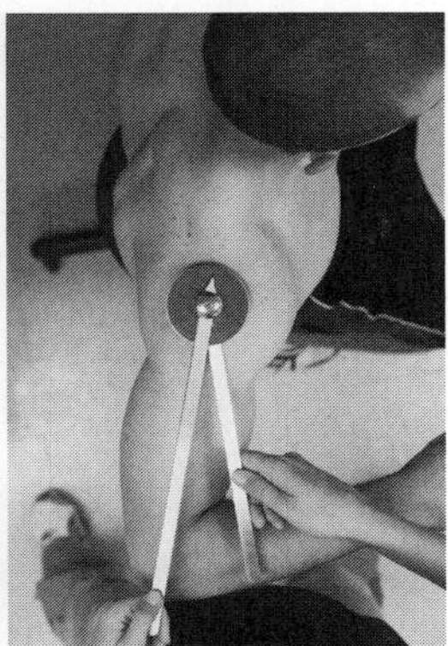

GH Horizontal Adduction 0° to 50°

Patient Position	Seated with the arm abducted to 90°; the elbow is flexed and the forearm is pronated.
Goniometer Alignment	
Fulcrum	Superior acromioclavicular joint
Proximal Arm	The stationary arm is perpendicular to the trunk.
Distal Arm	The movable arm is parallel to the longitudinal axis of the humerus.
Comment	To isolate glenohumeral motion during horizontal adduction, stabilize the scapula at its lateral border.

GH = glenohumeral.

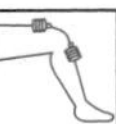

Manual Muscle Test 16-1
Shoulder Flexion and Extension

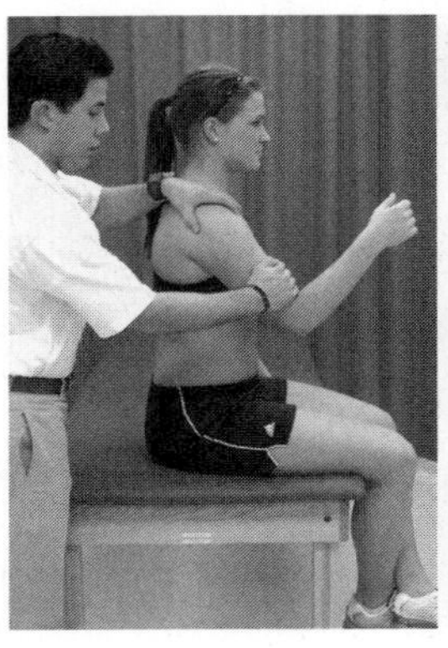

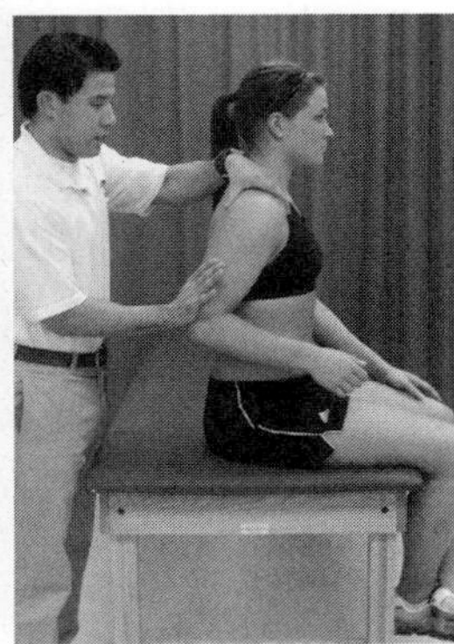

	Flexion	Extension
Patient Position	Seated	
Starting Position	The humerus in the neutral position	
Stabilization	Superior aspect of the shoulder	
Palpation	Anterior shoulder at anterior lateral aspect of clavicle	Latissimus dorsi: Inferior to inferior angle of scapula Teres major: Posterior axilla
Resistance	Distal anterior humerus, just proximal to the cubital fossa	Distal posterior humerus, just proximal to the olecranon
Primary Mover(s) (Innervation)	Anterior deltoid (C5, C6)	Latissimus dorsi (C6, C7, C8) Teres major (C5, C6, C7)
Secondary Mover(s) (Innervation)	Pectoralis major (clavicular portion) (C6, C7, C8, T1) Coracobrachialis (C6, C7) Middle deltoid (C5, C6) Biceps brachii (C5, C6) Lower trapezius (CN XI) Serratus anterior (C5, C6, C7)	Posterior deltoid (C5, C6) Triceps brachii (long head) (C6, C7, C8, T1)
Substitution	Trunk extension, scapular elevation	Scapular protraction (from pectoralis minor)
Comments	Not applicable	Maintain elbow extension to minimize contributions from the triceps.

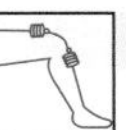

Manual Muscle Test 16-2
Shoulder Abduction and Adduction

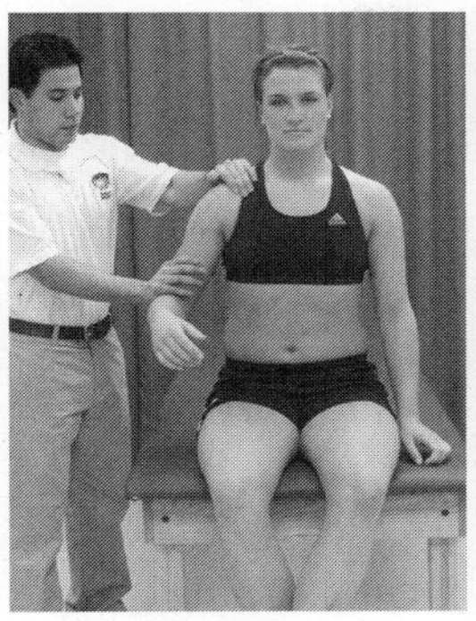

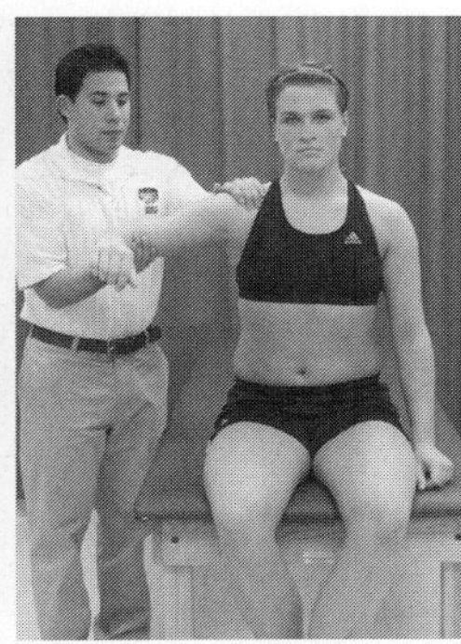

	Abduction	Adduction
Patient Position	Seated	Seated or supine
Starting Position	The humerus abducted to approximately 30°	
Stabilization	Scapula	
Palpation	Deltoid: Just lateral to tip of acromion.	Pectoralis major: Anterior axilla Latissimus dorsi: Inferior to inferior angle of scapula Teres major: Posterior axilla
Resistance	Distal humerus, just proximal to the lateral epicondyle	Distal humerus, just proximal to the medial epicondyle
Primary Mover(s) (Innervation)	Deltoid muscle group (C5, C6) Supraspinatus (C4, C5, C6)	Pectoralis major (C6, C7, C8, T1) Latissimus dorsi (C6, C7, C8) Teres major (C5, C6, C7)
Secondary Mover(s) (Innervation)	Biceps brachii (C5, C6) (greater than 90° abduction)	Coracobrachialis (C6, C7) Triceps brachii (C6, C7, C8, T1)
Substitution	Scapular elevation, external rotation, trunk lateral flexion to same or opposite side	Trunk lateral flexion to same side
Comments		The supine position is used for stabilization. Better isolation of the primary movers is achieved by testing shoulder extension and horizontal adduction.

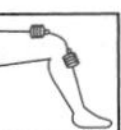

Manual Muscle Test 16-3
Shoulder Internal and External Rotation

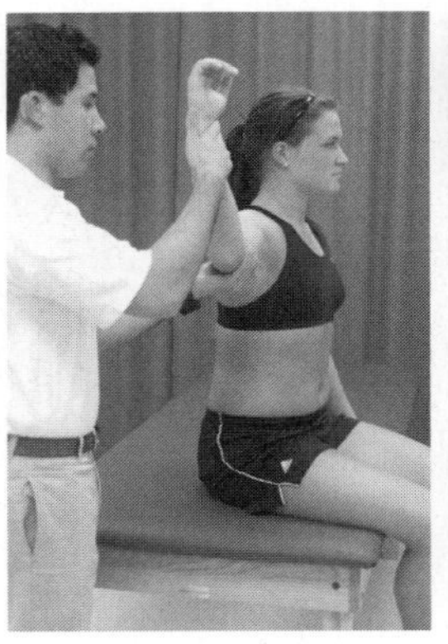

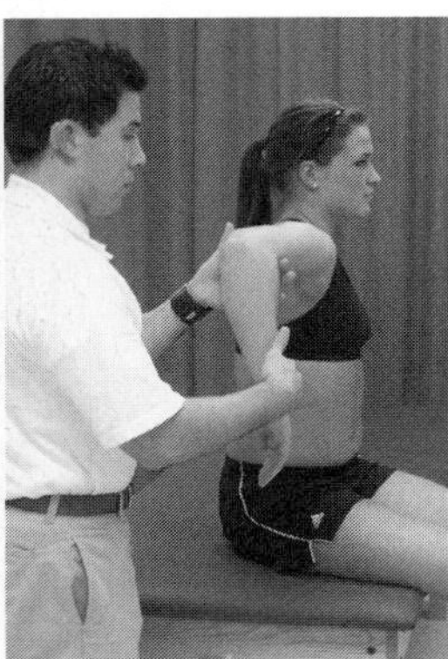

	Internal Rotation	External Rotation
Patient Position	Seated or prone. Stabilization is improved with the patient prone.	
Starting Position	The humerus is in neutral position or abducted to 90°. The elbow is flexed to 90°.	
Stabilization	The distal humerus is stabilized just proximal to the elbow.	
Palpation	Subscapularis: Too deep to palpate	Infraspinatus and teres minor: Inferior to spine of scapula
Resistance	Anterior distal forearm	Posterior distal forearm
Primary Mover(s) (Innervation)	Subscapularis (C5, C6, C7)	Infraspinatus (C5, C6) Teres minor (C5, C6)
Secondary Mover(s) (Innervation)	Teres major (C5, C6, C7) Pectoralis major (C6, C7, C8, T1) Latissimus dorsi (C6, C7, C8) Anterior deltoid (C5, C6)	Posterior deltoid (C5, C6)
Substitution	Elbow extension, scapular protraction	Elbow extension, scapular depression
Comments	Optimal isolation of the subscapularis occurs at 45° of internal rotation with the arm at the side.[85] The Gerber lift-off test is also used to assess subscapularis strength.	Optimal isolation of the infraspinatus occurs at 45° of internal rotation with the arm at the side.[85]

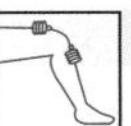

Manual Muscle Test 16-4
Horizontal Adduction and Abduction

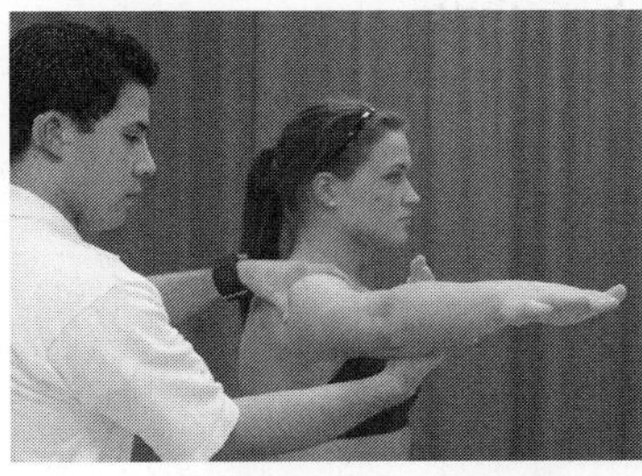

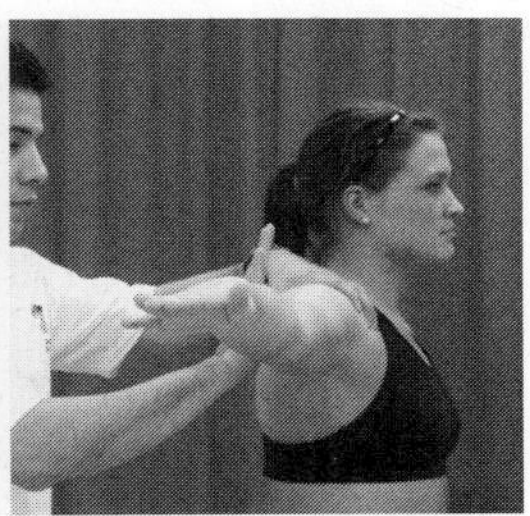

	Horizontal Adduction	Horizontal Abduction
Patient Position	Supine	Prone
Starting Position	The shoulder is abducted to 90°.	
Stabilization	Scapula	Scapula
Palpation	Anterior axilla	Inferior to lateral spine of the scapula
Resistance	Anterior portion of the distal humerus	Posterior portion of the distal humerus
Primary Mover(s) (Innervation)	Pectoralis major (C6, C7, C8, T1)	Posterior deltoid (C5, C6)
Secondary Mover(s) (Innervation)	Coracobrachialis (C6, C7) Anterior deltoid (C5, C6)	Infraspinatus (C5, C6) Teres minor (C5, C6)
Substitution	Trunk rotation	Scapular retraction, trunk rotation

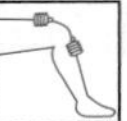

Manual Muscle Test 16-5
Scapular Retraction and Downward Rotation

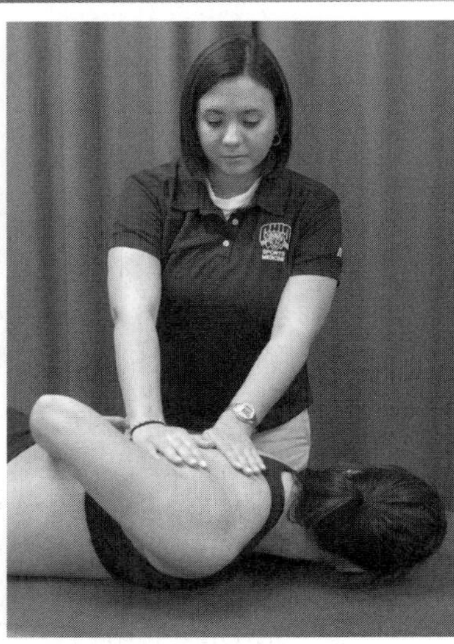

Patient Position	Prone
Starting Position	The arm being tested is behind the patient's back, with the humerus internally rotated.
Stabilization	Trunk
Palpation	Lateral to vertebral border of scapula
Resistance	Lateral scapula as the patient attempts to lift the hand off the back in an upward and lateral direction
Primary Mover(s) (Innervation)	Rhomboid major (C4, C5) Rhomboid minor (C4, C5)
Secondary Mover(s) (Innervation)	Middle trapezius (CN XI)
Substitution	Trunk rotation, glenohumeral extension, anterior tipping of scapula
Comments	Note the application of resistance on the scapula, which differentiates this from the Gerber lift-off test (see Special Test 16-2).

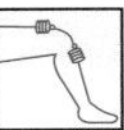

Manual Muscle Test 16-6
Scapular Retraction

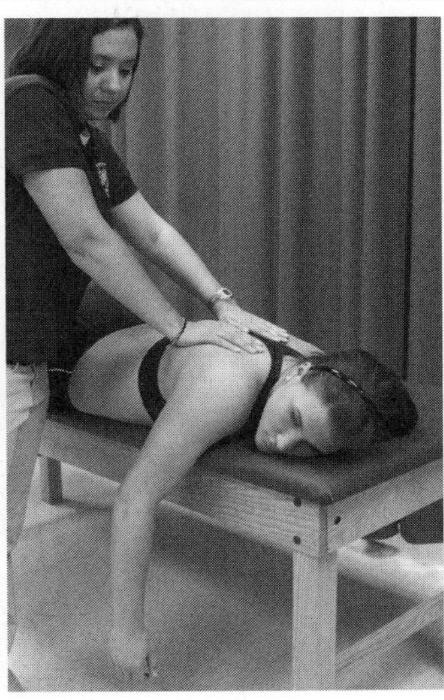

Patient Position	Prone
Starting Position	The elbow is extended and the humerus is flexed to 90°.
Stabilization	Trunk
Palpation	Between spine of scapula and spinous process
Resistance	Scapula
Primary Mover(s) (Innervation)	Middle trapezius (CN XI) Rhomboids (C4, C5)
Secondary Mover(s) (Innervation)	Upper and lower trapezius
Substitution	Trunk rotation, glenohumeral horizontal abduction

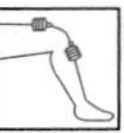

Manual Muscle Test 16-7
Scapular Protraction and Upward Rotation

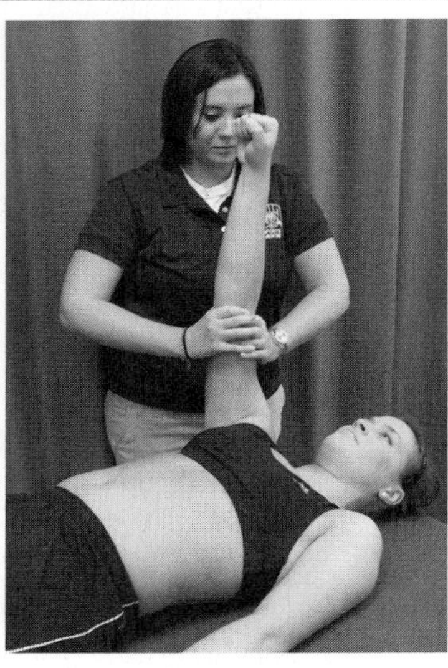

Patient Position	Supine
Starting Position	Test arm is flexed to 90°.
Stabilization	Trunk
Palpation	Lateral trunk
Resistance	Distal humerus, proximal to elbow. Instruct the patient to "punch the ceiling."
Primary Mover(s) (Innervation)	Serratus anterior (C5, C6, C7)
Secondary Mover(s) (Innervation)	Pectoralis minor (C7, C8, T1) Trapezius (CN XI)
Substitution	Glenohumeral adduction and horizontal adduction
Comments	Observe the patient performing a wall push-up to functionally assess the serratus anterior.

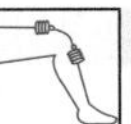

Manual Muscle Test 16-8
Scapular Depression and Retraction

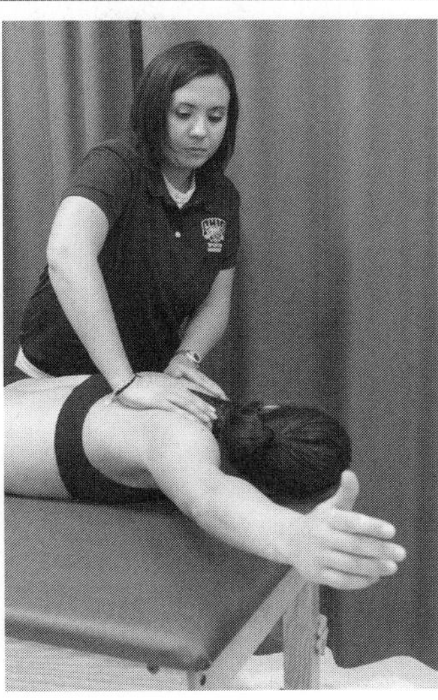

Patient Position	Prone
Starting Position	The arm being tested is abducted to 135° with the forearm supinated and the patient's head rotated to the side opposite that being tested.
Stabilization	Trunk
Palpation	Medial to inferior angle of scapula
Resistance	Scapula. Instruct the patient to "raise your arm."
Primary Mover(s) (Innervation)	Lower trapezius (CN XI)
Secondary Mover(s) (Innervation)	Middle trapezius (CN XI)
Substitution	Trunk rotation; glenohumeral extension
Comments	Patients suffering from impingement may be unable to achieve this test position. In this case, position the arm at the side and instruct the patient to bring the scapula "down and in."

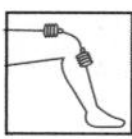

Manual Muscle Test 16-9
Scapular Elevation

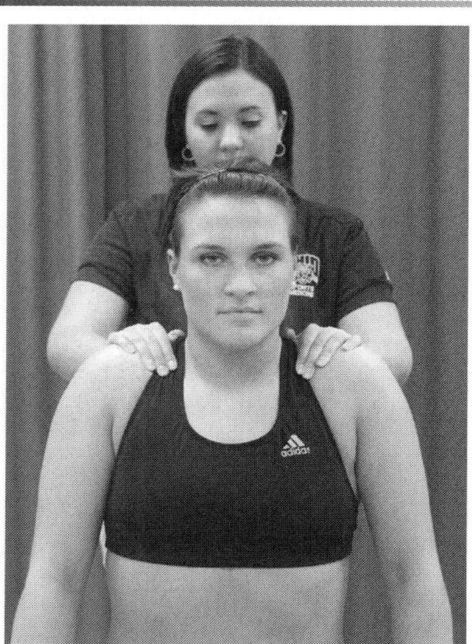

Patient Position	Seated
Starting Position	Seated
Stabilization	Trunk
Palpation	Superomedial to scapula
Resistance	Superior aspect of the shoulder. The patient assumes a shoulder shrug position which the examiner pushes down.
Primary Mover(s) (Innervation)	Upper trapezius (CN XI) Levator scapulae (C3, C4, C5)
Secondary Mover(s) (Innervation)	Not applicable
Substitution	Trunk rotation or side-bending

Special Test 16-1
Drop Arm Test for Rotator Cuff Tendinopathy

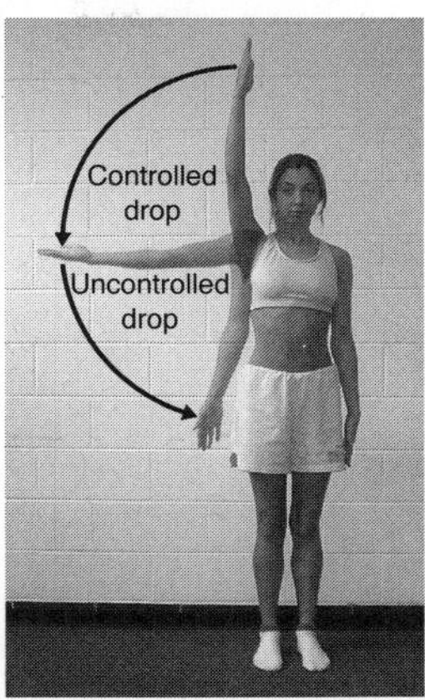

The drop arm test determines the patient's ability to control humeral motion via an eccentric contraction as the arm is slowly lowered from full abduction to adduction.

Patient Position	Standing or sitting The humerus fully abducted and externally rotated and the forearm supinated
Position of Examiner	Standing lateral to, or behind, the involved extremity
Evaluative Procedure	The patient slowly lowers the arm to the side.
Positive Test	The arm falls uncontrollably to the side from a position of approximately 90° abduction. Severe pain may also be described.
Implications	The inability to lower the arm in a controlled manner is indicative of lesions to the rotator cuff, especially the supraspinatus.
Modification	If the patient is able to lower the arm in a controlled manner through the ROM, a derivative of the drop arm test may be implemented: The patient holds the humerus in 90° abduction. The examiner applies gentle pressure on the distal forearm. A positive test result causes the arm to fall against the side of the body, indicating lesions to the rotator cuff.
Evidence	Positive likelihood ratio Not Useful — Useful Very Small · Small · Moderate · Large 0 1 2 3 4 5 6 7 8 9 10 Negative likelihood ratio Not Useful — Useful Very Small · Small · Moderate · Large 1.0 0.9 0.8 0.7 0.6 0.5 0.4 0.3 0.2 0.1 0

ROM = range of motion.

Special Test 16-2
Gerber Lift-off Test for Subscapularis Pathology

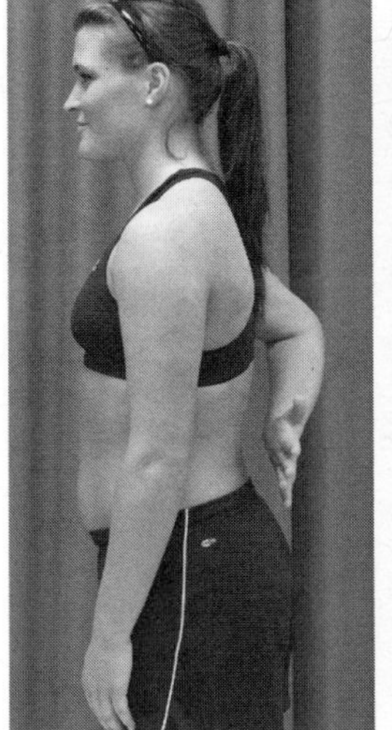

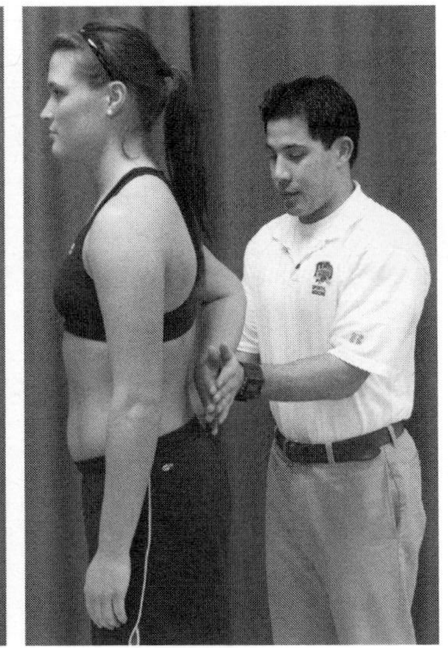

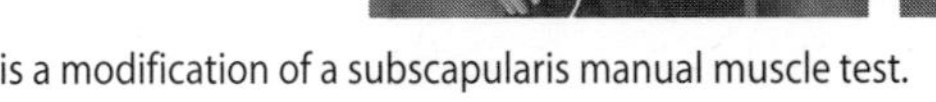

The Gerber lift-off test is a modification of a subscapularis manual muscle test.

Patient Position	Standing with the humerus internally rotated The dorsal surface of the hand placed against the midlumbar spine
Position of Examiner	Standing behind the patient
Evaluative Procedure	The patient attempts to actively lift the hand off the spine while the humerus stays in extension.

Positive Test	Inability to lift the hand off the back
Implications	Positive test findings are associated with tears or weakness of the subscapularis muscle. Possible C5, C6, C7 nerve root pathology
Modification	Resistance can be applied to the patient's palm.
Comments	Test should be performed only if the patient has sufficient internal rotation to reach sacral region or above. Do not allow compensatory motions such as GH extension. With the arm in this position, the subscapularis contributes almost 90% of the force when no resistance is applied. A MMT lower than grade 3 (lift off with no resistance) accurately identifies those with a subscapularis tear 85% of the time.[85]
Evidence	Positive likelihood ratio Not Useful — Useful Very Small · Small · Moderate · Large 0 1 2 3 4 5 6 7 8 9 10 Negative likelihood ratio Not Useful — Useful Very Small · Small · Moderate · Large 1.0 0.9 0.8 0.7 0.6 0.5 0.4 0.3 0.2 0.1 0

MMT = manual muscle test.

Table 16-2 Muscles Acting on the Scapula

Muscle	Action	Origin	Insertion	Innervation	Root
Latissimus Dorsi	Depression of shoulder girdle Internal humeral rotation Humeral extension Humeral adduction	Spinous processes of T6–T12 and the lumbar vertebrae via the lumbodorsal fascia. Posterior iliac crest	Intertubercular groove of the humerus	Thoracodorsal	C6, C7, C8
Levator Scapulae	Elevation Downward rotation Extension of cervical spine Rotation of the cervical spine	Transverse processes of cervical vertebrae C1–C4	Superior medial angle of the scapula	Dorsal scapular	C3, C4, C5
Rhomboid Major	Scapular retraction Scapular elevation Downward rotation of the scapula	Spinous processes of T2, T3, T4, and T5	Vertebral border of scapula (lower two thirds)	Dorsal scapular	C4, C5
Rhomboid Minor	Scapular retraction Scapular elevation	Inferior portion of the ligamentum nuchae Spinous processes C7 and T1	Vertebral border of scapula (near the medial border of the scapular spine)	Dorsal scapular	C4, C5
Serratus Anterior	Upward rotation Protraction Depression (lower fibers) Elevation (upper fibers)	Anterior portion of 1st–8th or 9th ribs Aponeuroses of the intercostal muscles	Costal surfaces of the: • Superior angle of scapula • Vertebral border of scapula Inferior angle of scapula	Long thoracic	C5, C6, C7

Trapezius (upper one third)	Fixation of the scapula to the thorax Elevation of scapula Upward rotation of scapula Rotation of C-spine to the opposite side Extension of C-spine	Occipital protuberance Superior nuchal line of the occipital bone Upper portion of the ligamentum nuchae Spinous process of C7	Distal/lateral one third of clavicle Acromion process Scapular spine	Accessory	CN XI
Trapezius (middle one third)	Retraction of scapula Fixation of thoracic spine	Lower portion of the ligamentum nuchae Spinous processes of the 7th cervical vertebra and T1–T5	Acromion process Spine of the scapula (superior, lateral border)	Accessory	CN XI
Trapezius (lower one third)	Depression of scapula Retraction of scapula Fixation of thoracic spine	Spinous processes and supraspinal ligaments of T8–T12	Spine of the scapula (medial portion)	Accessory	CN XI
Pectoralis Major	Depression of the shoulder girdle (clavicular fibers) Adduction of the humerus Horizontal adduction of the humerus Humeral flexion (clavicular segment) Internal humeral rotation	Medial one-half of the clavicle Anterolateral portion of the sternum	Greater tuberosity of the humerus—lateral lip of the bicipital groove.	Lateral and medial pectoral	C6, C7, C8, T1
Pectoralis Minor	Forward (anterior) tilting	Costal cartilages of ribs 6–7 Anterior portion of 3rd–5th ribs	Coracoid process of scapula	Lateral pectoral	C7, C8, T1

Table 16-3 Muscles Acting on the Humerus

Muscle	Action	Origin	Insertion	Innervation	Root
Biceps Brachii	Flexion Abduction	Long head: Supraglenoid tuberosity of scapula Short head: Coracoid process of scapula	Radial tuberosity and aponeurosis	Musculocutaneous	C5, C6
Coracobrachialis	Flexion Adduction	Coracoid process	Medial shaft of the humerus, adjacent to the deltoid tuberosity	Musculocutaneous	C6, C7
Deltoid (anterior one third)	Flexion Abduction Horizontal adduction Internal rotation	Lateral one third of the clavicle	Deltoid tuberosity	Axillary	C5, C6
Deltoid (middle one third)	Abduction Flexion	Acromion process	Deltoid tuberosity	Axillary	C5, C6
Deltoid (posterior one third)	Extension Horizontal abduction Abduction External rotation	Spine of the scapula	Deltoid tuberosity	Axillary	C5, C6
Infraspinatus	External rotation Horizontal abduction Humeral head stabilization	Infraspinous fossa of the scapula	Lateral portion of the greater tuberosity of the humerus GH joint capsule	Suprascapular	C5, C6
Latissimus Dorsi	Extension Internal rotation Adduction Depression of shoulder girdle	Spinous processes of T6–T12 and the lumbar vertebrae via the lumbodorsal fascia. Posterior iliac crest	Floor of the bicipital groove of the humerus	Thoracodorsal	C6, C7, C8

Pectoralis Major	Adduction of the humerus Horizontal adduction of the humerus Humeral flexion (clavicular segment) Internal humeral rotation Depression of the shoulder girdle (clavicular fibers)	Medial one half of the clavicle Anterolateral portion of the sternum Costal cartilages of ribs 6–7	Greater tuberosity of the humerus	Lateral and medial pectoral	C6, C7, C8, T1
Subscapularis	Internal rotation Humeral head stabilization	Anterior surface (subscapular fossa) and axillary border of the scapula	Lesser tuberosity of the humerus Ventral portion of the GH capsule	Upper and lower subscapular	C5, C6, C7
Supraspinatus	Abduction External rotation Humeral head stabilization	Supraspinous fossa (medial two thirds) of the scapula	Medial aspect of the greater tuberosity GH joint capsule	Suprascapular	C4, C5, C6
Teres Major	Extension Internal rotation Adduction	Inferior angle of scapula Lower one third of the axillary border of the scapula	Medial lip of the bicipital groove	Lower subscapular	C5, C6, C7
Teres Minor	External rotation Horizontal abduction	Lateral upper two thirds of axillary border of the scapula	Lateral aspect of the greater tuberosity	Axillary	C5, C6
Triceps Brachii	Extension (long head) Adduction	Long head: Infraglenoid tuberosity of scapula Lateral head: Lateral and posterior surface of the proximal one half of the humerus Medial head: Distal two thirds of medial and posterior humerus	Olecranon process of ulna	Radial	C6, C7, C8, T1

GH = glenohumeral.

Passive Range of Motion Tests

Flexion and Extension

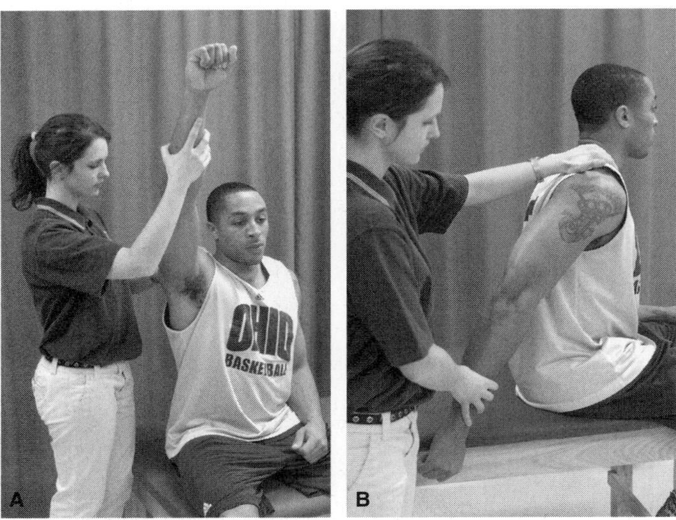

FIGURE 16-9 ■ Passive range of motion testing for (A) shoulder flexion and (B) shoulder extension.

Abduction and Adduction

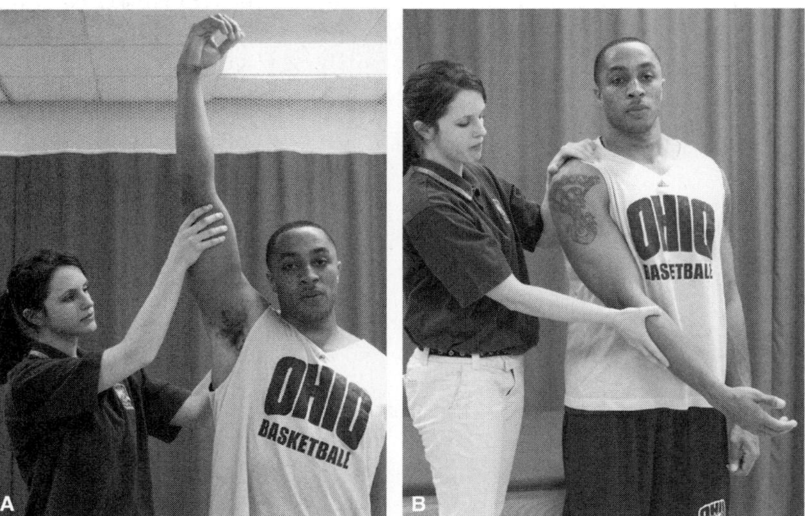

FIGURE 16-10 ■ Passive range of motion testing for shoulder abduction (A) and adduction (B).

Internal and External Rotation

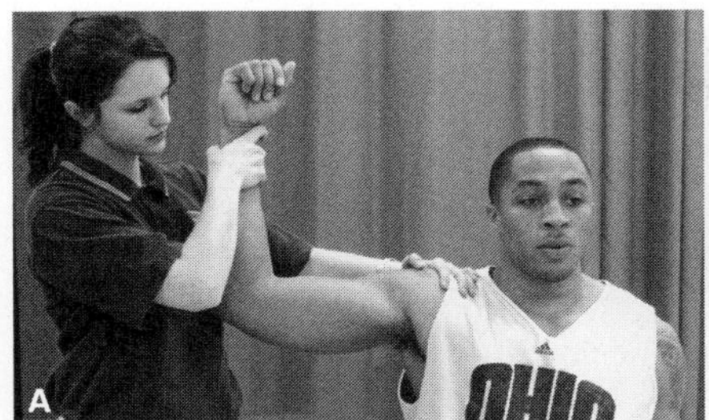

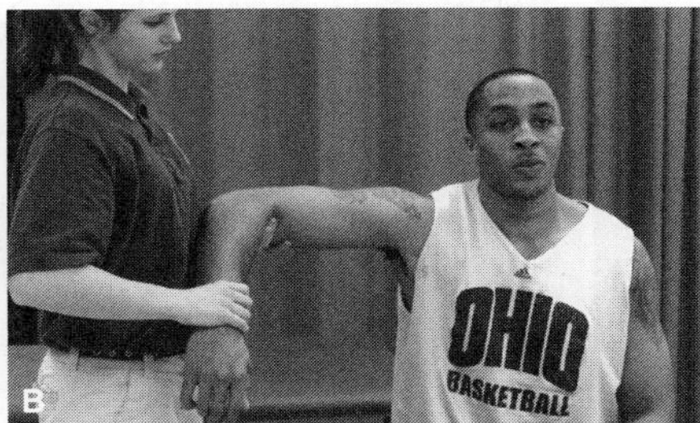

FIGURE 16-11 ■ Passive range of motion testing for shoulder external rotation **(A)** and internal rotation **(B)**.

Horizontal Adduction and Horizontal Abduction

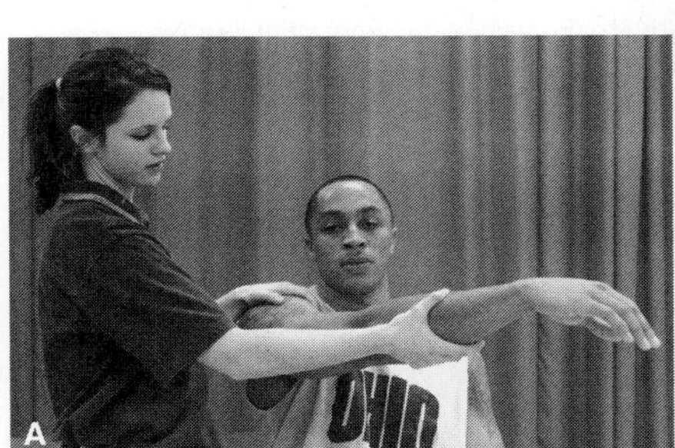

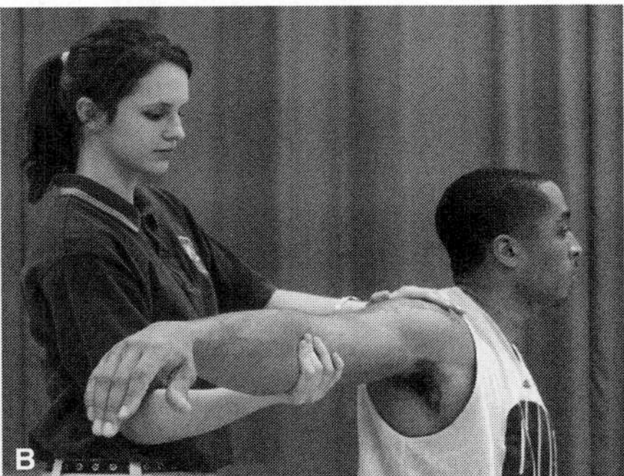

FIGURE 16-12 ■ Passive range of motion testing for **(A)** shoulder horizontal adduction and **(B)** shoulder horizontal abduction.

Joint Play 16-1
Sternoclavicular Joint Play

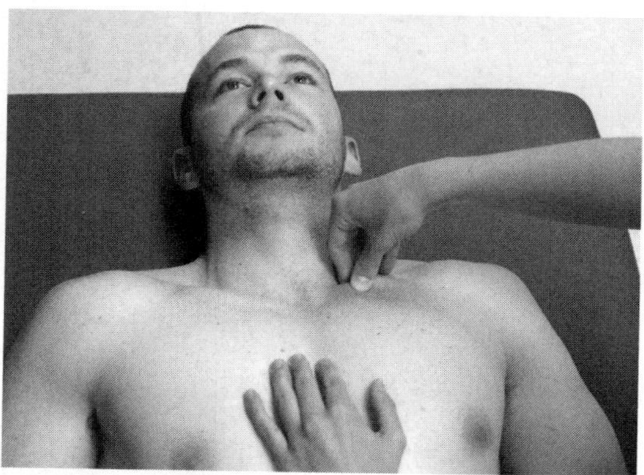

The proximal portion of the clavicle is manipulated to determine the amount of inferior, superior, anterior, and posterior motion available at the joint.

Patient Position	Supine or seated
Position of Examiner	Standing next to the patient, grasping the proximal clavicle
Evaluative Procedure	Apply a gliding pressure that forces the medial clavicle downward, upward, anteriorly, and posteriorly relative to the sternum, noting pain or laxity elicited.
Positive Test	Pain, hypermobility, or hypomobility
Implications	Hypermobility: Laxity and/or spasm Hypomobility: Joint adhesions

Clavicular Motion	Structures Stressed
Inferior	Interclavicular ligament
Superior	Costoclavicular ligament (anterior and posterior fibers)
Anterior	SC ligament (posterior fibers)
Posterior	SC ligament (anterior fibers)

SC = sternoclavicular.

Joint Play 16-2
Acromioclavicular Joint Play

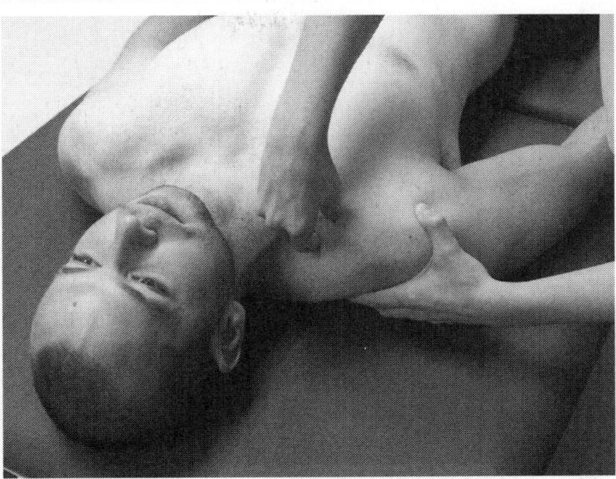

The distal portion of the clavicle is manipulated to determine the amount of inferior, superior, anterior, and posterior motion available at the acromioclavicular joint.

Patient Position	Seated or supine
Position of Examiner	Standing lateral to the patient, grasping the distal portion of the clavicle, just proximal to the AC joint The opposite hand is stabilizing the acromion process
Evaluative Procedure	Apply a gliding pressure that forces the distal clavicle downward, upward, anteriorly, and posteriorly relative to the scapula, noting pain or laxity elicited.

Clavicular Motion	Structures Stressed
Inferior	AC ligament (superior fibers)
Superior	Conoid ligament*
	Trapezoid ligament*
	AC ligament (inferior fibers)
Anterior	AC ligament
	Coracoclavicular ligament (in the absence of the AC ligament)
Posterior	Clavicle contacting acromion (posterior block)
	AC ligament

*Portions of the coracoclavicular ligament.

Positive Test	Pain, hypermobility, or hypomobility
Implications	Hypermobility: Laxity Hypomobility: Joint adhesions

AC = acromioclavicular.

Joint Play 16-3
Glenohumeral Joint Play

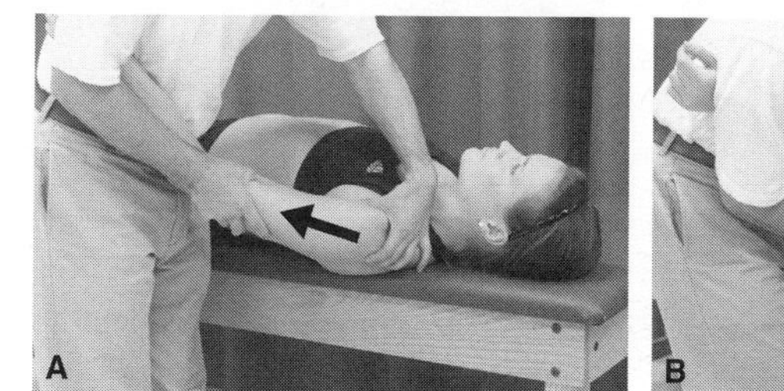

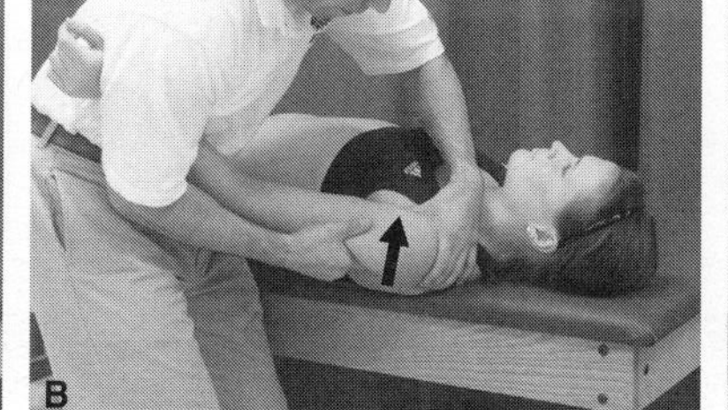

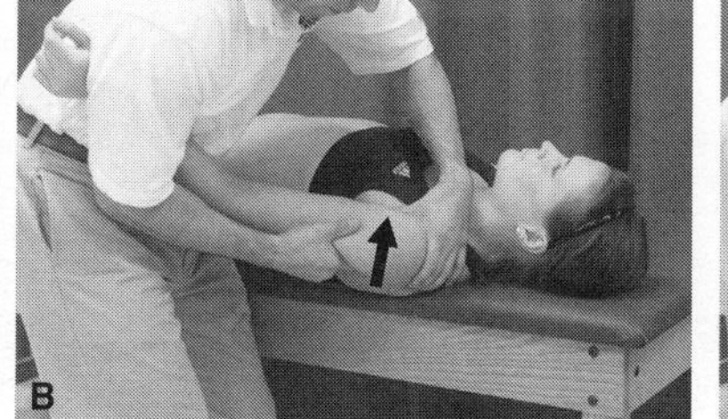

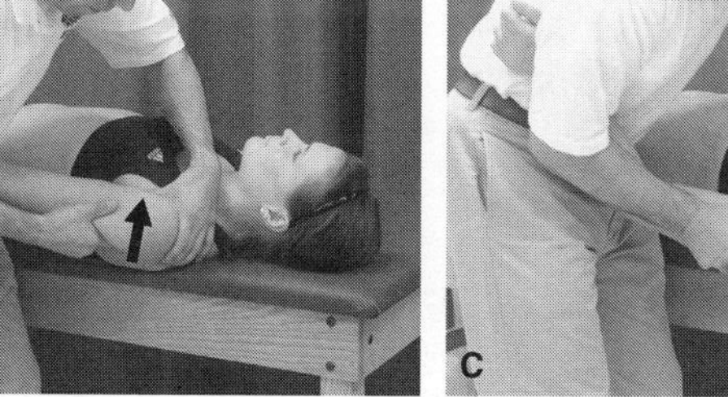

Glenohumeral joint play assesses the amount of mobility allowed by the joint capsule and ligaments.

Patient Position	Seated The patient's arm is placed in the resting position (GH joint abducted to approximately 55° and flexed to approximately 30°). The examiner maintains the patient's arm in this position to assure relaxation.
Position of Examiner	**(A) Inferior glide**: One hand supports the arm to maintain the resting position. The opposite hand cups the superior aspect of the humerus. **(B) Anterior glide**: One hand stabilizes the scapula anteriorly by applying pressure to the coracoid process, reaching under the axilla to the scapular body. The opposite hand applies force at the posterior aspect of the humerus. **(C) Posterior glide**: One hand stabilizes the scapula at the acromion process. The opposite hand applies force at the anterior aspect of the humeral head.
Evaluative Procedure	A gentle yet firm force is applied that distracts the joint (to take up the slack) and then moves the humeral head inferiorly, anteriorly or posteriorly.

Positive Test	Pain, increased mobility, or decreased mobility compared with the same direction on the opposite shoulder.
Implications	Hypermobility or hypomobility of the static stabilizers of the GH joint: **(A)** Inferior: Inferior joint capsule, superior GH ligament, coracohumeral ligament **(B)** Anterior: Coracohumeral ligament, superior and middle GH ligaments, anterior joint capsule, labral tear **(C)** Posterior: Posterior joint capsule, labral tear.
Modification	In the case of large patients, a second examiner can be used to assist in manually stabilizing the scapula or using straps. Load and shift test: Center the humeral head in the fossa by applying an axial load while the patient's humerus is in 20° of abduction and 20° of forward flexion and the scapula stabilized. Joint play is then assessed.
Comment	These results should be interpreted with caution and considered in light of the remaining exam because of the low inter-rater and intra-rater reliability.[86] It is difficult to detect subtle changes (e.g., grade 0 and grade 1). The difference between the inferior glide test and the sulcus sign (see Special Test Box 16-9) is that the sulcus sign is not performed in the resting position.

GH = glenohumeral.

Load and Shift Test Findings

Grade	Amount of Humeral Head Translation
Trace (0)	No translation of the humeral head
Grade I	Translation of the humeral head to the glenoid rim, but not over it
Grade II	Translation of the humeral head over the glenoid rim, but the head spontaneously reduces
Grade III	Dislocation of the humeral head without spontaneous reduction

Special Test 16-3
Acromioclavicular Traction Test

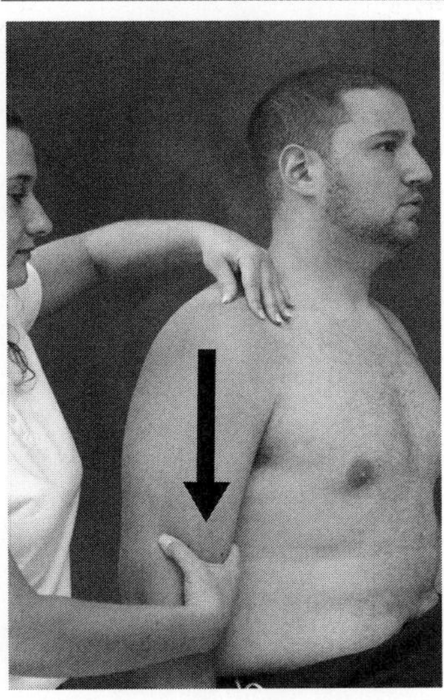

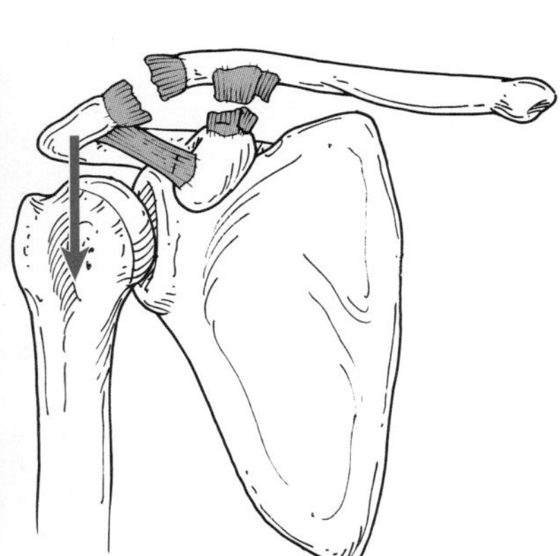

The principle behind the AC traction test is similar to a stress radiograph used to diagnose AC instability.

Patient Position	Sitting or standing The arm hanging naturally from the side
Position of Examiner	Standing lateral to the involved side The clinician grasps the patient's humerus proximal to the elbow. The opposite hand gently palpates the AC joint.
Evaluative Procedure	The examiner applies a downward traction on the humerus.
Positive Test	The humerus and scapula move inferior to the clavicle, causing a step deformity, pain, or both.
Implications	Sprain of the AC or costoclavicular ligaments
Comments	Patients displaying positive AC traction test results should be referred to a physician for follow-up radiographic stress testing and to rule out a clavicular fracture.
Evidence	Absent or inconclusive in the literature

AC = acromioclavicular.

Special Test 16-4
Acromioclavicular Compression Test

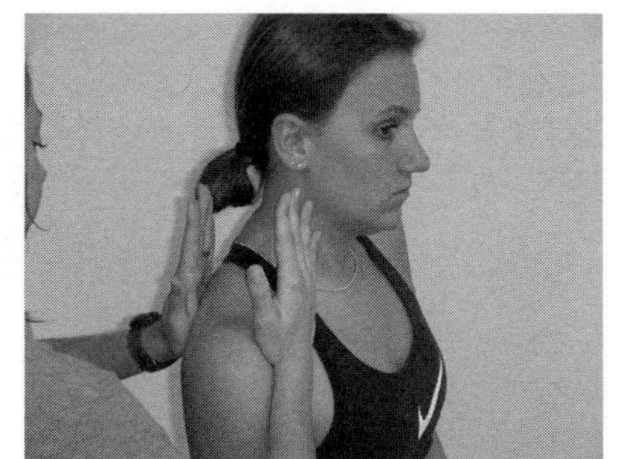

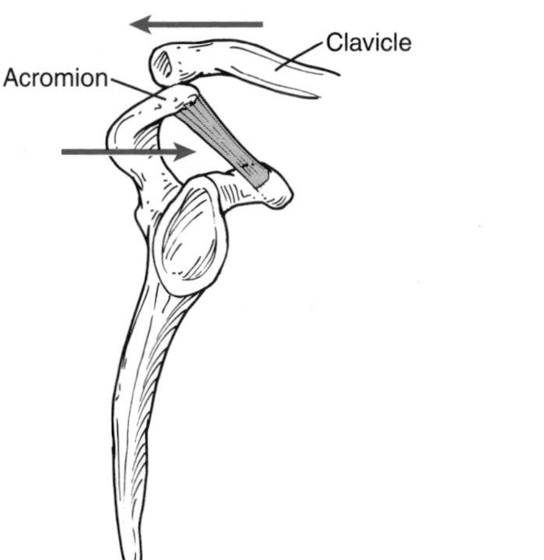

The AC compression test attempts to displace the clavicle over the acromion process, stressing the coracoclavicular ligament.

Patient Position	Sitting or standing with the arm hanging naturally at the side
Position of Examiner	Standing on the involved side with the hands cupped over the anterior and posterior joint structures
Evaluative Procedure	The examiner squeezes the hands together, compressing the AC joint.
Positive Test	Pain at the AC joint or excursion of the clavicle over the acromion process

Implications	Damage to the AC ligament and possibly the coracoclavicular ligament
Modification	Place a thumb on the posterolateral aspect of the acromion process and the index and middle fingers of the same or opposite hand on the midpoint of the clavicle.[87] An anterosuperior force is applied with the thumb and an inferior force on the clavicle. A positive test is marked by pain.
Evidence	Positive Likelihood Ratio Not Useful — Useful Very Small, Small, Moderate, Large 0 1 2 3 4 5 6 7 8 9 10 Negative Likelihood Ratio Not Useful — Useful Very Small, Small, Moderate, Large 1.0 0.9 0.8 0.7 0.6 0.5 0.4 0.3 0.2 0.1 0

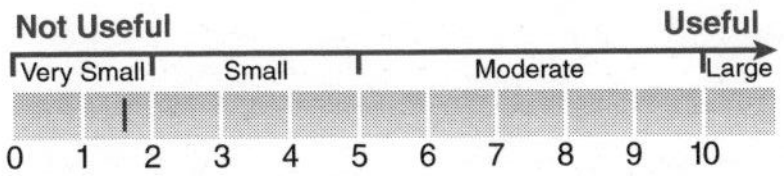

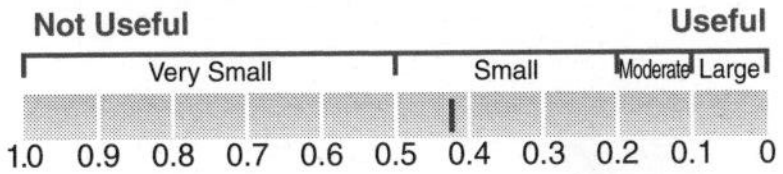

AC = acromioclavicular.

Special Test 16-5
Apprehension Test for Anterior Glenohumeral Laxity

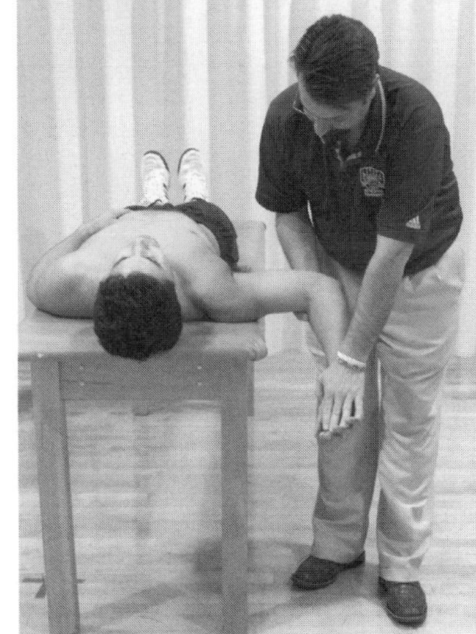

The apprehension test, passive external rotation of the glenohumeral joint, places the joint in the closed-pack position and replicates the mechanism of injury for anterior GH dislocations.

Patient Position	Supine, standing, or sitting The GH joint is abducted to 90° and the elbow is flexed to 90°.
Position of Examiner	Positioned in front of or beside the patient on the involved side The examiner supporting the humerus at midshaft while the forearm is grasped proximal to the wrist

Evaluative Procedure	While supporting the humerus at 90° abduction, the examiner passively externally rotates the GH joint by slowly applying pressure to the anterior forearm.
Positive Test	The patient displays apprehension that the shoulder may dislocate and resists further movement. Pain is centered in the anterior capsule of the GH joint.
Implications	The anterior capsule, inferior GH ligament, or glenoid labrum have been compromised, allowing the humeral head to dislocate or subluxate anteriorly on the glenoid fossa. Apprehension coupled with pain is often associated with instability secondary to rotator cuff pathology.[88] Pain in the deep posterior shoulder may be associated with internal impingement.[88]
Comments	Pressure should be applied gradually and the test terminated at the first sign of apprehension. Do not perform this test when there is obvious dislocation or subluxation of the GH joint. A positive apprehension test is typically followed by the relocation test. (See Special Text Box 16-6.)
Evidence	Positive likelihood ratio Not Useful / Useful Very Small / Small / Moderate / Large 18 – 48.18 0 1 2 3 4 5 6 7 8 9 10 Negative likelihood ratio Not Useful / Useful Very Small / Small / Moderate / Large 1.0 0.9 0.8 0.7 0.6 0.5 0.4 0.3 0.2 0.1 0

GH = glenohumeral.

Special Test 16-6
Relocation and Anterior Release Tests for Anterior Glenohumeral Laxity

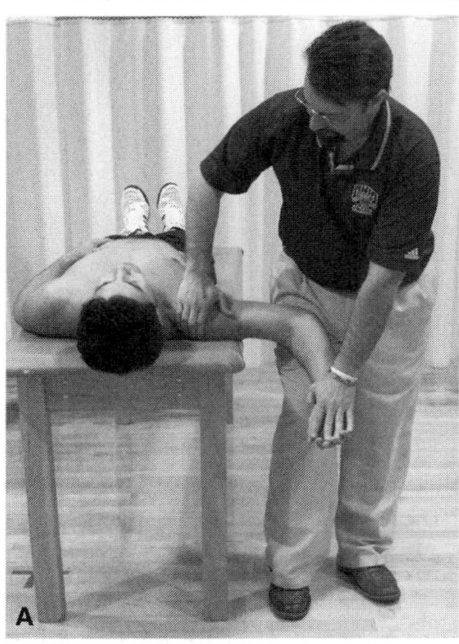

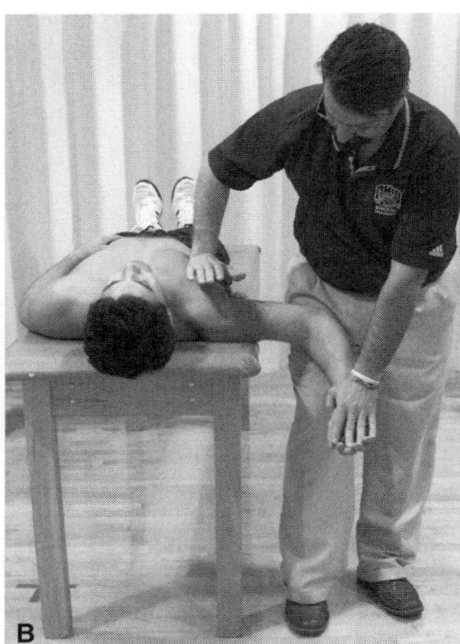

Performed after a positive apprehension test (Special Test 16-5), the relocation test uses manual pressure to maintain alignment and stability of the GH joint as it moves into external rotation **(A)**. The anterior release test determines apprehension when the pressure applied during the apprehension test is suddenly released ("surprise!") **(B)**. The anterior release test, also known as the surprise test, should be performed with caution.

Patient Position	Supine The GH joint is abducted to 90°. The elbow is flexed to 90°.
Position of Examiner	Standing beside the patient, inferior to the humerus on the involved side The forearm is grasped proximal to the wrist to provide leverage during external rotation of the humerus. The opposite hand is held over the humeral head.
Evaluative Procedure	**(A) Relocation test**: With the patient's arm in the original position, the examiner applies a posterior force to the head of the humerus and maintains that force while externally rotating the humerus. **(B) Anterior release test ("Surprise!" test)**: With the GH in external rotation during the relocation test, the examiner removes the hand applying the posterior pressure.
Positive Test	**Relocation test**: Decreased pain or increased ROM (or both) compared with the anterior apprehension test **Anterior release test**: Apprehension and/or pain when the anterior stabilizing pressure from the relocation test is removed.

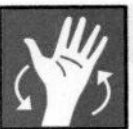

Special Test 16-6—cont'd
Relocation and Anterior Release Tests for Anterior Glenohumeral Laxity

Implications	**Relocation test**: Anterior pain may be the result of increased laxity in the anterior ligamentous and capsular structures or a tear of the labrum. Posterior pain may be from internal impingement of the posterior capsule or labrum. A positive test result supports the conclusion of increased laxity in the anterior capsule owing to capsular damage or labrum tears. The manual pressure applied by the examiner increases the stability of the anterior portion of the GH capsule, allowing more external rotation to occur. **Anterior release test**: Apprehension and/or pain when the anterior stabilizing pressure from the relocation test is removed.
Comments	The relocation test is usually performed after a positive anterior apprehension test. The anterior release test is usually performed after a positive relocation test. The apprehension test and the relocation test may also be positive in the presence of internal impingement. Positive findings with the relocation test (e.g., pain reduction) may also be associated with a SLAP lesion, as tension on the disrupted long head of the biceps tendon is reduced.[89,90] The relocation test adds little predictive value in detecting anterior shoulder instability. It has more predictive value when the posterior force reduces the feeling of apprehension rather than pain.
Evidence	***Relocation Test***

Positive likelihood ratio

Not Useful — Useful
Very Small | Small | Moderate | Large
0 1 2 3 4 5 6 7 8 9 10

Negative likelihood ratio

Not Useful — Useful
Very Small | Small | Moderate | Large
1.0 0.9 0.8 0.7 0.6 0.5 0.4 0.3 0.2 0.1 0

Anterior Release

Positive likelihood ratio

Not Useful — Useful
Very Small | Small | Moderate | Large
58.09
0 1 2 3 4 5 6 7 8 9 10

Negative likelihood ratio

Not Useful — Useful
Very Small | Small | Moderate | Large
1.0 0.9 0.8 0.7 0.6 0.5 0.4 0.3 0.2 0.1 0

GH = glenohumeral; ROM = range of motion; SLAP = superior labrum anterior to posterior.

Special Test 16-7
Posterior Apprehension Test for Glenohumeral Laxity

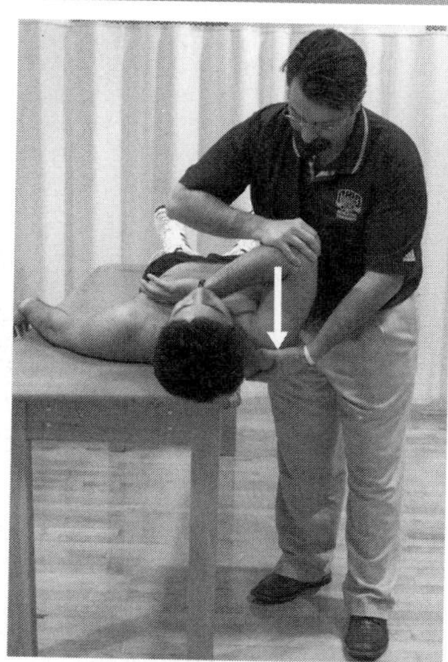

The humeral head is moved posteriorly on the glenoid fossa. In the presence of posterior glenohumeral laxity or instability the patient will abruptly stop the test.

Patient Position	Sitting or supine The shoulder is flexed to 90° and the elbow is flexed to 90°. The GH joint being tested is off to the side of the table.
Position of Examiner	Standing on the involved side One hand grasps the forearm. The opposite hand stabilizes the posterior scapula.
Evaluative Procedure	The examiner applies a longitudinal force to the humeral shaft, encouraging the humeral head to move posteriorly on the glenoid fossa. The examiner may choose to alter the amount of flexion and rotation of the humerus.
Positive Test	The patient displays apprehension and produces muscle guarding to prevent the shoulder from subluxating posteriorly.
Implications	Laxity in the posterior GH capsule, torn posterior labrum
Modification	Horizontally adduct the humerus so that the posterior force is directed perpendicular to the plane of the scapula.
Evidence	Absent or inconclusive in the literature

GH = glenohumeral.

Special Test 16-8
Jerk (Posterior Stress) Test for Labral Tears

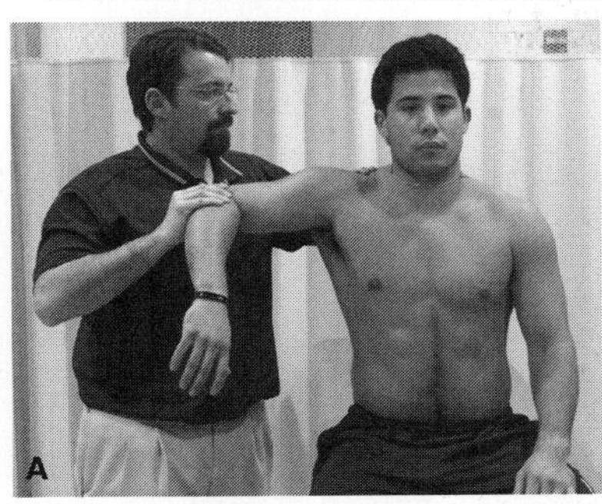

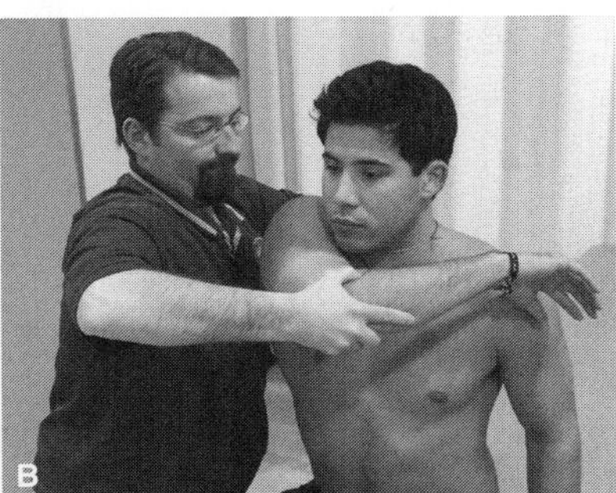

A posterior force is applied to the glenohumeral joint. Pain is associated with posteroinferior instability; a clunk is associated with a tear of the glenoid labrum.

Patient Position	Supine or seated. The supine position provides better scapular stabilization.
Position of Examiner	Behind the patient One hand stabilizes the scapula. The opposite hand holds the affected arm at 90° of flexion and internal rotation **(A)**.
Evaluative Procedure	The affected arm is passively horizontally adducted while the examiner applies a simultaneous axial load to the humerus **(B)**.
Positive Test	Clunk that may or may not be painful
Implications	Posteroinferior instability with or without posteroinferior labral tear
Comments	A painful clunk is frequently associated with a posteroinferior labral tear that must be surgically repaired. Patients with a painless clunk respond well to nonsurgical treatment.[91]
Evidence	Positive likelihood ratio Not Useful — Useful Very Small / Small / Moderate / Large 36.5 0 1 2 3 4 5 6 7 8 9 10 Negative likelihood ratio Not Useful — Useful Very Small / Small / Moderate / Large 1.0 0.9 0.8 0.7 0.6 0.5 0.4 0.3 0.2 0.1 0

Special Test 16-9
Sulcus Sign for Inferior Glenohumeral Laxity

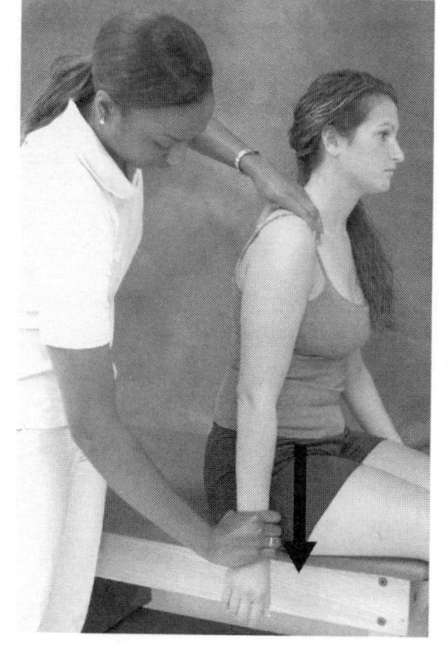

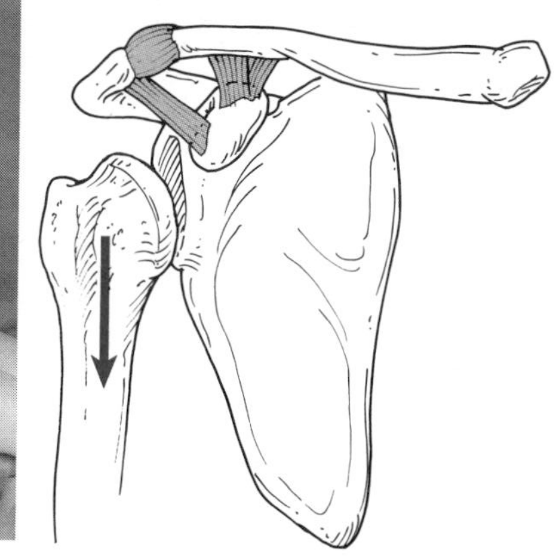

The sulcus sign determines the amount of inferior glide of the humeral head when traction is applied to the humerus.

Patient Position	Sitting Arm hanging at the side
Position of Examiner	Standing lateral to the involved side
Evaluative Procedure	The patient's arm is gripped distal to the elbow. A downward (inferior) traction force is applied to the humerus while the scapula is stabilized.

Positive Test	An indentation (sulcus) appears beneath the acromion process. To differentiate the results of this test from those of the AC traction test for AC joint instability, the movement of the humeral head is away from the scapula and clavicle in this test. In the AC traction test, the humerus and scapula move away from the clavicle.
Implications	The humeral head slides inferiorly on the glenoid fossa, indicating laxity in the superior GH ligament. The grade is based on the widening of the subacromial space:[92] Grade 1: 1 cm or less Grade 2: 1–2 cm Grade 3: Greater than 2 cm
Modification	A positive sulcus sign with the humerus flexed to 90° may indicate inferior instability.
Comments	The results of this test are more meaningful when the patient is anesthetized, indicating the influence of muscle tension on the findings.
Evidence	Positive likelihood ratio Not Useful — Useful Very Small / Small / Moderate / Large 0 1 2 3 4 5 6 7 8 9 10 Negative likelihood ratio Not Useful — Useful Very Small / Small / Moderate / Large 1.0 0.9 0.8 0.7 0.6 0.5 0.4 0.3 0.2 0.1 0

AC = acromioclavicular; GH = glenohumeral.

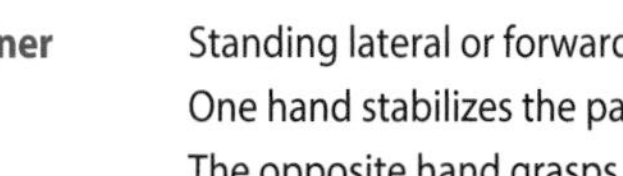

Special Test 16-10
The Neer Shoulder Impingement Test

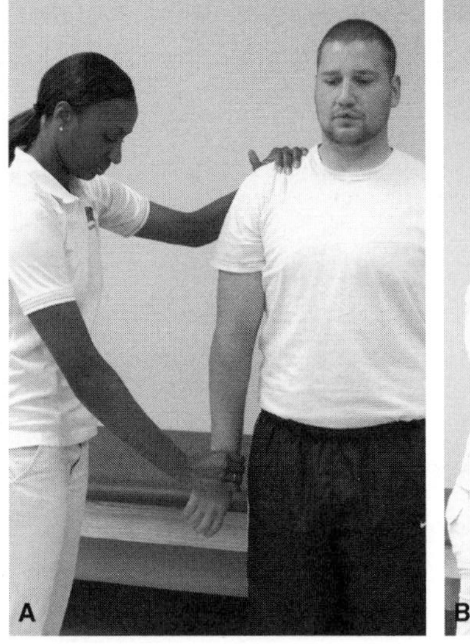

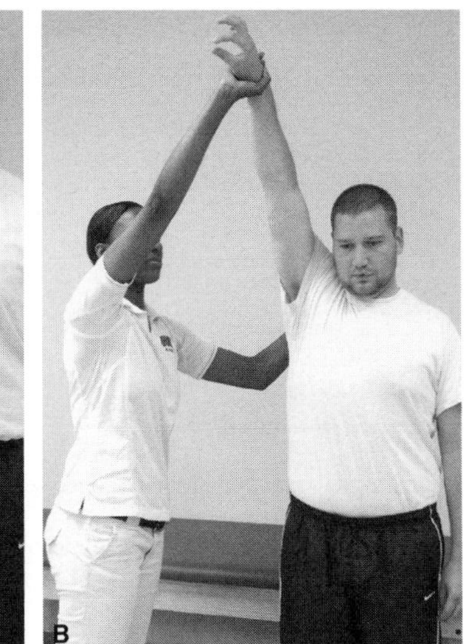

The patient's arm is passively moved through flexion to reproduce the symptoms of rotator cuff impingement, usually between 90° and 180° of flexion.

Patient Position	Standing or sitting The shoulder, elbow, and wrist begin in the anatomical position.
Position of Examiner	Standing lateral or forward of the involved side **(A)** One hand stabilizes the patient's scapula. The opposite hand grasps the patient's arm distal to the elbow joint.

Evaluative Procedure	With the elbow extended, the humerus is placed in internal rotation and the forearm is pronated. The GH joint is then forcefully moved through forward flexion as the scapula is stabilized **(B)**.
Positive Test	Pain in the anterior or lateral shoulder, in range of 90° to full elevation
Implications	Pathology is present in the rotator cuff group (especially the supraspinatus) or the long head of the biceps brachii tendon. The motion of the test impinges these structures between the greater tuberosity and the inferior side of the acromion process and AC joint.
Comments	Bursal involvement only (no rotator cuff damage); the sensitivity improves to 85.7% but the specificity decreases to 49.2% with a positive likelihood ratio of 1.69.[93]
Evidence	Positive likelihood ratio Not Useful — Useful Very Small · Small · Moderate · Large 0 1 2 3 4 5 6 7 8 9 10 Negative likelihood ratio Not Useful — Useful Very Small · Small · Moderate · Large 1.0 0.9 0.8 0.7 0.6 0.5 0.4 0.3 0.2 0.1 0

AC = acromioclavicular; GH = glenohumeral.

Special Test 16-11
The Hawkins Shoulder Impingement Test

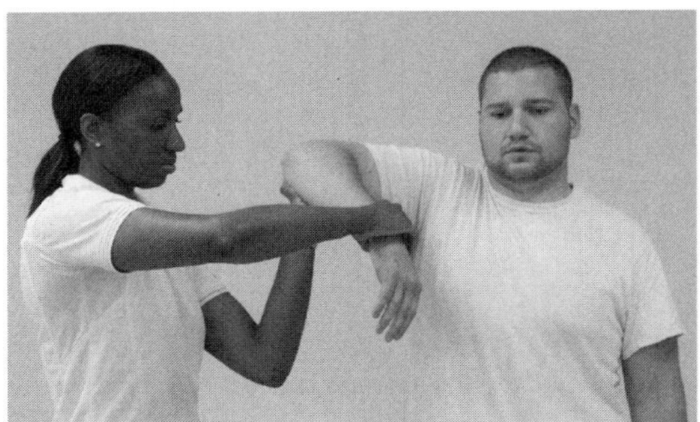

With the glenohumeral joint abducted to 90° in the scapular plane the humerus is internally rotated to reproduce the symptoms of rotator cuff impingement.

Patient Position

Sitting or standing

The shoulder, elbow, and wrist are in the anatomical position.

Position of Examiner

Standing lateral or forward of the involved side

Grasp the patient's arm at the elbow joint.

Evaluative Procedure

With the elbow flexed, the GH joint is elevated to 90° in the scapular plane. At this point, the humerus is passively internally rotated until painful or scapular rotation is felt or observed.

Positive Test

Pain with motion, especially near the end of the ROM

Implications

Pathology is present in the rotator cuff group (especially the supraspinatus) or the long head of the biceps brachii tendon. The motion of the test impinges these structures between the greater tuberosity and the inferior side of the acromion process.

Comments

If the humerus is brought in toward the sagittal plane, the chance of eliciting a false-positive result secondary to AC joint pathology increases.

Evidence

Positive likelihood ratio

Not Useful — Useful

Very Small | Small | Moderate | Large

0 1 2 3 4 5 6 7 8 9 10

Negative likelihood ratio

Not Useful — Useful

Very Small | Small | Moderate | Large

1.0 0.9 0.8 0.7 0.6 0.5 0.4 0.3 0.2 0.1 0

AC = acromioclavicular; GH = glenohumeral; ROM = range of motion.

Special Test 16-12
Empty Can Test for Supraspinatus Pathology

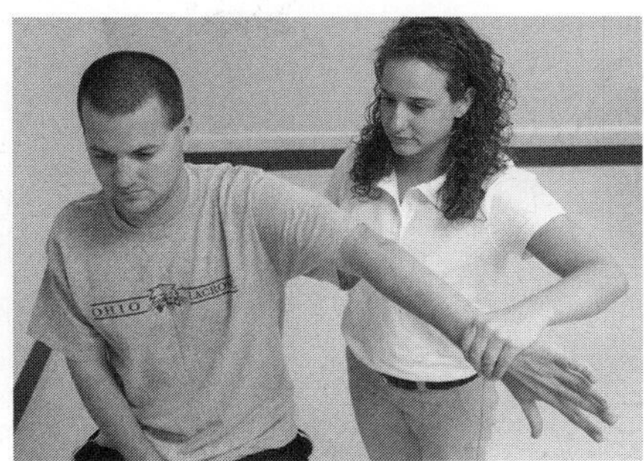

The empty can test is actually a manual muscle test for the supraspinatus muscle. A positive test often indicates subacromial impingement or a lesion to the musculotendinous unit.

Patient Position

Sitting or standing

The GH is abducted to 90° in the scapular plane, the elbow extended, and the humerus internally rotated and the forearm pronated so that the thumb points downward.

Position of Examiner

Standing facing the patient

One hand is placed on the superior portion of the midforearm to resist the motion of abduction in the scapular plane.

Evaluative Procedure

The evaluator resists abduction (applies a downward pressure).

Positive Test

Weakness or pain accompanying the movement

Implications

The supraspinatus tendon (1) is being impinged between the humeral head and the coracoacromial arch, (2) is inflamed, or (3) contains a lesion.

Modification

This test can be performed with the humerus externally rated and the forearm supinated so that the thumb is facing upward, the full can test.

Comments

The empty can and full can test are about equally accurate in detecting supraspinatus tears. Because the full can test is less pain provoking of impingement symptoms, its use is recommended.[94]

Pain alone does not help detect partial-thickness tears or tendinopathy.[95]

Evidence

Positive likelihood ratio

Not Useful — Useful

Very Small | Small | Moderate | Large

0 1 2 3 4 5 6 7 8 9 10

Negative likelihood ratio

Not Useful — Useful

Very Small | Small | Moderate | Large

1.0 0.9 0.8 0.7 0.6 0.5 0.4 0.3 0.2 0.1 0

GH = glenohumeral.

Special Test 16-13
Yergason's Test

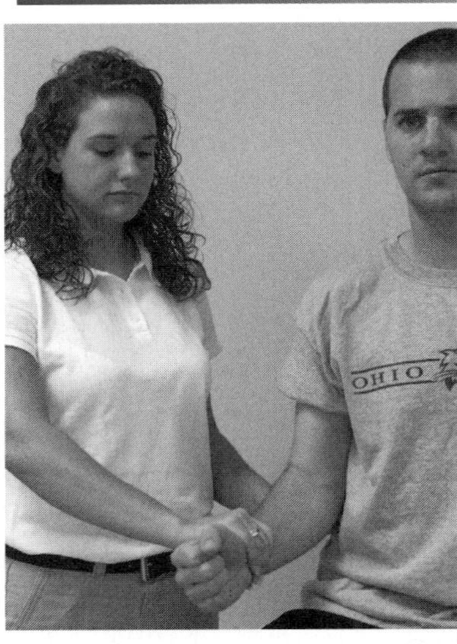

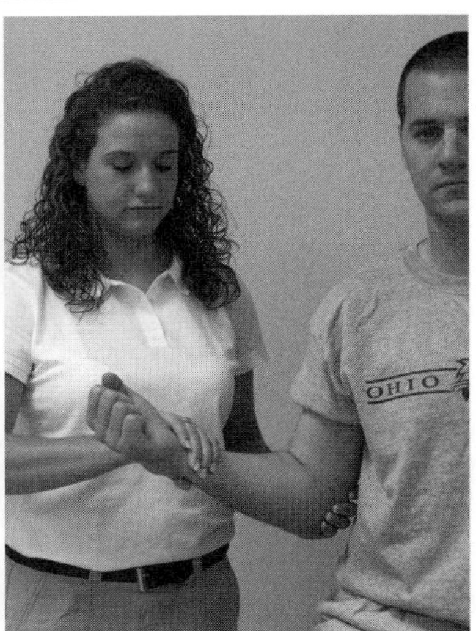

The Yergason test identifies the presence of pathology to the long head of the biceps tendon within the bicipital groove or the presence of a SLAP lesion. Palpate the tendon as it passes through the bicipital groove to identify lesions involving this area.

Patient Position	Sitting or standing GH joint in the anatomical position The elbow is flexed to 90°. The forearm is positioned so that the lateral border of the radius faces upward (neutral position).
Position of Examiner	Lateral to the patient on the involved side, lightly palpating the bicipital groove The olecranon is stabilized inferiorly and maintained close to the thorax. The forearm is stabilized proximal to the wrist.
Evaluative Procedure	The patient provides resistance while the examiner concurrently moves the GH joint into external rotation while resisting supination.
Positive Test	Pain or snapping (or both) in the bicipital groove Pain at the superior glenohumeral joint (SLAP lesion)
Implications	**Primary**: Snapping or popping in the bicipital groove indicates a tear or laxity of the transverse humeral ligament. This pathology prevents the ligament from securing the long head of the tendon in its groove. **Secondary**: Pain with no associated popping in the bicipital groove may indicate bicipital tendinopathy.

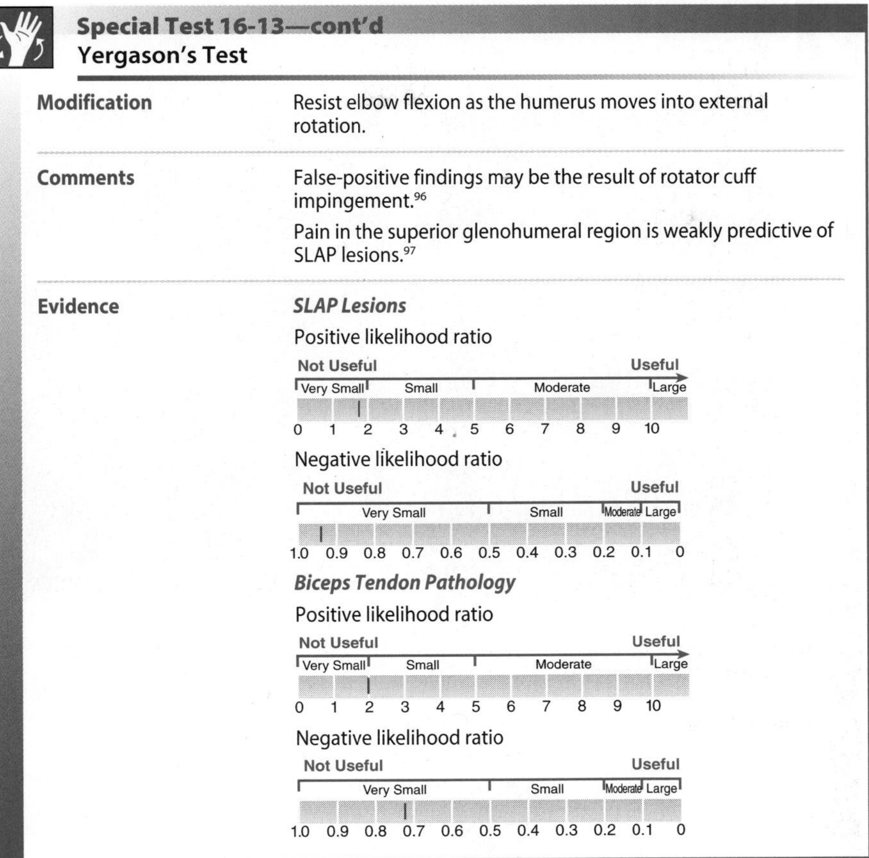

Special Test 16-13—cont'd
Yergason's Test

Modification

Resist elbow flexion as the humerus moves into external rotation.

Comments

False-positive findings may be the result of rotator cuff impingement.[96]

Pain in the superior glenohumeral region is weakly predictive of SLAP lesions.[97]

Evidence

SLAP Lesions

Positive likelihood ratio

Negative likelihood ratio

Biceps Tendon Pathology

Positive likelihood ratio

Negative likelihood ratio

GH = glenohumeral; SLAP = superior labrum anterior to posterior.

Special Test 16-14
Speed's Test for Long Head of the Biceps Brachii Tendinopathy

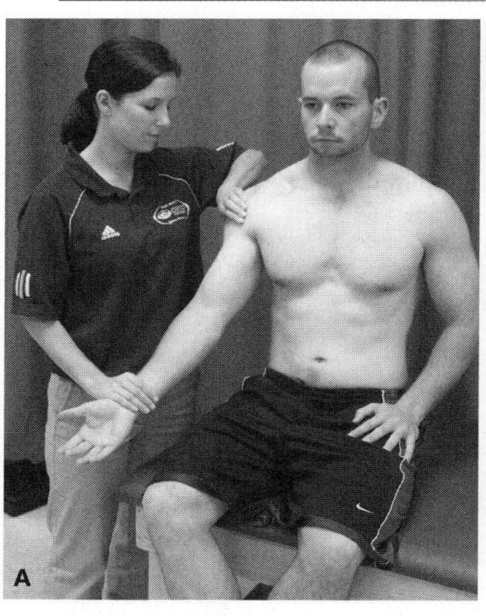

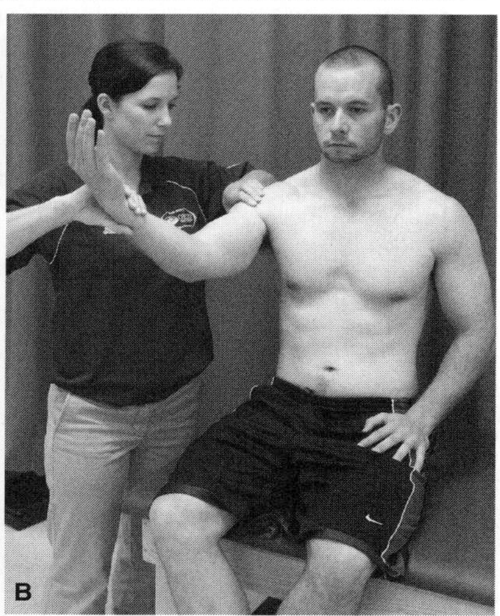

Resisted shoulder flexion with the elbow extended **(A)** or shoulder flexion and elbow flexion **(B)** elicit pain in the bicipital groove in the presence of long head of the biceps tendinopathy, a disruption of the transverse humeral ligament, or a SLAP lesion.

Patient Position	Sitting or standing The elbow is extended. The GH joint is in neutral position or slightly extended to stretch the biceps brachii.
Position of Examiner	Standing lateral to and in front of the involved limb The fingers of one hand are positioned over the bicipital groove while stabilizing the shoulder. The forearm is stabilized proximal to the wrist.
Evaluative Procedure	The clinician resists flexion of the GH joint and elbow while palpating for tenderness over the bicipital groove. Allow the patient to move through flexion range of motion.
Positive Test	Pain along the long head of the biceps brachii tendon, especially in the bicipital groove or at the superior shoulder
Implications	Inflammation of the long head of the biceps tendon as it passes through the bicipital groove Possible tear of the transverse humeral ligament with concurrent instability of the long head of the biceps tendon as it passes through the bicipital groove Pain at the superior shoulder (SLAP lesion)

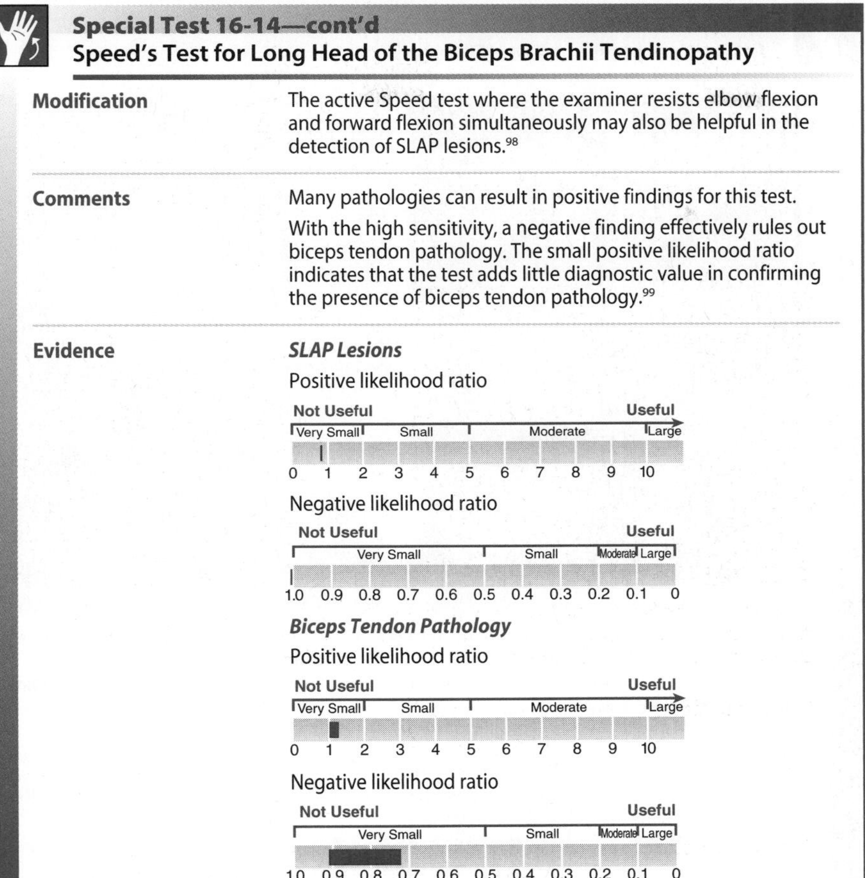

Special Test 16-14—cont'd
Speed's Test for Long Head of the Biceps Brachii Tendinopathy

Modification

The active Speed test where the examiner resists elbow flexion and forward flexion simultaneously may also be helpful in the detection of SLAP lesions.[98]

Comments

Many pathologies can result in positive findings for this test.

With the high sensitivity, a negative finding effectively rules out biceps tendon pathology. The small positive likelihood ratio indicates that the test adds little diagnostic value in confirming the presence of biceps tendon pathology.[99]

Evidence

SLAP Lesions

Positive likelihood ratio

Negative likelihood ratio

Biceps Tendon Pathology

Positive likelihood ratio

Negative likelihood ratio

GH = glenohumeral; SLAP = superior labrum anterior to posterior.

Special Test 16-15
Active Compression Test (O'Brien Test)

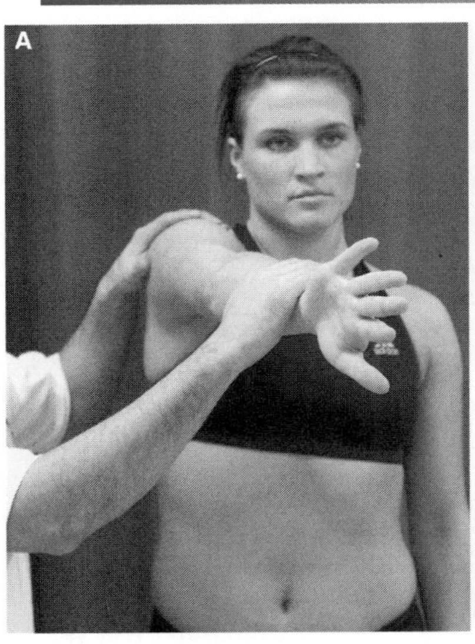

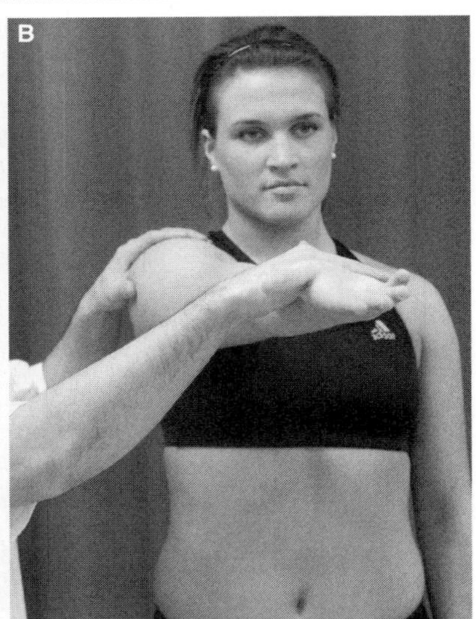

An isometric contraction with the humerus flexed to 90° and horizontally abducted once with the humerus internally rotated **(A)** and then again with the humerus externally rotated **(B)**. Depending on the positions pain is produced, a positive test may indicate a labral tear, AC joint pathology, or a SLAP lesion.

Patient Position	Standing The GH joint is flexed to 90° and horizontally adducted 15° from the sagittal plane. The humerus is in full internal rotation, elbow extended, and the forearm pronated **(A)**.
Position of Examiner	In front of the patient One hand is placed over the superior aspect of the patient's distal forearm.
Evaluative Procedure	The patient isometrically resists the examiner's downward force. The test is repeated with the humerus externally rotated and the forearm supinated **(B)**.
Positive Test	Pain that is experienced with the arm internally rotated but is decreased during external rotation: **1.** Pain or clicking within the GH joint may indicate a labral tear. **2.** Pain at the AC joint may indicate AC joint pathology. Positive SLAP lesion tests are confirmed with pain relief when the hand is supinated; pain with cross-armed horizontal adduction is used to confirm AC pathology.[92]
Implications	SLAP lesion AC joint pathology

Special Test 16-15—cont'd
Active Compression Test (O'Brien Test)

Comments

The presence of rotator cuff pathology and impingement may produce false-positive results.

Evidence

Inter-rater reliability

Not Reliable | Very Reliable
Poor | Moderate | Good
0 0.1 0.2 0.3 0.4 0.5 0.6 0.7 0.8 0.9 1.0

AC Joint Pathology

Positive likelihood ratio

Not Useful | Useful
Very Small | Small | Moderate | Large
29.41
0 1 2 3 4 5 6 7 8 9 10

Negative likelihood ratio

Not Useful | Useful
Very Small | Small | Moderate | Large
1.0 0.9 0.8 0.7 0.6 0.5 0.4 0.3 0.2 0.1 0

SLAP Lesions

Positive likelihood ratio

Not Useful | Useful
Very Small | Small | Moderate | Large
0 1 2 3 4 5 6 7 8 9 10

Negative likelihood ratio

Not Useful | Useful
Very Small | Small | Moderate | Large
1.0 0.9 0.8 0.7 0.6 0.5 0.4 0.3 0.2 0.1 0

Labral Tears

Positive likelihood ratio

Not Useful | Useful
Very Small | Small | Moderate | Large
0 1 2 3 4 5 6 7 8 9 10

Negative likelihood ratio

Not Useful | Useful
Very Small | Small | Moderate | Large
1.0 0.9 0.8 0.7 0.6 0.5 0.4 0.3 0.2 0.1 0

AC = acromioclavicular; GH = glenohumeral; SLAP = superior labrum anterior to posterior.

Special Test 16-16
Anterior Slide Test

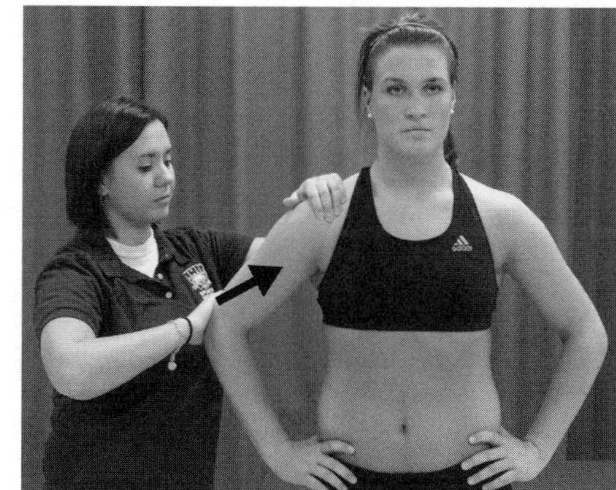

The anterior slide test creates an anteriorly and superiorly directed force that would result in humeral head translation if the superior labrum was torn.

Patient Position	Seated or standing Hands on hips with thumbs pointing posteriorly
Position of Examiner	Behind the patient One hand is placed over the shoulder with the index finger lateral to the acromion and over the glenohumeral joint. The opposite hand is behind the elbow on the test side.
Evaluative Procedure	An anterior and slightly superior force is applied longitudinally through the humerus. The patient resists, or pushes back, against this force.

Positive Test	Shoulder pain or pop or click under the examiner's index finger Patient report of reproduction of symptoms
Implications	SLAP lesion
Comments	A positive anterior slide test partnered with patient complaints of "popping" or "clicking" are strongly associated with a labral tear.[100]
Evidence	Inter-rater reliability Positive likelihood ratio Negative likelihood ratio

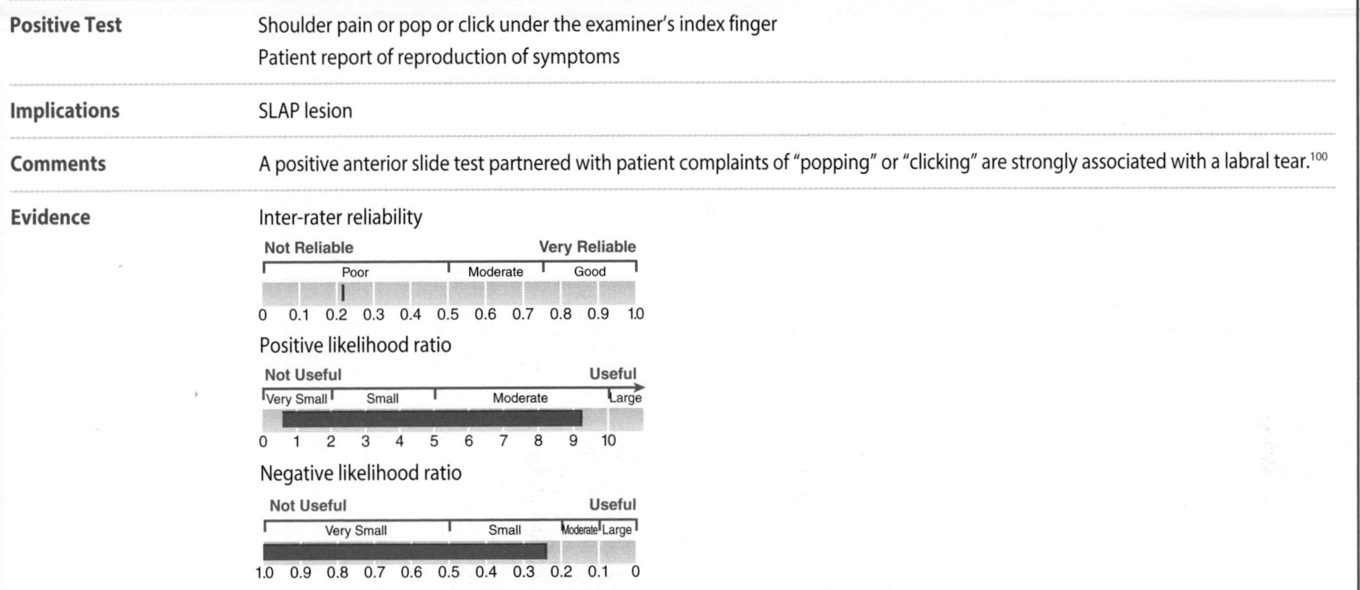

SLAP = superior labrum anterior to posterior.

Special Test 16-17
Compression–Rotation (Grind) Test

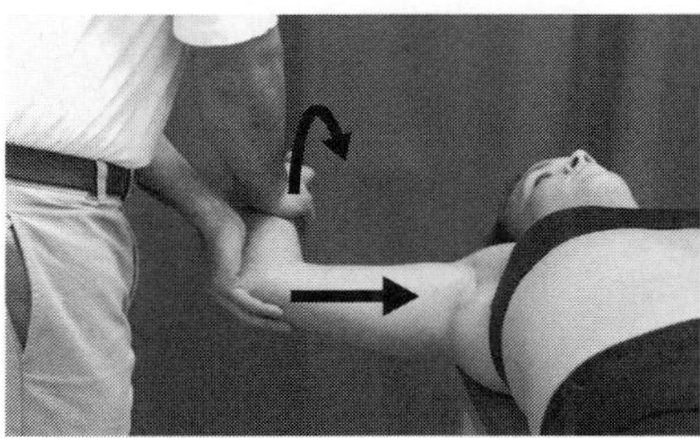

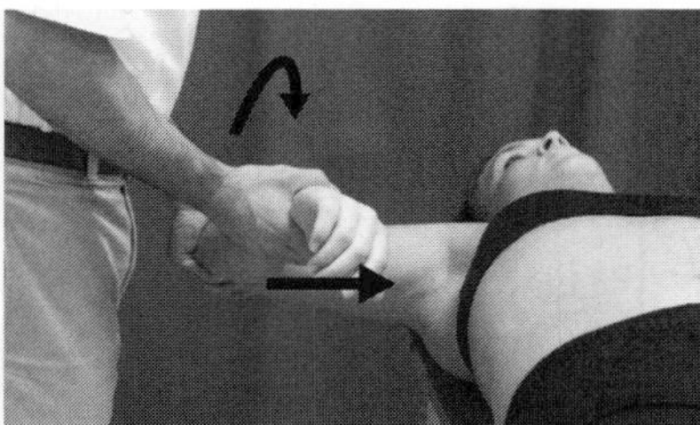

This test is designed to compress the labrum, resulting in reproduction of painful symptoms.

Patient Position	Supine The shoulder is abducted to 90°. The elbow is flexed to 90°.
Position of Examiner	At the test side of the patient
Evaluative Procedure	The examiner maintains an axial load on the humerus while internally and externally rotating it.
Positive Test	Reproduction of symptoms
Implications	SLAP lesion
Modification	The crank test incorporates a similar mechanism with the arm positioned in maximum forward flexion.
Evidence	Positive likelihood ratio Not Useful / Useful Very Small / Small / Moderate / Large 0 1 2 3 4 5 6 7 8 9 10 Negative likelihood ratio Not Useful / Useful Very Small / Small / Moderate / Large 1.0 0.9 0.8 0.7 0.6 0.5 0.4 0.3 0.2 0.1 0

SLAP = superior labrum anterior to posterior.

Referred Pain Patterns

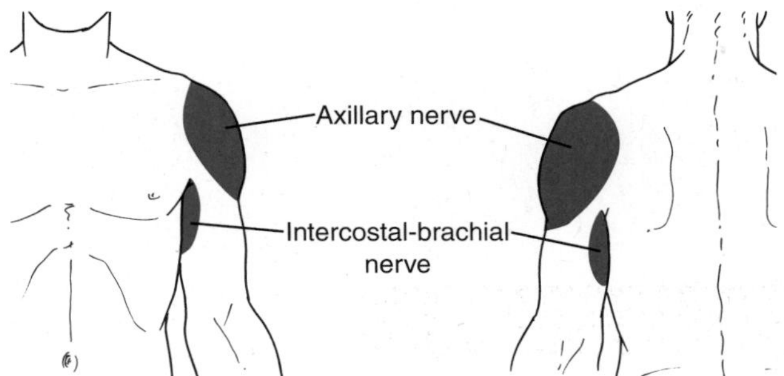

FIGURE 16-13 ■ Neuropathies of the shoulder and upper arm. Pain may also be referred to this area from the thorax (see Fig. 15-1) and the brachial plexus (see Neurological Screening Box 1-2).

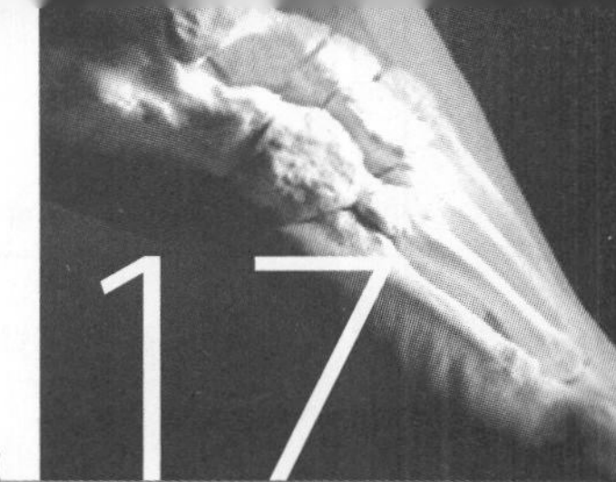

CHAPTER 17

Elbow and Forearm Pathologies

Examination Map

HISTORY

Past Medical History
General medical health

History of the Present Condition
Location and onset of symptoms

Mechanism of injury

INSPECTION

Functional Assessment

Inspection of the Anterior Structures
Carrying angle

Cubital fossa

Inspection of the Medial Structures
Medial epicondyle

Flexor muscle mass

Inspection of the Lateral Structures
Alignment of the wrist and forearm

Cubital recurvatum

Extensor muscle mass

Inspection of the Posterior Structures
Bony alignment

Olecranon process and bursa

PALPATION

Palpation of the Anterior Structures
Biceps brachii

Cubital fossa

Brachioradialis

Wrist flexor group
- Pronator teres
- Flexor carpi radialis
- Palmaris longus
- Flexor carpi ulnaris

Palpation of the Medial Structures
Medial epicondyle

Ulna

Ulnar collateral ligament

Palpation of the Lateral Structures
Lateral epicondyle

Radial head

Radial collateral ligament

Capitellum

Annular ligament

Lateral ulnar collateral ligament

Palpation of the Posterior Structures
Olecranon process

Olecranon fossa

Triceps brachii

Anconeus

Ulnar nerve

Wrist extensors
- Extensor carpi ulnaris
- Extensor carpi radialis brevis
- Extensor carpi radialis longus

Finger extensors
- Extensor digitorum
- Extensor digiti minimi

Thumb musculature
- Extensor pollicis brevis
- Abductor pollicis longus

Radial tunnel

JOINT AND MUSCLE FUNCTION ASSESSMENT

Goniometry
Flexion

Extension

Continued

Examination Map—cont'd

Pronation

Supination

Active Range of Motion

Flexion

Extension

Pronation

Supination

Manual Muscle Tests

Flexion

Extension

Pronation

Supination

Passive Range of Motion

Flexion

Extension

Pronation

Supination

JOINT STABILITY TESTS

Stress Testing

Valgus stress test

Varus stress test

Joint Play Assessment

Humeroulnar distraction

Radioulnar anterior–posterior

Radiohumeral

Humeroulnar

NEUROLOGIC EXAMINATION

Upper Quarter Screen

PATHOLOGIES AND SPECIAL TESTS

Elbow Dislocations

Elbow Fractures

Elbow Sprains

Ulnar collateral ligament

- Valgus extension overload
- Posterolateral rotatory instability

Radial collateral ligament

Epicondylalgia

Lateral epicondylalgia

- Tennis elbow test

Medial epicondylalgia

Distal Biceps Tendon Rupture

Osteochondritis Dissecans of the Capitellum

Nerve Pathology

Ulnar nerve pathology

Radial nerve pathology

Median nerve pathology

Forearm compartment syndrome

Table 17-1 Possible Pathology Based on the Location of Pain

	Location of Pain			
	Lateral	**Anterior**	**Medial**	**Posterior**
Soft Tissue Injury	Annular ligament sprain Radial collateral ligament sprain Radiocapitellar chondromalacia Lateral epicondylalgia (tennis elbow) Radial head dislocation Radial nerve pathology	Biceps brachii tendinopathy Rupture of the biceps brachii tendon Median nerve trauma Anterior capsule sprain	Ulnar collateral ligament sprain Medial epicondylalgia Ulnar nerve pathology	Olecranon bursitis Triceps brachii tendinopathy Triceps tendon rupture
Bony Injury	Avulsion of the common extensor tendon Lateral epicondyle fracture Radius fracture Radial head fracture Radial head dislocation	Osteochondral fracture Avulsion of the biceps brachii tendon	Avulsion of the common flexor tendon Medial epicondyle fracture Ulna fracture Osteophyte formation	Fracture of the olecranon process Osteophyte formation

Inspection of the Carrying Angle

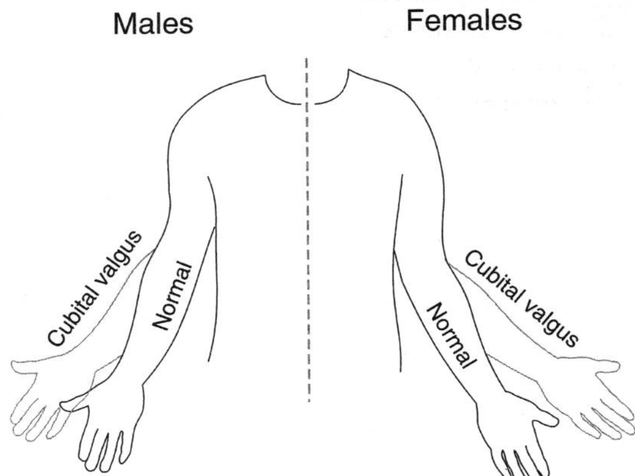

FIGURE 17-1 ■ Angular relationships at the elbow. On average, women have an increased angle between the midline of the forearm and the humerus (the "carrying angle") relative to men. Long term participation in overhand throwing sports increases this angle.[101]

PALPATION

Palpation of the Anterior Structures

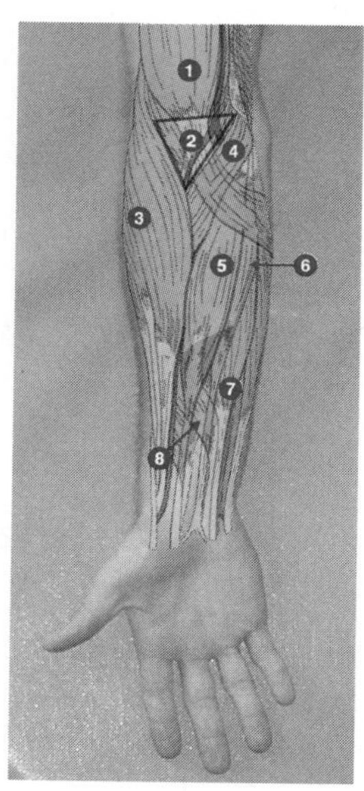

1 Biceps brachii

2 Cubital fossa

3 Brachioradialis

4 Pronator teres

5 Flexor carpi radialis

6 Palmaris longus

7 Flexor carpi ulnaris

8 Pronator quadratus

Identifying the Flexor Muscles

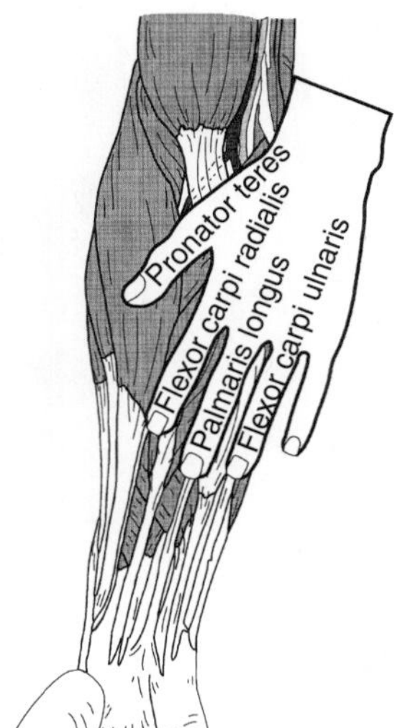

FIGURE 17-2 ■ Method of approximating the superficial muscles of the flexor forearm.

Palpation of the Medial Structures

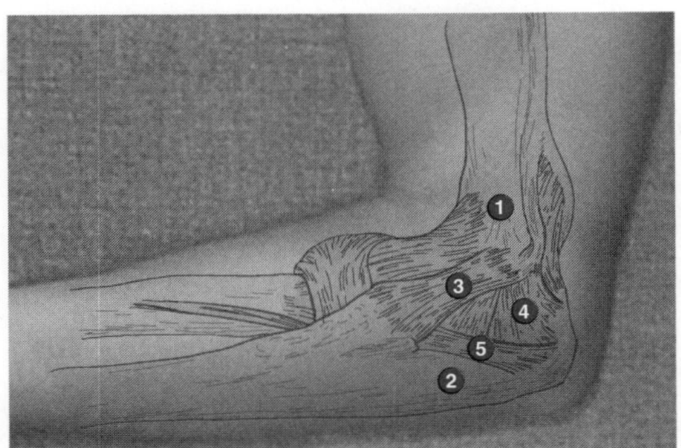

1 Medial epicondyle

2 Ulna

3 Anterior band—ulnar collateral ligament

4 Posterior bundle—ulnar collateral ligament

5 Transverse bundle—ulnar collateral ligament

Palpation of the Lateral Structures

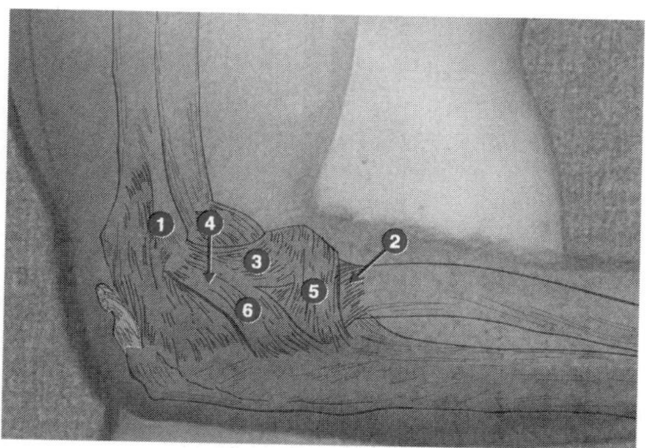

1 Lateral epicondyle

2 Radial head

3 Radial collateral ligament

4 Capitellum

5 Annular ligament

6 Lateral ulnar collateral ligament

Palpation of the Posterior Structures

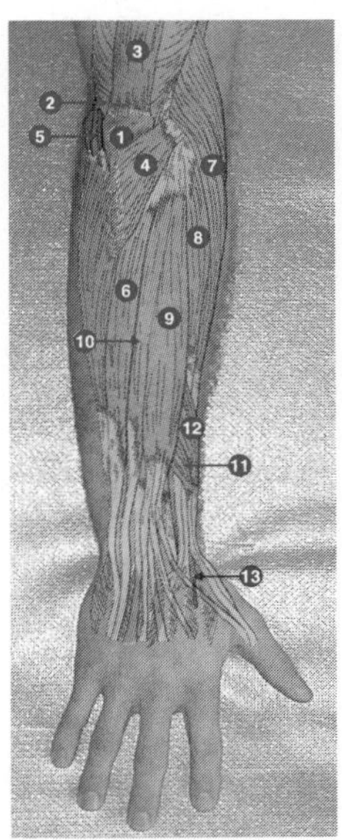

1 Olecranon process

2 Olecranon fossa

3 Triceps brachii

4 Anconeus

5 Ulnar nerve

6 Extensor carpi ulnaris

7 Extensor carpi radialis brevis

8 Extensor carpi radialis longus

9 Extensor digitorum

10 Extensor digiti minimi

11 Extensor pollicis brevis

12 Abductor pollicis longus

13 Radial tunnel

Table 17-2	Elbow: Ulnohumeral and Radiohumeral Joint Capsular Patterns and End-feels
Capsular Pattern: Flexion, Extension	
Extension	Hard
Flexion	Soft
Elbow: Superior Radioulnar Joints	
Capsular Pattern: Supination and Pronation Equally	
Radioulnar supination	Firm
Radioulnar pronation	Hard or firm

Active Range of Motion

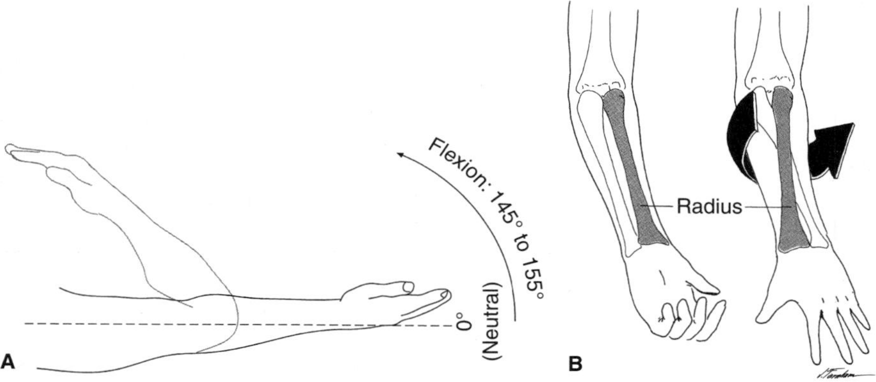

FIGURE 17-3 ■ Active range of motion at the elbow. **(A)** Elbow flexion and extension; **(B)** forearm pronation and supination. (**B**, Courtesy of Norkin, CC, and Levangie, PK: *Joint Structure and Function: A Comprehensive Analysis*, ed 2. Philadelphia: FA Davis, 1992.)

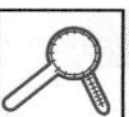

Goniometry Box 17-1
Elbow Goniometry: Flexion and Extension

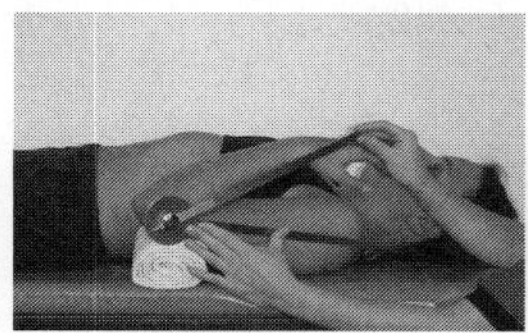

Flexion 0° to 145°– 155°

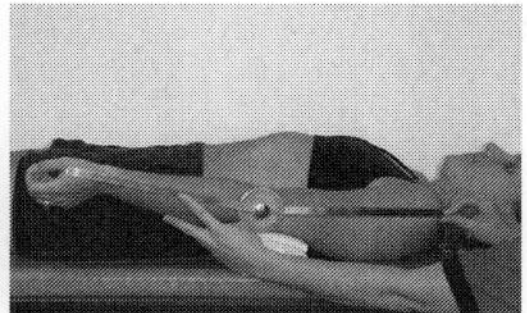

Extension 0°

Patient Position	Supine with the humerus close to the body, the shoulder in the neutral position, and the forearm supinated A bolster is placed under the distal humerus.
Goniometer Alignment	
Fulcrum	Centered over the lateral epicondyle
Proximal Arm	The stationary arm is aligned with the long axis of the humerus, using the acromion process as the proximal landmark.
Distal Arm	The movement arm is aligned with the long axis of the radius, using the styloid process as the distal landmark.

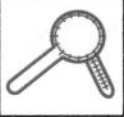

Goniometry Box 17-2
Elbow Goniometry: Pronation and Supination

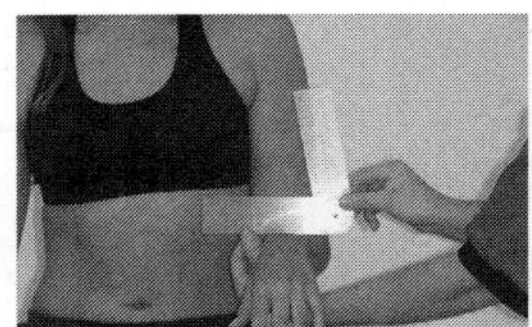

Pronation 0°–90°

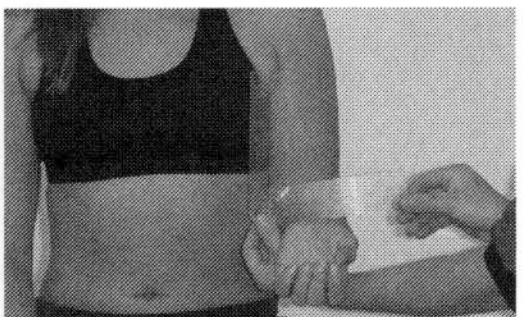

Supination 0°–90°

Patient Position	Sitting with the humerus held against the torso The elbow is flexed to 90°.	
Goniometer Alignment		
Fulcrum	Centered lateral to the ulnar styloid process	
Proximal Arm	Align the stationary arm parallel to the midline of the humerus.	
Distal Arm	The movement arm is positioned across the dorsal portion of the forearm, proximal to the radiocarpal joint.	The movement arm is positioned across the ventral portion of the forearm, proximal to the radiocarpal joint.
Modifications	The motion arm is aligned parallel to a pencil held in the hand, using the 3rd metacarpal as the axis.[102] This method captures a more functional range by incorporating movement at the wrist. Both measurement strategies demonstrate high inter- and intra-rater reliability.[103]	

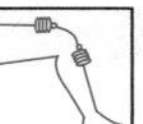

Manual Muscle Test 17-1
Elbow Flexion and Extension

	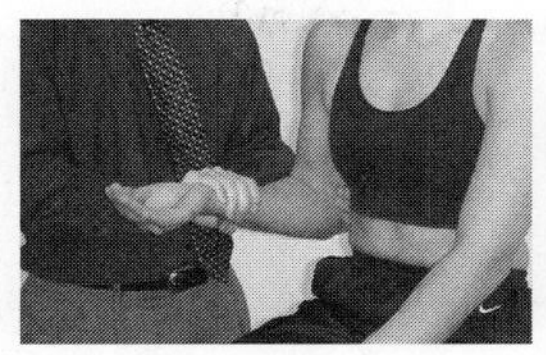 Flexion	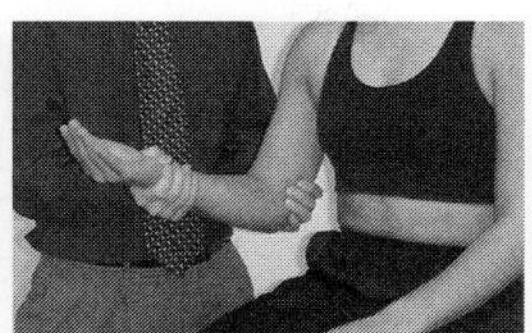 Extension
Patient Position	Sitting, standing, or supine.	Prone or sitting
Starting Position	The shoulder in the neutral position To isolate a specific muscle during the test: Forearm supinated Forearm pronated Forearm in midposition	The shoulder is abducted to 90°. The elbow is flexed and the forearm pronated.
Stabilization	Anterior humerus, being careful not to compress the involved muscles	Posterior humerus, being careful not to compress the involved muscles
Palpation	Over the corresponding muscle belly	Posterior upper arm
Resistance	Over the distal forearm	Over the posterior aspect of the distal forearm
Primary Mover(s) (Innervation)	Forearm supinated: Biceps brachii (C5, C6) Forearm pronated: Brachialis (C5, C6) Forearm neutral: Brachioradialis (C5, C6)	Triceps brachii (C7, C8)
Secondary Mover(s) (Innervation)	Flexor carpi ulnaris (C8, T1)	Anconeus (C7, C8)
Substitution	Wrist and finger flexion, shoulder elevation	Wrist and finger extension, glenohumeral horizontal abduction, scapular retraction.
Comments	The patient should keep the fingers relaxed.	An alternative test position is supine, with the shoulder flexed to 90° and the elbow flexed.

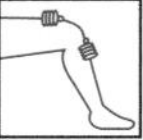

Manual Muscle Test 17-2
Pronation and Supination

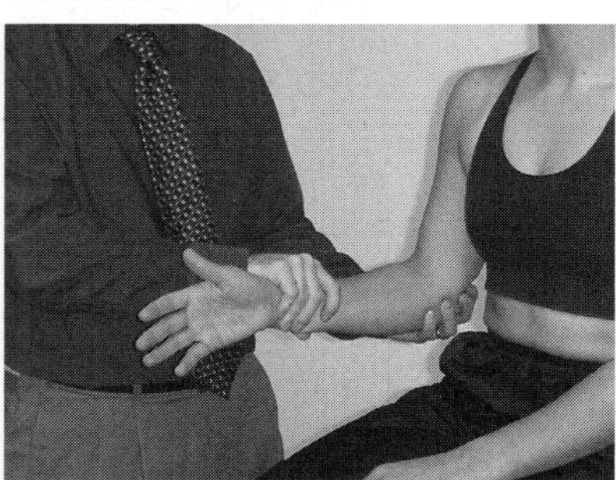

Pronation and Supination

Patient Position	Seated	
Starting Position	The shoulder in the neutral position and the elbow flexed to 90°. The thumb is facing upward.	
Stabilization	Proximal to the elbow to prevent abduction or adduction of the glenohumeral joint	
Palpation	Proximal anterior forearm	Anterior upper arm
Resistance	Resistance is applied to the ventral aspect of the forearm.	Resistance is applied to the dorsal surface of the forearm.
Primary Mover(s) (Innervation)	Pronator quadratus (C8, T1) Pronator teres (C6, C7)	Biceps brachii (C5, C6)
Secondary Mover(s) (Innervation)	Brachioradialis (C5, C6) Flexor carpi radialis (C6, C7)	Brachioradialis (C5, C6) Supinator (C6, C7, C8)
Substitution	Finger flexion, glenohumeral internal rotation	Wrist extension, glenohumeral external rotation
Comments	A more functional assessment of pronation and supination strength is performed by having the patient grip the examiner's hand and rotating. The brachioradialis assists in returning the forearm to neutral from a pronated or supinated position. Pronator weakness is commonly associated with C6 radiculopathy.[104]	

Alternate Method for Testing Pronation and Supination

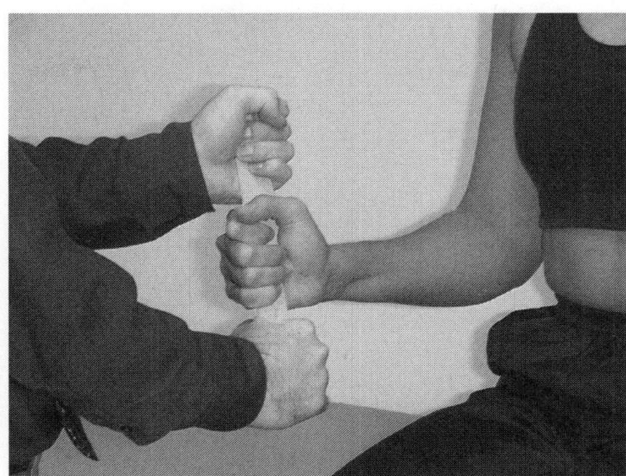

FIGURE 17-4 ■ Alternate method for muscle strength assessment pronation and supination.

Table 17-3 Muscles Acting on the Elbow and Forearm

Muscle	Action	Origin	Insertion	Innervation	Root
Anconeus	Elbow extension Stabilization of ulna during pronation and supination	Posterior surface of the lateral epicondyle	Lateral border of the olecranon process	Radial	C7, C8
Biceps Brachii	Elbow flexion Forearm supination Shoulder flexion	Long head: Supraglenoid tuberosity of scapula Short head: Coracoid process of scapula	Radial tuberosity	Musculocutaneous	C5, C6
Brachialis	Elbow flexion	Distal one half of anterior humerus	Coronoid process of ulna Ulnar tuberosity	Musculocutaneous	C5, C6
Brachioradialis	Elbow flexion Forearm pronation May assist with forearm supination	Lateral supracondylar ridge of humerus	Styloid process of radius	Radial	C5, C6
Extensor Carpi Radialis Brevis	Wrist extension Radial deviation	Lateral epicondyle via the common extensor tendon Radial collateral ligament	Base of the 3rd metacarpal	Radial	C6, C7
Extensor Carpi Radialis Longus	Wrist extension Radial deviation	Supracondylar ridge of humerus	Radial side of the 2nd metacarpal	Radial	C6, C7
Extensor Carpi Ulnaris	Wrist extension Ulnar deviation	Lateral epicondyle via the common extensor tendon	Ulnar side of the base of the 5th metacarpal	Deep radial	C6, C7, C8
Extensor Digitorum Communis	Wrist extension MCP extension PIP extension	Lateral epicondyle via the common extensor tendon	Into the dorsal surface of the base of the middle and distal phalanges of each of the four fingers	Deep radial	C6, C7, C8
Flexor Carpi Radialis	Forearm pronation Wrist flexion Radial deviation Elbow flexion	Medial epicondyle via the common flexor tendon	Palmar aspect of the bases of the 2nd and 3rd metacarpal bones	Median	C6, C7

Flexor Carpi Ulnaris	Wrist flexion Ulnar deviation Elbow flexion	Humeral head: Medial epicondyle via the common flexor tendon Ulnar head: Medial border of the olecranon; proximal two-thirds of the posterior ulna	Pisiform Hamate Palmar aspect of the base of the 5th metacarpal	Ulnar	C8, T1
Flexor Digitorum Profundus	DIP flexion PIP flexion Wrist flexion	Anteromedial proximal three fourths of the ulna and associated interosseous membrane	Bases of the distal phalanges of the second through fifth digits	Lateral: Median nerve Medial: Ulnar nerve	C8, T1
Flexor Digitorum Superficialis	PIP flexion MCP flexion Wrist flexion	Humeral head: Medial epicondyle via the common flexor tendon; ulnar collateral ligament Ulnar head: Coronoid process Radial head: Oblique line of radius	Middle phalanges of the second through fifth digits	Median	C7, C8, T1
Palmaris Longus	Wrist flexion	Medial epicondyle via the common flexor tendon	Flexor retinaculum Palmar aponeurosis	Median	C6, C7
Pronator Quadratus	Forearm pronation	Anterior surface of the distal one fourth of ulna	Lateral portion of the distal one fourth of the radius	Anterior interosseous nerve	C8, T1
Pronator Teres	Forearm pronation Elbow flexion	Humeral head: Proximal to the medial epicondyle of humerus Ulnar head: Coronoid process	Middle one third of the lateral radius	Median	C6, C7
Supinator	Forearm supination	Lateral epicondyle Radial collateral ligament Annular ligament Supinator crest of ulna	Proximal one third of radius	Deep radial	C6, C7, C8
Triceps Brachii	Elbow extension Shoulder extension	Long head: Infraglenoid tuberosity of scapula Lateral head: Posterolateral surface of the proximal one-half of the humeral shaft Medial head: Posteromedial surface of the humerus	Olecranon process of the ulna	Radial	C7, C8

DIP = distal interphalangeal; MCP = metacarpophalangeal; PIP = proximal interphalangeal.

Passive Range of Motion

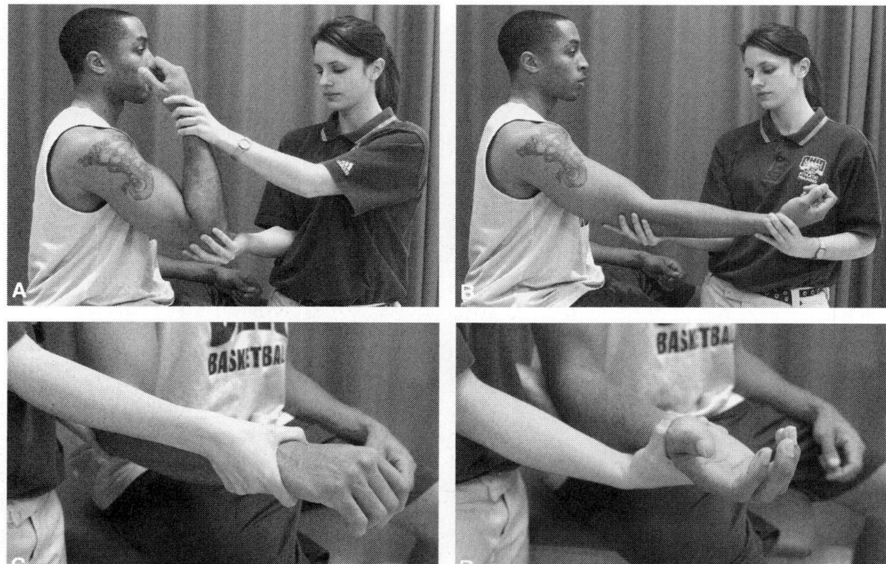

FIGURE 17-5 ■ Passive range of motion for (A) and (B) flexion and extension and (C) and (D) pronation and supination.

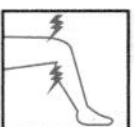

Stress Test 17-1
Valgus Stress Test

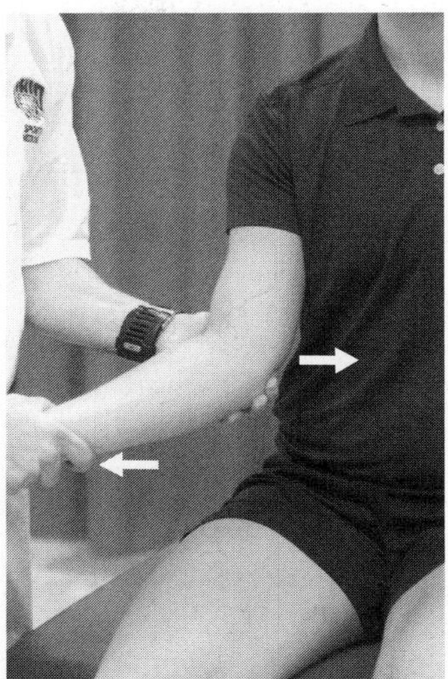

The valgus stress test determines the integrity of the ulnar collateral ligament. Also see the Moving Valgus Stress Test (Special Test 17-1).

Patient Position	Standing, sitting, or supine The elbow is flexed to 10°–25°. The humerus is internally rotated.
Position of Examiner	Standing lateral to the joint being tested One hand supports the lateral elbow with the fingers reaching behind the joint to palpate the medial joint. The opposite hand grasps the distal forearm.
Evaluative Procedure	A valgus force is applied to the joint. The procedure is repeated with the elbow in various degrees of flexion.
Positive Test	Increased laxity compared with the opposite side, or pain, or both
Implications	Sprain of the ulnar collateral ligament, especially the anterior oblique portion Laxity beyond 60° of flexion also implicates involvement of the posterior oblique fibers. Laxity in full extension is indicative of an olecranon or humeral fracture.
Modification	The patient can be positioned with the humerus in external rotation for better stabilization. This position should be avoided in patients with anterior glenohumeral instability.
Comments	Laxity may also indicate epiphyseal injury.

Continued

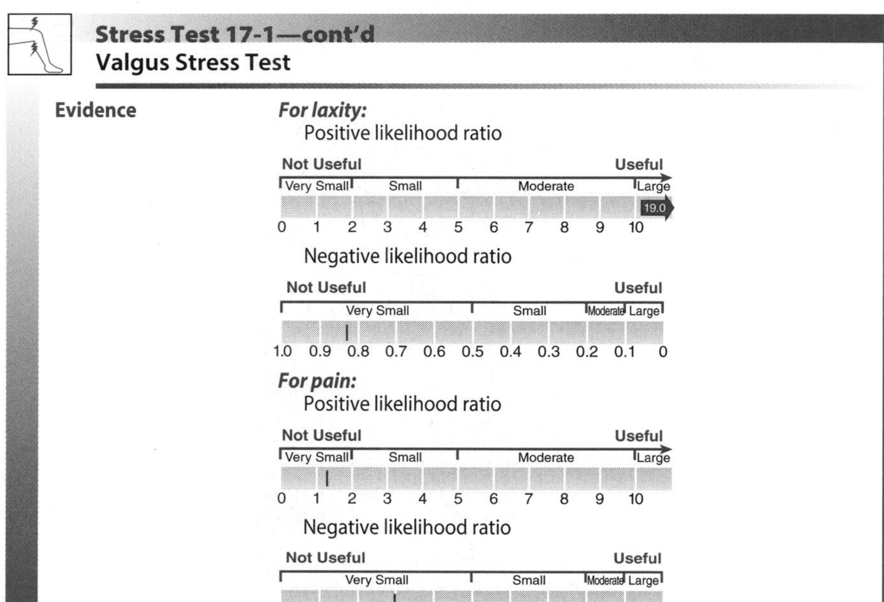
Stress Test 17-1—cont'd
Valgus Stress Test
Evidence
For laxity:
Positive likelihood ratio
Not Useful
Useful
Very Small
Small
Moderate
Large
19.0
0 1 2 3 4 5 6 7 8 9 10
Negative likelihood ratio
Not Useful
Useful
Very Small
Small
Moderate
Large
1.0 0.9 0.8 0.7 0.6 0.5 0.4 0.3 0.2 0.1 0
For pain:
Positive likelihood ratio
Not Useful
Useful
Very Small
Small
Moderate
Large
0 1 2 3 4 5 6 7 8 9 10
Negative likelihood ratio
Not Useful
Useful
Very Small
Small
Moderate
Large
1.0 0.9 0.8 0.7 0.6 0.5 0.4 0.3 0.2 0.1 0

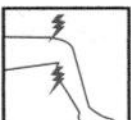

Stress Test 17-2
Varus Stress Test

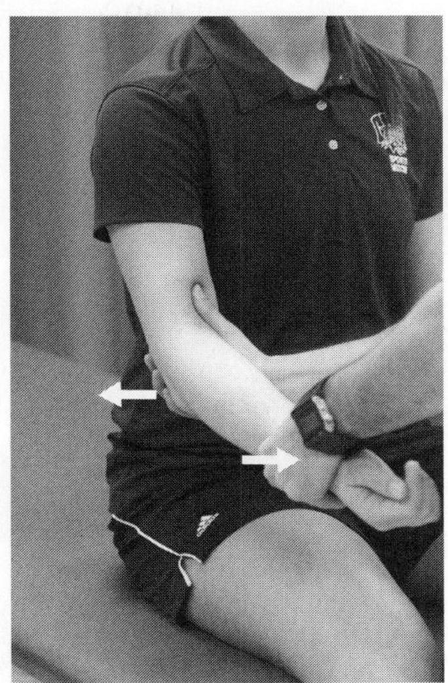

The varus stress test determines the integrity of the radial collateral ligament.

Patient Position	Standing or sitting The elbow is flexed to 25°. The humerus is in neutral.
Position of Examiner	Standing medial to the joint being tested One hand supports the medial elbow with the fingers reaching behind the joint to palpate the lateral joint line. The opposite hand grasps the distal forearm.
Evaluative Procedure	A varus force is applied to the elbow. This process is repeated with the joint in various degrees of flexion.
Positive Test	Increased laxity compared with the opposite side, and/or pain is produced.
Implications	Moderate laxity reflects trauma to the radial collateral ligament. Gross laxity may also indicate damage to the annular or accessory lateral collateral ligament, causing the radius to displace from the ulna.
Comments	Laxity may also indicate epiphyseal injury.
Evidence	Absent or inconclusive in the literature

Joint Play

Joint Play 17-1
Elbow Joint Play

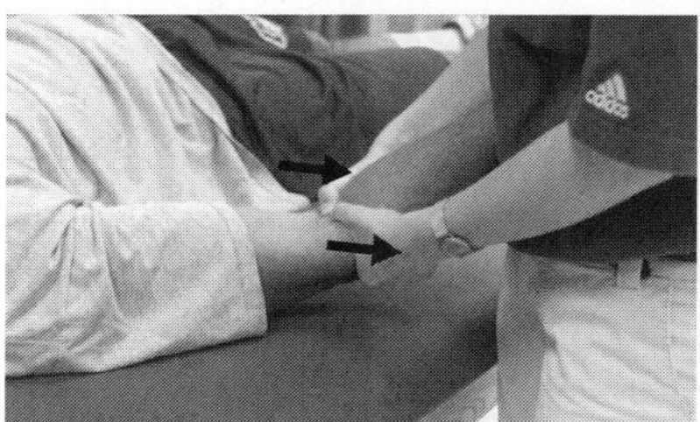

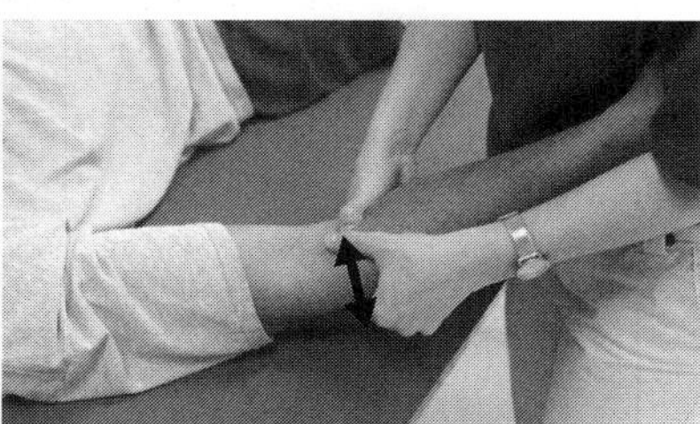

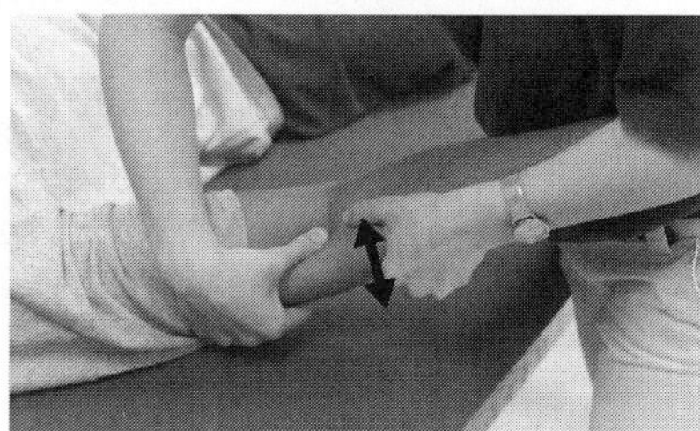

Joint play at the elbow assesses the amount of mobility allowed by the joint capsule and ligaments.

Patient Position	Humeroulnar: Supine; elbow in about 70° of flexion Radioulnar: Sitting or supine; elbow in 70° of flexion and 35° of supination Radiohumeral: Sitting or supine; elbow extended and forearm supinated
Position of Examiner	At the side of the patient
Evaluative Procedure	Humeroulnar: The examiner places thumbs on the proximal ulna while stabilizing distal forearm between his forearm and body. Applies a distracting force to the elbow Radioulnar: The examiner stabilizes the proximal ulna and applies an anterior and then posterior force at the humeral head. Radiohumeral: The examiner stabilizes the proximal ulna and applies an anterior and then posterior force at the humeral head.
Positive Test	Hypomobility or hypermobility
Implications	Restrictions in all articulations may accompany loss of physiologic elbow motion. Hypomobility at the radioulnar joint is associated with restricted supination and pronation.
Comments	Note that only the patient's position differs when assessing the radioulnar and radiohumeral articulations. The pressure needed to grasp the patient's radial head may be painful in noninjured patients. Joint movement is easier to detect in the posterior direction. Joint play of radial and ulnar deviation is performed as in valgus and varus stress testing of the elbow.

Special Test 17-1
Moving Valgus Stress Test

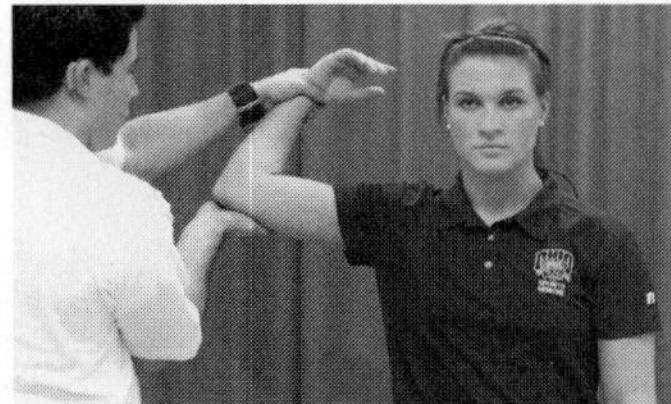

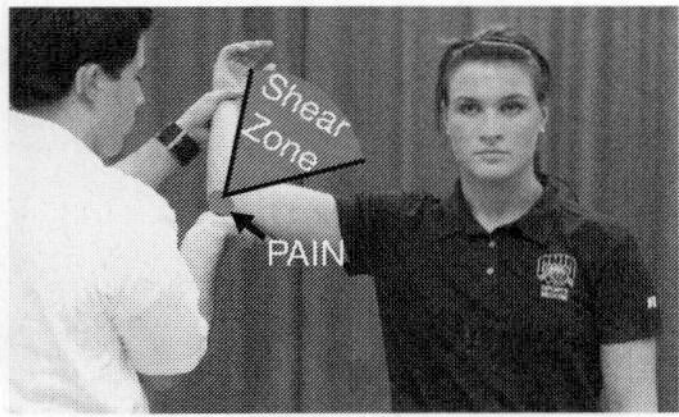

The moving valgus stress test places tensile forces on the ulnar collateral ligament through elbow flexion and extension to identify dynamic elbow instability.

Patient Position	Sitting The shoulder is abducted to 90°. The elbow is flexed to the end of the ROM.
Position of Examiner	Standing next to the patient One hand stabilizes the distal humerus. The opposite hand grasps the ulnar side of the distal forearm.
Evaluative Procedure	While applying a valgus force on the elbow, the examiner externally rotates the humerus. The examiner extends the elbow to approximately 30° while maintaining a valgus force on the joint, noting the position(s) that pain is evoked. The examiner then moves the elbow from extension into flexion while maintaining a valgus stress on the joint.
Positive Test	(1) Pain at the medial elbow that reproduces functional pain, often producing an apprehension response AND (2) Pain that occurs between 120° and 70° (representing the position of the late cocking and early acceleration throwing phases) A positive test is marked by the reproduction of pain at the same point in the ROM during both the flexion and extension segments of the examination.
Implications	Partial tear or attenuation of the UCL
Comments	Shoulder pathology may elicit pain during this procedure. Do not perform this test in the presence of known glenohumeral instability
Evidence	Positive likelihood ratio Not Useful — Useful Very Small / Small / Moderate / Large 0 1 2 3 4 5 6 7 8 9 10 Negative likelihood ratio Not Useful — Useful Very Small / Small / Moderate / Large 1.0 0.9 0.8 0.7 0.6 0.5 0.4 0.3 0.2 0.1 0

ROM = range of motion; UCL = ulnar collateral ligament.

Special Test 17-2
Posterolateral Rotatory Instability Test (Pivot Shift)

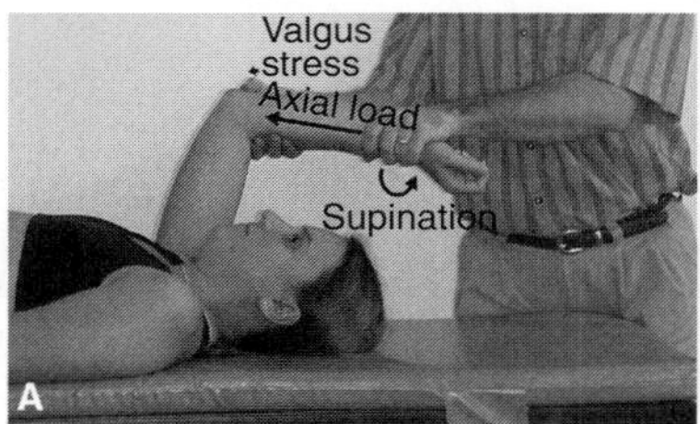

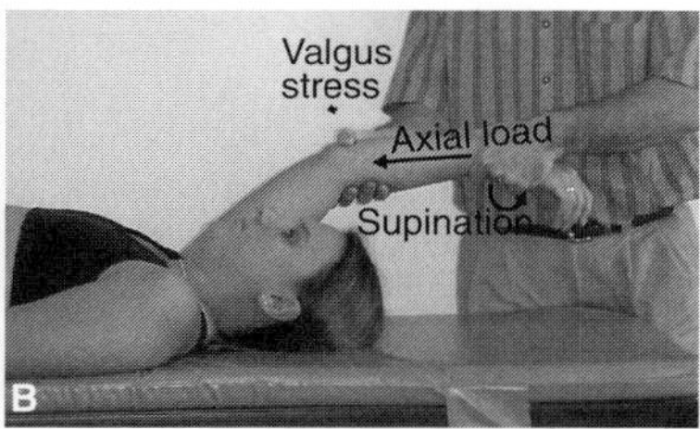

Test for posterolateral rotatory instability of the elbow consists of extending the elbow with a axial load, valgus stress, and forearm supination. The elbow subluxates as it nears full extension. A palpable reduction may be felt as the elbow is moved back into flexion.

Patient Position	Supine The shoulder and elbow are flexed to 90° and the forearm is fully supinated.
Position of Examiner	Standing at the head of the patient One hand grasps the proximal forearm and the other hand grasps the distal forearm at the wrist **(A).**
Evaluative Procedure	While applying a valgus stress and axial compression, the elbow is extended and the forearm is maintained in full supination **(B)**. The elbow then can be taken back into flexion (not shown).
Positive Test	The elbow subluxates as it is extended and can be felt to relocate as it is flexed.
Implications	Chronic instability of the elbow
Comments	When performed with the patient under anesthesia, the posterolateral rotatory instability test was positive only when the entire lateral collateral ligament was sectioned.[105]
Evidence	Absent or inconclusive in the literature

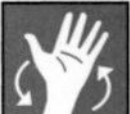

Special Test 17-3
Test for Lateral Epicondylalgia ("Tennis Elbow" Test)

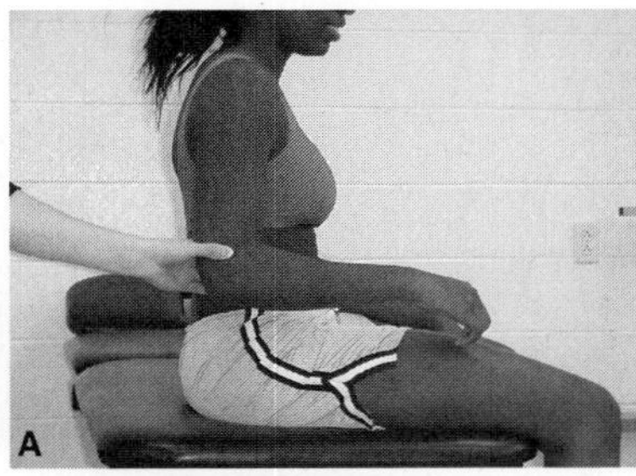

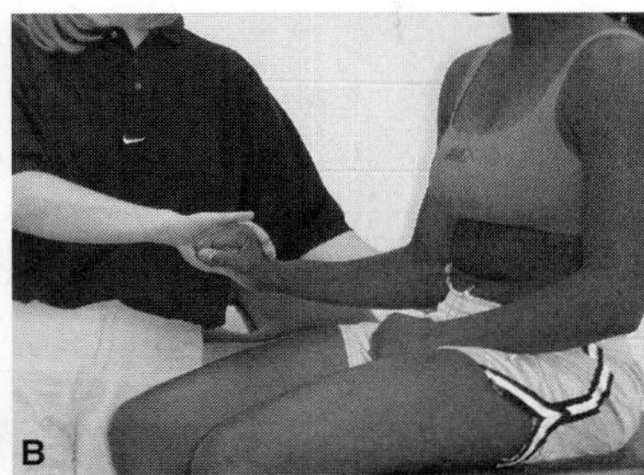

(A) The location of the thumb on the lateral epicondyle. **(B)** Resisted wrist extension.

Patient Position	Seated with the tested elbow flexed to 90°, the forearm pronated, and the fingers flexed
Position of Examiner	Standing lateral to the patient with one hand positioned over the dorsal aspect of the wrist and hand
Evaluative Procedure	The examiner resists wrist extension while palpating the lateral epicondyle and common attachment of the wrist extensors.
Positive Test	Pain in the lateral epicondyle
Implications	Lateral epicondylalgia ("tennis elbow")
Modification	This test may also be performed with the elbow in extension.
Comments	This is the manual muscle test for wrist extension performed through a full range of motion instead of midrange.
Evidence	Absent or inconclusive in the literature

Nerve Distribution in the Hand

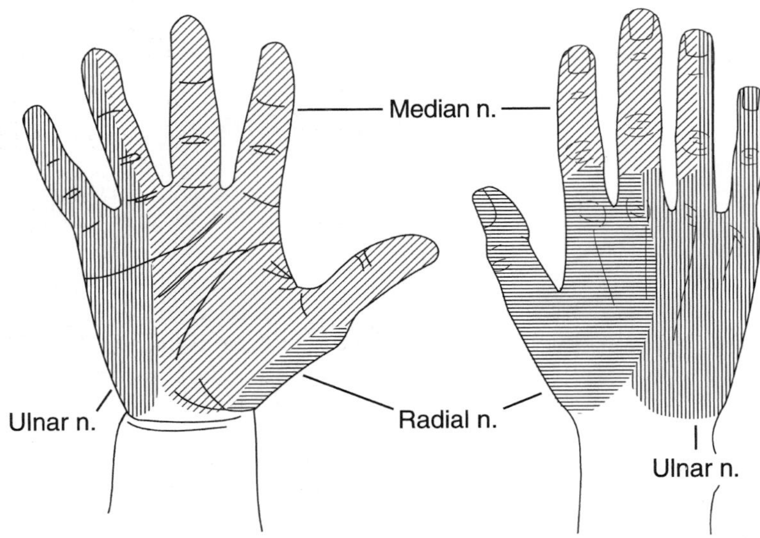

FIGURE 17-6 ■ The median, ulnar, and radial nerve sensory distribution in the hand. Note that texts differ on the exact delineation between the cutaneous distribution of the individual nerves.

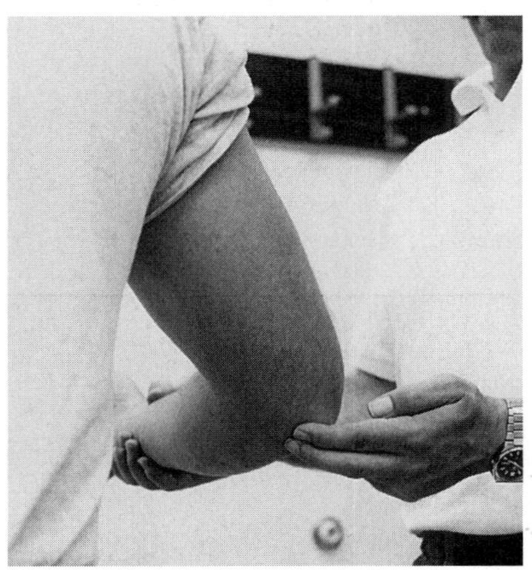

FIGURE 17-7 ■ Tinel's sign for neuropathy. In the presence of neuropathy, tapping on the ulnar (shown) or radial nerve results in a burning sensation in the hand.

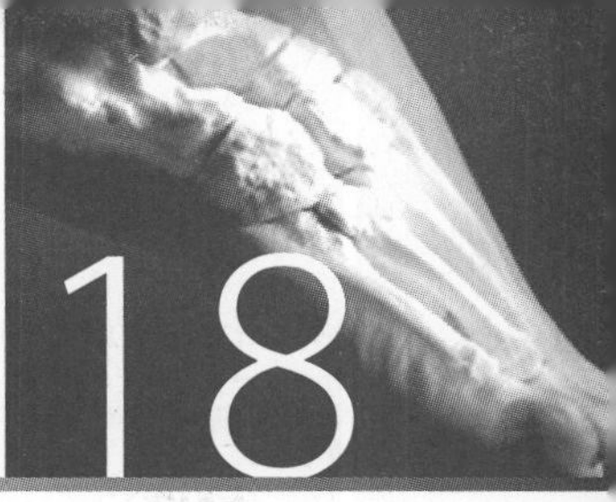

CHAPTER 18

Wrist, Hand, and Finger Pathologies

Examination Map

HISTORY

Past Medical History
Previous injury history

General medical health

History of the Present Condition
Location of pain

Mechanism of injury

Onset and severity of symptoms

Changes in activity

INSPECTION

Functional Assessment

General Inspection
Wrist and hand posture

Gross deformity

Palmar creases

Lacerations or scars

- Russell's sign

Inspection of the Wrist and Hand
Continuity of the radius and ulna

Continuity of the carpals and metacarpals

Alignment of the MCP and IP joints

Ganglion cyst

Inspection of the Thumb and Fingers
Skin and fingernails

Subungual hematoma

Felon

Paronychia

Alignment of fingernails

Muscle contour

Finger posture

PALPATION

Palpation of the Wrist and Finger Flexor Muscle Group
Medial epicondyle

Flexor carpi ulnaris

Flexor digitorum profundus

Flexor digitorum radialis

Flexor carpi radialis

Palmaris longus

Carpal tunnel

Palpation of the Wrist and Finger Flexor Muscle Group
Lateral epicondyle

Extensor digitorum communis

Extensor pollicis longus

Abductor pollicis longus

Extensor pollicis brevis

Abductor pollicis longus

Palpation of the Hand
Metacarpals

MCP joint collateral ligaments

Phalanges

IP joint collateral ligaments

Thenar compartment

- Opponens pollicis
- Abductor pollicis brevis
- Flexor pollicis brevis

Thenar webspace

- Adductor pollicis

Central compartment

Hypothenar compartment

Continued

Examination Map—cont'd

Palpation of the Wrist

Ulna

Ulnar styloid process

Ulnar collateral ligament

Radius

Radial styloid process

Lister's tubercle

Radial collateral ligament

Palpation of the Carpals

Scaphoid

Lunate

Triquetrum

Pisiform

Trapezium

Trapezoid

Capitate

Hamate

- Anatomic snuffbox

JOINT AND MUSCLE FUNCTION ASSESSMENT

Goniometry

Wrist

- Flexion
- Extension
- Radial deviation
- Ulnar deviation

Finger

- Flexion
- Extension
- MCP abduction

Thumb

- CMC flexion
- CMC extension
- CMC abduction

Active Range of Motion

Wrist

- Flexion
- Extension
- Radial deviation
- Ulnar deviation

Finger

- Flexion
- Extension
- Abduction
- Adduction

Thumb

- CMC flexion
- CMC extension
- CMC abduction
- CMC adduction
- Opposition
- Reposition

Manual Muscle Tests

Wrist

- Flexion and radial deviation
- Flexion and ulnar deviation
- Extension and radial deviation
- Flexion and ulnar deviation

Thumb

- MCP flexion
- MCP extension
- IP flexion
- IP extension
- CMC abduction
- CMC adduction
- Opposition

Finger (MCP, PIP, and DIP)

- Flexion
- Extension
- MCP abduction
- MCP adduction

Grip dynamometry

Passive Range of Motion

Wrist

- Flexion
- Extension
- Radial deviation
- Ulnar deviation

Finger (MCP, PIP, and DIP)

- Flexion
- Extension
- MCP abduction
- MCP adduction

Thumb

- CMC flexion
- CMC extension
- CMC abduction
- CMC adduction
- Opposition
- Reposition

JOINT STABILITY TESTS

Stress Testing

Wrist

- Radial collateral ligament
- Ulnar collateral ligament

Finger (PIP and DIP)

- Radial collateral ligament
- Ulnar collateral ligament

Examination Map—cont'd

Joint Play Assessment

Wrist
- Radial glide
- Ulnar glide
- Dorsal glide
- Palmar glide

Hand
- Intermetacarpal glide

NEUROLOGIC EXAMINATION

Upper Quarter Screen

Tinel Sign

PATHOLOGIES AND SPECIAL TESTS

Wrist Pathologies

Distal forearm fracture
- Colles' fracture
- Smith's fracture

Scaphoid fracture
- Scaphoid compression test

Preiser's disease

Hamate fracture

Perilunate/lunate dislocation
- Dissociative carpal instability
- Kienböck's disease

Wrist sprains
- Watson test

Triangular fibrocartilage complex injury

Carpal tunnel syndrome

Hand Pathologies

Metacarpal fractures

Finger Pathologies

Collateral ligament injuries

Boutonniere deformity
- Pseudo-boutonniere deformity

Finger fractures

Tendon ruptures and avulsion fractures

Thumb Pathologies

De Quervain's syndrome

Thumb sprains

MCP joint dislocations

Thumb fractures

Inspection Findings 18-1
Pathological Hand and Finger Postures

	Ape Hand	Bishop's Deformity	Claw Hand
	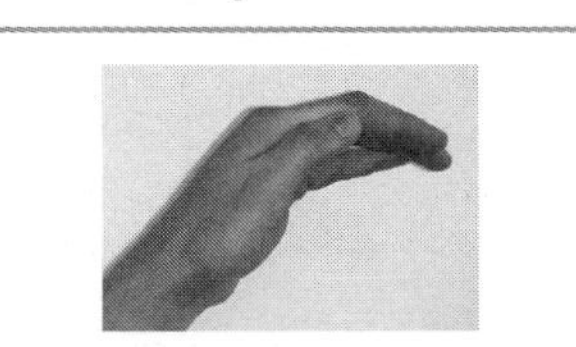		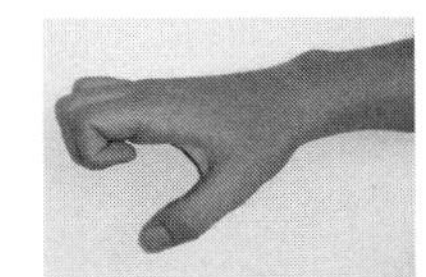
Impairments	Weakness and atrophy of the muscles of the thenar eminence results in overemphasis of the extensor muscles, which pull the thumb parallel with the fingers. Opposition and flexion of the MCP and IP are weakened.	Weakness and atrophy of the hypothenar, interossei, and medial two lumbricals causes the medial fingers to assume a resting posture of flexion in the PIP and DIP joints. Extension of these joints is limited.	Weakness and atrophy of the hand intrinsic muscles results in extension of the MCP joint and flexion of the PIP and DIP joints.
Pathology	Median nerve neuropathy	Inhibition of the ulnar nerve; also known as "Benediction deformity"	Ulnar and median nerve involvement

	Dupuytren's Contracture	Swan-Neck Deformity	Volkmann's Ischemic Contracture
	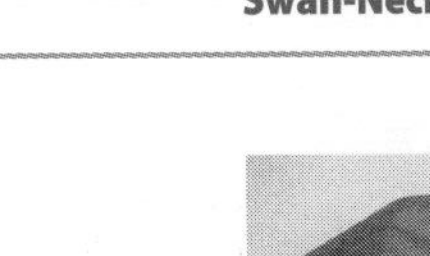	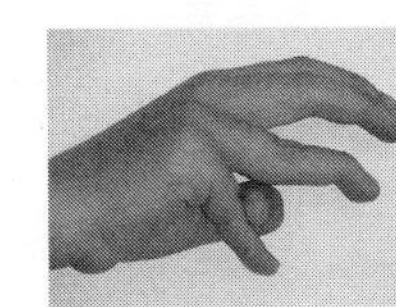 	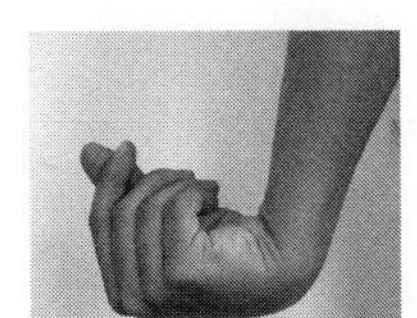
Impairments	Involved finger(s) assume excessively flexed resting position. Inability to passively or actively extend the MCP and PIP joints of the involved finger	Characterized by flexion of the MCP and DIP joints and hyperextension of the PIP joint	Flexion contraction of the wrist and fingers (claw fingers) resulting in limited extension at these joints
Pathology	Flexion contracture of the MCP and PIP joints is caused by a shortening or adhesion (or both) of the palmar fascia. This hereditary condition most commonly affects the 4th and 5th fingers.	Can be caused by a wide range of pathologies, including volar plate injuries, malunion fractures of the middle phalanx, trauma to the finger flexor or extensor muscles, or rheumatoid arthritis.	A decrease in the blood supply to the forearm muscles; Volkmann's contracture can occur after a forearm fracture, fracture or dislocation of the elbow, or forearm compartment syndrome.

DIP = distal interphalangeal; MCP = metacarpophalangeal; PIP = proximal interphalangeal.

Inspection Findings 18-2
Finger Deformities

	Jersey Finger	Mallet Finger*	Boutonnière Deformity*
Observation			
Illustration	FDP FDS		Boutonnière Deformity Pseudo-Boutonnière Deformity Volar plate
Pathology	Avulsion of the flexor digitorum profundus tendon	Avulsion of the extensor digitorum longus tendon	Boutonnière deformity: A rupture of the central extensor tendon Pseudo-boutonnière deformity: A rupture of the volar plate
Impairment	Inability to actively flex the DIP joint	Inability to actively extend the distal phalanx, which assumes the posture of 25°–35° of flexion	Extension of the MCP and DIP joints and flexion of the PIP joint; acutely, the PIP joint can be passively extended in those with boutonnière deformities but active PIP extension is absent. In pseudo-boutonnière deformities, passive and active PIP extension are limited.

DIP = distal interphalangeal; MCP = metacarpophalangeal; PIP = proximal interphalangeal.
*Courtesy of Stanley BG and Tribuzi SM: *Concepts in Hand Rehabilitation*. Philadelphia: FA Davis, 1992.

Finger Fracture

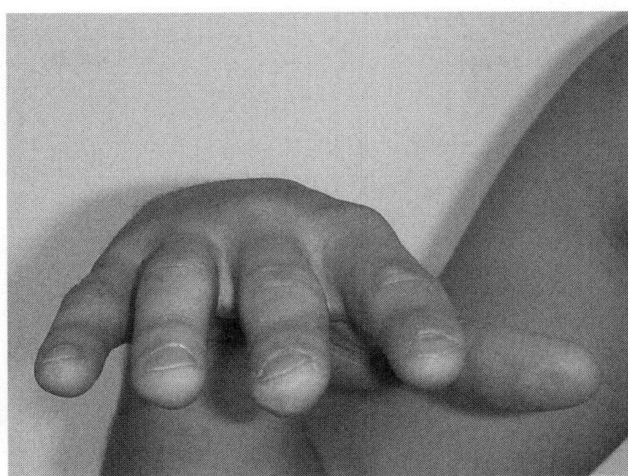

FIGURE 18-1 ■ Rotational malalignment associated with a spiral fracture of the phalanx or metacarpal. Note the rotational displacement of the third fingernail.

PALPATION

Palpation of the Hand

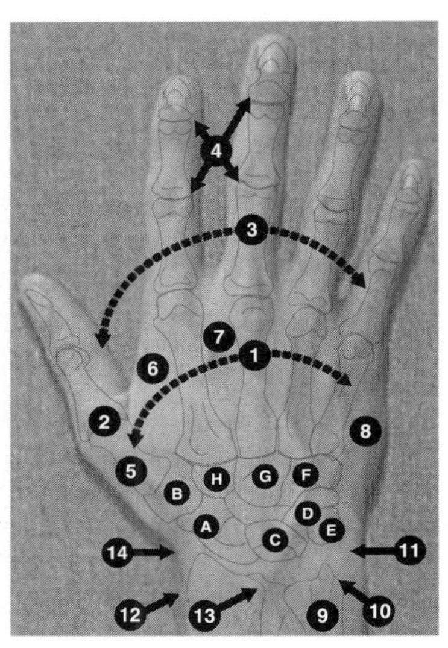

1 Metacarpals

2 Collateral ligaments of the metacarpophalangeal joints

3 Phalanges

4 Collateral ligaments of the IP joints

5 Thenar compartment

6 Thenar webspace

7 Central compartment

8 Hypothenar compartment

9 Ulna

10 Ulnar styloid process

11 Ulnar collateral ligament

12 Distal radius and styloid process

13 Lister's tubercle

14 Radial collateral ligament

Palpation of the Carpals

A Scaphoid

B Trapezius

C Lunate

D Triquetrum

E Pisiform

F Hamate

G Capitate

H Trapezoid

Anatomical Snuffbox

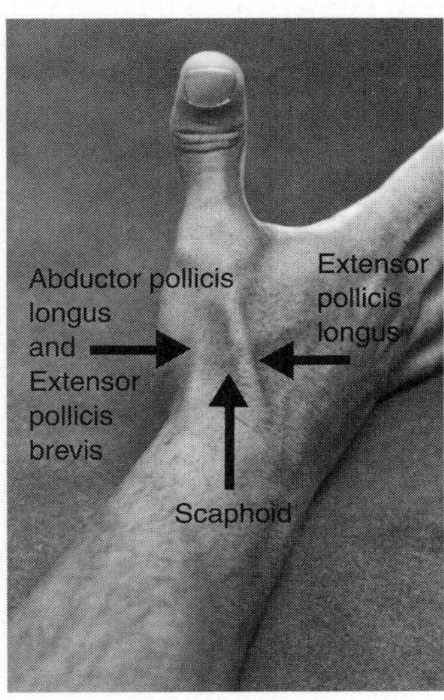

FIGURE 18-2 ■ Borders of the anatomical snuffbox.

Table 18-1 Normal End-Feels Obtained During Passive Range-of-Motion Testing

Area	Motion	End-Feel	Tissues
Wrist	Flexion	Firm	Dorsal radiocarpal ligament and joint capsule
	Extension	Firm	Palmar radiocarpal ligament and joint capsule
	Radial deviation	Hard	Scaphoid striking styloid process of radius
	Ulnar deviation	Firm	Radiocarpal ligaments and tendons
Thumb (CMC)	Flexion	Soft	Approximation of thenar eminence and the palm
	Extension	Firm	Palmar joint capsule, flexor pollicis brevis, opponens pollicis, first interossei
	Abduction	Firm	Stretching of the webspace
	Adduction	Soft	Approximation of thenar eminence and palm
Fingers and Thumb (MCP)	Flexion	Hard	Proximal phalanx contacts the metacarpal
	Extension	Firm	Tension in the volar plate
	Abduction	Firm	Stretching of the collateral ligaments and webspace
	Adduction	Firm	Stretching of the collateral ligaments and webspace
Fingers (PIP)	Flexion	Hard	Proximal and middle phalanges contact
	Extension	Firm	Stretching of the volar plate
Fingers (DIP) and Thumb (IP)	Flexion	Firm	Tension in dorsal joint capsule and collateral ligaments
	Extension	Firm	Stretching of palmar joint capsule and volar plate

CMC = carpometacarpal; DIP = distal interphalangeal; IP = interphalangeal; MCP = metacarpophalangeal; PIP = proximal interphalangeal.

Active Range of Motion, Wrist

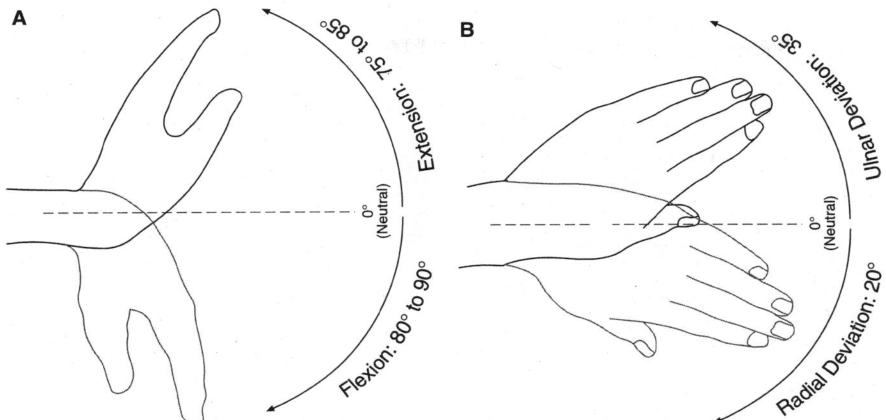

FIGURE 18-3 ■ **(A)** Active range of motion for wrist flexion and extension. **(B)** Active range of motion for radial and ulnar deviation of the wrist.

Active Range of Motion, Thumb

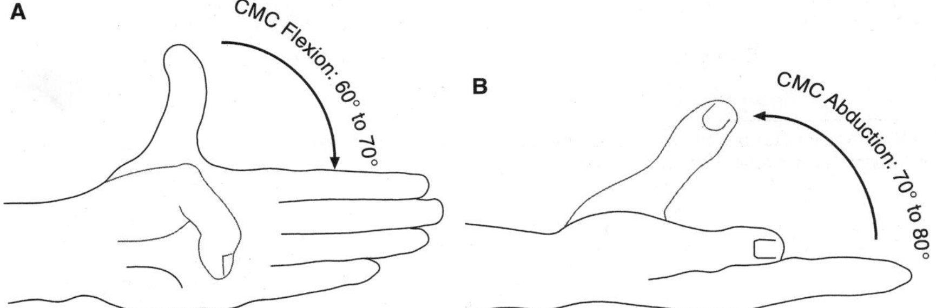

FIGURE 18-4 ■ Active range of motion of the first carpometacarpal joint: **(A)** flexion/extension (extension is placing the hand in the hitchhiker's position); **(B)** abduction/adduction (abduction is holding a can).

Active Range of Motion, Finger

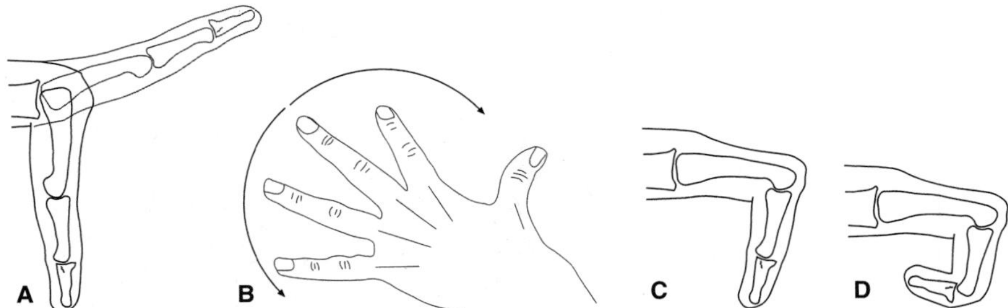

FIGURE 18-5 ■ Finger range of motion: **(A)** metacarpophalangeal flexion and extension; **(B)** metacarpophalangeal abduction; **(C)** flexion of the proximal interphalangeal joint; **(D)** flexion of the proximal and distal interphalangeal joints.

Goniometry

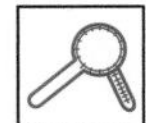

Goniometry Box 18-1
Wrist

	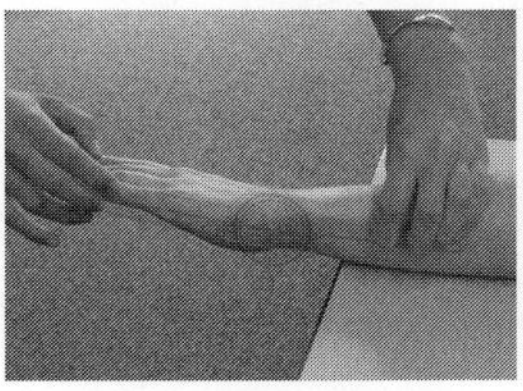 **Flexion and Extension 0° to 90°; 0° to 85°**	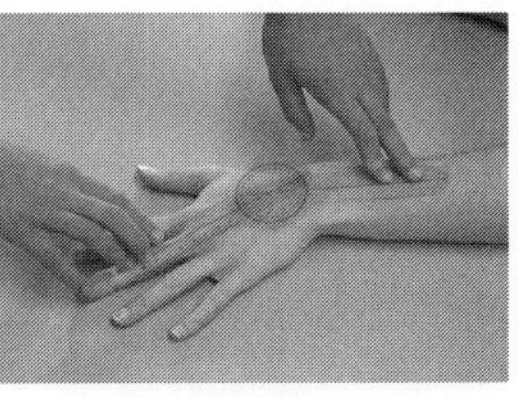 **Radial and Ulnar Deviation 0° to 20°; 0° to 35°**
Patient Position	Forearm is pronated with the hand resting on the table. Elbow is flexed to 90°. During wrist flexion, the fingers are allowed to extend. During wrist extension, the fingers are allowed to flex.	Forearm is pronated with the hand off the edge of the table. Elbow is flexed to 90°.
Goniometer Alignment		
Fulcrum	Aligned with the ulnar styloid process	Aligned with the capitate on the dorsal aspect of the wrist
Proximal Arm	The stationary arm is centered on the midline of the ulnar shaft.	The stationary arm is centered over the midline of the forearm.
Distal Arm	The movement arm is parallel to the longitudinal axis of the fifth metacarpal.	The movement arm is centered over the third metacarpal.
Comments	During measurement of PROM, apply the overpressure evenly at the dorsum of the metacarpals to avoid rotation at the wrist.	Avoid wrist extension during the measurement. Popping during ulnar deviation may be indicative of tear of the triangular fibrocartilage complex.

PROM = passive range of motion.

Goniometry Box 18-2
Finger

	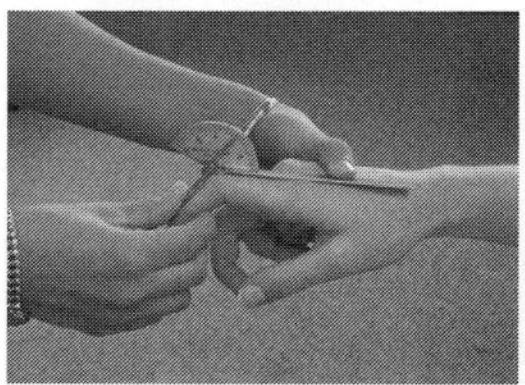 **Flexion/Extension (MCP, PIP, and DIP)**	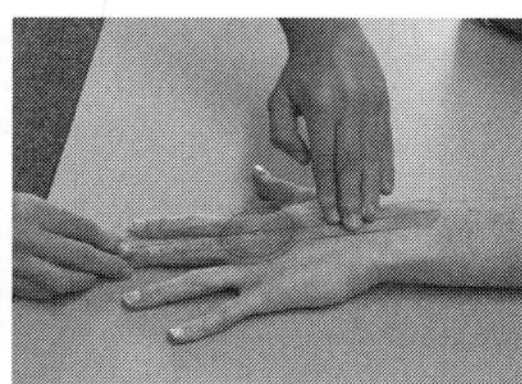 **Abduction and Adduction (MCP)**
Patient Position	The patient is sitting with the elbow flexed to 90° and the forearm in midposition. The forearm and hand are supported on the table. The wrist is in its neutral position.	The patient is sitting with the elbow flexed to 90° and the forearm pronated with the hand flat on the table. The wrist is in its neutral position.
Goniometer Alignment		
Fulcrum	Flexion: Positioned over the dorsal aspect of the joint being tested. Extension: Positioned over the palmar aspect of the joint being tested	Positioned over the dorsal aspect of the MCP joint
Proximal Arm	The stationary arm is centered on the midline of the bone proximal to the joint being tested.	The stationary arm is aligned over the metacarpal of the joint being tested.
Distal Arm	The movement arm is centered on the midline of the bone distal to the joint being tested.	The movement arm is centered over the proximal phalanx of the joint being tested.
Comments	Stabilize the joints proximal to the joint being measured. Flexion and extension of the MCP of the index finger may be measured on the radial aspect. The same positioning is used to measure MCP and IP flexion and extension of the thumb.	Other fingers may need to be moved to permit full adduction.

DIP = distal interphalangeal; MCP = metacarpophalangeal; PIP = proximal interphalangeal.

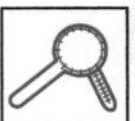

Goniometry Box 18-3
Thumb

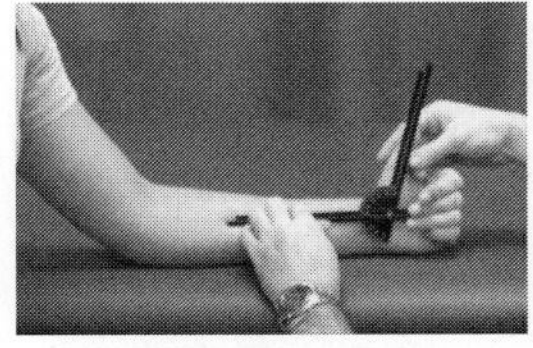
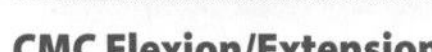
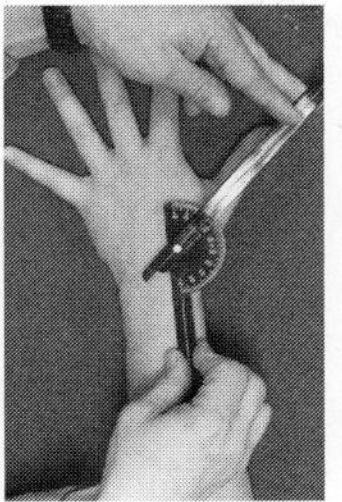

	CMC Flexion/Extension	CMC Abduction
Patient Position	The patient is sitting with the elbow flexed to 90° and the forearm in midposition. The forearm and hand are supported on the table. The wrist is in its neutral position.	The patient is seated with the forearm pronated. The palm is flat on the table.
Goniometer Alignment		
Fulcrum	The axis is centered at the palmar aspect of the CMC.	The axis is centered at the dorsal aspect of the CMC, where the bases of the first and second metacarpals meet.
Proximal Arm	The stationary arm is aligned parallel to the shaft of the radius.	The stationary arm is aligned parallel to the shaft of the second metacarpal.
Distal Arm	The movement arm is aligned parallel to the shaft of the first metacarpal.	The movement arm is aligned parallel to the shaft of the first metacarpal.
Comments	Flexion and extension occur in the frontal plane. When measuring PROM, apply overpressure at the distal metacarpal instead of the proximal phalanx. The initial position of the goniometer is considered the start or zero position.	When measuring PROM, apply overpressure at the distal metacarpal instead of the proximal phalanx. Stabilize the 2nd metacarpal. The initial position of the goniometer is considered the start or zero position.

CMC = carpometacarpal; PROM = passive range of motion.

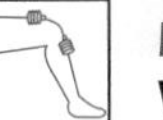

Manual Muscle Test 18-1
Wrist Flexion and Extension

	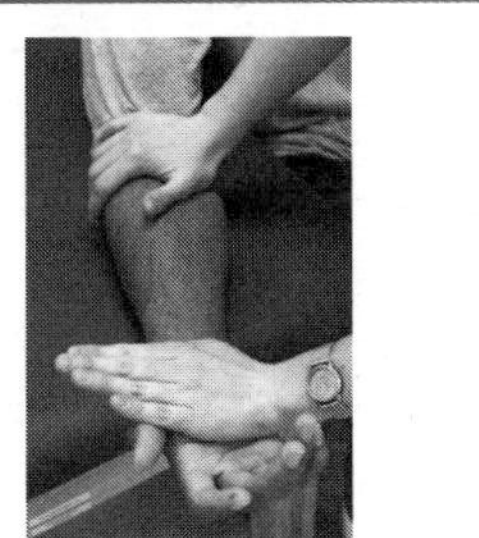 **Flexion and Radial Deviation** **Flexion and Ulnar Deviation (Shown)**	**Extension and Radial Deviation** **Extension and Ulnar Deviation (Shown)**
Patient Position	Seated	Seated
Starting Position	The elbow is flexed to 90°, the forearm is supinated, and the wrist is flexed off the end of the table and ulnarly deviated (FCR) or radially deviated (FCU).	The elbow is flexed to 90°. The forearm is pronated and the wrist is extended and ulnarly deviated (ECRB/ECRL) or radially deviated (ECU), with the fingers in a relaxed position.
Stabilization	Anterior portion of the mid-forearm	Posterior portion of the mid-forearm
Palpation	FCR: Anterior lateral wrist in line with second web space[106] FCU: Anterior medial wrist just proximal to pisiform.	ECRL/ECRB: ECRL—dorsal base of 2nd metacarpal; ECRB—dorsal base of 3rd metacarpal. ECU: dorsal wrist between base of 5th metacarpal and distal ulna.
Resistance	FCR: Thenar eminence FCU: Hypothenar eminence	Dorsal surface of the hand

Primary Mover(s) (Innervation)	***Flexion and radial deviation:*** Flexor carpi radialis (median: C6, C7) ***Flexion and ulnar deviation:*** Flexor carpi ulnaris (ulnar: C8, T1)	***Extension and radial deviation:*** Extensor carpi radialis longus (radial: C6, C7) Extensor carpi radialis brevis (radial: C6, C7) ***Extension and ulnar deviation:*** Extensor carpi ulnaris (DR: C6, C7, C8)
Secondary Mover(s) (Innervation)	***Flexion and radial deviation:*** Flexor carpi ulnaris (ulnar: C8, T1) Palmaris longus (median: C6, C7) Flexor digitorum profundus (PI: C8, T1) Flexor digitorum superficialis (median: C7, C8, T1) Flexor pollicis longus (PI: C8, T1) ***Flexion and ulnar deviation:*** Flexor carpi radialis (median: C6, C7) Palmaris longus (median: C6, C7) Flexor digitorum profundus (ulnar: C8, T1) Flexor digitorum superficialis (median: C7, C8, T1) Flexor pollicis longus (PI: C8, T1)	***Extension and radial deviation:*** Extensor carpi ulnaris (DR: C6, C7, C8) Extensor digitorum communis (DR: C6, C7, C8) Extensor pollicis longus (DR: C6, C7, C8) ***Extension and ulnar deviation:*** Extensor carpi radialis longus (radial: C6, C7) Extensor carpi radialis brevis (radial: C6, C7) Extensor digitorum communis (DR: C6, C7, C8) Extensor pollicis longus (DR: C6, C7, C8)
Substitution	***Flexion and radial deviation:*** Ulnar deviation, finger flexion ***Flexion and ulnar deviation:*** Radial deviation, finger flexion	***Extension and radial deviation:*** Ulnar deviation, finger extension ***Extension and ulnar deviation:*** Radial deviation, finger extension
Comments	To minimize contributions from the FDS and FDP, the fingers should not flex during the test.	To minimize contributions from the extensor pollicis longus and extensor digitorum communis, instruct the patient to keep the fingers relaxed during the test.

DR = deep radial nerve; PI = palmar interosseous nerve.

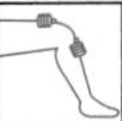

Manual Muscle Test 18-2
Thumb: MCP and IP Flexion and Extension

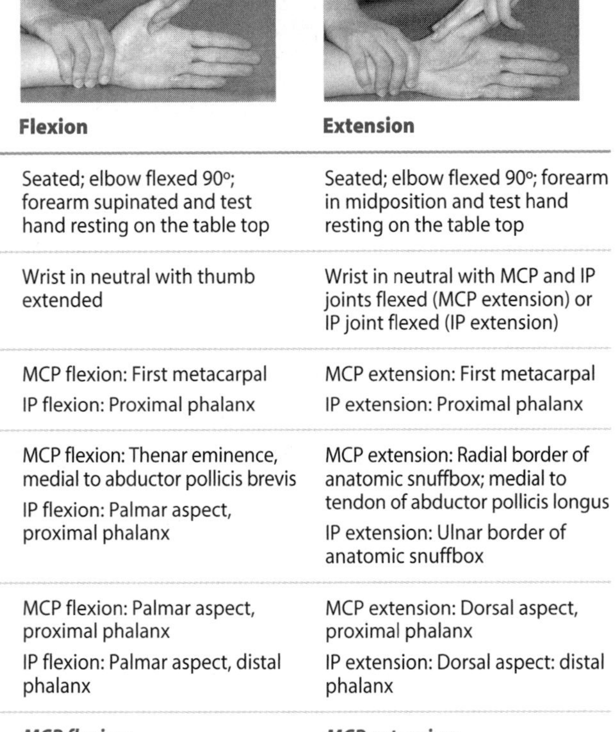

	Flexion	Extension
Patient Position	Seated; elbow flexed 90°; forearm supinated and test hand resting on the table top	Seated; elbow flexed 90°; forearm in midposition and test hand resting on the table top
Starting Position	Wrist in neutral with thumb extended	Wrist in neutral with MCP and IP joints flexed (MCP extension) or IP joint flexed (IP extension)
Stabilization	MCP flexion: First metacarpal IP flexion: Proximal phalanx	MCP extension: First metacarpal IP extension: Proximal phalanx
Palpation	MCP flexion: Thenar eminence, medial to abductor pollicis brevis IP flexion: Palmar aspect, proximal phalanx	MCP extension: Radial border of anatomic snuffbox; medial to tendon of abductor pollicis longus IP extension: Ulnar border of anatomic snuffbox
Resistance	MCP flexion: Palmar aspect, proximal phalanx IP flexion: Palmar aspect, distal phalanx	MCP extension: Dorsal aspect, proximal phalanx IP extension: Dorsal aspect: distal phalanx
Primary Mover(s) (Innervation)	***MCP flexion:*** Flexor pollicis brevis (DPB: C6, C7, C8, T1) ***IP flexion:*** Flexor pollicis longus (PI: C8, T1)	***MCP extension:*** Extensor pollicis brevis (DR: C6, C7) ***IP extension:*** Extensor pollicis longus (DR: C6, C7, C8)
Secondary Mover(s) (Innervation)	***MCP flexion:*** Flexor pollicis longus (PI: C8, T1) IP flexion: None	***MCP extension:*** Extensor pollicis longus (DR: C6, C7, C8) IP extension: None
Substitution	MCP flexion: Do not allow IP joint flexion.	MCP extension: Do not allow IP joint extension.

DPB = deep palmar branch (median nerve); DR = deep radial nerve; IP = interphalangeal; MCP = metacarpophalangeal; PI = palmar interosseous nerve.

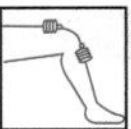

Manual Muscle Test 18-3
First Carpometacarpal Joint Abduction and Adduction

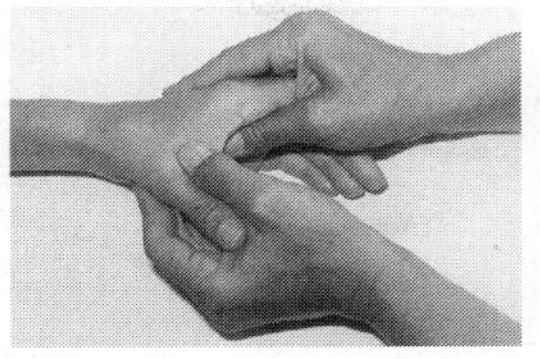

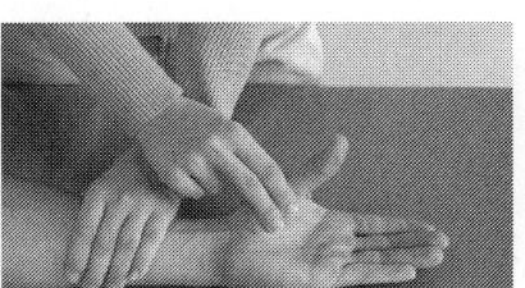

	Abduction	Adduction
Patient Position	Seated; elbow flexed to 90°; forearm supinated with hand resting on table top	Seated; the elbow flexed to 90°; forearm supinated with hand resting on table top
Starting Position	Neutral hand position	Thumb in palmar abduction with MCP and IP joints flexed
Stabilization	Wrist and lateral four metacarpals	Wrist and lateral four metacarpals
Palpation	Lateral aspect of first metacarpal	Palmar surface at thenar eminence between 1st and 2nd metacarpal
Resistance	Lateral aspect of proximal phalanx	Medial border of the proximal phalanx
Primary Mover(s) (Innervation)	Abductor pollicis brevis (median: C6, C7)	Adductor pollicis (DPB: C8, T1)
Secondary Mover(s) (Innervation)	Abductor pollicis longus (median: C6, C7) Extensor pollicis brevis (DR: C6, C7)	Flexor pollicis brevis (DPB: C6, C7, C8, T1)
Substitution	Radial abduction	Not applicable
Comments	Provide resistance to abduction with the thumb at a 45° angle from the sagittal plane to better isolate the abductor pollicis longus. This is sometimes called radial abduction.	Maintain IP and MCP flexion during the test.

DPB = deep palmar branch (median nerve); DR = deep radial nerve; IP = interphalangeal; MCP = metacarpophalangeal.

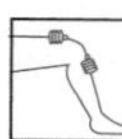

Manual Muscle Test 18-4
Opposition (First and Fifth Carpometacarpal Joint Flexion)

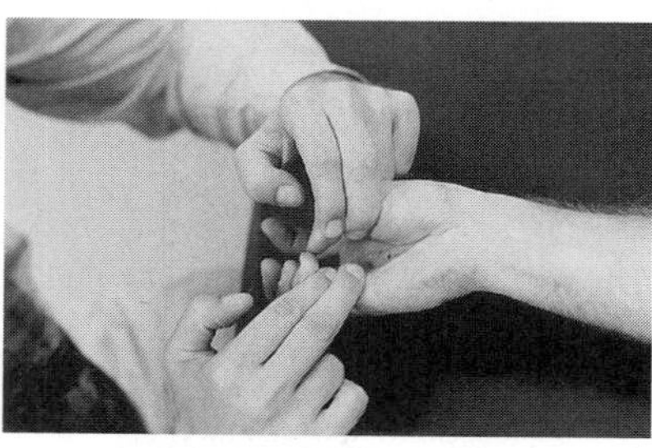

Patient Position	Seated; elbow flexed to 90º; forearm supinated with hand resting on table top
Starting Position	The thumb and 5th fingers opposed
Stabilization	Not applicable
Palpation	Thenar and hypothenar eminences
Resistance	The examiner attempts to separate the fingers, applying resistance at the distal 1st and 5th metacarpals.
Primary Mover(s) (Innervation)	Opponens pollicis (median: C6, C7) Opponens digiti minimi (ulnar: C8, T1)
Secondary Mover(s) (Innervation)	Abductor pollicis brevis (median: C6, C7) Flexor pollicis brevis (DPB: C6, C7, C8, T1)
Substitution	IP joint and wrist flexion

DPB = deep palmar branch (median nerve); IP = interphalangeal.

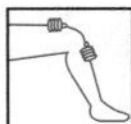

Manual Muscle Test 18-5
PIP and DIP Flexion

	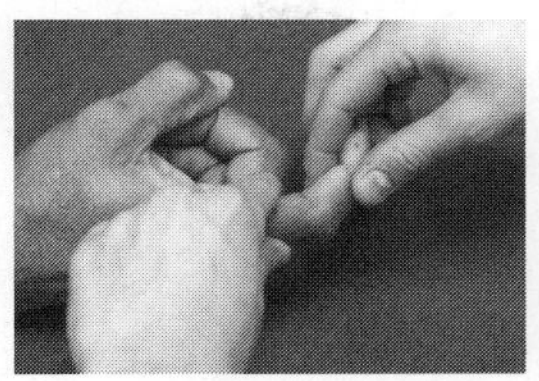 PIP Flexion	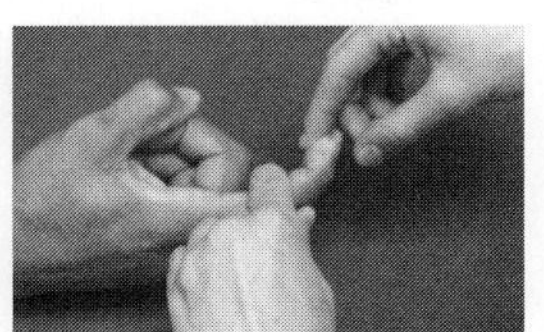 DIP Flexion
Patient Position	Seated; forearm in supination and resting on table	Seated; forearm in supination and resting on table
Starting Position	Test finger in extension	Test finger in extension
Stabilization	Proximal phalanx	Middle phalanx
Palpation	Palmar surface, proximal phalanx	Palmar surface
Resistance	Palmar surface, middle phalanx	Palmar surface, distal phalanx
Primary Mover(s) (Innervation)	Flexor digitorum superficialis (C7, C8, T1)	Flexor digitorum profundus (C8, T1)
Secondary Mover(s) (Innervation)	Flexor digitorum profundus (C8, T1)	None
Substitution	DIP flexion (FDP)	None
Comments	Maintain nontest fingers in extension to limit contribution from the FDP.[106]	

DIP = distal interphalangeal; FDP = flexor digitorum profundus; PIP = proximal interphalangeal.

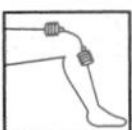

Manual Muscle Test 18-6
MCP Abduction and Adduction

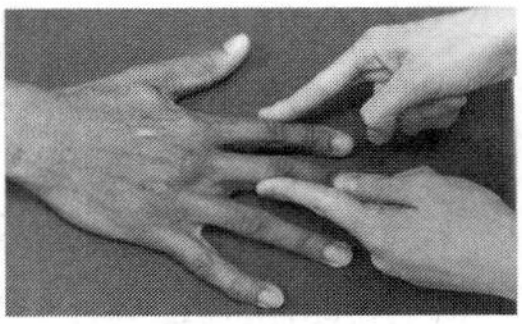

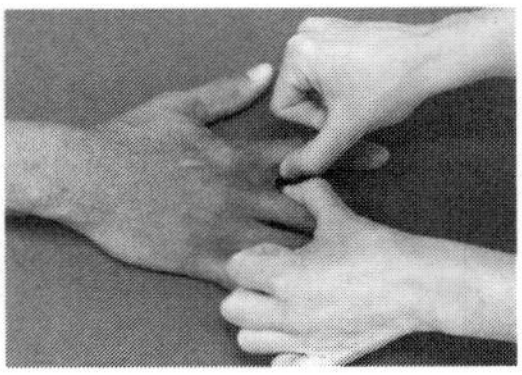

	Abduction	Adduction
Patient Position	Seated; elbow flexed to 90°; forearm pronated and hand resting on table	Seated; elbow flexed to 90°; forearm supinated and hand resting on table
Starting Position	The joint being tested is placed in the neutral position	The fingers are abducted.
Stabilization	Dorsum of hand	Dorsum of hand
Palpation	1st DI: radial aspect, 2nd metacarpal Abductor digiti minimi: ulnar aspect, 5th metacarpal	Cannot be palpated.
Resistance	Proximal phalanx of test finger	Proximal phalanx of test finger
Primary Mover(s) (Innervation)	Dorsal interossei (C8, T1) Abductor digiti minimi (5th finger) (C8, T1)	Palmar interossei (C8, T1)
Secondary Mover(s) (Innervation)	None	None
Substitution	MCP flexion	None
Comments	To test all four dorsal interossei, apply resistance to abduction at the ulnar aspect of the ring finger, at the radial and ulnar aspect of the middle finger and at the radial aspect of the index finger.	To test the three palmar interossei, apply resistance to adduction at the radial aspect of the little finger, the radial aspect of the ring finger, and the radial aspect of the index finger.

MCP = metacarpophalangeal.

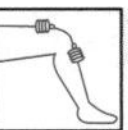

Manual Muscle Test 18-7
Finger MCP Extension and Flexion with IP Extension

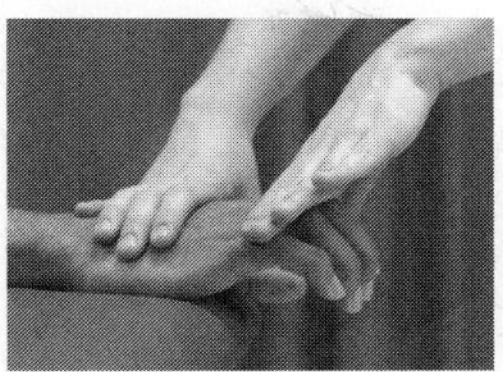

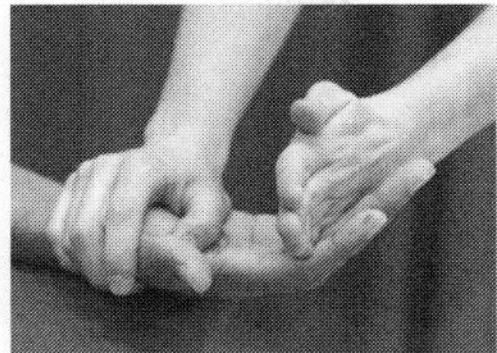

	MCP Extension	Flexion with IP Extension
Patient Position	Seated; elbow in 90° of flexion; forearm pronated; wrist in neutral	Seated; elbow in 90° of flexion; forearm supinated and resting on the table
Starting Position	MCP and IP joints flexed over the end of the table	MCP joints extended and adducted; IP joints flexed
Stabilization	Metacarpals	Metacarpals
Palpation	The tendon to each finger is palpated on the dorsum of the hand. The extensor indicis is medial to the extensor digitorum communis tendon to the index finger. The extensor digiti minimi is lateral to the extensor digitorum communis tendon of the little finger.	Cannot be palpated.
Resistance	Dorsal aspect, proximal phalanx of the test finger	Palmar aspect, proximal phalanx (to resist MCP flexion); dorsal aspect, middle phalanx (to resist PIP extension)
Primary Mover(s) (Innervation)	Extensor digitorum communis (C6, C7, C8) Extensor indicis (radial: C6, C7, C8) Extensor digiti minimi (radial: C6, C7, C8)	Lumbricales (C6, C7, C8, T1)
Secondary Mover(s) (Innervation)	None	Flexor digiti minimi (ulnar: C8, T1) Dorsal interossei (C8, T1) Palmar interossei (C8, T1)
Substitution	Wrist extension	Wrist flexion
Comments	Test MCP extension of all fingers at the same time. IP joint flexion should be maintained during the test. To assess for extensor digitorum communis tendon rupture, have the patient attempt to actively extend the involved joint while stabilizing the proximal segment.	Resist PIP extension and MCP flexion simultaneously. MCP flexion also occurs via the interossei. The flexor digiti minimi can be tested by resisting MCP flexion of the little finger.

IP = interphalangeal; MCP = metacarpophalangeal; PIP = proximal interphalangeal.

Table 18-2 Extrinsic Muscles Acting on the Wrist and Hand

Muscle	Action	Origin	Insertion	Innervation	Root
Abductor Pollicis Longus	1st CMC joint abduction 1st CMC joint extension Assists in radial deviation of the wrist	Posterior surface of the distal ulna Posterior surface of the distal radius Adjoining interosseous membrane	Radial side of the base of the 1st metacarpal	Median	C6, C7
Extensor Carpi Radialis Brevis	Wrist extension Radial deviation	Lateral epicondyle via the common extensor tendon Radial collateral ligament	Base of the 3rd metacarpal	Radial	C6, C7
Extensor Carpi Radialis Longus	Wrist extension Radial deviation	Supracondylar ridge of humerus	Radial side of the base of the 2nd metacarpal	Radial	C6, C7
Extensor Carpi Ulnaris	Wrist extension Ulnar deviation	Lateral epicondyle via the common extensor tendon	Ulnar side of the base of the 5th metacarpal	Deep radial	C6, C7, C8
Extensor Digiti Minimi	5th MCP joint extension 5th DIP and PIP extension, working with the lumbricales and interossei	Lateral epicondyle via the common extensor tendon Deep antebrachial fascia	To the middle and distal phalanx of the 5th finger via the extensor digitorum longus tendon	Radial	C6, C7, C8
Extensor Digitorum Communis	Wrist extension MCP extension IP extension Radial deviation of the wrist	Lateral epicondyle via the common extensor tendon	Dorsal surface of the proximal base of the middle and distal phalanges of each of the four fingers	Deep radial	C6, C7, C8
Extensor Indicis	2nd MCP extension (index finger) 2nd DIP and PIP extension, working with the lumbricales and interossei	Posterior surface of the ulna, distal to the extensor pollicis longus Interosseous membrane	To the middle and distal phalanx of the index finger via the extensor digitorum longus tendon	Radial	C6, C7, C8
Extensor Pollicis Brevis	1st MCP joint extension 1st CMC joint extension 1st CMC joint abduction Assists in wrist radial deviation	Posterior surface of the distal radius Adjoining interosseous membrane	Dorsal surface of the base of the proximal phalanx of the thumb	Deep radial	C6, C7
Extensor Pollicis Longus	1st IP joint extension 1st MCP joint extension	Posterior surface of the middle one third of the ulna	Dorsal surface of the base of the distal phalanx of the thumb	Deep radial	C6, C7, C8

	1st CMC joint extension Assists in wrist extension Assists in wrist radial deviation	Adjoining interosseous membrane			
Flexor Carpi Radialis	Wrist flexion Forearm pronation Radial deviation	Medial epicondyle via the common flexor tendon	Bases of the 2nd and 3rd metacarpals	Median	C6, C7
Flexor Carpi Ulnaris	Wrist flexion Ulnar deviation	Humeral head • Medial epicondyle via the common flexor tendon Ulnar head • Medial border of the olecranon • Proximal two thirds of the posterior ulna	Pisiform Hamate 5th metacarpal	Ulnar	C8, T1
Flexor Digitorum Profundus	DIP flexion PIP flexion Wrist flexion	Anteromedial proximal three fourths of ulna and associated interosseous membrane	Bases of the medial phalanges of digits II–V	Palmar interosseous	C8, T1
Flexor Digitorum Superficialis	PIP flexion MCP flexion Wrist flexion	Humeral head • Medial epicondyle via the common flexor tendon • Ulnar collateral ligament Ulnar head • Coronoid process Radial head • Oblique line of radius	Sides of the middle phalanges of digits II–V	Median	C7, C8, T1
Flexor Pollicis Longus	1st IP joint flexion 1st MCP joint flexion Assists in wrist flexion	Anterior surface of the radius Adjoining interosseous membrane Coronoid process of ulna	Palmar surface of the base of the distal phalanx of the thumb	Palmar interosseous	C8, T1
Palmaris Longus	Wrist flexion	Medial epicondyle via the common flexor tendon	Flexor retinaculum Palmar aponeurosis	Median	C6, C7

CMC = carpometacarpal; DIP = distal interphalangeal; IP = interphalangeal; MCP = metacarpophalangeal; PIP = proximal interphalangeal.

Table 18-3 Intrinsic Muscles Acting on the Hand

Muscle	Action	Origin	Insertion	Innervation	Root
Abductor Digiti Minimi	Abduction of the 5th finger Assists in opposition	Tendon of flexor carpi ulnaris Pisiform	By two slips into the 5th finger • Ulnar side of the base of the proximal phalanx • Ulnar border of the extensor expansion	Ulnar	C8, T1
Abductor Pollicis Brevis	1st CMC joint abduction 1st MCP joint abduction Assists in opposition	Flexor retinaculum Trapezium Scaphoid	Radial surface of the base of the proximal phalanx of the thumb Via a slip into the extensor expansion	Median	C6, C7
Adductor Pollicis	1st CMC joint adduction 1st MCP joint adduction 1st MCP joint flexion Assists in opposition	Capitate bone Bases of 2nd and 3rd metacarpals Palmar surface of 3rd metacarpal	Ulnar surface of the base of the proximal phalanx of the thumb Via a slip into the extensor expansion	Deep palmar branch	C8, T1
Dorsal Interossei	Abduction of the 3rd, 4th and 5th fingers Assists in MCP flexion Assists in extension of the IP joints	Thumb • Ulnar border of 1st metacarpal • Radial border of 2nd metacarpal 2nd, 3rd, and 4th fingers • Adjacent sides of metacarpals	Thumb • Radial border of the 2nd finger 2nd • Radial side of the 3rd finger 3rd • Ulnar side of 3rd finger 4th • Ulnar side of 4th finger	Deep palmar branch	C8, T1
Flexor Digiti Minimi	5th MCP joint flexion Assists in opposition	Hook of the hamate bone Flexor retinaculum	Ulnar border of the proximal phalanx of the 5th finger	Ulnar	C8, T1
Flexor Pollicis Brevis	1st MCP joint flexion 1st CMC joint flexion Assists in opposition	Flexor retinaculum Trapezoid Capitate	Radial surface of the base of the proximal phalanx Via a slip into the extensor expansion	Median Deep palmar branch	C6, C7 C8, T1

Lumbricales	Flexion of the 2nd through 5th MCP joints Extension of the PIP and DIP joints	1st and 2nd • Radial surface of flexor profundus tendons 3rd • Adjacent sides of flexor profundus tendons of 3rd and 4th fingers 4th • Adjacent sides of flexor profundus tendons of the 4th and 5th fingers	Radial border of the extensor tendons of the respective digits	1st and 2nd: Median 3rd and 4th: Deep palmar branch	C6, C7 C8, T1
Opponens Digiti Minimi	Opposition of the 5th finger	Hook of the hamate bone Flexor retinaculum	Ulnar border of the length of the 5th metacarpal	Ulnar	C8, T1
Opponens Pollicis	Thumb opposition	Flexor retinaculum Trapezium	Length of the 1st metacarpal	Median	C6, C7
Palmar Interossei	Adducts 1st, 2nd, 4th, and 5th fingers Assists in flexion of the MCP joints	Thumb • Ulnar border of the 1st metacarpal 2nd • Ulnar border of the 2nd metacarpal 3rd • Radial border of the 4th metacarpal 4th • Radial border of the 5th metacarpal	Thumb • Ulnar border of thumb 2nd • Ulnar side of 2nd finger 3rd • Radial side of ring finger • Radial side of little finger	Deep palmar branch	C8, T1

CMC = carpometacarpal; DIP = distal interphalangeal; IP = interphalangeal; MCP = metacarpophalangeal; PIP = proximal interphalangeal.

Passive Range of Motion, Wrist

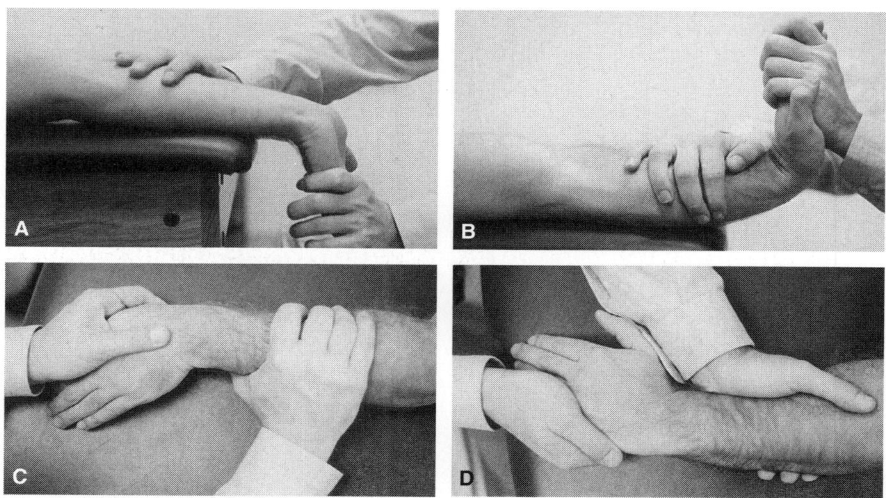

FIGURE 18-6 ■ Passive range of motion of the wrist: **(A)** flexion; **(B)** extension; **(C)** radial deviation; **(D)** ulnar deviation.

Passive Range of Motion, Thumb

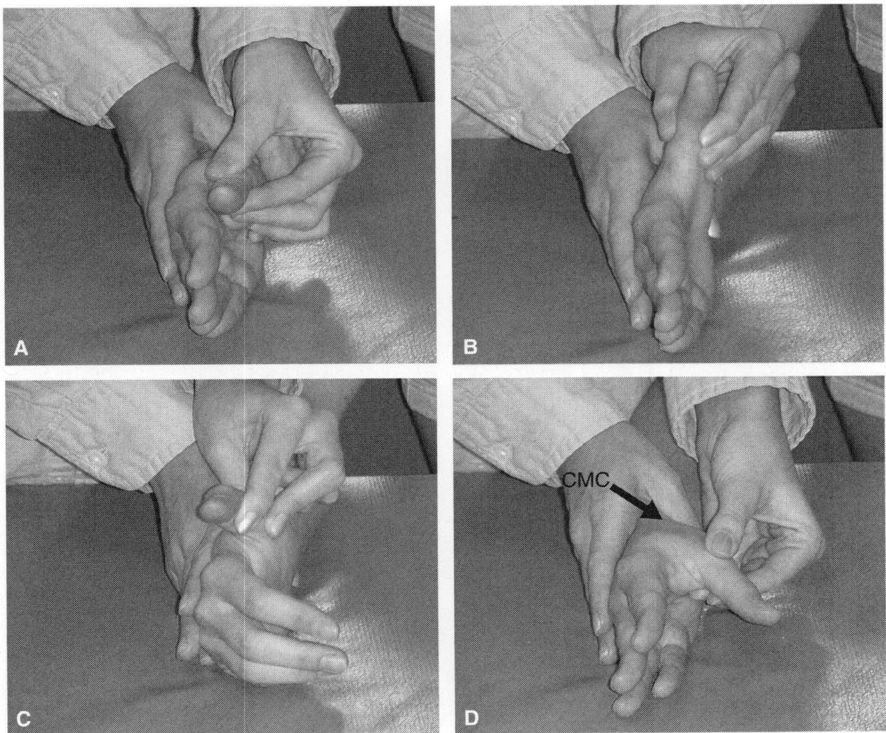

FIGURE 18-7 ■ Passive range of motion of the first carpometacarpal joint: **(A)** flexion, **(B)** extension, **(C)** adduction, **(D)** abduction. Do not confuse CMC motion with motion produced by the MP joint.

Passive Range of Motion, Finger

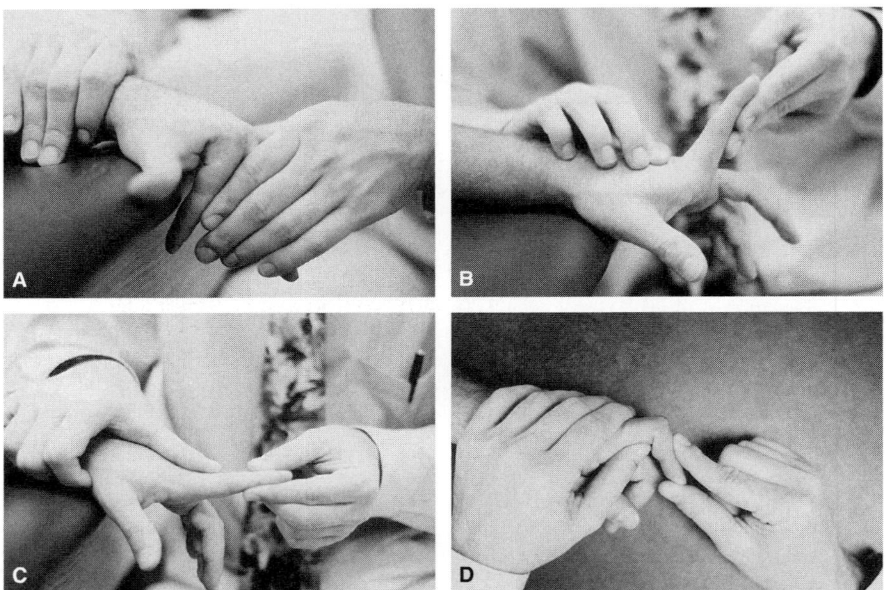

FIGURE 18-8 ■ Passive finger range of motion: **(A)** flexion and **(B)** extension of the metacarpophalangeal joint; **(C)** extension of the proximal interphalangeal joint; **(D)** flexion of the proximal interphalangeal joint.

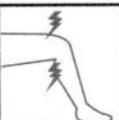

Stress Test 18-1
Radial Collateral and Ulnar Collateral Ligament Stress Tests of the Wrist

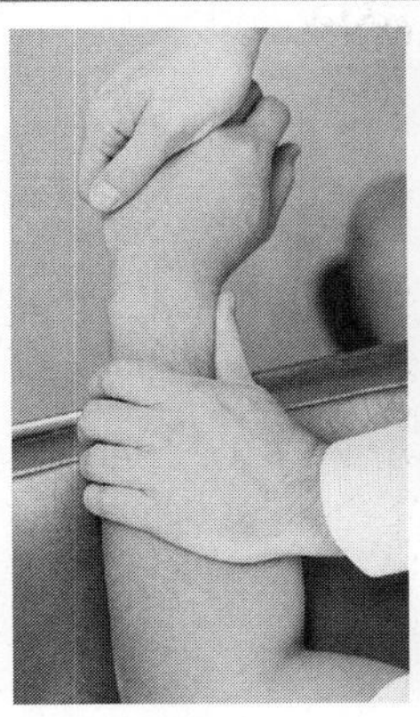

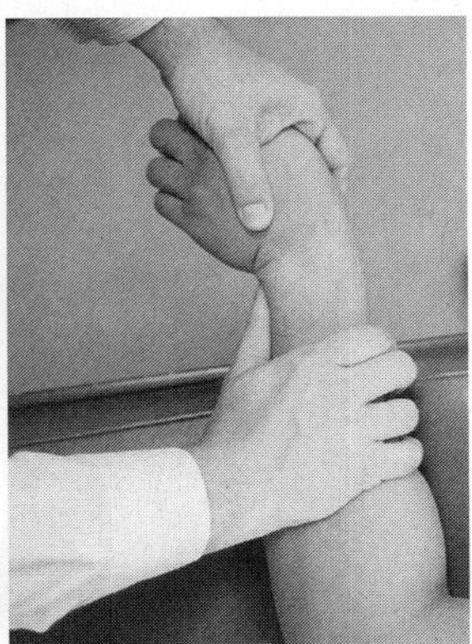

Although of limited clinical use, a valgus stress assesses the ulnar collateral ligament. A varus test stresses the radial collateral ligament of the wrist.

Patient Position	Sitting The elbow flexed to 90°, the forearm pronated, and the fingers assuming the relaxed position of flexion
Position of Examiner	Sitting or standing lateral to the wrist being tested One hand grips the distal forearm and the other grasps the hand across the metacarpals.
Evaluative Procedure	UCL: A valgus stress is applied, radially deviating the wrist. RCL: A varus stress is applied, ulnarly deviating the wrist.
Positive Test	Pain or laxity (or both) compared with the same ligament on the opposite wrist
Implications	Sprain of the UCL or RCL
Comments	Pain may be elicited in the presence of trauma to the triangular fibrocartilage, scaphoid fractures, or the palmar or dorsal radiocarpal or ulnocarpal ligaments. These tests are rarely positive for hypermobility.
Evidence	Absent or inconclusive in the literature

RCL = radial collateral ligament; UCL = ulnar collateral ligament.

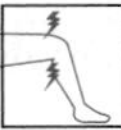

Stress Test 18-2
Valgus and Varus Testing of the Interphalangeal Joints

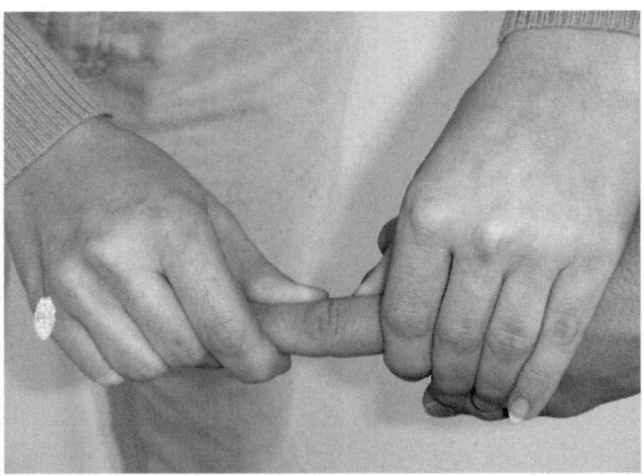

Stress testing the ulnar collateral ligament of the PIP joint. This test should be repeated using varus stress for the radial collateral ligament.

Patient Position	Sitting or standing The joint being tested is in extension.
Position of Examiner	Standing in front of the patient, stabilizing the phalanx proximal to the joint being tested
Evaluative Procedure	The examiner grasps the phalanx distal to the joint being tested and applies a valgus stress to the joint. A varus stress is then applied to the joint.
Positive Test	Increased gapping, compared with the same motion on the same finger of the opposite hand Pain
Implications	Collateral ligament sprain Avulsion fracture
Comments	Except in the case of a complete disruption of the ligament, the degree of injury to the ligament cannot be established. Avoid placing the stabilizing finger over the ligament.
Evidence	Absent or inconclusive in the literature

PIP = proximal interphalangeal.

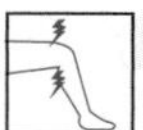

Stress Test 18-3
Test for Laxity of the Thumb MCP Collateral Ligaments

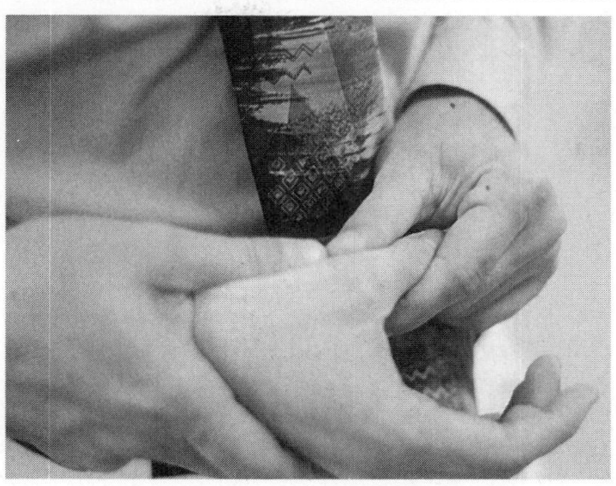

A valgus and varus stress is applied to the MCP joint to determine the integrity of the ulnar collateral and radial collateral ligaments.

Patient Position	Sitting or standing
Position of Examiner	Standing in front of the patient
Evaluative Procedure	The examiner stabilizes the first metacarpal with one hand and its proximal phalanx with the other. While stabilizing the first metacarpal with the thumb slightly abducted and extended, the examiner applies a valgus stress to the ulnar collateral ligament. In extension, the test stresses the accessory collateral ligament. In full flexion, the collateral ligament proper is stressed.
Positive Test	The ulnar side of the first MCP joint gaps farther than the uninjured side or the patient describes pain (or both).
Implications	Sprain of the ulnar collateral ligament Avulsion fracture
Comments	Avoid stabilizing over the MCP ligament stressed.
Evidence	Absent or inconclusive in the literature

MCP = metacarpophalangeal.

Joint Play Tests

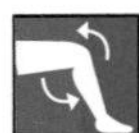

Joint Play 18-1
Radiocarpal and Midcarpal Joint Play

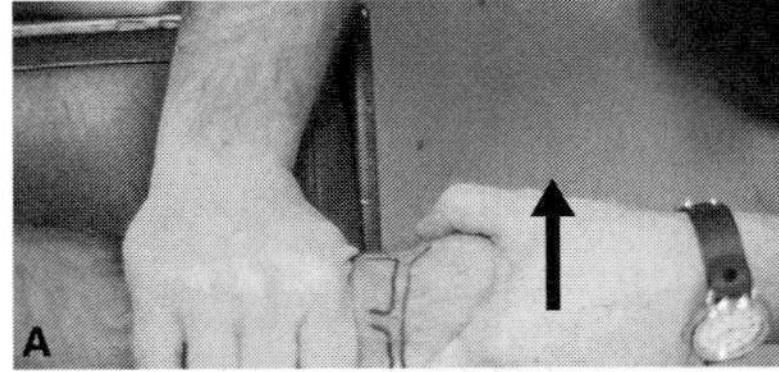

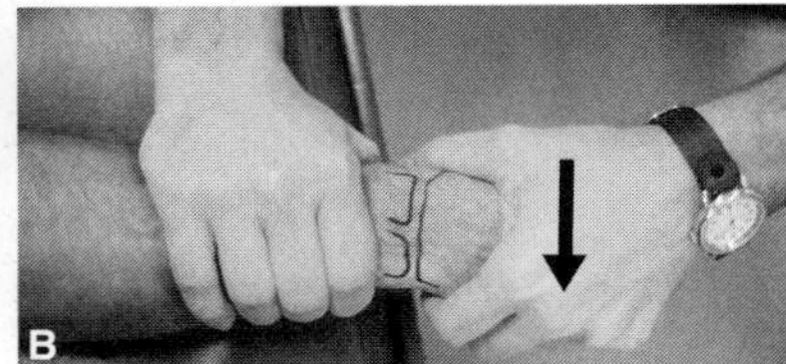

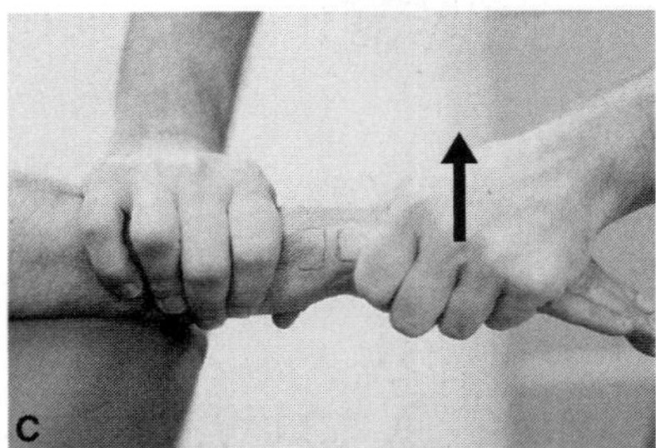

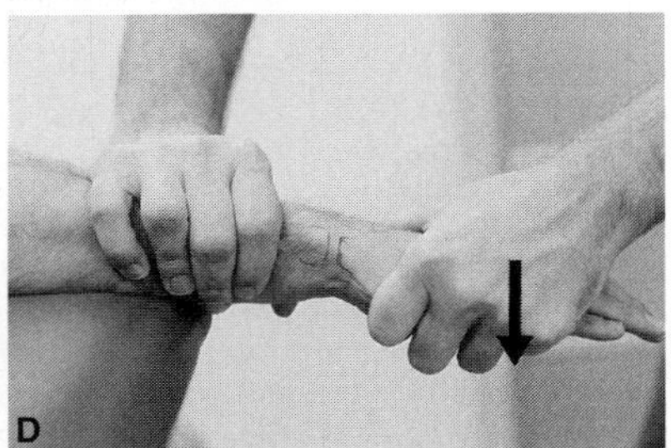

Joint play of the radiocarpal joint: radial glide **(A)**; ulnar glide **(B)**; dorsal glide **(C)**; and palmar glide **(D)**. Note that the hands are spread to allow visualization of the bones in the photographs. When performed clinically the hands should almost be touching.

Patient Position	Sitting The elbow is flexed to 90°, the forearm pronated, and the fingers in a relaxed position.
Position of Examiner	Sitting or standing lateral to the wrist being tested Radiocarpal joint: One hand grips the distal radius and the other hand grasps the proximal carpal row. Midcarpal joint: The proximal hand stabilizes the proximal carpal row, immediately distal to the radius. The other hand is immediately distal to the proximal row.
Evaluative Procedure	A shear force is applied to the wrist by gliding the distal segment in a radial and ulnar direction and then in a dorsal and palmar direction.
Positive Test	Pain or significant change in glide compared with the opposite side
Implications	Sprain of the collateral or intercarpal ligaments or trauma to the triangular fibrocartilage. Decreased glide may indicate adhesions and capsular stiffness after injury or surgery.
Comment	Radial and ulnar glide stresses both collateral ligaments; the determination of which ligament is involved is based on the location of pain.
Evidence	Absent or inconclusive in the literature

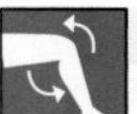

Joint Play 18-2
Intercarpal Joint Play

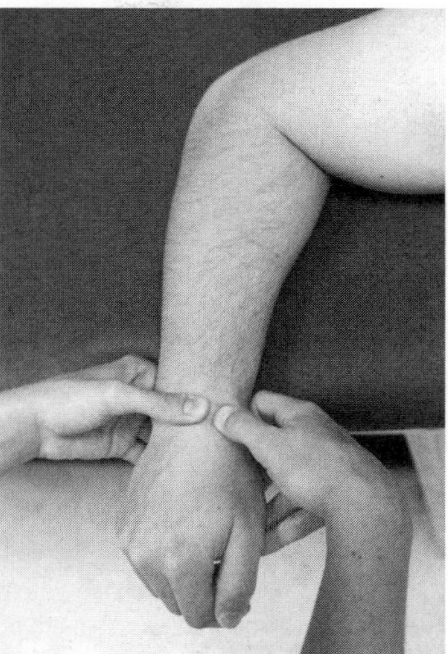

Joint play of the intercarpal articulations. Joint play of the scapholunate articulation is shown above.

Patient Position	Sitting The elbow is flexed to 90°, the forearm pronated, and the fingers in a relaxed position.
Position of Examiner	Sitting or standing lateral to the wrist being tested The thumb and index finger of one hand stabilize one carpal, with the thumb and index finger of the other hand stabilizing the other (or the radius).
Evaluative Procedure	A dorsal or palmar shear force is applied to one carpal while stabilizing the other.
Positive Test	Pain or significant change in glide compared with the opposite side
Implications	Tear or stretching of the intercarpal ligaments. Decreased glide may indicate adhesions and capsular stiffness after injury or surgery.
Modification	Apply slight traction to the wrist during the test.
Comment	A systematic approach to testing each intercarpal articulation is required.
Evidence	Absent or inconclusive in the literature

Special Test 18-1
Grip Dynamometry

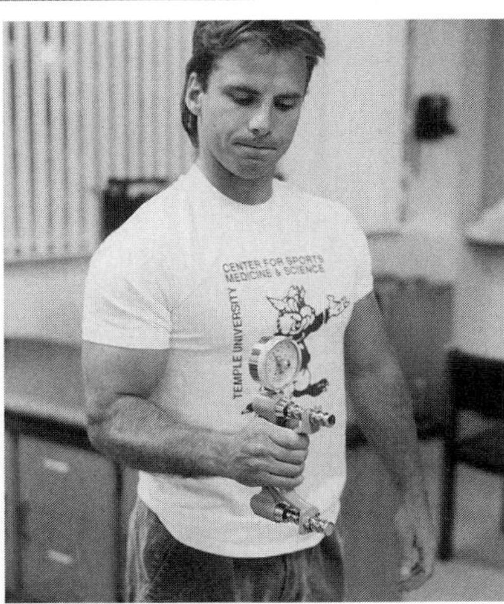

Use of a grip dynamometer provides a qualitative assessment of grip strength.

Patient Position	Holding the grip dynamometer with the elbow flexed to 90° and the radioulnar joint in its neutral position
Position of Examiner	Standing in front of the patient, viewing the dynamometer's gauge
Evaluative Procedure	The dynamometer is set at one of five specified settings (1, 1.5, 2, 2.5, and 3 inches). The patient squeezes the dynamometer's handle with maximum force at every setting, with adequate recovery time allowed between bouts. The values are recorded and the test is repeated on the opposite hand.
Positive Test	***Injured nondominant hand:*** More than 10% bilateral strength deficit compared with the dominant hand ***Injured dominant hand:*** More than 5% bilateral strength deficit compared with the nondominant hand
Implications	Pathology that inhibits grip strength; the underlying cause of the weakness must be determined.
Comments	Because of the wide range of variation in grip strength, the outcome of each of these tests is most meaningful when compared with a baseline measure. This test can be repeated three times at any one setting and the results averaged.
Evidence	Inter-rater reliability: **Not Reliable** **Very Reliable** Poor Moderate Good 0 0.1 0.2 0.3 0.4 0.5 0.6 0.7 0.8 0.9 1.0

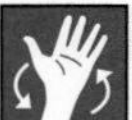

Special Test 18-2
Watson Test for Scapholunate Instability

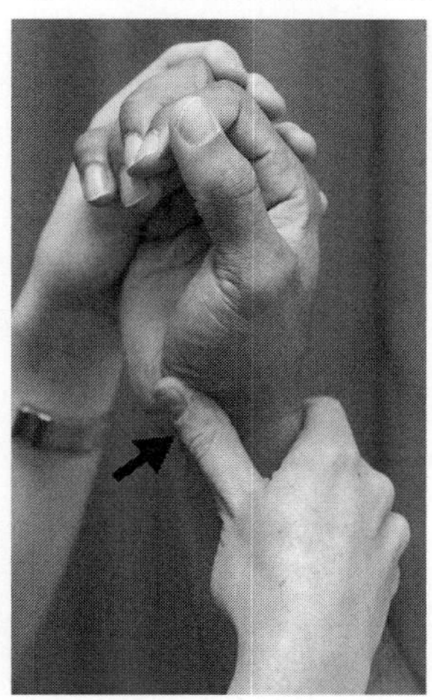

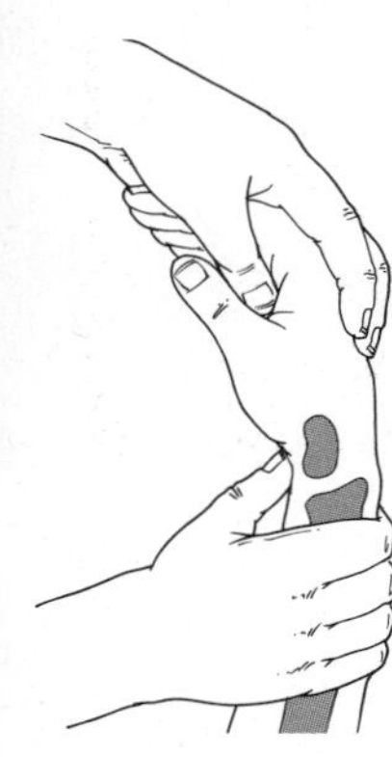

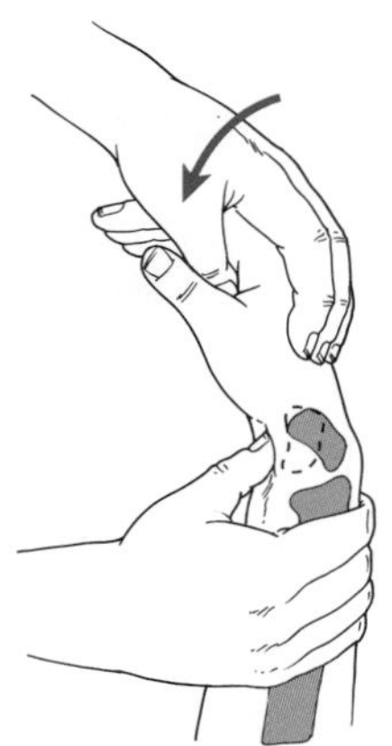

Application of a dorsally directed force attempts to shift the scaphoid from the lunate.

Patient Position	Seated with the elbow flexed and supported on the table and the forearm and hand pointing up, resembling the starting position for arm wrestling The wrist is ulnarly deviated.
Position of Examiner	In front of the patient
Evaluative Procedure	The examiner's thumb applies dorsal pressure to the distal pole of the scaphoid and then moves the patient's wrist from ulnar to radial deviation.
Positive Test	Reproduction of pain and notable pop at the scapholunate articulation
Implications	Scapholunate dissociation
Comments	This test may be difficult to perform on the acutely injured patient. Bilateral comparison is important because many patients have nonpathologic but positive findings.[107]
Evidence	Positive likelihood ratio Not Useful — Useful Very Small / Small / Moderate / Large 0 1 2 3 4 5 6 7 8 9 10 Negative likelihood ratio Not Useful — Useful Very Small / Small / Moderate / Large 1.0 0.9 0.8 0.7 0.6 0.5 0.4 0.3 0.2 0.1 0

Special Test 18-3
Phalen's Test for Carpal Tunnel Syndrome

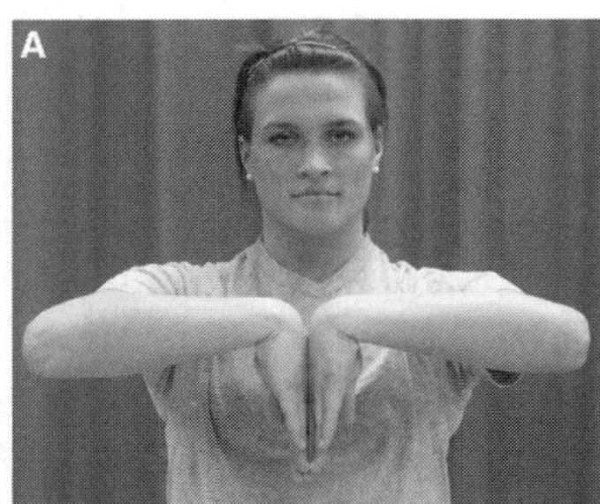

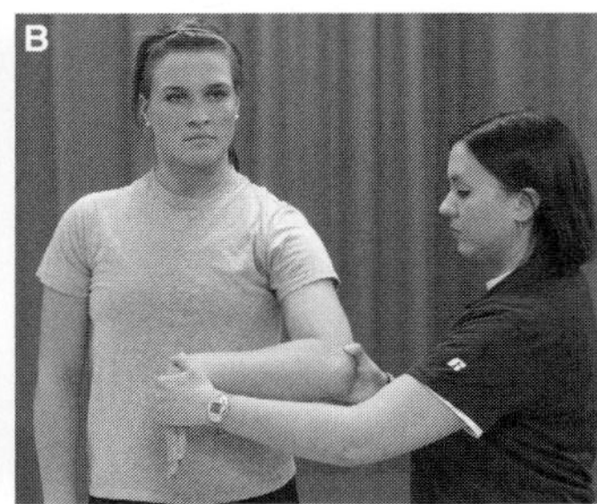

(A) Original test as described by Phalen. **(B)** Modification of Phalen's test (described below).

Patient Position	Standing or seated
Position of Examiner	Standing in front of the patient
Evaluative Procedure	The examiner applies overpressure during passive wrist flexion and holds the position for 1 minute. Repeat this procedure for the opposite extremity.
Positive Test	Tingling develops or increases in the distribution of the median nerve distal to the carpal tunnel.
Implications	Median nerve compression
Modification	The traditional version of this test, in which the patient maximally flexes the wrists by pushing the dorsal aspects of the hands together, is not recommended because the patient may shrug the shoulders, causing compression of the median branch of the brachial plexus as it passes through the thoracic outlet. Reverse Phalen's, with the wrist positioned in maximum extension, is an alternate position to stress the median nerve, with approximately the same diagnostic value.[108,109]
Comments	Patients with numbness may not have an exacerbation of symptoms with this test, leading to a false-negative result.[108]
Evidence	Inter-rater reliability Not Reliable — Very Reliable Poor / Moderate / Good 0 0.1 0.2 0.3 0.4 0.5 0.6 0.7 0.8 0.9 1.0 Positive likelihood ratio Not Useful — Useful Very Small / Small / Moderate / Large 0 1 2 3 4 5 6 7 8 9 10 Negative likelihood ratio Not Useful — Useful Very Small / Small / Moderate / Large 1.0 0.9 0.8 0.7 0.6 0.5 0.4 0.3 0.2 0.1 0

Test for Lunotriquetral Stability

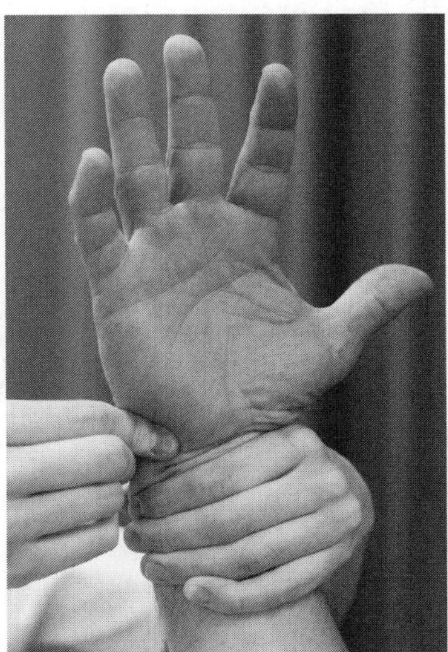

FIGURE 18-9 ■ A compressive force placed on the ulnar side of the triquetrum, compressing the proximal carpal row radially and a palmar to dorsal force applied over the lunotriquetral joint stress the lunotriquetral ligament.

Special Test 18-4
Finkelstein's Test for De Quervain's Syndrome

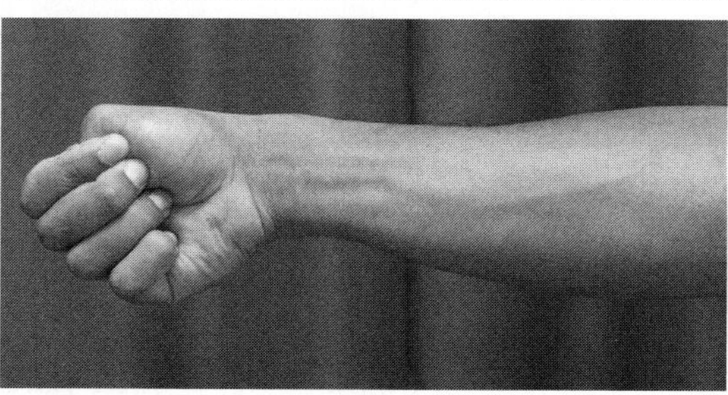

The patient ulnarly deviates the wrist while the thumb is clasped by the fingers.

Patient Position	Seated or standing
Position of Examiner	Standing in front of the patient
Evaluative Procedure	The patient tucks the thumb under the fingers by making a fist. The patient then ulnarly deviates the wrist.
Positive Test	Increased pain in the area of the radial styloid process and along the length of the extensor pollicis brevis and abductor pollicis longus tendons
Implications	De Quervain's syndrome (tenosynovitis of the extensor pollicis brevis and abductor pollicis longus tendons)
Comments	This test often produces false-positive results, so the results must be correlated with other findings of the evaluation.
Evidence	Absent or inconclusive in the literature

Nerve Distribution

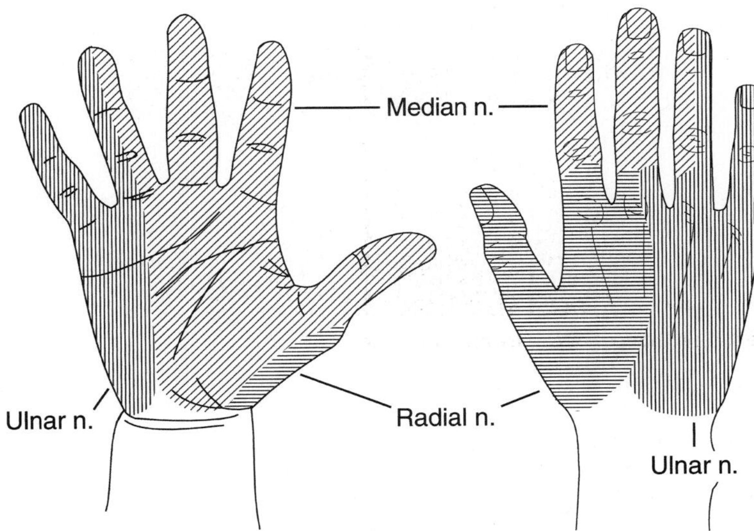

FIGURE 18-10 ■ Nerve distribution in the hand.

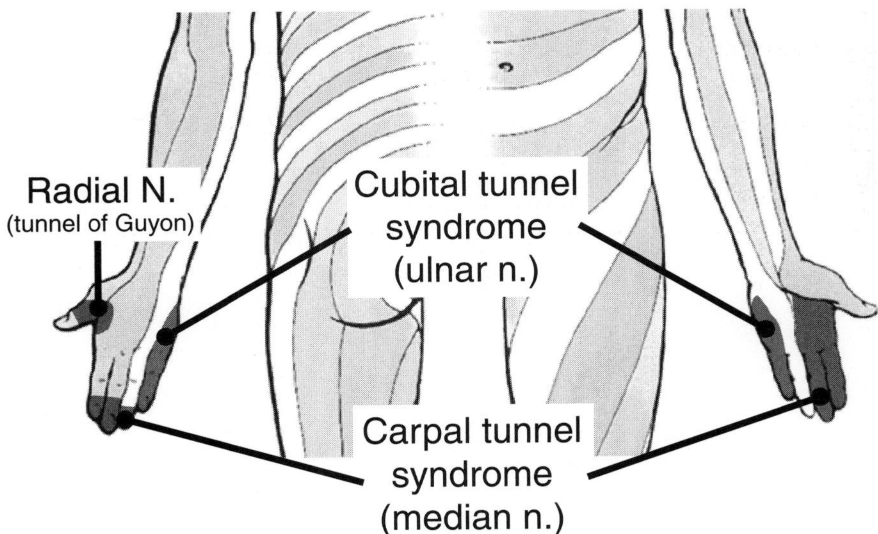

FIGURE 18-11 ■ Local neuropathies of the hand. Correlate these findings with those of an upper quarter neurologic screen (see Neurologic Screening Box 1-2).

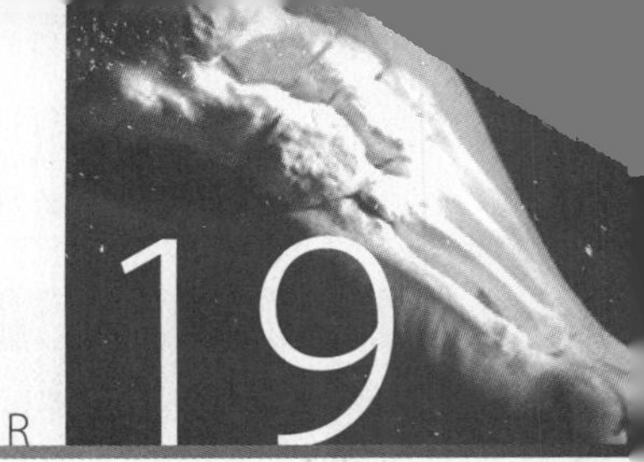

CHAPTER 19

Eye Pathologies

Examination Map

HISTORY

Past Medical History
Prior vision assessment
Mental health status

History of the Present Condition
General health status
Location of pain
Radicular symptoms
Mechanism of injury
Onset of condition

INSPECTION

Periorbital Area
Discoloration
Gross deformity

Inspection of the Globe
General appearance
- Eyelids
- Cornea
- Conjunctiva
- Sclera
- Iris
- Pupil shape and size

PALPATION

Orbital Margin
Frontal Bone
Nasal Bone
Zygomatic Bone
Soft Tissue

FUNCTIONAL ASSESSMENT

Vision Assessment
Pupillary Reaction to Light

NEUROLOGIC EXAMINATION

CN III, IV, VI

PATHOLOGIES AND SPECIAL TESTS

Orbital Fractures
Blowout fractures
Corneal Abrasion
Corneal Laceration
Iritis
Hyphema
Retinal Detachment
Ruptured Globe
Conjunctivitis
Foreign Bodies

Table 19-1 Blunt Eye Trauma and the Resulting Eye Pathology*

Size Relative to the Orbit	Elastic Property	Resulting Pathology
Larger	Hard	Orbital fracture, periorbital contusion
Larger	Elastic	Blow-out fracture, ruptured globe, corneal abrasion, traumatic iritis, periorbital contusion
Smaller	Hard	Ruptured globe, corneal abrasion, corneal laceration, traumatic iritis
Smaller	Elastic	Ruptured globe, blow-out fracture, corneal abrasion, traumatic iritis

*All of these mechanisms of injury can result in subconjunctival hemorrhage and retinal pathology.

Table 19-2 Findings that Warrant an Immediate Referral to an Ophthalmologist

History	Inspection	Palpation	Functional Tests	Neurological Tests
Loss of all or part of the visual field Persistent blurred vision Diplopia Photophobia Throbbing or penetrating pain around or within the eye Description of mechanism for a ruptured globe Air escaping from the eyelid or pain when blowing the nose	Foreign body protruding into the eye Laceration involving the margin of the eyelid Deep laceration of the lid Inability to open the eyelid because of swelling Protrusion of the globe (or other obvious displacement) Injected conjunctiva with a small pupil Loss of corneal clarity Hyphema Pupillary distortion Unilateral pupillary dilation or constriction	Crepitus of the orbital rim	Restricted eye movement Double vision occurring with eye movement	Numbness or paresthesia over the lateral nose and cheek Pupillary reaction abnormality

Eyelid Laceration

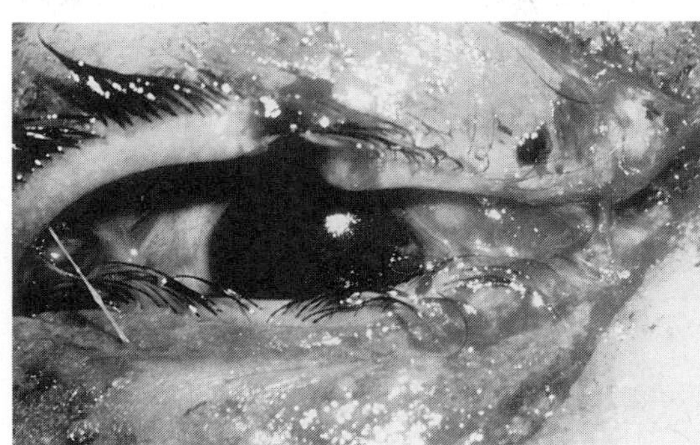

FIGURE 19-1 ■ This injury may also conceal underlying eye trauma.

Hyphema

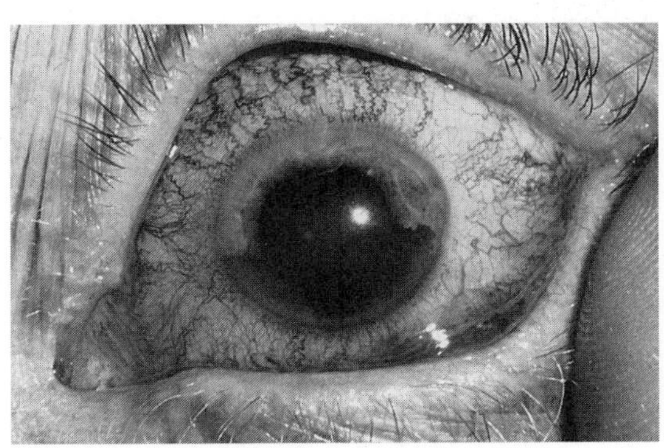

FIGURE 19-2 ■ A collection of blood within the anterior chamber of the eye.

Inspection of the Eye

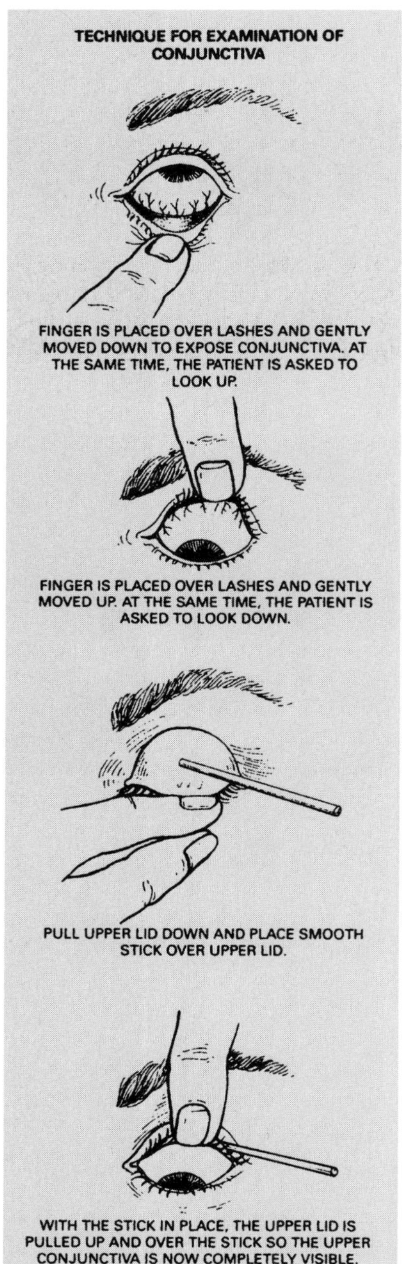

FIGURE 19-3 ■ The upper eyelid is inverted around a cotton-tipped applicator to expose the upper portion of the sclera and conjunctiva. (From Venes D, Ed: *Taber's cyclopedic medical dictionary*, ed 21, Beth Anne Willert, MS, medical illustrator. Philadelphia: FA Davis, 2009.)

Subconjunctival Hemorrhage

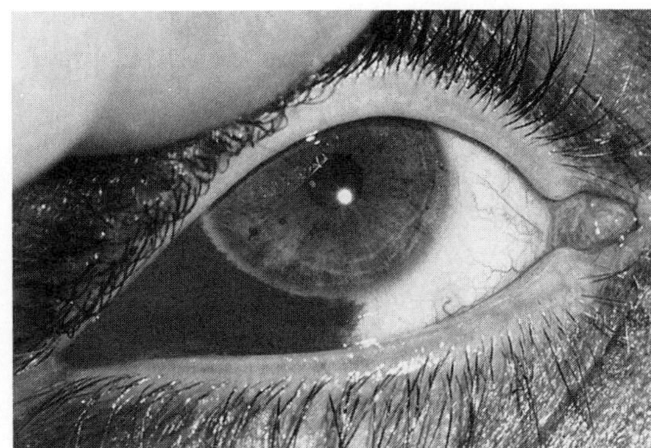

FIGURE 19-4 ■ Subconjunctival hemorrhage. This condition by itself is usually benign but may conceal underlying pathology.

Teardrop Pupil

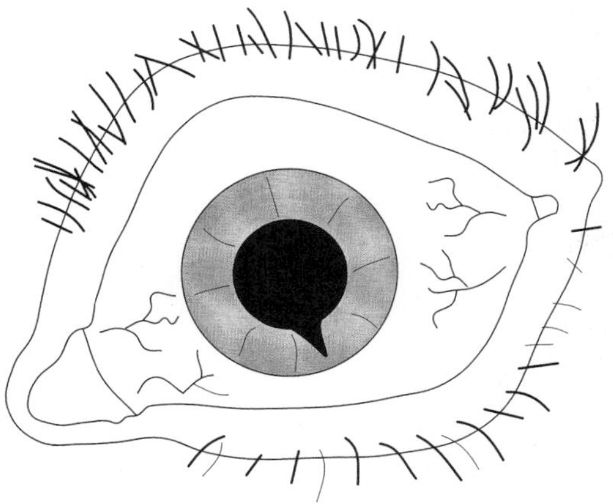

FIGURE 19-5 ■ This condition, or any other deviation in the normally round shape of the pupil, indicates serious underlying pathology such as a corneal laceration or ruptured globe.

Blow-out Fracture

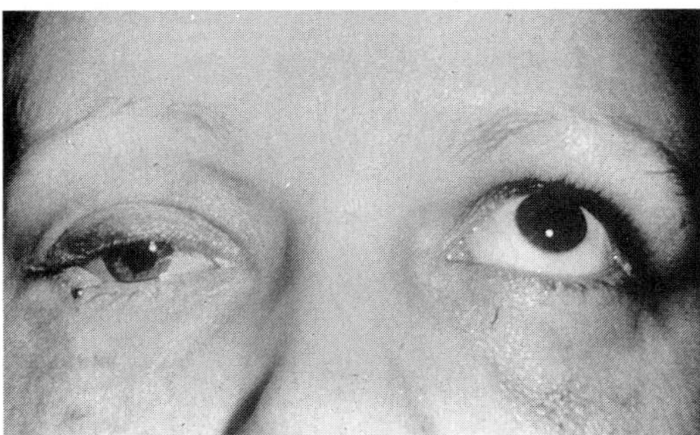

FIGURE 19-6 ■ Restriction of eye motion following a blow-out fracture of the orbital floor. The person's right eye is unable to gaze upward, indicating an entrapment of the inferior rectus muscle.

PALPATION

Palpation of the Orbital Area

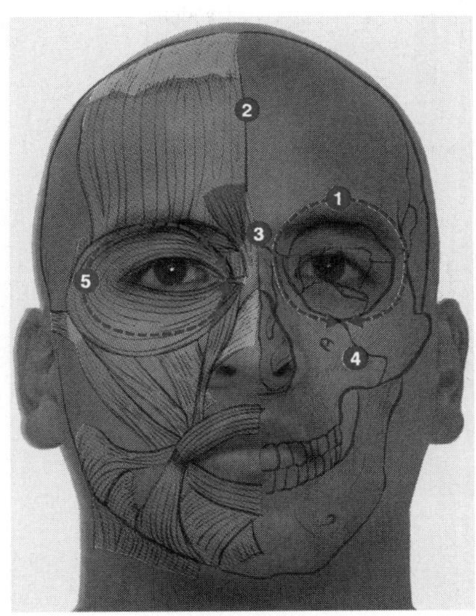

1 Orbital margin

2 Frontal bone

3 Nasal bone

4 Zygomatic bone

5 Periorbital area

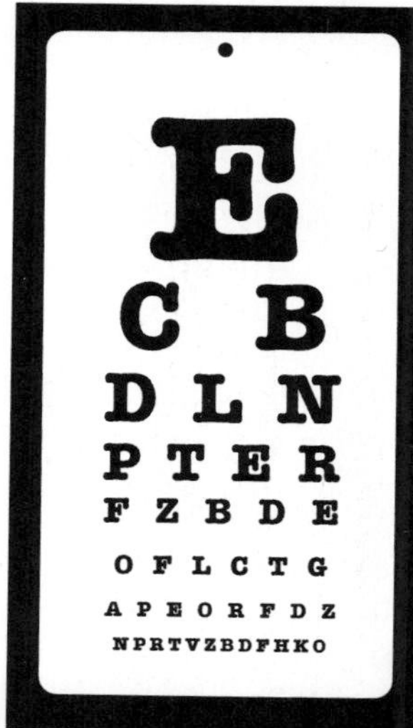

FIGURE 19-7 ■ Snellen-type chart. This device is commonly used to determine an individual's visual acuity.

Eye Motion

Table 19-1 Extrinsic Muscles Acting on the Eye

Muscle	Action	Origin	Insertion	Innervation	Root
Inferior Rectus	Downward rotation of the globe	From a tendinous ring on the posterior aspect of the orbit	Middle of the inferior aspect of the anterior globe	Oculomotor	CN III
Superior Rectus	Upward rotation of the globe	From a tendinous ring on the posterior aspect of the orbit	Middle of the superior aspect of the anterior globe	Oculomotor	CN III
Medial Rectus	Medial rotation of the globe	From a tendinous ring on the posterior aspect of the orbit	Middle of the medial aspect of the anterior globe	Oculomotor	CN III
Lateral Rectus	Lateral rotation of the globe	From a tendinous ring on the posterior aspect of the orbit	Middle of the lateral aspect of the anterior globe	Abducens	CN VI
Inferior Oblique	Adduction of the globe Elevation of the globe Rotation of the globe when abducted	From the periosteum of the maxilla	Inferolateral quadrant of the globe	Oculomotor	CN III
Superior Oblique	Abduction of the globe Depression of the globe Rotation of the globe when adducted	Greater wing of the sphenoid	Superolateral quadrant of the globe	Trochlear	CN IV

CN = cranial nerve.

Special Test 19-1
Pupillary Reaction Assessment

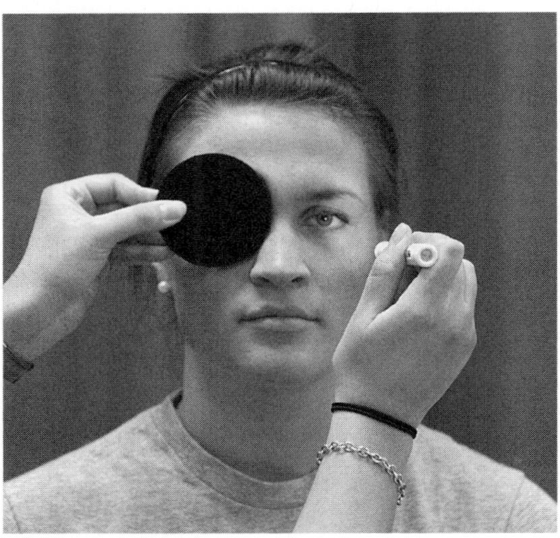

Checking for normal pupil reaction to light. If a penlight is not available, the eye tested can be covered and the pupil observed for constriction when the eye is exposed to light.

Patient Position	Sitting or standing
Position of Examiner	Standing in front of the patient
Evaluative Procedure	A card, an occluder, or the patient's hand is held in front of the eye not being tested. A penlight is used to shine light into the pupil for 1 s and then removed. The examiner observes for the pupil constricting when the light is applied and dilating when the light is removed. This process is repeated for the opposite eye.
Positive Test	A pupil that is unresponsive to light, reacts sluggishly compared with the opposite eye, or paradoxically dilates or constricts.
Implications	***Afferent lesion (retina or optic nerve):*** The involved pupil enlarges as the light is moved from the unaffected side to the affected side (paradoxical dilation). ***Efferent lesion (CN III or pupillary muscle lesion):*** The involved pupil does not react to light.[110]
Evidence	Absent or inconclusive in the literature

CN = cranial nerve.

Special Test 19-2
Assessment of Eye Motility

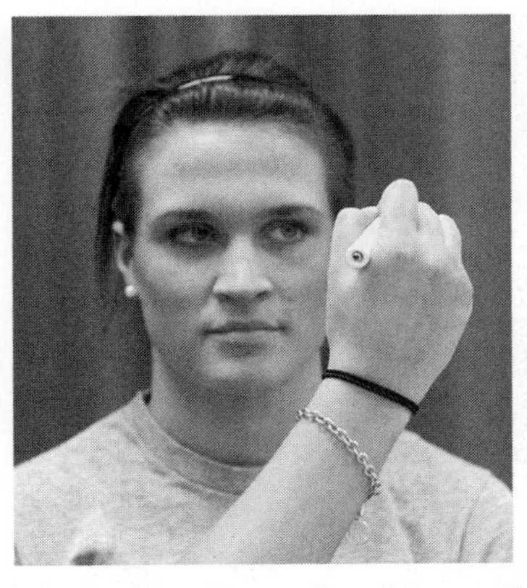

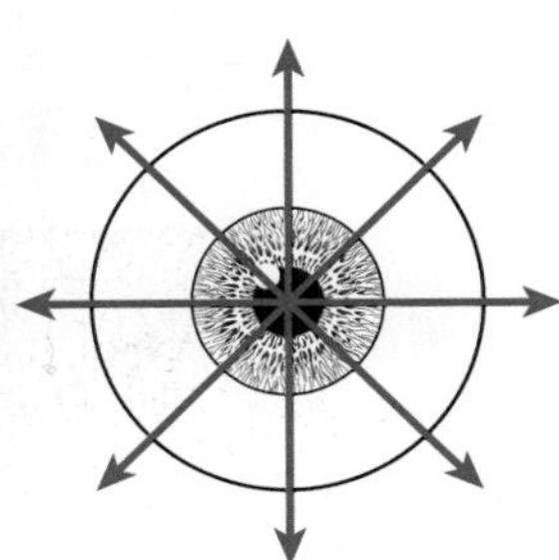

Checking the range of motion, motility, of the eye. The eyes should track smoothly and travel an equal distance.

Patient Position	Sitting or standing
Position of Examiner	Standing in front of the patient, holding a finger approximately 2 ft. from the patient's nose
Evaluative Procedure	The patient focuses on the examiner's finger and is instructed to report any double vision experienced during test. The examiner moves the finger upward, downward, left, and right relative to the starting point. The patient follows this motion using only the eyes and is allowed to fix the gaze at the terminal end of each movement. The finger is then moved through the diagonal fields of gaze.
Positive Test	Asymmetrical tracking of the eyes or double vision produced at the end of the ROM.
Implications	Decreased motility of the eyes as the result of neurologic or muscular trauma or decreased vision.
Evidence	Absent or inconclusive in the literature

ROM = range of motion.

Special Test 19-3
Fluorescent Dye Test for Corneal Abrasions

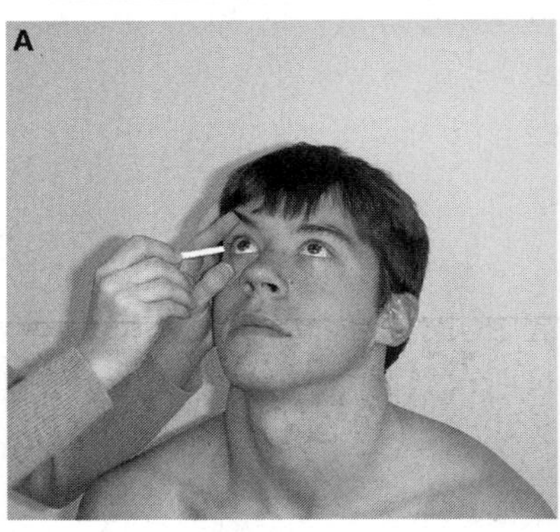

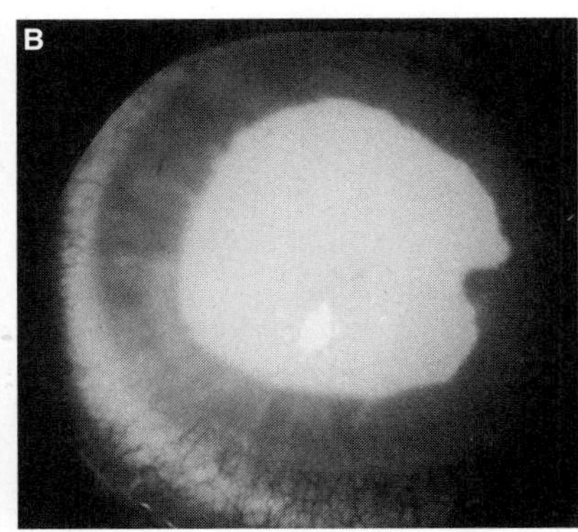

(A) A fluorescein strip is lightly touched to the conjunctiva. **(B)** A cobalt-blue light is shined into the eye to highlight the abraded area.

Patient Position	Seated or supine
Position of Examiner	Standing in front of or beside the patient
Evaluative Procedure	Soak the fluorescein strip with sterile saline solution. Lightly touch the wet fluorescein strip to the conjunctiva of the lower eyelid for a few seconds. Avoid placing the strip directly on the cornea. Ask the patient to blink the eye a few times to spread the solution. Darken the room and use a cobalt blue light to illuminate the eye.
Positive Test	When viewed with the cobalt blue light, corneal abrasions appear as a bright yellow-green pattern on the eye.
Implications	A corneal abrasion
Evidence	Absent or inconclusive in the literature

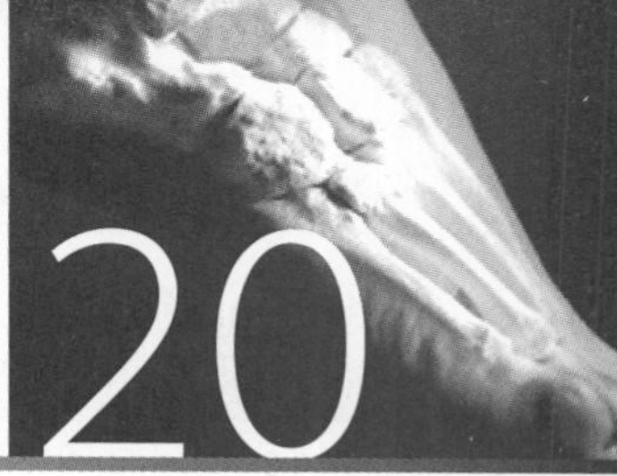

CHAPTER 20

Face and Related Structures Pathologies

Examination Map

HISTORY

Location of Pain
Onset
Activity and Injury Mechanism
Symptoms

INSPECTION

Inspection of the Ear
Auricle
Tympanic membrane
Periauricular area

Inspection of the Nose
Alignment
Epistaxis
Septum and mucosa
Eyes and face

Inspection of the Nose
Respiration
Thyroid and cricoid cartilage

Inspection of the Face and Jaw
Bleeding
Ecchymosis
Symmetry
Muscle tone

Inspection of the Oral Cavity
Lips
Teeth
Tongue
Lingual frenulum
Gums

PALPATION

Palpation of the Anterior Structures
Nasal bone
Nasal cartilage
Zygoma
Maxilla
Temporomandibular joint
Periauricular area
External ear
Teeth
Mandible
Hyoid bone
Cartilages

Palpation of the Lateral Structures
Temporalis
Masseter
Buccinator

FUNCTIONAL ASSESSMENT

Ear
Hearing
Balance

Nose
Smell

Temporomandibular Joint
Range of motion
Tracking

NEUROLOGIC EXAMINATION

Cranial Nerve Assessment

Continued

Examination Map—cont'd

PATHOLOGIES AND SPECIAL TESTS

Ear Pathologies
Auricular hematoma

Tympanic membrane rupture

Otitis externa

Otitis media

Nasal Pathologies

Throat Pathologies

Facial Pathologies
Mandibular fracture

Zygoma fracture

Maxillary fracture

LeFort fracture

Dental Conditions
Tooth fracture

Tooth luxation

Dental caries

Temporomandibular Joint Dysfunction

Inspection Findings 20-1
Use of an Otoscope for Inspection of the Ear and Nose

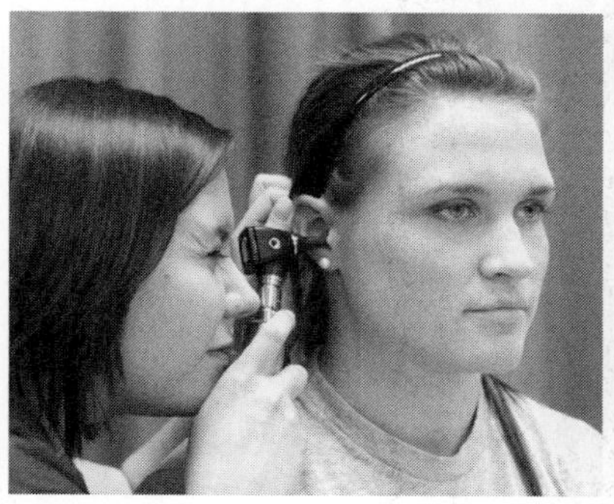

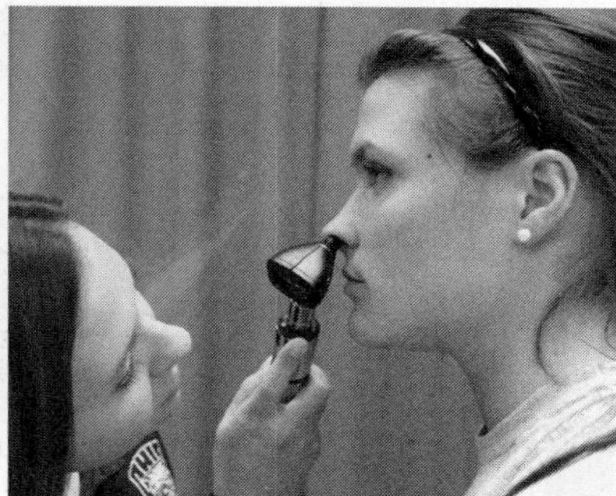

An otoscope with a speculum that fits snugly within the ear canal, without causing pain, is used to inspect the tympanic membrane. The speculum needs to be placed only slightly into the ear canal to view the structures. Visualization is improved when the pinna is pulled upward and backward (some clinicians prefer to pull the earlobe downward).

An otoscope is used to visualize the tympanic membrane and nasal passage.

Patient Position	Seated or standing
Position of Examiner	Position to easily access the patient's ear or nose.
Evaluative Procedure	Select and fit a speculum on the otoscope that will fit snugly into the opening. When inspecting the ear, open the auditory canal by gently pulling upward and backward on the pinna or downward on the earlobe. Look through the otoscope and insert it gently into the canal. Deep penetration is not necessary.
Positive Test	***Ear:*** Reddened and/or bulging tympanic membrane; fluid buildup behind the tympanic membrane; fluid in the ear canal; ruptured tympanic membrane ***Nose:*** Deviation or deformity of the nasal passage(s)
Implications	***Ear:*** Reddened and/or bulging tympanic membrane is indicative of middle ear infection (acute otitis media). Fluid behind the tympanic membrane (otitis media effusion) is not necessarily indicative of an infection. Fluid in the ear canal may represent otorrhea, or leakage of cerebrospinal fluid, and is associated with a skull fracture. A ruptured tympanic membrane may result from a blow to the ear ***Nose:*** Fracture, deviated septum
Comments	Cerumen may obscure the tympanic membrane. To clear cerumen, gently flush the ear with hydrogen peroxide or warm water. Do not do this if a tympanic membrane rupture is suspected.
Evidence	Absent or inconclusive in the literature

External Ear Laceration

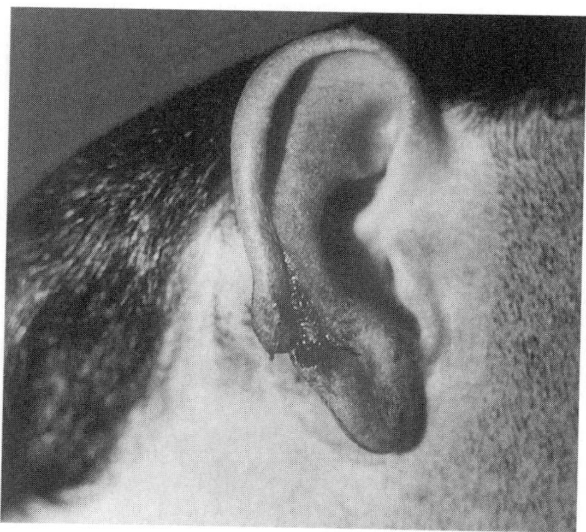

FIGURE 20-1 ■ Laceration of the external ear. This injury requires suturing to prevent permanent deformity of the ear.

Auricular Hematoma

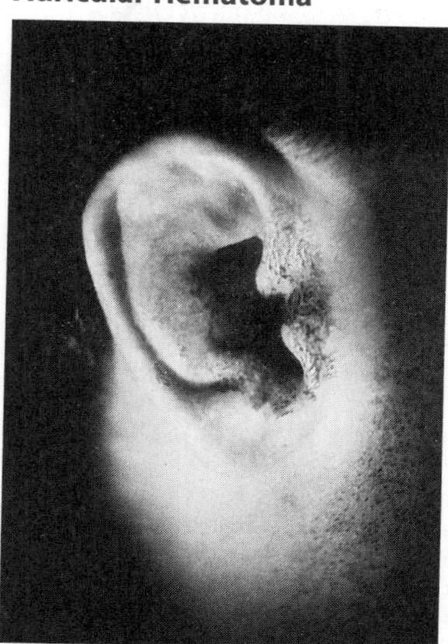

FIGURE 20-2 ■ Auricular hematoma, or "cauliflower ear." This condition is shown in its acute stage. If the hematoma is allowed to develop, the underlying cartilage is destroyed, resulting in permanent deformity of the external ear. Hearing acuity is affected secondary to the decreased ability to funnel sound waves into the middle ear.

Suborbital Hematoma

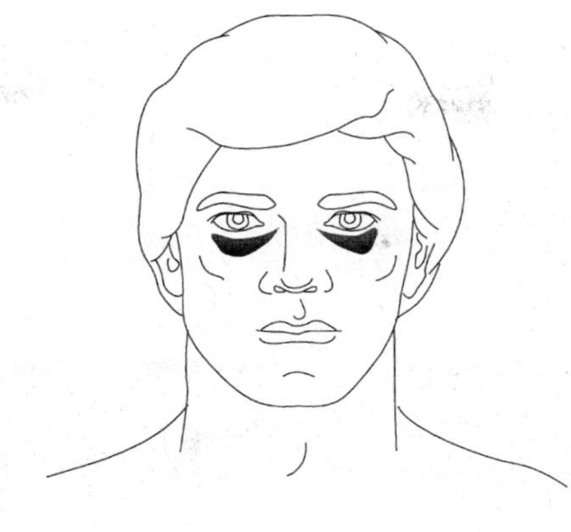

FIGURE 20-3 ■ Raccoon eyes. After a nasal fracture, blood lost because of hemorrhage follows the contour of the face and pools beneath the eyes. This condition can also result from a skull fracture.

Inspection of the Oral Cavity

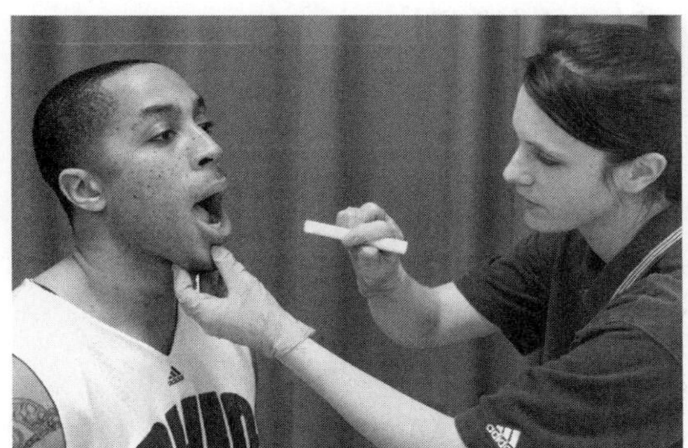

FIGURE 20-4 ■ Inspection of the oral cavity to rule out tooth fractures and to locate the source of bleeding.

Inspection of the Lingual Frenulum

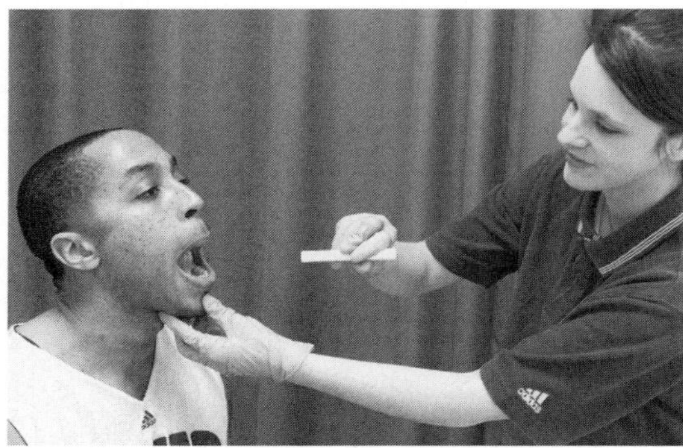

FIGURE 20-5 ■ Inspection of the lingual frenulum. The patient is asked to lift the tongue to the roof of the mouth.

Observation for Malocclusion of the Teeth

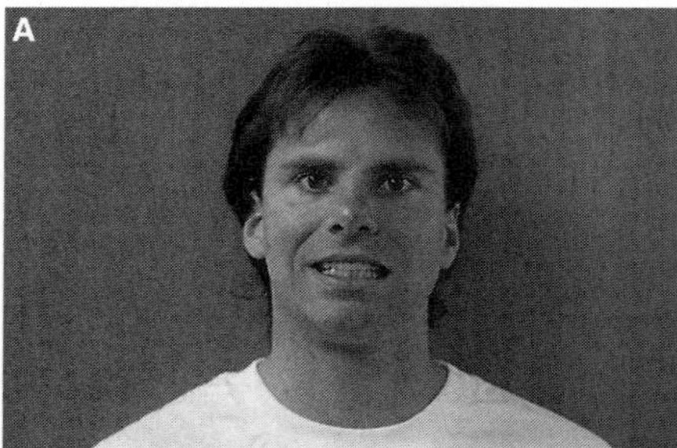

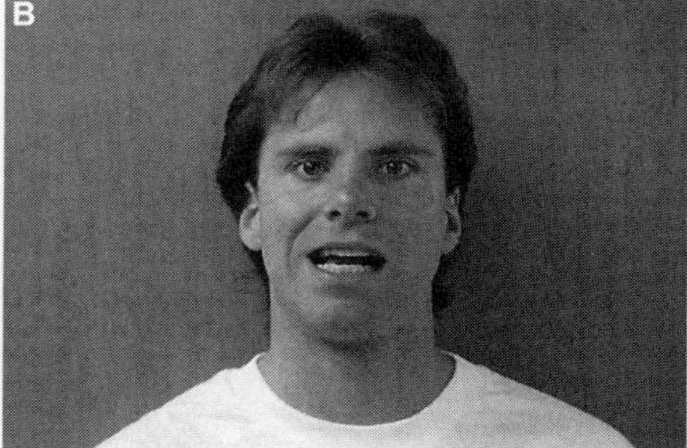

FIGURE 20-6 ■ **(A)** Normally, the mandible travels in a straight line. **(B)** Trauma to the temporomandibular joint or a fracture of the mandible causes the jaw to track laterally and results in a malalignment of the teeth.

Numbering System for Referencing the Teeth

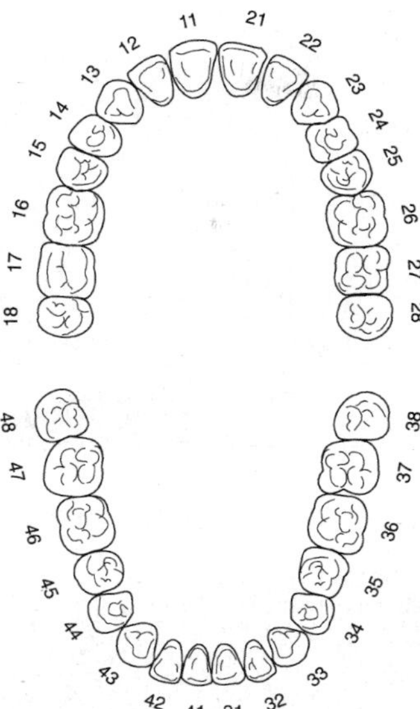

FIGURE 20-7 ■ The upper right teeth are numbered by 10s, the upper left by 20s, the lower left by 30s, and the lower right by 40s.

Tooth Fractures

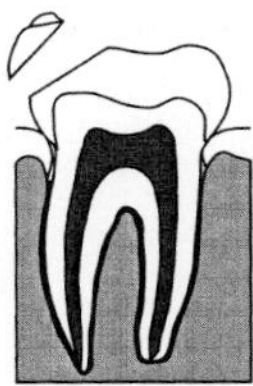

Class I

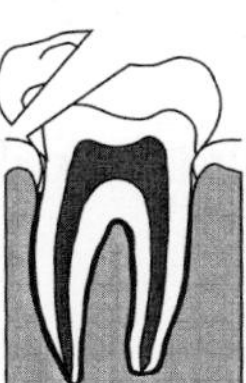

Class II

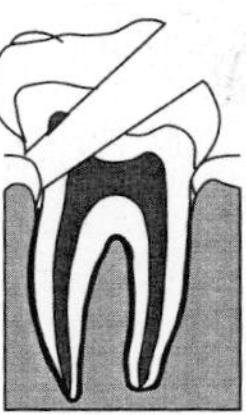

Class III

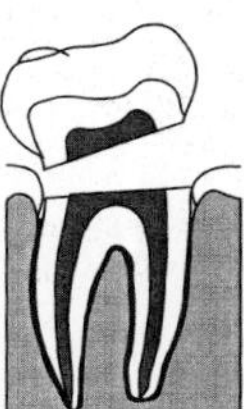

Class IV

FIGURE 20-8 ■ Classification scheme for tooth fractures.

Tooth Luxations

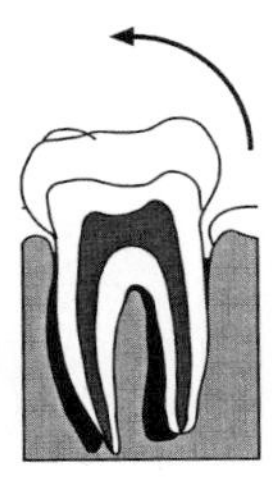

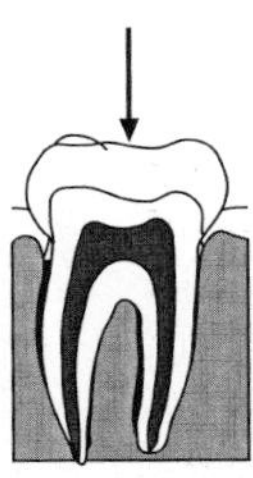

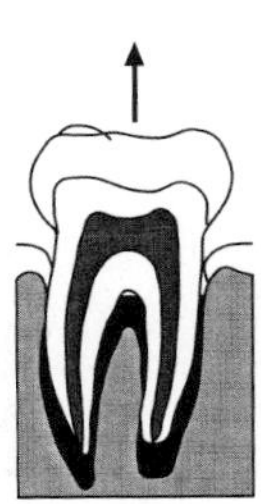

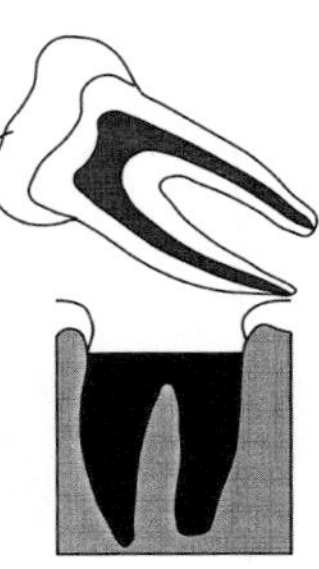

FIGURE 20-9 ■ Classification scheme for tooth luxations.

Root Fractures

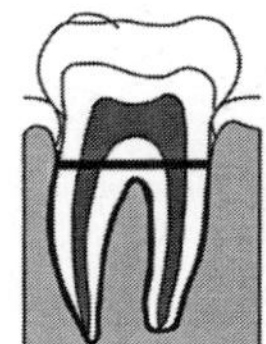

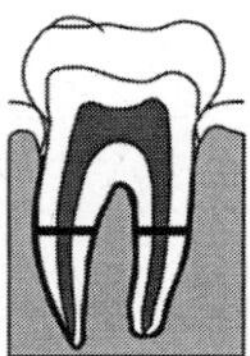

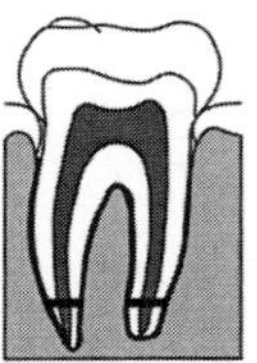

FIGURE 20-10 ■ Classification scheme for root fractures.

PALPATION

Palpation of the Anterior Structures

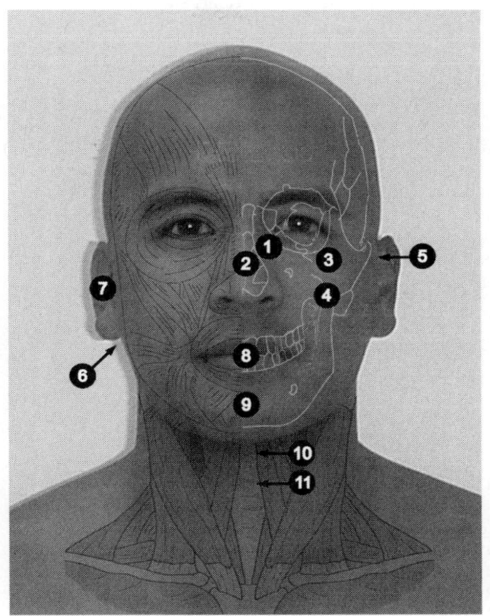

1 Nasal bone

2 Nasal cartilage

3 Zygoma

4 Maxilla

5 Temporomandibular joint

6 Periauricular area

7 External ear

8 Teeth

9 Mandible

10 Hyoid bone

11 Cartilages

Palpation of the Lateral Structures

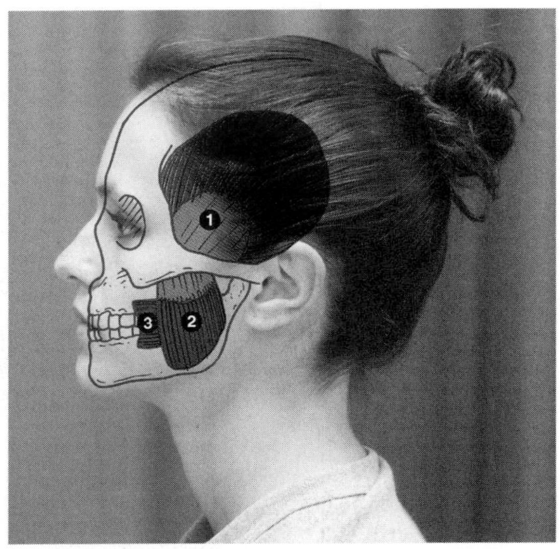

1 Temporalis

2 Masseter

3 Buccinator

Palpation of the External Temporomandibular Joint

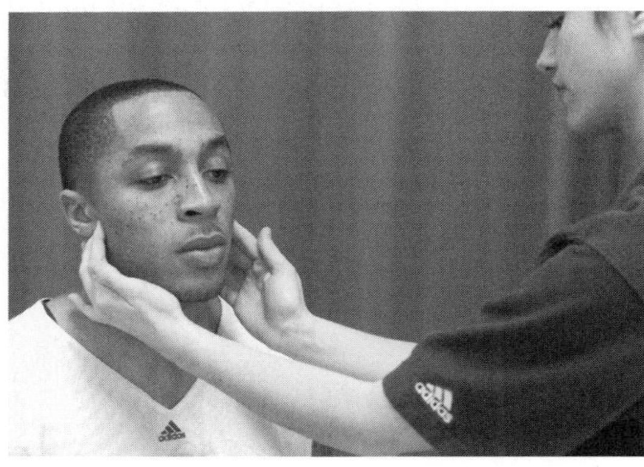

FIGURE 20-11 ■ The temporomandibular joint is palpated while the mouth is opened and closed. Asymmetry of movement and clicking or locking of the joint are noted.

Palpation of the Internal Temporomandibular Joint

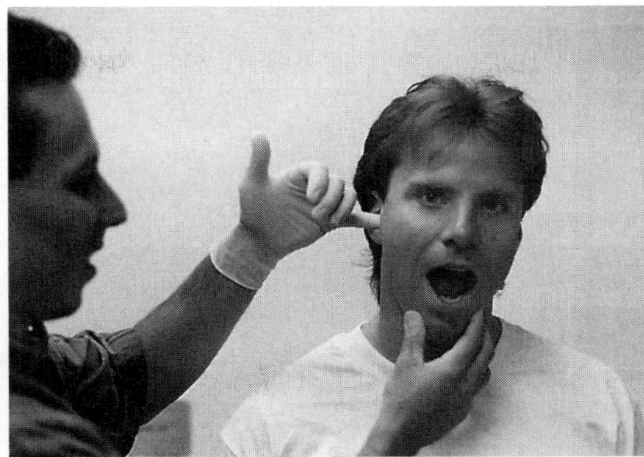

FIGURE 20-12 ■ Wearing gloves, the examiner lightly places a finger in the outermost portion of the auditory canal to further palpate the mechanics of the temporomandibular joint as the mouth is opened and closed.

Palpation of the Teeth

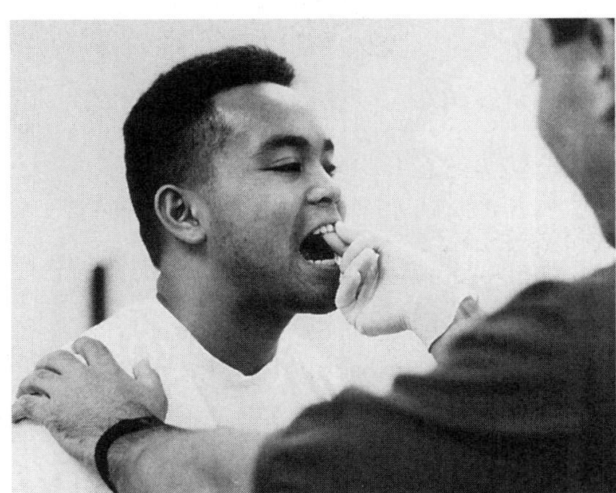

FIGURE 20-13 ■ Because of the possibility of exposure to bloodborne pathogens, gloves must be worn during this process.

Special Test 20-1
Temporomandibular Joint Range of Motion

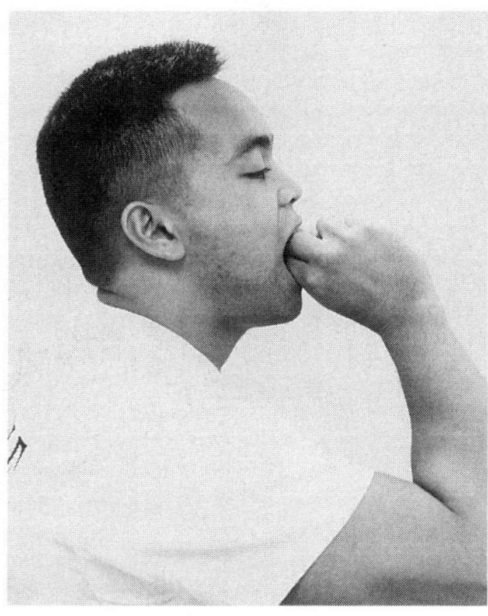

The temporomandibular joint should provide enough motion to allow two fingers to be inserted into the mouth.

Patient Position	Seated or standing
Position of Examiner	In front of the patient
Evaluative Procedure	The patient attempts to place as many flexed knuckles as possible between the upper and lower teeth.
Positive Test	The patient is unable to place a minimum of two knuckles within the mouth.
Implications	***Less than two fingers:*** TMJ hypomobility ***Three or more fingers:*** TMJ hypermobility
Evidence	Absent or inconclusive in the literature

TMJ = temporomandibular joint.

Special Test 20-2
Tongue Blade Test

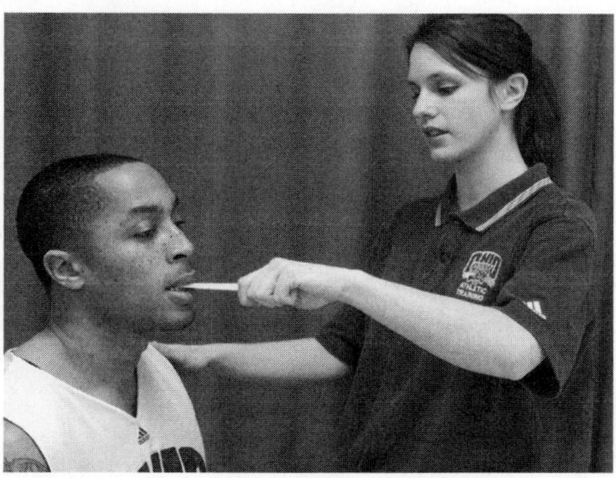

In the presence of a fractured mandible, the patient will not be able to bite down hard on the tongue depressor.

Patient Position	Seated
Position of Examiner	Standing in front of the patient
Evaluative Procedure	A tongue blade (tongue depressor) is placed in the patient's mouth. As the patient attempts to hold the tongue blade in place, the examiner rotates (twists) the blade.
Positive Test	The patient is unable to maintain a firm bite or pain is elicited.
Implications	Possible mandibular fracture
Evidence	Absent or inconclusive in the literature

Table 20-1 Muscles of Expression (Partial List)

Muscle	Action	Origin	Insertion	Innervation	Root
Buccinator	Depresses the cheeks	Alveolar process of the maxilla and mandible.	Angle of the mouth	Facial	CN VII
Depressor Anguli Oris	Draws the angle of the mouth downward (frowning)	Oblique line of the mandible	Angle of the mouth	Facial	CN VII
Depressor Labii Inferioris	Lowers the mouth	Oblique line of the mandible	Lower lip	Facial	CN VII
Digastric	Opens mouth	Inferior border of the mandible	Superior aspect of the hyoid bone	Trigeminal	CN V
Geniohyoid	Opens mouth	Median ridge of the mandible	Body of the hyoid bone	Ansa cervicalis	CN I, CN II
Levator Anguli Oris	Raises each side of the mouth (a bilateral muscle)	Just superior to the canine teeth	Angle of the mouth	Facial	CN VII
Masseter	Aids in biting	Superficial portion: Zygomatic process of maxilla; anterior two-thirds of zygomatic arch Profundus portion: Posterior one-third of the zygomatic arch	Superficial portion: Inferior one-half of the lateral ramus of the mandible Profundus portion: Superior one-half of the ramus and coronoid process of the mandible	Trigeminal	CN V
Mentalis	Elevates the skin of the chin.	Incisive fossa of the mandible	Point of the mandible	Facial	CN VII
Mylohyoid	Opens mouth	Inferior border of the mandible	Superior aspect of the hyoid bone	Trigeminal	CN V
Orbicularis Oris	"Puckers" lips	Originates off of the muscles surrounding the mouth	Skin surrounding the lips	Facial	CN VII
Procerus	Wrinkles the nose	Lower portion of the nasal bone Lateral nasal cartilage	Lower portion of the forehead between the eyebrow	Facial	CN VII
Temporalis	Aids in biting	Temporal fossa	Coronoid process and ramus of the mandible	Trigeminal	CN V
Zygomaticus Major	Used for smiling	Zygomatic bone	Angle of the mouth	Facial	CN VII

CN = cranial nerve.

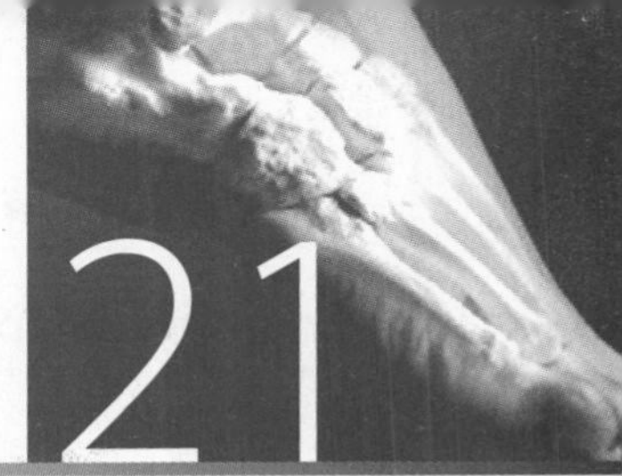

CHAPTER 21

Head and Cervical Spine Pathologies

Examination Map

EVALUATION OF ATHLETE'S POSITION

DETERMINATION OF CONSCIOUSNESS

Level of Consciousness

Primary Survey

Secondary Survey

HISTORY

Location of Symptoms

Cervical pain

Head pain

Mechanism of Injury

Coup

Contrecoup

Repeated subconcussive forces

Rotational/shear force

Cervical spine mechanism

- Flexion/axial loading
- Extension
- Lateral bending/rotation

Loss of consciousness

History of concussion

Weakness

Persistent symptoms

INSPECTION

Inspection of the Bony Structures

Position of the head

Cervical vertebrae

Mastoid process

Skull and scalp

Inspection of the Eyes

General

Nystagmus

Pupil size

Pupil reaction to light

Inspection of the Nose and Ears

Fluid escaping

PALPATION

Palpation of the Bony Structures

Spinous processes

Transverse processes

Skull

Palpation of Soft Tissue

Musculature

Throat

FUNCTIONAL ASSESSMENT

Neurocognitive Function

Behavior

Analytical skills

Information processing

Memory

- Test for retrograde amnesia
- Test for anterograde amnesia

Neuropsychological testing

Balance and Coordination

Romberg test

Tandem walk test

Balance error scoring system

Vital Signs

Respiration

Pulse

Continued

Examination Map—cont'd

Blood pressure

Pulse pressure

NEUROLOGIC EXAMINATION

Cranial Nerve Function

Eyes

Face

Ears

Shoulder and neck

Spinal Nerve Root Evaluation

Upper quarter screen

Lower quarter screen

PATHOLOGIES AND SPECIAL TESTS

Head Trauma

Mild Traumatic Brain Injury

Standardized assessment of concussion

Concussion rating systems

Postconcussion Syndrome

Second Impact Syndrome

Intracranial Hemorrhage

Epidural hematoma

Subdural hematoma

Skull Fractures

Cervical Spine Trauma

Cervical fracture/dislocation

Transient quadriplegia

Table 21-1 Signs and Symptoms of a Head or Cervical Spine Injury to Note Throughout the Evaluation

Area	Signs and Symptoms
Brain	Amnesia (retrograde and anterograde) Confusion Disorientation Irritability Incoordination Dizziness Headache
Ocular	Blurred vision Photophobia Nystagmus
Ears	Tinnitus Dizziness
Stomach	Nausea Vomiting
Systemic	Unusually fatigued

Table 21-2 Early and Late Signs and Symptoms of Postconcussion Syndrome

Early	Late
Disorientation	Lack of concentration
Confusion	Poor memory
Headache	Irritability
Dizziness	Depression
Blurred vision	Anxiety
Nausea	Fatigue
Drowsiness	Headache
Sleep disturbance	Sleep disturbance

Table 21-3	Progression of Symptoms Associated with an Epidural Hematoma

Patient is unconscious or has other signs of a concussion (these are not prerequisite findings).
The patient has a period of very lucid consciousness, perhaps eliminating the suspicion of a serious concussion.
Patient appears to become disoriented, confused, and drowsy.
Complaints of a headache that increases in intensity with time
Signs and signals of cranial nerve disruption
Onset of coma
If untreated, death or permanent brain damage occurs.

Table 21-4 Respiration Patterns

Type	Characteristics	Implications
Apneustic	Prolonged inspirations unrelieved by attempts to exhale	Trauma to the pons
Biot's	Periods of apnea followed by hyperapnea	Increased intracranial pressure
Cheyne-Stokes	Periods of apnea followed by breaths of increasing depth and frequency	Frontal lobe or brain stem trauma
Slow	Respiration consisting of fewer than 12 breaths per minute	CNS disruption
Thoracic	Respiration in which the diaphragm is inactive and breathing occurs only through expansion of the chest; normal abdominal movement is absent	Disruption of the phrenic nerve or its nerve roots

Table 21-5 Pulse Patterns

Type	Characteristics	Implication
Accelerated	Pulse >150 beats per minute (bpm) (>170 bpm usually has fatal results)	Pressure on the base of the brain; shock
Bounding	Pulse that quickly reaches a higher intensity than normal, then quickly disappears	Ventricular systole and reduced peripheral pressure
Deficit	Pulse in which the number of beats counted at the radial pulse is less than that counted over the heart itself	Cardiac arrhythmia
High Tension	Pulse in which the force of the beat is increased; an increased amount of pressure is required to inhibit the radial pulse	Cerebral trauma
Low Tension	Short, fast, faint pulse having a rapid decline	Heart failure; shock

Table 21-6 Clinical Assessment of Blood Pressure via Palpation

Palpable Pulse	Minimum Systolic Blood Pressure, mm Hg
Carotid artery	60
Femoral artery	70
Radial artery	90

Inspection Findings 21-1
Postures Assumed After Spinal Cord Injury

Decerebrate Posture

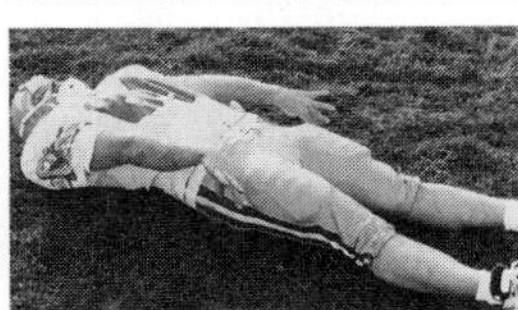

Description	Extension of the extremities and retraction of the head
Pathology	Lesion of the brain stem; also possible secondary to heat stroke

Decorticate Posture

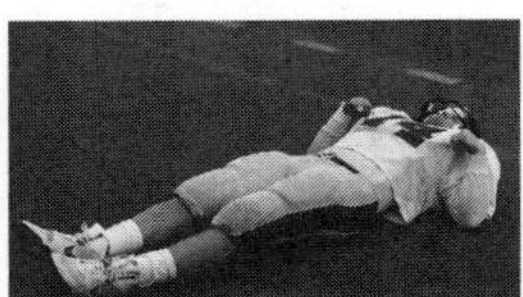

Description	Flexion of the elbows and wrists, clenched fists, and extension of the lower extremity
Pathology	Lesion above the brain stem

Flexion Contracture

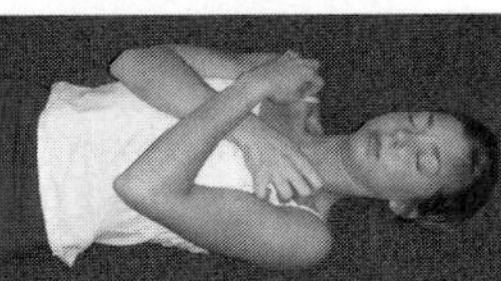

Description	Arms flexed across the chest
Pathology	Spinal cord lesion at the C5–C6 level

Table 21-7 Behavioral Signs and Symptoms of Concussion

Sign	Behavior
Vacant Stare	Confused or blank facial expression
Delayed Verbal and Motor Responses	Slow to answer questions or follow instructions
Inability to Focus Attention	Easily distracted; unable to complete normal activities
Disorientation	Walking in the wrong direction; time, date, and place disorientation
Slurred or Incoherent Speech	Rambling, disjointed, incomprehensible statements
Gross Incoordination	Stumbling; inability to walk a straight line
Heightened Emotions	Appearing distraught, crying for no apparent reason, emotional responses that are out of proportion to the circumstances
Memory Deficits	As evidenced by the retrograde and anterograde memory tests

Table 21-8 Dysfunction Guide for Evaluating the Extent of Cerebral Concussions

Function	Slight	Severe	Comments
Consciousness	No loss of consciousness	Unconscious for 10 seconds to 1 minute or altered consciousness for less than 2 minutes	Institutional standard operating procedures should identify the minimum duration of unconsciousness required to activate emergency medical services.
Memory	The patient is initially unable to remember the immediate events leading to the trauma	Retrograde amnesia: Inability to remember events before the mechanism of injury Anterograde amnesia: Inability to remember events after the injury	Transitory loss of memory of the injurious contact is to be expected and often associated with a brief loss of consciousness ("seeing stars" or "blacking out").
Cognitive Function	Slight transient mental confusion ("What happened?")	Disorientation to person, place, or time Demonstration of violent, aggressive, and otherwise inappropriate behavior or language Inability to process information "normally"	These traits may be expected immediately after the injury. Their continued presence is correlated with the severity of the injury.
Balance and Coordination	Slight unsteadiness or unsteadiness that rapidly subsides	Profound disruption of balance and coordination; inability to walk without assistance and difficulty performing basic manual skills	These functions are based not only on the results of Romberg's test and the heel–toe walk but also on general observation.
Tinnitus	None or transitory	Prolonged tinnitus or tinnitus worsening over time	Ringing in the ears may be described immediately after the blow but should subside with time.
Pupil Size	Equal; both pupils responsive to light	Dilated pupil that is unresponsive to light	Pupillary change indicates increased intracranial pressure on CN III, indicative of intracranial bleeding. Unequal pupil size (anisocoria) may be normally present.
Nystagmus	Absent	Present	Nystagmus indicates increased intracranial pressure or inner ear dysfunction. This may be a normal finding.
Vision	Normal or initially blurred, which quickly subsides	Persistent blurred or double vision	The athlete's normal vision should be taken into account (i.e., if the athlete wears glasses).
Nausea	None or slight	Vomiting	Cumulative effect
Pulse	Within normal limits, possible decreasing with rest	Abnormally increasing or decreasing	Abnormal changes in pulse indicate intracranial hemorrhage.
Blood Pressure	Within normal limits	Rapidly rising or falling	Rapid blood pressure changes suggest intracranial hematoma.
Respirations	Normal	Abnormal	See Table 21-4.

CN = cranial nerve.

Table 21-9 Postconcussion Symptom Scale

Symptom	Preseason Baseline	Time of Injury	2 to 3 Hours Postinjury
Headache	0	2	4
Nausea	0	3	2
Vomiting	0	0	2
Dizziness	0	4	2
Poor Balance	0	4	2
Sensitivity to Noise	0	1	2
Ringing in the Ears	0	5	1
Sensitivity to Light	0	3	3
Blurred Vision	1	3	2
Poor Concentration	0	2	3
Memory Problems	0	2	2
Drowsiness	0	4	4
Fatigue	1	5	4
Sadness/Depression	1	5	4
Irritability	0	4	5
Neck Pain	0	0	0
TOTAL SCORE	3	47	42

Each symptom is graded on a scale of 0 (none) to 6 (severe). Columns are summed to demonstrate the patient's current state.

Table 21-10 Concussion Rating Systems

Rating System	Signs and Symptoms		
	Grade I	**Grade II**	**Grade III**
American Academy of Neurology[111]	No loss of consciousness Transient confusion Concussion symptoms resolve in less than 15 minutes	No loss of consciousness Transient confusion Concussion symptoms or mental status abnormalities on examination resolve in more than 15 minutes	Any loss of consciousness either brief (seconds) or prolonged (minutes)
American College of Sports Medicine Guidelines[111]	None or transient retrograde amnesia None to slight mental confusion No loss of coordination Transient dizziness Rapid recovery	Retrograde amnesia; memory may return slight to moderate mental confusion Moderate dizziness Transitory tinnitus Slow recovery	Sustained retrograde amnesia; anterograde is possible with intracranial hemorrhage Severe mental confusion Profound loss of coordination Obvious motor impairment Prolonged tinnitus Delayed recovery
Cantu Concussion Rating Guidelines[112]	No loss of consciousness Concussion symptoms resolving in less than 15 minutes Posttraumatic amnesia for less than 30 minutes	Loss of consciousness for less than 5 minutes Posttraumatic amnesia for more than 30 minutes but less than 24 hours	Loss of consciousness for more than 5 minutes Posttraumatic amnesia for more than 24 hours
Colorado Medical Society Concussion Rating Guidelines[113]	No loss of consciousness Transient confusion No amnesia	No loss of consciousness Transient confusion Amnesia	Loss of consciousness
Zurich Group[114]	Simple Injury resolves over 7–10 days	Complex Persistent symptoms, specific, specific sequelae, prolonged loss of consciousness (>1 minute) or prolonged cognitive impairment	

NOTE: Current guidelines recommend that concussion grading schemes NOT be used; the individual either has concussion or does not. Therefore any patient graded as I, II, or III above would be described as suffering from a concussion.

Table 21-11 The Glasgow Coma Scale

Response	Points	Action
Eye Opening		
Spontaneously	4	Reticular system is intact; patient may not be aware
To verbal command	3	Opens eyes when told to do so
To pain	2	Opens eyes in response to pain
None	1	Does not open eyes to any stimuli
Verbal		
Oriented, converses	5	Relatively intact CNS; aware of self and surroundings
Disoriented, converses	4	Well articulated, organized, but disoriented
Inappropriate words	3	Random, exclamatory words
Incomprehensible	2	No recognizable words
No response	1	No audible sounds or intubated
Motor		
Obeys verbal commands	6	Readily moves limbs when told to
Localizes painful stimuli	5	Moves limb in an effort to avoid pain
Flexion withdrawal	4	Pulls away from pain with a flexion motion
Abnormal flexion	3	Exhibits decorticate rigidity
Extension	2	Exhibits decerebrate rigidity
No response	1	Demonstrates dypotonicity, flaccid: Suggests loss of medullary function or spinal cord injury

CNS = central nervous system.

Special Test 21-1
Halo Test

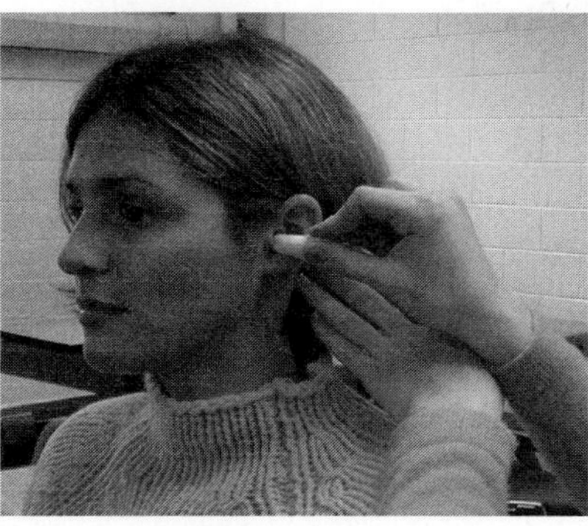

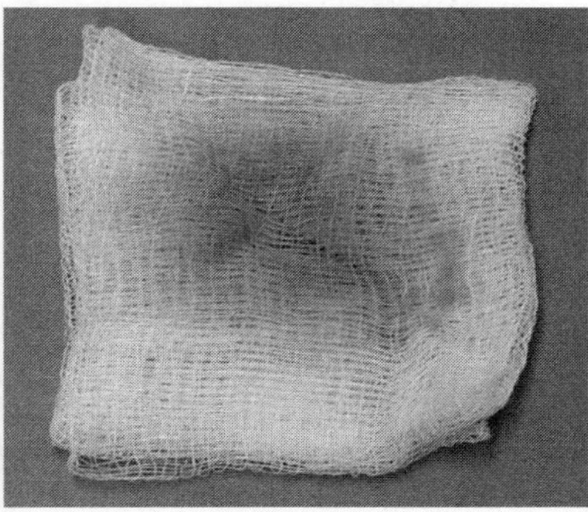

The halo test determines the presence of cerebrospinal fluid in any fluid escaping from the ears or nose.

Patient Position	Lying or sitting
Position of Examiner	Lateral to the patient's ear
Evaluative Procedure	Fold a piece of sterile gauze into a triangle. Using the point of the gauze, collect a sample of the fluid leaking from the ear or nose and allow it to be absorbed by the gauze.
Positive Test	A pale yellow "halo" will form around the sample on the gauze.
Implications	Cerebrospinal fluid (CSF) leakage, indicative of a skull fracture. The frontal bone and ethmoid bone are most commonly involved.[115]
Comments	CSF leakage from the intracranial space to the nose significantly increases the risk of infection.[115]
Evidence	Absent or inconclusive in the literature

Special Test 21-2
Determination of Retrograde Amnesia

Patient Position	Standing, sitting, or lying down
Position of Examiner	In a position to hear the patient's response
Evaluative Procedure	The patient is asked a series of questions beginning with the time of the injury. Each successive question progresses backward in time, as described by the following set of questions: What happened? What play were you running? (or other applicable question regarding the patient's activity at the time of injury) Where are you? Who am I? Who are you playing? What quarter is it (or what time is it)? What did you have for a pregame meal (or what did you have to eat for lunch)? Who did you play last week?
Positive Test	The patient has difficulty remembering or cannot remember events occurring before the injury.
Implications	Retrograde amnesia, the severity of which is based on the relative amount of memory loss demonstrated by the inability to recall events Not remembering events from the day before is more significant than not remembering more recent events The same set of questions should be repeated to determine whether the memory is returning, deteriorating, or remaining the same. Further deterioration of the memory or acutely profound memory loss that does not return in a matter of minutes warrants the immediate termination of the evaluation and transportation to an emergency medical facility.
Comments	Try to ask questions that you know the answers to or can otherwise verify. Record the patient's responses. Retrograde and/or anterograde memory loss is a common deficit associated with concussion.[116]
Evidence	Absent or inconclusive in the literature

Special Test 21-3
Determination of Anterograde Amnesia

Patient Position	Sitting or lying
Position of Examiner	In a position to hear the patient's response
Evaluative Procedure	The athlete is given a list of four unrelated items with instructions to memorize them, for example: Hubcap Film Dog tags Ivy The list is immediately repeated by the patient to ensure that it has been memorized. The patient is asked to repeat the list to the examiner every 5 minutes.
Positive Test	The inability to recite the list completely
Implications	Anterograde amnesia, possibly the result of intracranial bleeding or concussion
Comment	This test is usually performed after the test for retrograde amnesia.
Evidence	Absent or inconclusive in the literature

Special Test 21-4
Romberg Test

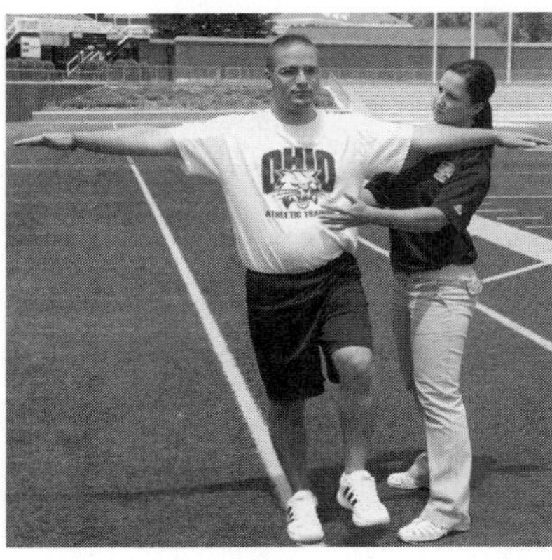
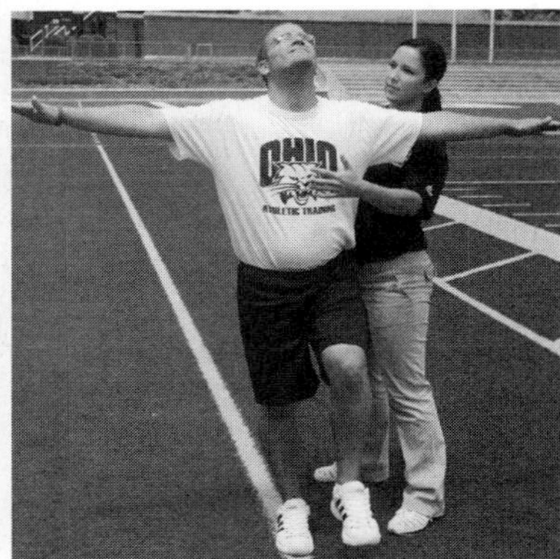

The Romberg test is used to determine the patient's balance and coordination.

Patient Position	Standing with the feet shoulder width apart
Position of Examiner	Standing lateral or posterior to the patient, ready to support the patient as needed
Evaluative Procedure	The patient shuts the eyes and abducts the arms to 90° with the elbows extended. The patient tilts the head backward and lifts one foot off the ground while attempting to maintain balance. If this portion of the examination is adequately completed, the patient is asked to touch the index finger to the nose (with the eyes remaining closed).
Positive Test	The patient displays gross unsteadiness.
Implications	Lack of balance and/or coordination indicating cerebellar or cranial nerve VIII dysfunction
Comments	Changes in balance as measured by clinical balance equipment are commonly associated with concussions.[117]
Evidence	Absent or inconclusive in the literature

Special Test 21-5
Tandem Walking

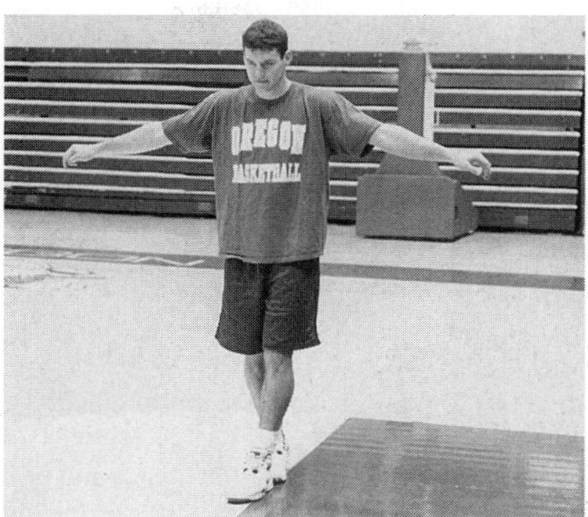

The tandem walk test determines the patient's balance.

Patient Position	Standing with the feet straddling a straight line (e.g., sideline)
Position of Examiner	Beside the patient ready to provide support
Evaluative Procedure	The patient walks heel-to-toe along the straight line for approximately 10 yards. The patient returns to the starting position by walking backward.
Positive Test	The patient is unable to maintain a steady balance.
Implications	Cerebral or inner ear dysfunction that inhibits balance
Evidence	Absent or inconclusive in the literature

Special Test 21-6
Balance Error Scoring System

Firm Surface Bout			Soft Surface Bout		
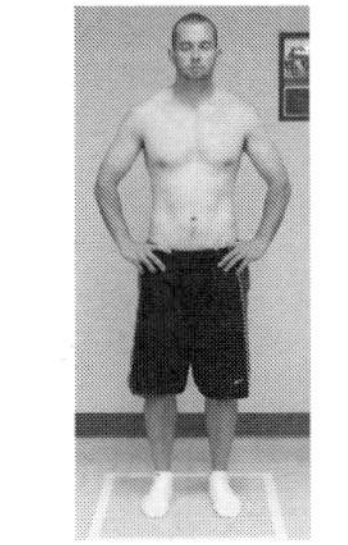 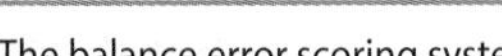 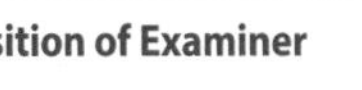	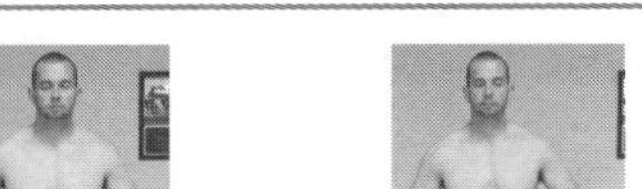	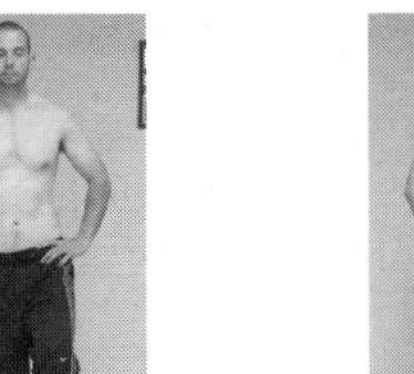	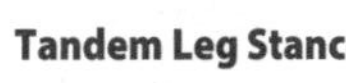 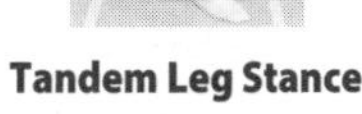 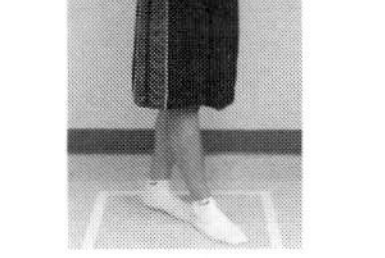	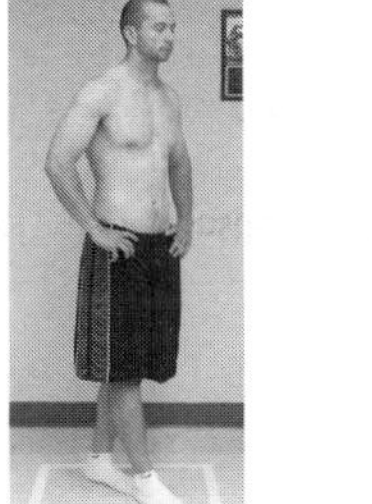 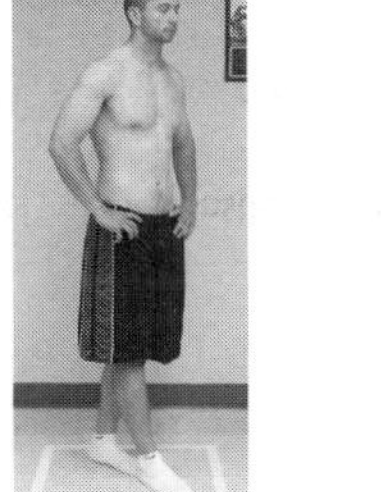 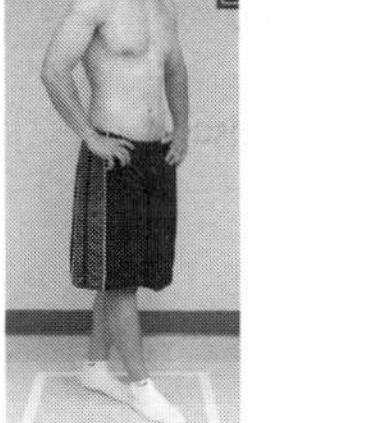 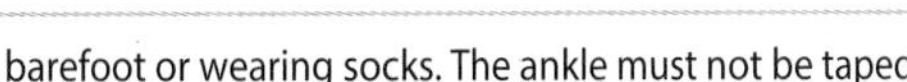	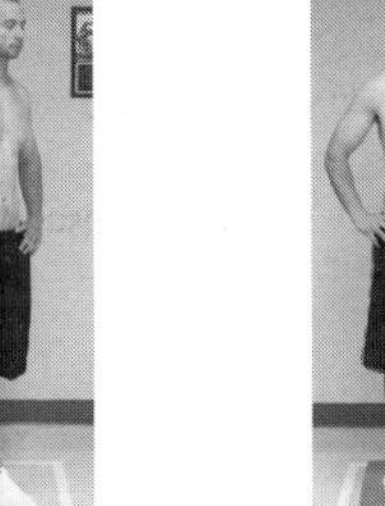
Double Leg Stance	**Single Leg Stance**	**Tandem Leg Stance**	**Double Leg Stance**	**Single Leg Stance**	**Tandem Leg Stance**

The balance error scoring system involves three different stances, each completed twice, once while standing on a firm surface and again while standing on a foam surface.

Patient Position	The patient is barefoot or wearing socks. The ankle must not be taped during the test. The patient assumes the following stances for each phase of the test: ***Phase 1:*** Double leg stance ***Phase 2:*** Single leg stance—standing on the nondominant leg. The non–weight-bearing hip is flexed to 20°–30° and the knee is flexed to 40°–50°. ***Phase 3:*** Tandem leg stance—The nondominant leg is placed behind the dominant leg and the patient stands in a heel–toe manner. The patient's hands are placed on the iliac crests. The eyes are closed during the test.
Position of Examiner	The examiner stands in front of the athlete. A stopwatch is required to time the trials. A second clinician acts as a spotter.
Evaluative Procedure	The first battery of tests is performed with the patient standing on a firm surface. The patient assumes the double leg stance and attempts to hold the position for 20 seconds.

	The test is repeated using the single leg stance and then the tandem leg stance. The second battery of tests is performed with the patient standing on a piece of medium density foam (60 kg/m^3) that is 45 cm × 45 cm and 13 cm thick. The trial is incomplete if the patient cannot hold the testing position for a minimum of 5 seconds.
Scoring	One point is scored for each of the following errors: Lifting hands off the iliac crest Opening the eyes Stepping, stumbling, or falling Moving the hip into more than 30° of flexion or abduction Lifting the foot or heel Remaining out of the testing position for more than 5 seconds If more than one error occurs simultaneously, only one error is recorded. Patients who are unable to hold the testing position for 5 seconds are assigned the score of 10.
Positive Test	Scores that are 25% above the patient's baseline or the norm[118] An increase in 3 BESS errors represents a clinically significant change. Performance on the BESS improves with repeated testing, a practice effect.[118,119]
Implications	Impaired cerebral function
Modification	Not applicable
Comments	To improve accuracy, BESS pretests and postinjury tests should be administered in the same environmental conditions (e.g., athletic training facility, sideline).[120] BESS scores correlate well with scores acquired from more sophisticated balance equipment.[121]
Evidence	Intra-rater reliability: Not Reliable — Very Reliable Poor — Moderate — Good 0 0.1 0.2 0.3 0.4 0.5 0.6 0.7 0.8 0.9 1.0

Special Test 21-7
Standardized Assessment of Concussion

Orientation (1 point each)

	Correct
Month	☐
Date	☐
Day of week	☐
Year	☐
Time (within 1 hour)	☐
Score	___/5

Immediate Memory (1 point for each correct response)

	Trial 1	Trial 2	Trial 3
Word 1	☐	☐	☐
Word 2	☐	☐	☐
Word 3	☐	☐	☐
Word 4	☐	☐	☐
Word 5	☐	☐	☐
Score	☐	☐	___/15

Concentration

Reverse Digits (1 point each for each string length)

		Correct
3–8–2	5–1–8	☐
2–7–9–3	2–1–6–8	☐
5–1–8–6–9	9–4–1–7–5	☐
6–9–7–3–5–1	4–2–8–9–3–7	☐

Delayed Recall (1 point each)

	Correct
Word 1	☐
Word 2	☐
Word 3	☐
Word 4	☐
Word 5	☐
Score	___/5

Summary of Total Scores

Orientation	___/5
Immediate memory	___/15
Concentration	___/5
Delayed recall	___/5
TOTAL SCORE	___/30

The following are performed between the Immediate Memory and Delayed Recall portions of the SAC, along with tests for memory, cerebral function, and strength.

Neurologic Screening

Recollection of the injury:

Strength:

Sensation:

Coordination:

Months of the Year in Reverse Order (1 point for entire sequence correct)	Correct	Exertional Maneuvers (when appropriate)
		1 40-yard sprint
Dec–Nov–Oct–Sept–Aug–July		5 sit-ups
June–May–Apr–Mar–Feb–Jan	☐	5 push-ups
Score	___/5	5 knee bends

Procedures

(Administration time is approximately 5 minutes): Proper training is required for appropriate use.

Orientation	Patient is asked to identify the current place in time and receives 1 point for each correct response.
Immediate Memory	The patient is asked to memorize a list of 5 random words. The list of words is repeated 3 times in succession, with 1 point being awarded for each correct response for a maximum total of 15 points. This list of words will be used for the delayed memory testing, but do not inform the patient as such.
Neurologic Screening	The patient is evaluated for loss of consciousness, amnesia, etc.
Concentration	***Reverse digits:*** The patient is given a sequence of numbers and asked to repeat them in reverse order (i.e., 2–8–3 would be recited as 3–8–2). If the patient correctly responds on the first attempt, progress to the next string length. If the patient incorrectly responds on the first attempt, use a second set of digits for the second attempt. If the patient incorrectly responds on the second attempt, move on to months of the year. ***Months of year:*** The patient is asked to recite the months of the year in reverse order.
Delayed Recall	Approximately 5 minutes after the "Immediate Memory" test, the patient is asked to recall the list of words that were used for the immediate memory test. One point is awarded for each correct response.
Total	The scores for each of the four sections are totaled to yield an overall index of impairment. A decrease from baseline of 2 points is clinically significant.[118]
Comments	Normal females score higher on the SAC than males.
Evidence	Absent or inconclusive in the literature

Table 21-12 Cranial Nerve Function

Number	Name	Type	Function
I	Olfactory	Sensory	Smell
II	Optic	Sensory	Vision
III	Oculomotor	Motor	Effect on pupillary reaction and size Elevation of upper eyelid Eye adduction and downward rolling
IV	Trochlear	Motor	Upward eye rolling
V	Trigeminal	Mixed	Motor: Muscles of mastication Sensation: Nose, forehead, temple, scalp, lips, tongue and lower jaw
VI	Abducens	Motor	Lateral eye movement
VII	Facial	Mixed	Motor: Muscles of expression Sensory: Taste
VIII	Vestibulocochlear	Sensory	Equilibrium Hearing
IX	Glossopharyngeal	Mixed	Motor: Pharyngeal muscles Sensory: Taste
X	Vagus	Mixed	Motor: Muscles of pharynx and larynx Sensory: Gag reflex
XI	Accessory	Motor	Trapezius and sternocleidomastoid muscles
XII	Hypoglossal	Motor	Tongue movement

Clinical Application

Function	Cranial Nerves	How Tested
Eye Assessment	II, III, IV, VI	Visual acuity, pupillary reaction, and tracking
Balance	VIII	Romberg test, BESS
Speaking/Hearing	VIII, IX, X, XII	Speaking to the patient; the patient speaking
Facial Expression	V, VII, XII	Smile, frown, stick out tongue
Smelling	I	Based on self-reported symptoms (often a "foul odor")
Shoulder Shrug	XI	Resist shoulder girdle raise

Table 21-13 Landmarks Used During Palpation

Upper Extremity		Lower Extremity	
Area	**Dermatome**	**Area**	**Dermatomes**
Superior shoulder	C4	Lateral thigh	L1, L2, L3
Lateral humerus	C5	Lateral lower leg and foot	L5, S1
Lateral forearm	C6	Medial lower leg and foot	L4
Middle finger	C7		
Medial forearm	C8		
Medial humerus	T1		

Table 21-14 Neuropsychological Assessment Tests Used for Mild Head-Injured Athletes

Test and Publisher	Description
Trail Making Test A & B (Reitan Neuropsychological Laboratory, Tucson, AZ)	**Description:** The patient sequentially connects a series of numbers (Trail Making A) or series of alternating letters and numbers (Trail Making B). **Measurement:** The time required for successful completion **Assessment:** Visual conceptual, visuomotor tracking, general brain function
Wechsler Digit Span Test (WDST) (Psychological Corporation, San Antonio, TX)	**Description:** The patient is presented with a random list of single-digit numbers (0–9 with no repetition) and asked to repeat the list in the same order (Digits Forward) or reverse order (Digits Backwards). The first bout begins with 3 numbers and the next has 4 numbers, progressing up to 10. **Measurement:** The number of successful trials is recorded for each part. **Assessment:** Short-term memory, auditory attention, concentration
Stroop Color Word Test (Stoelting Co., Wood Dale, IL)	**Description:** Patients are presented with a list of 100 words (5 columns x 20 words each). The test itself consists of three trials, each 45 seconds in length. In the first trial, the patient is asked to read through the list as quickly as possible and read aloud the words "red," "green," and "blue," which are written in black ink. During the second trial, words are replaced with "XXXX" written in red, green, or blue ink, which the patient must identify the proper color. In the third trial, the words "red," "green," and "blue" are written in a color other than their own (e.g., "red" is written in blue ink and "blue" is written in green ink). The patient must identify the color the word is printed in, not the word itself. **Measurement:** Sum total of the number of correct responses in each subset **Assessment:** Cognitive processing speed, concentration ability to filter out distractions (inhibition)

Continued

Table 21-14 Neuropsychological Assessment Tests Used for Mild Head-Injured Athletes—cont'd

Test and Publisher	Description
Hopkins Verbal Learning Test (Johns Hopkins University, Baltimore, MD)	**Description:** The patient is read a list of 12 words grouped into 3 semantic categories of 4 words each 3 times. After each reading, the patient is asked to recall as many words as possible. After a 20-minute break, the patient is read a list of 24 words, 12 words from the original list, 6 words that are closely related, and 6 unrelated words. **Measurement:** The number of incorrect responses from the fourth trial subtracted from the total number of correct responses from the first three trials **Assessment:** Language function, short-term memory
Symbol Digit Modalities Test (Western Psychological Services, Los Angeles, CA)	**Description:** Patients are given 30 seconds to memorize a list of nine symbols and their corresponding symbols. In one version of the test, the patient is asked to repeat the symbols corresponding to a four-digit number. An alternate form has the patient write the number that corresponds to a specific symbol. **Measurement:** The number of correct responses divided by the total number of completed responses **Assessment:** Psychomotor speed, concentration, visual speed, and visual perception
Controlled Oral Word Association Test (COWAT) (Psychological Assessment Resources, Inc. Odessa, FL)	**Description:** The patient is given three word naming trials based on two groups of letters, "C–F–L" and "P–R–W." In the first session, the patient is then asked to say as many words as possible that begins with that letter of the alphabet, starting with the first letter within the first code group and then progressing to the subsequent letter. The second code group is used in the second session. Proper names, numbers, and different variations of the same word (e.g., "count," "counting," "counted") are not allowed. This is repeated for three trials. **Measurement:** The raw score based on the total number of acceptable words produced in the three trials. The publisher of the COWAT provides formulas that allow the score to be adjusted based on the patient's age, gender, and level of education. **Assessment:** Verbal fluency

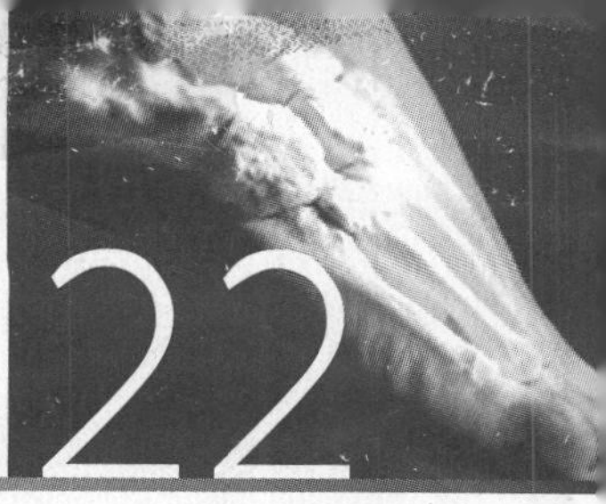

CHAPTER 22

Environment-Related Conditions

Examination Map

HISTORY

Past Medical History
Weight loss
Recent history of illness
Sickle cell trait
Inadequate nutrition
Prior environmental illness or injury

History of the Present Condition
Mechanism of injury
Environmental conditions
Thirst
Conditioning level
Body build
Drug and alcohol use

INSPECTION

Skin color
Muscle tone
Pupils

PALPATION

Skin temperature

REVIEW OF SYSTEMS

Cardiovascular
- Pulse
- Blood pressure
- Core temperature

Respiration
Neurologic
Genitourinary
- Urine specific gravity

PATHOLOGIES AND SPECIAL TESTS

Heat Illness
Heat cramps
Heat syncope
Heat exhaustion
Heat stroke
Exertional hyponatremia

Cold Injuries
Hypothermia
Frostbite

Heat Illness

Table 22-1 Conditions Predisposing to Heat Illness

Predisposing Condition	Rationale
Large Body Mass	Large muscle mass increases the body's heat production. Large layers of adipose tissue decrease the heat exchange mechanism.
Age	The heat exchange mechanism of the young and old does not efficiently remove heat.
Conditioning Level	Individuals who are poorly conditioned or conditioned athletes who are not acclimated to the environment produce increased levels of metabolic heat and are less efficient at dissipating the heat.
Poor Hydration	Internal fluids are required for maximum efficiency of the heat transfer mechanism. Illnesses, especially those involving vomiting or diarrhea, dehydrate the body. Lack of hydration before, during, and after exercise.
History of Heat Illness	A history of heat-related illness can indicate a chronically inadequate level of hydration or nutrition. An athlete with a recent history of heat-related illness may not have sufficient time to rehydrate.
Medications and Other Substances	Diuretic and laxative medications and alcohol promote fluid loss via urination and defecation. Creatine and anabolic steroids increase muscle mass and tend to increase the level of intramuscular fluids. Antihistamines, decongestants (pseudoephedrine), and amphetamines increase metabolism, cause vasoconstriction, or otherwise increase the risk of heat illness.

Table 22-2 Prevention of Heat Illness

Technique	Rationale
Acclimation	Improves the efficiency of muscle contraction, improves the efficiency of the cardiovascular system, lowers sweat threshold, and improves kidney function.
Proper Nutrition and Hydration	Provides the body with the fluids and electrolytes to maintain homeostasis during exercise.
Avoidance of Environmental Extremes	When practical, exercise in less hot or humid environments to maximize heat transfer from the body.
Wearing Appropriate Clothing	Allows evaporation of perspiration to promote heat loss from the body when appropriate clothing is worn; therefore, full pads practices should not be conducted in extreme heat or humidity
Rest Periods	Allows recovery and rehydration for athletes; includes activities such as cooling off in a cool area, consuming fluids, and allowing clothing changes during breaks

Table 22-3 Guidelines for Modification of Athletic Competition in Hot or Humid Environments

Dry Bulb Temperature (°F)	Wet Bulb Temperature (°F)	Humidity (%)	Consequences
80–90	68	<70	No extraordinary precautions are required for athletes not predisposed to heat illness. Athletes who are predisposed (e.g., unconditioned, unacclimated, or losing more than 3% of body weight from water loss) require close observation.
80–90	69–79	>70	Regular rest breaks are necessary.
90–100		<70	Loose, breathable clothing should be worn, and wet uniforms require regular changing.
90–100	>80	>70	Practice should be shortened and modified. The use of protective equipment covering the body should be curtailed.
>100	>82		Practice should be canceled.

Table 22-4 Signs and Symptoms of Dehydration

Initial Stages	Thirst Irritability General discomfort
Late Stages	Headache Weakness Dizziness Cramps Chills Vomiting Nausea Decreased performance

Table 22-5 Rehydration Strategies

Strategy	Comments
Pre-exercise Hydration	At 2–3 hours before competition: Consume 500–600 mL (17–20 fl oz.) of water or sports drink. At 10–20 minutes before competition: Consume 200–300 mL (7–10 fl oz.) of water or sports drink.
Hydration Maintenance	Every 10–20 minutes: Consume 200–300 mL (7–10 fl oz.) of water or sports drink. Prevent the athlete from losing more than 2% of body weight through water loss.
Post-exercise Hydration	Within 2 hours: Replace water, carbohydrates, and electrolytes lost during activity.

Examination Findings 22-1
Heat Illness

Evaluative Finding	Heat Cramps	Heat Syncope	Heat Exhaustion	Heat Stroke
Hydration Status	Dehydrated	Dehydrated	Dehydrated	Dehydrated
Core Temperature*	WNL**	WNL	102°F–104°F (38.9°C–40°C)	Greater than 104°F (40°C)
Skin Color and Temperature	WNL	Pale	Cool/clammy Pale	Hot Red
Sweating	Moderate to profuse	WNL	Profuse	Slight to profuse The skin may be wet or dry
Pulse	WNL	Decreased	Rapid and weak	Increased
Blood Pressure	WNL	A sudden, imperceptible drop in blood pressure, which rapidly returns to normal	Low	High
Respiration	WNL	WNL	Hyperventilation	Rapid hyperventillation
Mental State	WNL Possible fatigue	Fatigue Dizziness Fainting	Dizziness Fatigue Slight confusion	Dizziness Drowsiness Confusion/disorientation Irritability Emotional instability Violent behavior
Neuromuscular Changes	Cramping in one or more muscles		Muscle cramps Weakness	Weakness Decerebrate posture
Gastrointestinal and Urinary Changes			Intestinal cramping Nausea Vomiting Diarrhea Decreased urinary output	Nausea Vomiting Diarrhea

Continued

Examination Findings 22-1—cont'd
Heat Illness

Evaluative Finding	Heat Cramps	Heat Syncope	Heat Exhaustion	Heat Stroke
Central Nervous System			Syncope Headache	Headache Unconsciousness Seizures Coma
Other Findings	Thirst	"Tunnel vision" may be reported.	Thirst Loss of appetite (anorexia) Chills	Dilated pupils

WNL = within normal limits.
*As determined by the rectal temperature.
**Within normal limits for an exercising athlete.

Table 22-6 Calculation of the Wind Chill Factor

Wind Speed, MPH	Actual Thermometer Reading (°F)											
	50	40	30	20	10	0	-10	-20	-30	-40	-50	-60
	Wind Chill Factor (°F)											
Calm	50	40	30	20	10	0	-10	-20	-30	-40	-50	-60
5	48	37	27	16	6	-5	-15	-26	-36	-47	-57	-68
10	40	28	16	4	-9	-24	-33	-46	-58	-70	-83	-95
15	36	22	9	-5	-18	-32	-45	-58	-72	-85	-99	-112
20	32	18	4	-10	-25	-39	-53	-67	-82	-96	-110	-124
25	30	16	0	-15	-29	-44	-59	-74	-88	-104	-118	-133
30	28	13	-2	-18	-33	-48	-63	-79	-94	-109	-125	-140
35	27	11	-4	-20	-35	-51	-67	-82	-98	-113	-129	-145
40	26	10	-6	-21	-37	-53	-69	-85	-100	-116	-132	-148
	Little danger				Moderate danger			Extreme danger				
					Skin freezes within 1 min			Skin freezes rapidly (<1 min)				

Table 22-7 National Collegiate Athletic Association's Recommended Guidelines for Reducing Cold Stress[122]

Guideline	Comments
Layering Clothing	Wearing several thin layers of clothing is best to retain body heat; layers may be added or removed as needed.
Covering the Head	As much as 50% of the body's heat is lost through the head.
Protecting the Hands	The use of mittens rather than gloves is recommended to protect the fingers from frostbite.
Staying Dry	Water increases the rate of heat loss from the body. Rather than wearing clothes made of cotton, wearing those made of polypropylene, wool, or other material that wicks moisture away from the skin is recommended.
Staying Hydrated	Fluids are needed to maintain the body's core temperature and are as important in preventing cold injuries as heat injuries.
Maintaining Energy Level	A negative energy balance increases the risk of hypothermia. Proper eating and consuming "energy snacks" and sports drinks helps maintain a positive energy balance.
Warming Up Thoroughly	A thorough warm-up is required before competition to elevate the core temperature.
Warming Incoming Air	The use of a scarf or mask across the mouth warms incoming air.
Avoiding Alcohol, Nicotine, and Other Drugs	These agents cause vasoconstriction or vasodilation of the superficial blood vessels, hindering regulation of the core temperature.
Never Training Alone	An injury that prevents the athlete from walking may be catastrophic in cold climates.

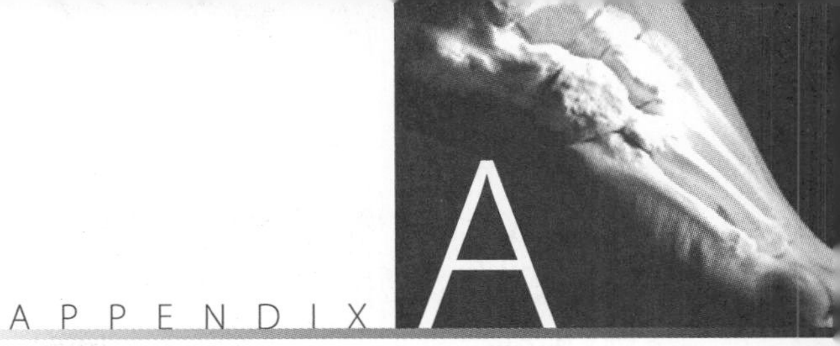

APPENDIX A

Reflex Testing

Grade	Response
0	No reflex elicited
1+	Hyporeflexia: Reflex elicited with reinforcement (precontracting the muscle)
2+	Normal response
3+	Hyperreflexia (brisk)
4+	Hyperactive with clonus

Facilitating the Reflex

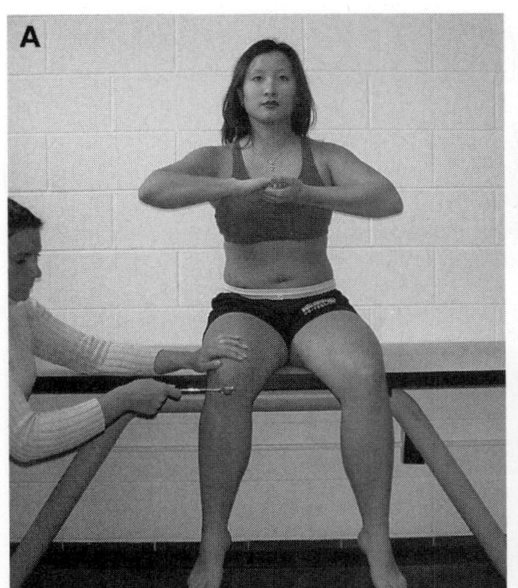

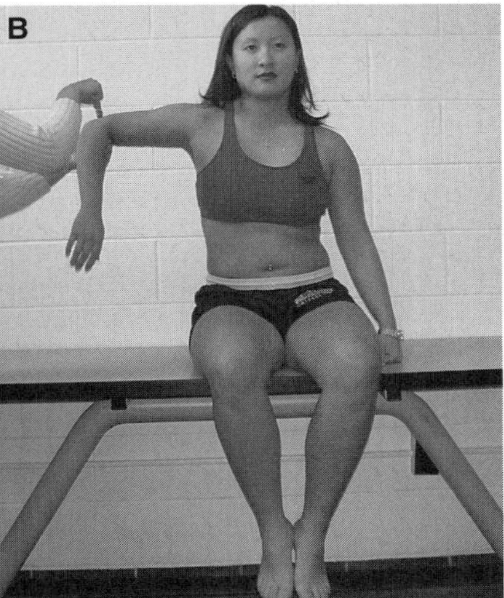

FIGURE A-1 ■ The Jendrassik maneuvers. **(A)** To facilitate muscle function during lower extremity reflex testing, have the patient attempt to pull the hands apart as shown. **(B)** Muscle facilitation during upper extremity reflex testing. The patient presses the medial aspects of the feet against each other.

Box A-1

C5 Nerve Root Reflex

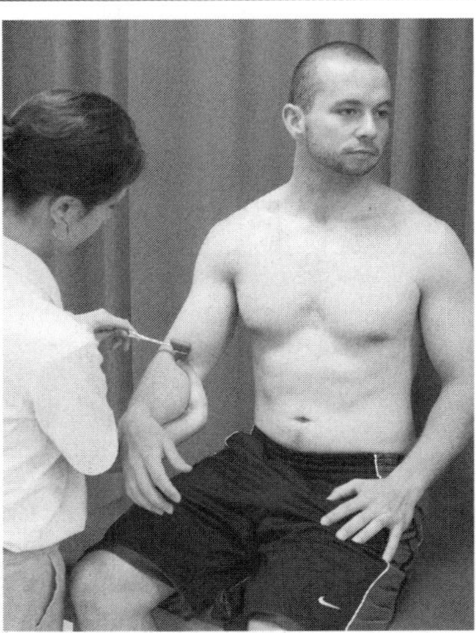

Muscle	Biceps brachii
Patient Position	Seated looking away from the tested side
Position of Examiner	Standing to the side of the patient, cradling the forearm with the thumb placed over the tendon
Evaluative Procedure	The thumb is tapped with the reflex hammer.
Innervation	Musculocutaneous nerve
Nerve Root	C5, C6

Box A-2
C6 Nerve Root Reflex

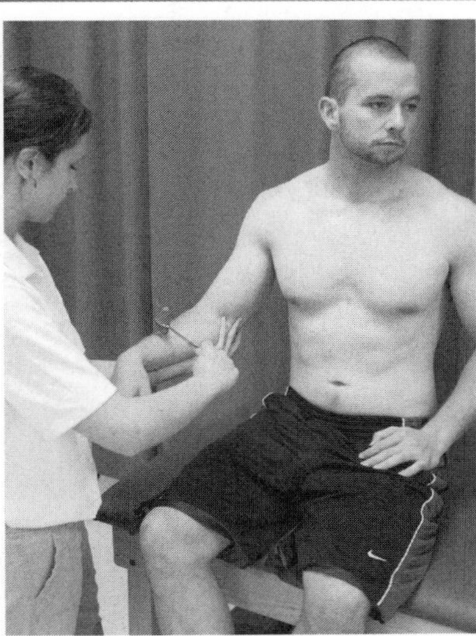

Muscle	Brachioradialis
Patient Position	Seated looking away from the tested side The elbow is passively flexed to between 60° and 90°
Position of Examiner	Cradling the patient's arm
Evaluative Procedure	The distal portion of the brachioradialis tendon is tapped with the reflex hammer. The proximal tendon may also be used.
Innervation	Radial nerve
Nerve Roots	C5, C6

Box A-3
C7 Nerve Root Reflex

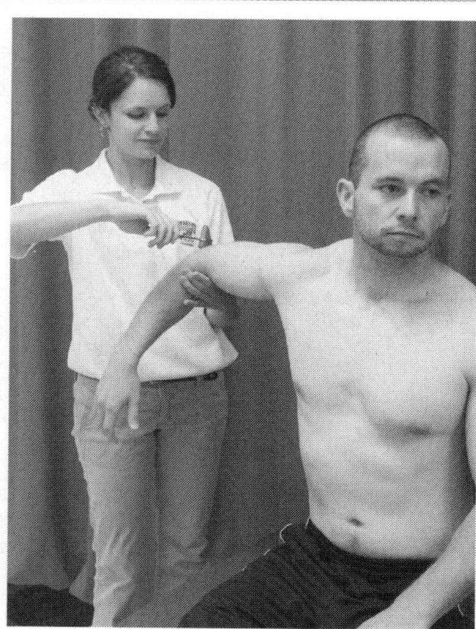

Muscle	Triceps brachii
Patient Position	Seated looking away from the tested side
Position of Examiner	Supporting the patient's shoulder abducted to 90° and the elbow flexed to 90°
Evaluative Procedure	The distal triceps brachii tendon is tapped with the reflex hammer.
Innervation	Radial nerve
Nerve Roots	(C6), C7, C8

Box A-4
L4 Nerve Root Reflex

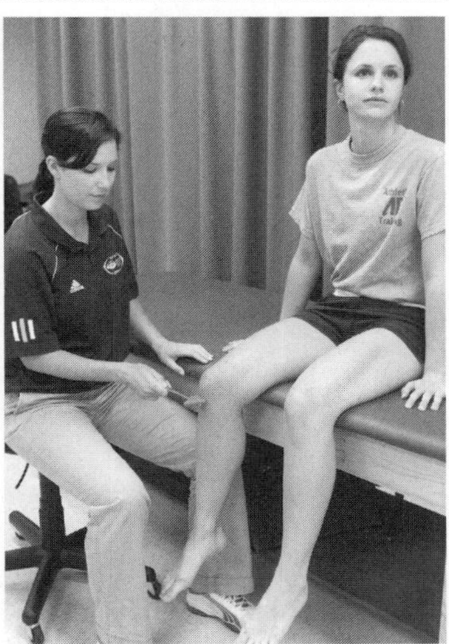

Muscle	Patellar tendon (quadriceps femoris)
Patient Position	Sitting with the knees flexed over the end of the table looking away from the tested side
Position of Examiner	Standing or seated to the side of the patient
Evaluative Procedure	The patellar tendon is tapped with the reflex hammer.
Innervation	Femoral nerve
Nerve Roots	(L2), L3, L4

Box A-5
L5 Nerve Root Reflex

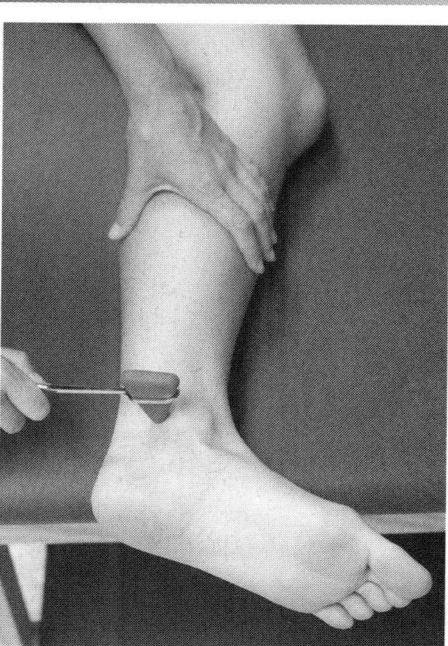

Muscle	Tibialis posterior
Patient Position	Sidelying on test side The test foot is off the edge of the table.
Position of Examiner	Standing or seated to the side of the patient
Evaluative Procedure	The tibialis posterior tendon is tapped with the reflex hammer posteriorly and just proximal to the medial malleolus.
Innervation	Tibial nerve
Nerve Roots	L5, (L4, S1)

Box A-6
L5 Nerve Root Reflex

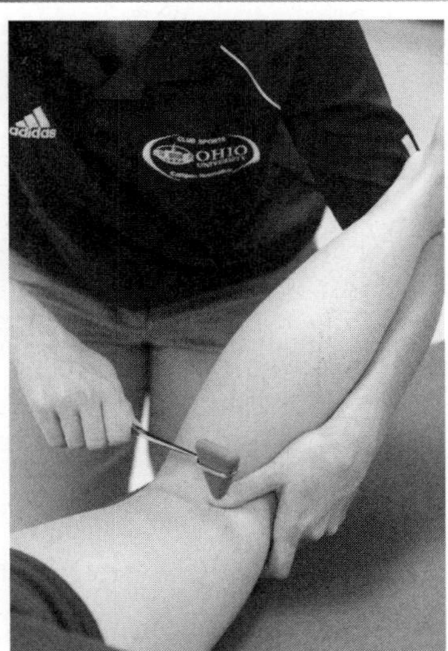

Muscle	Medial hamstrings (semitendinosus)
Patient Position	Supine with the knee slightly flexed looking away from the tested side
Position of Examiner	Standing or seated to the side of the patient. The thumb or finger is placed over the semitendinosus tendon immediately superior to the medial joint line.
Evaluative Procedure	The finger is tapped with the reflex hammer.
Innervation	Tibial nerve
Nerve Roots	L5, S1, (S2)

Box A-7
S1 Nerve Root Reflex

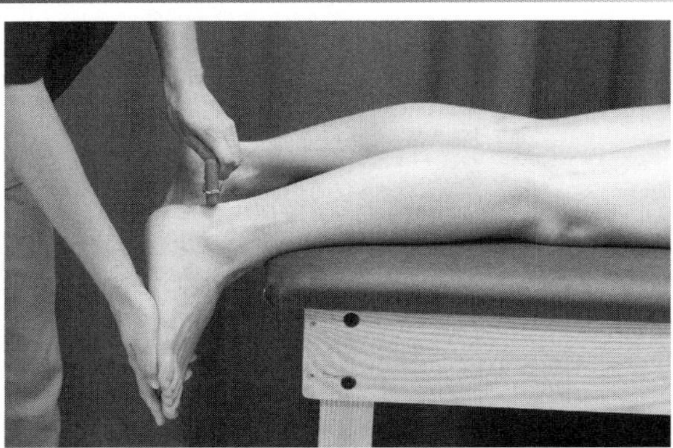

Muscle	Achilles tendon (triceps surae muscle group)
Patient Position	Prone with the feet off the edge of the table.
Position of Examiner	Seated or standing next to the patient, supporting the foot in its neutral position
Evaluative Procedure	The Achilles tendon is tapped with a reflex hammer.
Innervation	Tibial
Nerve Roots	S1, S2

Box A-8
S2 Nerve Root Reflex

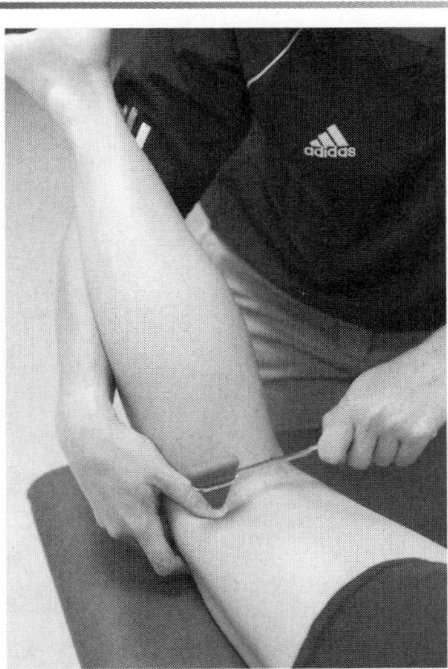

Muscle	Biceps femoris
Patient Position	Prone with the knee flexed to approximately 20°
Position of Examiner	Standing next to the patient The thumb is placed over the biceps femoris tendon just proximal to the joint line
Evaluative Procedure	The thumb is tapped with a reflex hammer.
Innervation	Tibial, common peroneal
Nerve Roots	L5, S1, S2, (S3)

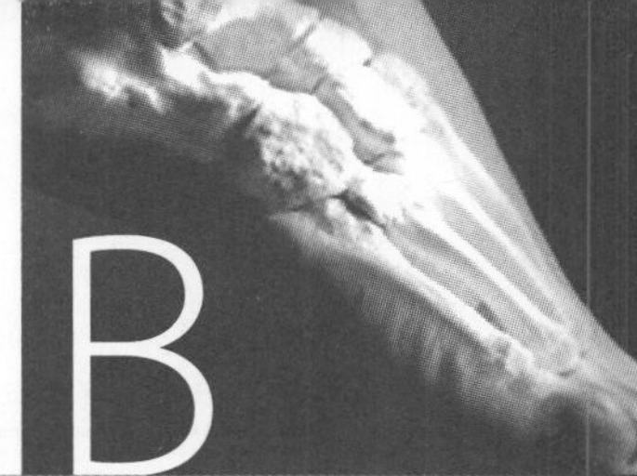

APPENDIX B

Lower Extremity Functional Assessment

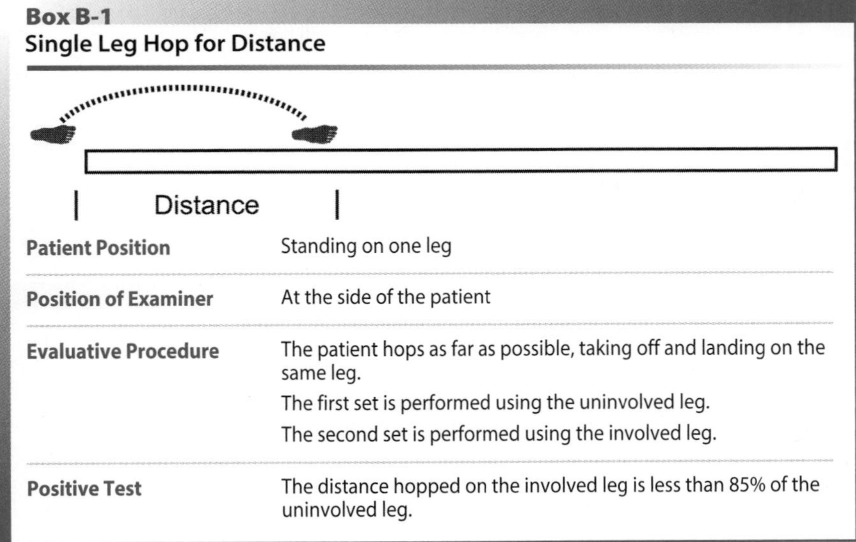

Box B-1
Single Leg Hop for Distance

Patient Position	Standing on one leg
Position of Examiner	At the side of the patient
Evaluative Procedure	The patient hops as far as possible, taking off and landing on the same leg. The first set is performed using the uninvolved leg. The second set is performed using the involved leg.
Positive Test	The distance hopped on the involved leg is less than 85% of the uninvolved leg.

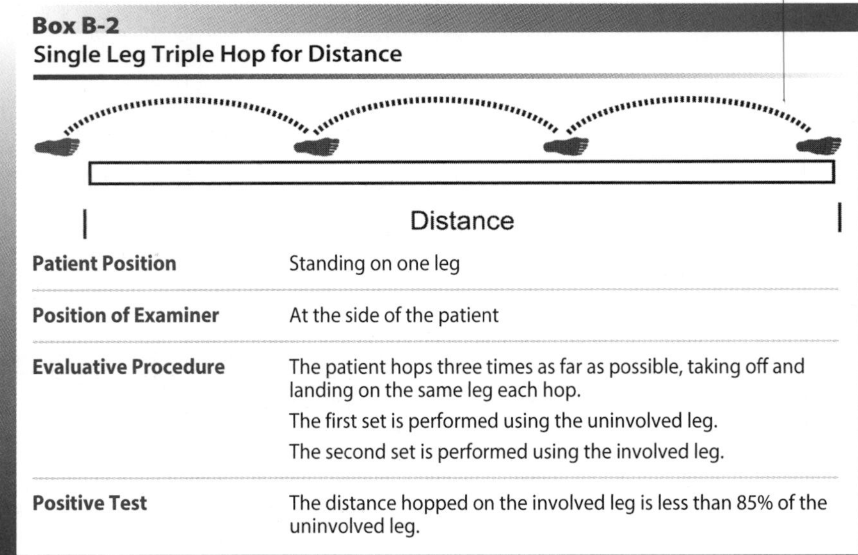

Box B-2
Single Leg Triple Hop for Distance

Patient Position	Standing on one leg
Position of Examiner	At the side of the patient
Evaluative Procedure	The patient hops three times as far as possible, taking off and landing on the same leg each hop. The first set is performed using the uninvolved leg. The second set is performed using the involved leg.
Positive Test	The distance hopped on the involved leg is less than 85% of the uninvolved leg.

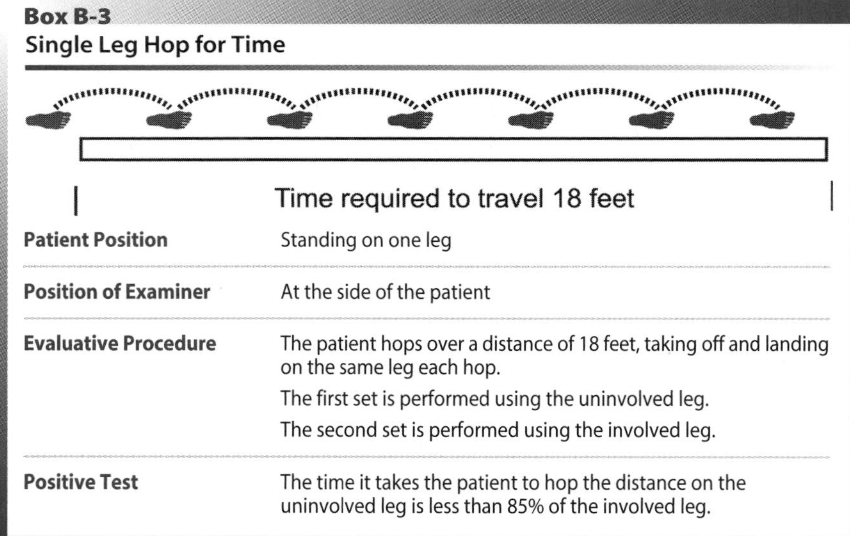

Box B-3
Single Leg Hop for Time

Patient Position	Standing on one leg
Position of Examiner	At the side of the patient
Evaluative Procedure	The patient hops over a distance of 18 feet, taking off and landing on the same leg each hop. The first set is performed using the uninvolved leg. The second set is performed using the involved leg.
Positive Test	The time it takes the patient to hop the distance on the uninvolved leg is less than 85% of the involved leg.

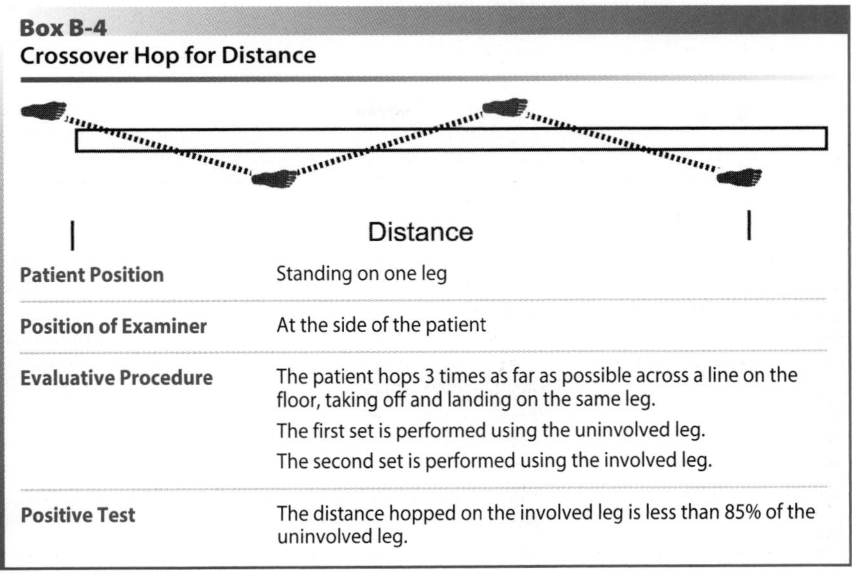

Box B-4
Crossover Hop for Distance

Patient Position	Standing on one leg
Position of Examiner	At the side of the patient
Evaluative Procedure	The patient hops 3 times as far as possible across a line on the floor, taking off and landing on the same leg. The first set is performed using the uninvolved leg. The second set is performed using the involved leg.
Positive Test	The distance hopped on the involved leg is less than 85% of the uninvolved leg.

REFERENCES

1. Ageberg, E, et al: Balance in single-limb stance in patients with anterior cruciate ligament injury: Relation to knee laxity, proprioception, muscle strength, and subjective function. *Am J Sports Med,* 33:1527, 2005.
2. Mawdsley, RH, Hoy, DK, and Erwin, PM: Criterion-related validity of the figure-of-eight method of measuring ankle edema. *J Orthop Sport Phys Ther,* 30:149, 2000.
3. Petersen, EJ, et al: Reliability of water volumetry and the figure of eight method on subjects with ankle joint swelling. *J Orthop Sports Phys Ther,* 29:609, 1999.
4. Tatro-Adams, D, McGann, SF, and Carbone, W: Reliability of the figure-of-eight method of ankle measurement. *J Orthop Sports Phys Ther,* 22:161, 1995.
5. Dewey, WS, et al: The reliability and concurrent validity of the figure-of-eight method of measuring hand edema in patients with burns. *J Burn Care Res,* 28:157, 2007.
6. Leard, JS, et al: Reliability and concurrent validity of the figure-of-eight method of measuring hand size in patients with hand pathology. *J Orthop Sports Phys Ther,* 34:335, 2004.
7. 2005 Baseball Rules: Indianapolis: The National Collegiate Athletic Association, 2005.
8. Bilk, E, and Jacob, B, prep: 2004 Basketball Men's and Women's Rules and Interpretations. Indianapolis, The National Collegiate Athletic Association, 2003.
9. The International Hockey Federation: Rules of Hockey-Including Explanations. Brussels, Belgium: The International Hockey Federation, 2004.
10. Adams, JR, prep: 2005 Football Rules and Interpretations. Indianapolis, The National Collegiate Athletic Association, 2005.
11. Duffy, PJ, prep: 2004 Ice Hockey Rules and Interpretations. Indianapolis, The National Collegiate Athletic Association, 2003.
12. McCrath, CC, prep: 2004 Men's and Women's Soccer Rules. Indianapolis, The National Collegiate Athletic Association, 2004.
13. Abrahamson, D, prep: 2005 Softball Rules. Indianapolis, The National Collegiate Athletic Association, 2004.
14. USTA Regulations: Part 3, Section W. 2005.
15. Bubb, RG, prep: 2005 Wrestling Rules and Interpretations. Indianapolis, The National Collegiate Athletic Association, 2004.
16. Spain, D: Casting acute fractures. Part 1—Commonly asked questions. *Aust Fam Physician,* 29:853, 2000.
17. Clanion, TO, and Coupe, KJ: Hamstrings strains in athletes: Diagnosis and treatment. *J Am Acad Orthop Surg,* 6:237, 1998.
18. Wilson, JJ, and Best, TM: Common overuse tendon problems: A review and recommendations for treatment. *Am Fam Phys,* 72:811, 2005.
19. Gross, MT: Chronic tendinitis: Pathomechanics of injury, factors affecting the healing response, and treatment. *J Orthop Sports Phys Ther,* 16:248, 1992.
20. Flegal, KM, et al: Overweight and obesity in the United States: Prevalence and trends, 1960–1994. *Int J Obes Relat Metab Disord,* 22:39, 1998.
21. Prentice, AM, and Jebb, SA: Beyond body mass index. *Obesity Rev,* 2:141, 2001.
22. Gurney, B: Leg length discrepancy. *Gait and Posture,* 15:195, 2002.
23. Defrin, R, et al: Conservative correction of leg-length discrepancies of 10 mm or less for the relief of chronic low back pain. *Arch Phys Med Rehabil,* 86:2075, 2005.
24. Nijs, J, et al: Clinical assessment of scapular positioning in patients with shoulder pain: State of the art. *J Manip Phys Ther,* 30:68, 2007.
25. Borstad, JD: Resting position variables at the shoulder: Evidence to support a posture-impairment association. *Phys Ther,* 86:549, 2006.
26. Naudie, DDR, Amendola, A, and Fowler, PJ: Opening wedge high tibial osteotomy for symptomatic hyperextension-varus thrust. *Am J Sports Med,* 32:60, 2004.
27. Culham, E, and Peat, M: Spinal and shoulder complex posture: Measurement using the 3S pace isotrak. *Clin Rehabil,* 7:309, 1993.
28. Harrison, AL, Barry-Greb, T, and Wojtowicz, G: Clinical measurement of head and shoulder posture variables. *J Orthop Sports Phys Ther,* 23:353, 1996.

29. Garrett, TR, Youdas, JW, and Madison, TJ: Reliability of measuring forward head posture in a clinical setting. *J Orthop Sports Phys Ther,* 17:155, 1993.
30. Mann, RA: Disorders of the first metatarsophalangeal joint. *J Am Acad Orthop Surg,* 3:34, 1995.
31. Buchanan, KR, and Davis, I: The relationship between forefoot, midfoot, and rearfoot static alignment in pain-free individuals. *J Orthop Sports Phys Ther,* 35:559, 2005.
32. Glascoe, WM, et al: Criterion-related validity of a clinical measure of dorsal first ray mobility. *J Orthop Sports Phys Ther,* 35:589, 2005.
33. Elveru, RA, et al: Methods for taking subtalar joint measurements. *Phys Ther,* 68:678, 1988.
34. Glascoe, WM, et al: Comparison of two methods used to assess first-ray mobility. *Foot Ankle Int,* 23:248, 2002.
35. Mueller, MJ, Host, JV, and Norton, BJ: Navicular drop as a composite measure of excessive pronation. *J Am Podiatr Med Assoc,* 83:198, 1993.
36. Picciano, AM, Rowlands, MS, and Worrell, T: Reliability of open and closed kinetic chain subtalar joint neutral positions and navicular drop test. *J Orthop Sport Phys Ther,* 18:553, 1993.
37. Sell, KE, et al: Two measurement techniques for assessing subtalar joint position: A reliability study. *J Orthop Sports Phys Ther,* 19:162, 1994.
38. Menz, HB, and Munteanu, SE: Validity of 3 clinical techniques for the measurement of static foot posture in older people. *J Orthop Sport Phys Ther,* 35:279, 2005.
39. De Garceau, D, et al: The association between diagnosis of plantar fasciitis and windlass test. *Foot Ankle Int,* 24:251, 2003.
40. Kinoshita, M, et al: The dorsiflexion-eversion test for diagnosis of tarsal tunnel syndrome. *J Bone Joint Surg,* 83(A):1835, 2001.
41. Vela, L, Tourville, TW, and Hertel, J: Physical examination of acutely injured ankles: An evidence-based approach. *Athletic Therapy Today,* 8:13, 2003.
42. Leddy, JJ, et al: Prospective evaluation of the Ottawa ankle rules in a university sports medicine center. With a modification to increase specificity for identifying malleolar fractures. *Am J Sports Med,* 26:158, 1998.
43. Bachmann, LM, et al: Accuracy of Ottawa ankle rules to exclude fractures of the ankle and mid-foot: Systematic review. *Br J Med,* 326:417, 2003.
44. Nugent, PJ: Ottawa Ankle Rules accurately assess injuries and reduce reliance on radiographs. *J Fam Pract,* 53:785, 2004.
45. Lynch, SA: Assessment of the injured ankle in the athlete. *J Athl Train,* 37:406, 2002.
46. Corazza, F, et al: Mechanics of the anterior drawer test at the ankle: The effects of ligament viscoelasticity. *J Biomech,* 38:2118, 2005.
47. Tohyama, H, et al: Anterior drawer test for acute anterior talofibular ligament injuries of the ankle: How much load should be applied during the test? *Am J Sports Med,* 31:226, 2003.
48. Alonso, A, Khoury, L, and Adams R: Clinical tests for ankle syndesmosis injury: reliability and prediction of return to function. *J Orthop Sports Phys Ther,* 27:276, 1998.
49. Beumer, A, Swierstra, BA, and Mulder, PG: Clinical diagnosis of syndesmotic ankle instability. Evaluation of stress tests behind the curtains. *Acta Orthop Scand,* 73:667, 2002.
50. Hertel, J, et al: Talocrural and subtalar instability after lateral ankle sprain. *Med Sci Sports Exer,* 31:1501, 1999.
51. Wuest, TK: Injuries to the distal lower extremity syndesmosis. *J Am Acad Orthop Surg,* 5:172, 1997.
52. Hislop, HJ, and Montgomery, J: *Muscle Testing: Techniques of Manual Examination.* Philadelphia: W.B. Saunders, 2002, p 187.
53. Wind, WM, Bergfeld, JA, and Parker, RD: Evaluation and treatment of posterior cruciate ligament injuries. *Am J Sports Med,* 32:1765, 2004.
54. Davies, H, Unwin, A, and Aichroth, P: The posterolateral corner of the knee. Anatomy, biomechanics and management of injuries. *Injury, Int J Care Injured,* 35:68, 2004.
55. Indelicato, PA: Isolated medial collateral ligament injuries of the knee. *J Am Acad Orthop Surg,* 3:9, 1995.

56. Cosgarea, AJ, and Jay, PR: Posterior cruciate ligament injuries: Evaluation and management. *J Am Acad Orthop Surg,* 9:297, 2001.
57. Stannard, JP, et al: The posterolateral corner of the knee. Repair versus reconstruction. *Am J Sports Med,* 33:881, 2005.
58. Covey, DC: Injuries of the posterolateral corner of the knee. *J Bone Joint Surg,* 83(A):106, 2001.
59. Loomer, RL: A test for knee posterolateral rotatory instability. *Clin Orthop,* (264):235, 1991.
60. Hughston, JC, and Norwood, LA: The posterolateral drawer test and external rotational recurvatum test for posterolateral rotatory instability of the knee. *Clin Orthop,* 147:82, 1980.
61. Karachalios, T, et al: Diagnostic accuracy of a new clinical test (the Thessaly test) for early detection of meniscal tears. *J Bone Joint Surg,* 87A:955, 2005.
62. Reese, NB, and Bandy, WD: Use of an inclinometer to measure flexibility of the iliotibial band using the Ober test and modified Ober test: Differences in the magnitude and reliability of measurements. *J Orthop Sports Phys Ther,* 33:326, 2003.
63. Gajdosik, RL, Sandler, MM, and Marr, HL: Influence of knee positions and gender on the Ober test for length of the iliotibial band. *Clin Biom,* 18:77, 2003.
64. Bicos, J, Fulkerson, JP, and Amis, A: Current concepts review: The medial patellofemoral ligament. *Am J Sports Med,* 35:484, 2007.
65. Fulkerson, J, et al: 1991 AAOS Instructional Course Lecture on Patellofemoral Pain, American Academy of Orthopaedic Surgeons, 1991.
66. Livingston, LA, and Spaulding, SJ: OPTOTRAK measurement of the quadriceps angle using standardized foot positions. *J Athl Train,* 37:252, 2002.
67. Guerra, JP, Arnold, MJ, and Gajdosik, RL: Q angle: Effects of isometric quadriceps contraction and body postion. *J Orthop Sport Phys Ther,* 19:200, 1992.
68. Greene, CC, et al: Reliability of the quadriceps angle measurement. *Am J Knee Surg,* 14:97, 2001.
69. Tanner, SM, et al: A modified test for patellar instability: The biomechanical basis. *Clin J Sport Med,* 13:327, 2003.
70. Nijs, J, et al: Diagnostic value of five clinical tests in patellofemoral pain syndrome. *Manual Ther,* 11:69, 2006.
71. Tonnis, D, and Heinecke, A: Current concepts review – Acetabular and femoral anteversion: Relationship with osteoarthritis of the hip. *J Bone Jt Surg [Am],* 81:1747, 1999.
72. Winters, MV, et al: Passive versus active stretching of hip flexor muscles in subjects with limited hip extension: A randomized clinical trial. *Phys Ther,* 84:800, 2004.
73. Reese, NB, and Bandy, WD: *Joint Range of Motion and Muscle Length Testing.* Philadelphia: W.B Saunders Co., 2002.
74. Westbrook, A, et al: The mannequin sign. *Spine,* 30:E115, 2005.
75. Fritz, JM: Lumbar intervertebral disc injuries in athletes. *Athletic Therapy Today,* March:27, 1999.
76. Coppieters, MW, et al: Strain and excursion of the sciatic, tibial, and plantar nerves during a modified straight leg raising test. *J Orthop Res,* 24:1883, 2006.
77. Reese, NB: *Muscle and Sensory Testing.* St. Louis, MO: Elsevier Saunders, 2005, p 203.
78. Chiu, TTW, Law, EYH, and Chiu, THF: Performance of craniocervical flexion test in subjects with and without chronic neck pain. *J Orthop Sports Phys Ther,* 35:567, 2005.
79. Walsh, MT: Upper limb neural tension testing and mobilization: Fact, fiction, and a practical approach. *J Hand Ther,* 18:241, 2005.
80. Wainer, RS, et al: Reliability and diagnostic accuracy of the clinical examination and patient self-report measures for cervical radiculopathy. *Spine,* 28:52, 2003.
81. Tong, HC, Haig, AJ, and Yamakawa, K: The Spurling Test and cervical radiculopathy. *Spine,* 27:156, 2002.
82. McAlister, FA, and Straus, SE: Measurement of blood pressure: An evidence based review. *BMJ,* 322:908, 2001.
83. Kaplan, NM, Deveraux, RB, and Miller, HS: Task force 4: systemic hypertension. *J Am Coll Cardiol,* 24:885, 1994.
84. Karnath, G, and Boyars, MC: Pulmonary auscultation. *Hosp Physician,* 22, 2002.

85. Kelly, BT, Kadrmas, WR, and Speer, KP: The manual muscle examination for rotator cuff strength. An electromyographic investigation. *Am J Sports Med,* 24:581, 1996.
86. Levy, AS, et al: Intra- and interobserver reproducibility of the shoulder laxity examination. *Am J Sports Med,* 58:272, 1999.
87. Walton, J, et al: Diagnostic values of tests for acromioclavicular joint pain. *J Bone Jt Surg,* 86-A:807, 2004.
88. Meister, K: Injuries to the shoulder in the throwing athlete. Part One: Biomechanics/Pathophysiology/Classification of injury. *Am J Sports Med,* 28:265, 2000.
89. Tripp, BL, et al: Functional multijoint position reproduction acuity in overhead throwing athletes. *J Athl Train,* 41:146, 2006.
90. Parentis, MA, et al: An evaluation of the provocative tests for superior labral anterior posterior lesions. *Am J Sports Med,* 34:265, 2006.
91. Kim, SH, et al: Painful jerk test: A predictor of success in nonoperative treatment of posteroinferior instability of the shoulder. *Am J Sports Med,* 32:1849, 2004.
92. Baker, CL, and Merkley, MS: Clinical evaluation of the athlete's shoulder. *J Athl Train,* 35:256, 2000.
93. Park, HB, et al: Diagnostic accuracy of clinical tests for the different degrees of subacromial impingement syndrome. *J Bone Joint Surg,* 87-A:1446, 2005.
94. Itoi, E, et al: Which is more useful, the "full can test" or the "empty can test" in detecting the torn supraspinatus tendon? *Am J Sports Med,* 27:65, 1999.
95. Holtby, R, and Razmjou, H: Validity of the supraspinatus test as a single clinical test in diagnosing patients with rotator cuff pathology. *J Orthop Sports Phys Ther,* 34:194, 2004.
96. Çaliş, M, et al: Diagnostic values of clinical diagnostic tests in subacromial impingement syndrome. *Ann Rheum Dis,* 59:44, 2000.
97. Holtby, R, and Razmjou, H: Accuracy of the Speed's and Yergason's tests in detecting biceps pathology and SLAP lesions: comparison with arthroscopic findings. *Arthroscopy,* 20:231, 2004.
98. Wilk, KE, et al: Current concepts in the recognition and treatment of superior labral (SLAP) lesions. *J Orthop Sports Phys Ther,* 35:273, 2005.
99. Bennett, WF: Specificity of the Speed's test: arthroscopic technique for evaluating the biceps tendon at the level of the bicipital groove. *Arthroscopy,* 14:789, 1998.
100. Walsworth, MK, et al: Reliability and diagnostic accuracy of history and physical examination for diagnosing glenoid labral tears. *Am J Sports Med,* e-pub, 2007.
101. King, JW, Brelsford, HJ, and Tullos, HS: Analysis of the pitching arm of the professional baseball pitcher. *Clin Orthop,* 67:116, 1969.
102. Gajdosik, RL: Comparison and reliability of three goniometric methods for measuring forearm supination and pronation. *Percept Mot Skills,* 93:353, 2001.
103. Karagiannopoulos, C, Sitler, M, and Michlovitz, S: Reliability of 2 functional goniometric methods for measuring forearm pronation and supination active range of motion. *J Orthop Sports Phys Ther,* 33:523, 2003.
104. Rainville, J, et al: Assessment of forearm pronation strength in C6 and C7 radiculopathies. *Spine,* 32:72, 2007.
105. Dunning, CE, et al: Ligamentous stabilizers against posterolateral rotatory instability of the elbow. *J Bone Joint Surg,* 83(A):1823, 2001.
106. Clarkson, HM: *Musculoskeletal Assessment. Joint Range of Motion and Manual Muscle Strength.* (ed 2). Philadelphia: Lippincott Williams & Wilkins, 2000.
107. Rettig, AC: Athletic injuries of the wrist and hand. Part I: Traumatic injuries of the wrist. *Am J Sports Med,* 31:1038, 2003.
108. MacDermid, JC, and Wessel, XX: Clinical diagnosis of carpal tunnel syndrome. A systematic review. *J Hand Ther,* 17:309, 2004.
109. Aird, J, et al: The impact of wrist extension provocation on current perception thresholds in patients with carpal tunnel syndrome: A pilot study. *J Hand Ther,* 19:299, 2006.
110. Rodriguez, JO, Lavina, AM, and Agarwal, A: Prevention and treatment of common eye injuries in sports. *Am Fam Physician,* 67:1481, 2003.

111. Practice parameter: The management of concussion in sports (summary statement). *Neurology,* 48:581, 1997.
112. LeBlanc, KE: Concussions in sports: Guidelines for return to competition. *Am Fam Physician,* 50:801, 1994.
113. Colorado Medical Society: *Report of the Sports Medicine Committee: Guidelines for the Management of Concussion in Sports* (revised). Paper presented at the Colorado Medical Society, Denver, CO, 1991.
114. McCrory, P, et al: Summary and agreement statement of the 2nd International Conference on Concussion in Sport, Prague 2004. *Clin J Sport Med,* 15:48, 2005.
115. Abuabara, A: Cerebrospinal fluid rhinorrhea: Diagnosis and management. *Med Oral Patol Oral Cir Bucal,* 12:E397, 2007.
116. Miller, JR, et al: Comparison of preseason, midseason, and postseason neurocognitive scores in uninjured collegiate football players. *Am J Sports Med,* 35:1284, 2007.
117. Broglio, SP, Macciocchi, SN, and Ferrara, MS: Sensitivity of the concussion assessment battery. *Neurosurgery,* 60:1050, 2007.
118. Valovich, TCV, et al: Psychometric and measurement properties of concussion assessment tools in youth sports. *J Athl Train,* 41:399, 2006.
119. Valovich, TC, Perrin, DH, and Gansneder, BM: Repeat administration elicits practice effect with the Balance Error Scoring System but not with the Standardized Assessment of Concussion in high school athletes. *J Athl Train,* 38:51, 2003.
120. Onate, JA, Beck, BC, and Van Lunen, BL: On-field testing environment and Balance Error Scoring System Performance during preseason screening of healthy collegiate baseball players. *J Athl Train,* 42:446, 2007.
121. Riemann, BL, and Guskiewicz, KM: Effects of mild head injury on postural stability as measured through clinical balance testing. *J Athl Train,* 35:19, 2000.
122. National Collegiate Athletics Association: Sports Medicine Handbook 2008-09 (ed 20). Retrieved from http://www.ncaa.org/wps/ncaa?ContentID=1446 (Accessed October 22, 2008).

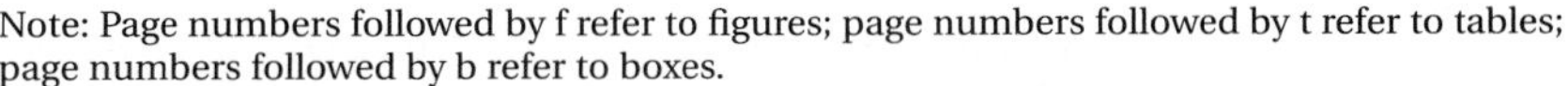

INDEX

Note: Page numbers followed by f refer to figures; page numbers followed by t refer to tables; page numbers followed by b refer to boxes.

A

D

E

F

G

H

Q

R

S

U

V

W

Y